Complications in Vascular Surgery

Complications in Vascular Surgery

Second Edition, Revised and Expanded

edited by

Jonathan B. Towne
Medical College of Wisconsin
Milwaukee, Wisconsin, U.S.A.

Larry H. Hollier
Louisiana State University
   Health Sciences Center School of Medicine
New Orleans, Louisiana, U.S.A.

MARCEL DEKKER, INC.   NEW YORK · BASEL

The first edition was published as *Complications in Vascular Surgery*, Victor M. Bernhard and Jonathan B. Towne, eds., 1991, by Quality Medical Publishing, Inc., St. Louis, Missouri.

Library of Congress Cataloging-in-Publication Data
A catalog record for this book is available from the Library of Congress.

ISBN: 0-8247-4776-3

This book is printed on acid-free paper.

Headquarters
Marcel Dekker, Inc.
270 Madison Avenue, New York, NY 10016, U.S.A.
tel: 212-696-9000; fax: 212-685-4540

Distribution and Customer Service
Marcel Dekker, Inc.
Cimarron Road, Monticello, New York 12701, U.S.A.
tel: 800-228-1160; fax: 845-796-1772

Eastern Hemisphere Distribution
Marcel Dekker AG
Hutgasse 4, Postfach 812, CH-4001 Basel, Switzerland
tel: 41-61-260-6300; fax: 41-61-260-6333

World Wide Web
http://www.dekker.com

The publisher offers discounts on this book when ordered in bulk quantities. For more information, write to Special Sales/Professional Marketing at the headquarters address above.

To Jesse Thompson, M.D. Dr. Thompson was our teacher, mentor, and role model. He played a significant role during our vascular fellowships and has been a friend and mentor throughout our careers.

Preface to the Second Edition

Under the best of circumstances, confident vascular surgeons will encounter a myriad of complications in the management of their patients. These problems reflect the complexity of the surgical care that must be provided to individuals who are usually beyond their sixth decade and are afflicted with a variety of associated diseases involving major organ systems, which places them at high risk. In 1980, 1985, and in 1991, we published a volume entitled *Complications in Vascular Surgery*. These initial three volumes were produced in collaboration with Victor M. Bernhard, M.D. Larry H. Hollier, M.D., has helped with the editorship of the present edition. The most significant changes in vascular surgery since 1991 have to do with the emergence of endovascular treatments and their increasing use in peripheral vascular surgery. A section on these techniques has been added to this book so as to make it more timely and helpful to the practicing vascular surgeon. The contributing authors are experts in their fields and were kind enough to share their experiences. Most physicians are reluctant to discuss complications; therefore these chapters represent significant contributions.

We thank Roberta Sutton for her help with editorial review and oversight of manuscript preparation.

Jonathan B. Towne
Larry H. Hollier

Preface to the First Edition

Under the best of circumstances, competent vascular surgeons will encounter a myriad of complications in the management of their patients. These problems reflect the complexity of surgical care that must be provided to individuals who are usually beyond their sixth decade and who are afflicted with a variety of associated diseases involving major organ systems, which places them at high risk. In 1980, and again in 1985, we asked a group of colleagues to participate in symposia specifically directed toward the management of vascular surgery complications. It was our perception that frank, objective, and timely appraisals of these problems would lead to more opportune and accurate diagnosis and effective therapy and would point the way to methods of prevention. Since the last symposium, many new procedures have been added to the armamentarium of the vascular surgeon. These procedures have in some instances replaced certain forms of therapy or have altered our perspective in the design of the most appropriate management course. It is well established that these interventions, as well as the more classic methods of management, may result in a variety of adverse outcomes due to the nature of the procedure itself or to the manner in which it is performed. Continued scrutiny of old and new techniques provides the basis for scientific management of these problems and offers a wider opportunity to develop and explore alternate forms of therapy.

Six years have passed since the last symposium, and we believed that the time was ripe for reassessment of the current status of vascular surgery complications in light of our broader understanding of the disease processes encountered and recent advances in technology. As in the past, we have invited experienced senior vascular surgeons whose published experiences identify them as experts in the field. It is our hope that this volume, which embodies the discussions at our third symposium, will serve as a useful reference for the clinical practitioner.

We wish to thank Ann Hopkins, who supervised the details of organization and took major responsibility for overseeing manuscript preparation and editorial review. We would also like to thank Lynne Mascarella of the Office of Continuing Medical Education at the University of Arizona College of Medicine for her help in organizing this symposium.

Victor M. Bernhard
Jonathan B. Towne

Contents

CONTENTS

Endovascular Stent-Graft Complication in Aneurysm Repair

Contributors

Mark B. Adams, M.D.   Professor of Surgery and Chair, Department of Surgery, Medical College of Wisconsin, Milwaukee, Wisconsin, U.S.A.

Ramtin Agah, M.D.   Division of Cardiology and Program in Human Molecular Biology and Genetics, University of Utah, Salt Lake City, Utah, U.S.A.

Gary M. Ansel, M.D., F.A.C.C.   Director, Peripheral Vascular Intervention, Department of Cardiology, Riverside Methodist Hospital, Columbus, Ohio, U.S.A.

Enrico Ascher, M.D.   Professor of Surgery and Director, Division of Vascular Surgery, Maimonides Medical Center, Brooklyn, New York, U.S.A.

William H. Baker, M.D.   Professor Emeritus, Division of Vascular Surgery, Department of Surgery, Loyola University Medical Center, Maywood, Illinois, U.S.A.

Dennis F. Bandyk, M.D., R.V.T.   Professor of Surgery, Division of Vascular and Endovascular Surgery, University of South Florida College of Medicine, Tampa, Florida, U.S.A.

Hugh G. Beebe, M.D.   Director Emeritus, Jobst Vascular Center, Toledo, Ohio, and Adjunct Professor of Surgery, Dartmouth–Hitchcock Medical Center, Hanover, New Hampshire, U.S.A.

Thomas M. Bergamini, M.D.   Associate Clinical Professor of Surgery, Department of Surgery, University of Louisville School of Medicine, and Surgical Care Associates, Louisville, Kentucky, U.S.A.

John J. Bergan, M.D., F.A.C.S., F.R.C.S.(Hon.), Eng.   Professor, Department of Surgery, University of California, San Diego, School of Medicine, San Diego, California, and Professor of Surgery, Uniformed Services University of the Health Sciences, Bethesda, Maryland, U.S.A.

Joshua Bernheim, M.D.   Vascular Surgery Fellow, Division of Vascular Surgery, New York Presbyterian Hospital–The University Hospitals of Columbia and Cornell, New York, New York, U.S.A.

David C. Brewster, M.D.   Clinical Professor of Surgery, Massachusetts General Hospital and Harvard Medical School, Boston, Massachusetts, U.S.A.

David A. Bull, M.D., F.A.C.S.   Associate Professor of Surgery, Division of Cardiothoracic Surgery, University of Utah Health Sciences Center, Salt Lake City, Utah, U.S.A.

Richard P. Cambria, M.D.   Chief, Division of Vascular and Endovascular Surgery, and Visiting Surgeon, Massachusetts General Hospital, and Professor of Surgery, Harvard Medical School, Boston, Massachusetts, U.S.A.

Robert A. Cambria, M.D.   Associate Professor of Surgery, Division of Vascular Surgery, Medical College of Wisconsin, Milwaukee, Wisconsin, U.S.A.

Jeffry D. Cardneau, M.D.   Fellow, Vascular Surgery and Interventional Radiology, Division of Vascular Surgery, University of California, San Francisco, San Francisco, California, U.S.A.

Alfio Carroccio, M.D.   Assistant Professor, Division of Vascular Surgery, Mount Sinai School of Medicine, New York, New York, U.S.A.

Gregory S. Cherr, M.D.   Assistant Professor, Department of Surgery, State University of New York at Buffalo, Buffalo, New York, U.S.A.

Kenneth J. Cherry, M.D.   Professor of Surgery, Division of Vascular Surgery, Department of Surgery, Mayo Clinic, Rochester, Minnesota, U.S.A.

G. Patrick Clagett, M.D.   Professor and Chairman, Division of Vascular Surgery, and Jan and Bob Pickens Distinguished Professorship in Medical Science, in memory of Jerry Knight Rymer and Annette Brannon Rymer and Mr. and Mrs. W. L. Pickens, University of Texas Southwestern Medical Center, Dallas, Texas, U.S.A.

W. Darrin Clouse, M.D. *   Fellow in Vascular Surgery, Massachusetts General Hospital and Harvard Medical School, Boston, Massachusetts, and Assistant Professor of Surgery, F. Edward Hébert School of Medicine, Uniformed Services University of the Health Sciences, Bethesda, Maryland, U.S.A.

Alexander W. Clowes, M.D.   Professor and Chief of Vascular Surgery, Department of Surgery, University of Washington, Seattle, Washington, U.S.A.

Current affiliation: Division of Vascular Surgery, Wilford Hall Medical Center, Lackland AFB, Texas, U.S.A.

Jeffery B. Dattilo, M.D.   Assistant Professor of Surgery, Division of Vascular Surgery, Vanderbilt University Medical Center, Nashville, Tennessee, U.S.A.

Sukru Dilege, M.D.   Assistant Professor of Surgery, Department of General Surgery, Istanbul Medical Faculty, Istanbul, Turkey

Hector M. Dourron, M.D.*   Fellow, Division of Vascular Surgery, Henry Ford Hospital, Detroit, Michigan, U.S.A.

John M. Draus, Jr.   General Surgery Resident, Department of Surgery, University of Louisville School of Medicine, Louisville, Kentucky, U.S.A.

Mark T. Eginton, M.D.   Division of Vascular Surgery, Medical College of Wisconsin, Milwaukee, Wisconsin, U.S.A.

Sharif H. Ellozy, M.D.   Division of Vascular Surgery, Mount Sinai School of Medicine, New York, New York, U.S.A.

Michael J. Englesbe, M.D.   Department of Surgery, University of Washington, Seattle, Washington, U.S.A.

Abigail Falk, M.D.   Assistant Professor, Department of Radiology, Mount Sinai Medical Center, New York, New York, U.S.A.

Mark A. Farber, M.D.   Assistant Professor, Division of Vascular Surgery, Department of Surgery, University of North Carolina, Chapel Hill, North Carolina, U.S.A.

Matthew I. Foley, M.D.   Vascular Surgery Resident, Division of Vascular Surgery, Department of General Surgery, Oregon Health & Science University, Portland, Oregon, U.S.A.

Julie A. Freishchlag, M.D.   William Stewart Halsted Professor and Director, Department of Surgery, Johns Hopkins School of Medicine, Baltimore, Maryland, U.S.A.

Peter Gloviczki, M.D.   Professor of Surgery, Mayo Medical School, Chair, Division of Vascular Surgery, and Director, Gonda Vascular Center, Department of Surgery, Mayo Clinic, Rochester, Minnesota, U.S.A.

Mitchel P. Goldman, M.D.   Associate Professor of Dermatology, University of California, San Diego, School of Medicine, San Diego, California, U.S.A.

Patricia Gum, M.D.   Department of Cardiovascular Medicine, The Cleveland Clinic Foundation, Cleveland, Ohio, U.S.A.

**Current affiliation*: Vascular Surgeon, Vascular Surgical Associates, P.C., Austell, Georgia, U.S.A.

Kimberly J. Hansen, M.D. Professor of Surgery and Head, Section of Vascular Surgery, Division of Surgical Sciences, Wake Forest University School of Medicine, Winston-Salem, North Carolina, U.S.A.

Anil Hingorani, M.D. Associate Professor of Surgery and Attending, Division of Vascular Surgery, Maimonides Medical Center, Brooklyn, New York, U.S.A.

John R. Hoch, M.D. Associate Professor, Section of Vascular Surgery, Department of Surgery, University of Wisconsin Medical School, Madison, Wisconsin, U.S.A.

Larry H. Hollier, M.D., F.A.C.S., F.A.C.C., F.R.C.S. (Eng) Professor of Surgery and Dean, Louisiana State University Health Sciences Center School of Medicine, New Orleans, Louisiana, U.S.A.

Glenn C. Hunter, M.D., F.R.C.S.(E), F.R.C.S.C. Professor, Department of Surgery, University of Texas Medical Branch, Galveston, Texas, U.S.A.

Tikva S. Jacobs, M.D. General Surgery Resident, Division of Vascular Surgery, Mount Sinai School of Medicine, New York, New York, U.S.A.

Gary M. Jacobson, M.D.* Fellow in Vascular Surgery, Henry Ford Hospital, Detroit, Michigan, U.S.A.

Christopher P. Johnson, M.D. Professor of Surgery, Department of Transplant Surgery, Medical College of Wisconsin, Milwaukee, Wisconsin, U.S.A.

Manju Kalra, M.D. Gonda Vascular Center, Department of Surgery, Mayo Clinic, Rochester, Minnesota, U.S.A.

Richard Kempczinski, M.D. Professor Emeritus, Department of Surgery, University of Cincinnati, Cincinnati, Ohio, U.S.A.

K. Craig Kent, M.D. Chief, Division of Vascular Surgery, New York Presbyterian Hospital–The University Hospitals of Columbia and Cornell, New York, New York, U.S.A.

Sashi Kilaru, M.D. Vascular Surgery Fellow, Division of Vascular Surgery, New York Presbyterian Hospital–The University Hospitals of Columbia and Cornell, New York, New York, U.S.A.

Gregory J. Landry, M.D. Assistant Professor of Surgery, Division of Vascular Surgery, Oregon Health & Science University, Portland, Oregon, U.S.A.

Evan C. Lipsitz, M.D., F.A.C.S. Assistant Professor of Surgery, Division of Vascular Surgery, Department of Surgery, Montefiore Medical Center and Albert Einstein College of Medicine, Bronx, New York, U.S.A.

Current affiliation: Vascular Surgical Associates, P.C., Marietta, Georgia, U.S.A.

David R. Lorelli, M.D., R.V.T. Attending Vascular Surgeon, Department of Vascular Surgery, St. John Hospital and Medical Center, Detroit, Michigan, U.S.A.

Thomas Maldonado, M.D. Fellow, Peripheral Vascular Surgery, Department of Surgery, New York University Medical Center, New York, New York, U.S.A.

Michael L. Marin, M.D. Professor and Chief, Division of Vascular Surgery, and Henry Kaufman Professor of Vascular Surgery, Mount Sinai School of Medicine, New York, New York, U.S.A.

Kenneth E. McIntyre, Jr., M.D. Professor of Surgery and Chief, Division of Vascular Surgery, University of Nevada School of Medicine, Las Vegas, Nevada, U.S.A.

Robert Mendes, M.D. Division of Vascular Surgery, Department of Surgery, University of North Carolina, Chapel Hill, North Carolina, U.S.A.

Louis M. Messina, M.D. Professor of Surgery, Division of Vascular Surgery, Edwin J. Wylie Endowed Chair in Surgery, and Vice Chair, Department of Surgery, University of California, San Francisco, San Francisco, California, U.S.A.

Gregory L. Moneta, M.D. Professor and Chief, Division of Vascular Surgery, Department of General Surgery, Oregon Health & Science University, Portland, Oregon, U.S.A.

Nicholas J. Morrissey, M.D. Assistant Professor, Division of Vascular Surgery, Mount Sinai School of Medicine, New York, New York, U.S.A.

Kyle Mueller, M.D. Surgical Resident, Division of Vascular Surgery, The Feinberg School of Medicine, Northwestern University, Chicago, Illinois, U.S.A.

Peter Neglén, M.D., Ph.D. River Oaks Hospital, Jackson, Mississippi, U.S.A.

Takao Ohki, M.D., Ph.D. Chief of Endovascular Programs, Division of Vascular Surgery, Department of Surgery, Montefiore Medical Center, and Associate Professor of Surgery, Albert Einstein College of Medicine, Bronx, New York, U.S.A.

Kenneth Ouriel, M.D. Chairman, Department of Vascular Surgery, The Cleveland Clinic Foundation, Cleveland, Ohio, U.S.A.

William H. Pearce, M.D. Violet R. and Charles A. Baldwin Professor of Vascular Surgery, Division of Vascular Surgery, The Feinberg School of Medicine, Northwestern University, Chicago, Illinois, U.S.A.

Daniel J. Reddy, M.D., F.A.C.S. D. Emerick and Eve Szilagyi Chair in Vascular Surgery, Department of Surgery, Henry Ford Hospital, Detroit, Michigan, U.S.A.

David Rigberg, M.D. Assistant Professor of Vascular Surgery, Department of Surgery, UCLA Medical Center, Los Angeles, California, U.S.A.

Thomas S. Riles, M.D.   The George David Stewart Professor and Chair, Department of Surgery, New York University School of Medicine, New York, New York, U.S.A.

Caron Rockman, M.D., F.A.C.S.   Assistant Professor of Surgery, Department of Surgery, New York University School of Medicine, New York, New York, U.S.A.

Robert J. Rosen, M.D.   Director, Interventional Radiology and Endovascular Surgery, Department of Radiology, New York University Medical Center, New York, New York, U.S.A.

Allan M. Roza, M.D.   Professor, Division of Transplant Surgery, Department of Surgery, Medical College of Wisconsin, Milwaukee, Wisconsin, U.S.A.

Gary R. Seabrook, M.D.   Professor of Surgery, Division of Vascular Surgery, Medical College of Wisconsin, Milwaukee, Wisconsin, U.S.A.

Maureen Sheehan, M.D.   Chief Surgical Resident, Division of Vascular Surgery, Department of Surgery, Loyola University Medical Center, Maywood, Illinois, U.S.A.

Alexander D. Shepard, M.D.   Senior Staff Surgeon, Department of Surgery, and Medical Director, Vascular Lab, Henry Ford Hospital, Detroit, Michigan, U.S.A.

Lloyd M. Taylor, Jr., M.D.   Professor of Surgery, Division of Vascular Surgery, Oregon Health & Science University, Portland, Oregon, U.S.A.

Jonathan B. Towne, M.D.   Professor of Surgery and Chairman, Division of Vascular Surgery, Medical College of Wisconsin, Milwaukee, Wisconsin, U.S.A.

Frank J. Veith, M.D.   Professor and Vice Chairman, The William J. von Liebig Chair in Vascular Surgery, Department of Surgery, Montefiore Medical Center and Albert Einstein College of Medicine, Bronx, New York, U.S.A.

Jay S. Yadav, M.D., F.A.C.C., F.S.C.A.I.   Director, Vascular Intervention, Department of Cardiovascular Medicine, The Cleveland Clinic Foundation, Cleveland, Ohio, U.S.A.

William R. Yorkovich, R.P.A.   Physician Assistant, Division of Vascular Surgery, Maimonides Medical Center, Brooklyn, New York, U.S.A.

1

Pitfalls of Noninvasive Vascular Testing

Dennis F. Bandyk

University of South Florida College of Medicine, Tampa, Florida, U.S.A.

Diagnostic testing of patients with vascular disease requires a thorough understanding of the instrumentation, arterial and venous anatomy, and hemodynamics of blood circulation. Although physical examination and vascular imaging studies—such as contrast arteriography, magnetic resonance angiography, and contrast-enhanced computed tomography—are indispensable in the management of peripheral vascular disease, noninvasive vascular testing retains a prominent role in patient evaluation both prior to and following intervention. Methods that use Doppler ultrasound—in particular duplex ultrasonography—and plethysmography form the cornerstone of noninvasive vascular testing. Testing is used to detect and grade the severity of cerebrovascular, peripheral arterial, and peripheral venous disease and thereby assists in disease management. The accuracy of duplex ultrasonography coupled with indirect physiological testing methods is superior to clinical evaluation alone and in many patients provides sufficient anatomical information of disease extent and severity to proceed with surgical or endovascular intervention without confirmatory imaging studies. Newer enhancements of duplex ultrasonography—such as power Doppler angiography, sonographic composite imaging, and the use of contrast agents—have further improved anatomic resolution, which allows better characterization of the extent and morphology of vascular disease.

Noninvasive vascular testing methods measure biophysical properties of the circulation (e.g., pressure, pulse contour, blood-flow velocity, turbulence-disturbed flow); these measurements can be used for disease localization and classification of severity. The diagnostic accuracy of each technique depends on the precision and reproducibility of the measurements. The measurements of blood pressure and velocity recorded by vascular laboratory instrumentation should not always be assumed to be accurate, since testing can be affected by a number of factors, including biological variability, instrumentation employed for testing, the skill and bias of the examiner, the pathological process being studied, and conditions under which the measurements are recorded. Interpretation of noninvasive testing studies requires an appreciation of the limitations, pitfalls, and artifacts associated with the various diagnostic techniques. Errors in any of these areas can result in an incorrect diagnosis and subsequent clinical decision making. In this chapter, the common pitfalls of noninvasive vascular testing related to instrumentation, testing protocols, and diagnostic interpretation are reviewed and techniques to minimize their occurrence are outlined.

I. CLASSIFICATION OF THE PITFALLS OF NONINVASIVE TESTING

Diagnostic errors associated with noninvasive vascular testing can result from procedural, interpretative, or statistical pitfalls. *Procedural pitfalls* can be due to the instrumentation, to deviations from the testing protocol, or to biological variability of the measurement. *Interpretative pitfalls* can decrease diagnostic accuracy when the measurement or physician's interpretation does not agree with a recognized "gold standard," such as arteriography. Interpretative errors can occur despite the recording of a precise and reproducible measurement. For example, the use of velocity criteria to grade internal carotid artery stenosis not previously validated by comparison with angiographic results can cause consistent over-classification of disease severity.

The accuracy of diagnostic testing is commonly expressed in terms of descriptive statistical parameters such as sensitivity, specificity, and positive and negative predictive values (PPV and NPV). These parameters are useful to compare the diagnostic accuracy between different testing methods or threshold criteria, but they are subject to *statistical pitfalls* introduced by the reliability of the gold standard used for correlation as well as disease prevalence and clinical status (symptomatic, asymptomatic) of the study population. For example, the sensitivity (ability to detect the presence of a disease state) and specificity (ability to recognize the absence of a disease state) of a specific test are not affected the prevalence of the particular disease state in the study population used to calculate diagnostic accuracy. But predictive values (PPV, NPV), which are better measures of clinical usefulness in the management of an individual patient, are highly dependent on disease prevalence. It is recommended that testing with the highest sensitivity be used to screen patients to rule out a particular disease state (1). For an individual patient, a test with a high (>90%) NPV can be used to exclude the disease state. Similarly, testing with high specificity and PPV should be used to confirm the presence of disease or to proceed with intervention—i.e., performing carotid endarterectomy based on duplex ultrasonography. It is impossible to eliminate all sources of measurement error associated with noninvasive vascular testing because of inherent variability in instrumentation, anatomy, and the examination technique. Despite this caveat, noninvasive vascular diagnostics, in particular duplex ultrasonography, demonstrate sufficient accuracy to permit medical, surgical, or endovascular intervention with a high degree of clinical certainty.

The noninvasive vascular laboratory typically employs a number of different instruments for testing in the areas of cerebrovascular, peripheral arterial, peripheral venous, and abdominal visceral disease. The most widely used instrumentation relies on ultrasound to interrogate vessels for patency and flow. Duplex ultrasonography is necessary instrumentation in an accredited vascular laboratory, and the clinical applications of this technique are numerous in the evaluation cerebrovascular, peripheral venous, peripheral arterial, and visceral vascular disease (Table 1). Plethysmographic instruments, such as the pulse volume recorder or photoplethysmograph, coupled with the pressure transducer (aneroid manometer), provide indirect hemodynamic measurements of peripheral arterial and venous flow and pressure. Compared with duplex ultrasound, these indirect techniques are vulnerable to their own unique diagnostic pitfalls.

Table 1 Clinical Applications of Duplex Ultrasonography

Cerebrovascular Testing
  Extracranial carotid and vertebral artery ultrasonography
  Duplex detection of plaque morphology
  Transcranial Doppler/duplex ultrasonography
Peripheral arterial testing
  Lower/upper limb arterial duplex mapping
  Infrainguinal graft surveillance
  Evaluation of stent-graft aortic aneurysm exclusion
  Dialysis access graft/fistula surveillance
Peripheral venous testing
  Diagnosis of lower/upper limb deep venous thrombosis
  Duplex evaluation of venous reflux—chronic venous insufficiency
  Preoperative saphenous/arm vein mapping
Visceral vascular testing
  Renal duplex ultrasonography
  Mesenteric duplex ultrasonography
  Evaluation of renal/liver organ transplants

II. PROCEDURAL PITFALLS

A. Instrumentation

Instrumentation in good operating condition and calibration is required for noninvasive vascular testing. Measurements of limb blood pressure (ankle-brachial systolic pressure index, or ABI), treadmill walking time, pulsatility index, and duplex-acquired velocity spectral parameters (peak systolic velocity, end-diastolic velocity) demonstrate reproducibility comparable to that of other common clinical (pulse rate, hemoglobin, serum creatinine) measurements. At a 95% confidence level, a significant change between two measurements has been found to be greater than 14% for ABI, greater than 120 for treadmill walking time, greater than 0.4 for pulsatility index, and greater than 20% for duplex-acquired velocity spectra and volume flow values (2).

Use of pressure cuffs of improper width relative to limb girth or noncalibrated manometers can result in erroneous measurement of segmental limb systolic blood pressure. The interpretation of the high-thigh pressure measurement to evaluate aortoiliac and common femoral artery inflow occlusive disease is highly dependent on the size of the limb to relative to the width of the cuff used. Theoretically, cuff width should be 20% greater than the diameter of the limb (3). When a narrow (10- to 12-cm) thigh cuff is used, normal high-thigh pressure is at least 20–30 mmHg higher than brachial pressure because of the artifact produced by the relatively narrow cuff (e.g., normal high-thigh systolic pressure index is >1.2; while the normal value of ankle-brachial systolic pressure index is >0.95) (1).

Careful attention to instrument calibration is particularly important when plethysmographic techniques are used for pulse volume recordings (PVR air plethysmography) or to measure lower limb venous outflow (air or impedance plethysmography). Standardization of cuff inflation pressure (approximately 65 mmHg) is mandatory to obtain reliable, reproducible air plethysmographic waveforms for the detection of arterial occlusive disease. Fortunately, modern computer-based PVR instruments include an *internal* calibration system that virtually eliminates operator errors in cuff application and technique. Improper cuff or photocell application can also produce artifacts and contribute to erroneous measurements of digital pressure and venous recovery time.

When ultrasound is used to image blood vessels or interrogate blood flow patterns within them, a variety of pitfalls can result in erroneous data or a study that cannot be interpreted. These problems can be minimized if the operator has a thorough understanding of ultrasound physics and the design features of the ultrasound system. A number of factors relating to the scan-head design, Doppler system, frequency analyzer, and display devices can affect imaging resolution and velocity spectral data (Table 2). Inappropriate selection of the transducer's ultrasound frequency is a common pitfall of duplex ultrasonography. High (7- to 15-MHz) B-mode imaging frequencies allow superior lateral and depth resolution but are strongly attenuated by tissue, thereby limiting imaging to only superficial (1- to 5-cm) vessels. Selection of an optimum transducer frequency should be based on the depth of the vessel examined and the composition of overlying tissue. Table 3 lists the transducer ultrasound frequency to obtain the strongest Doppler signal from vessels imaged through different tissues; these frequencies are based on equations that account for ultrasound scatter, tissue attenuation, and vessel depth (4). For example, duplex testing of the carotid artery in an obese patient that lies under fat and muscle at a depth of 7 cm may require a transducer frequency of 3 MHz to record a strong Doppler signal.

Variation in beam pattern and focusing can result in lateral image and refractive distortion. Because ultrasound is a wave, the shape of the beam varies at distance from the transducer. By increasing the transducer bandwidth, unwanted variations in the beam pattern are smoothed out. Adjusting the focus (focal point) to just below the area of interest is important to minimize lateral image distortion. In general, steering the ultrasound beam perpendicular to vessel walls provides superior depth resolution. Refractive distortion results when the ultrasound travels through and crosses a boundary from one tissue to another with a different ultrasound propagation speed. This can result in errors in dimensions and the number of objects in the lateral direction of any ultrasound image. Duplication of the

Table 2 Factors Affecting Ultrasonic Imaging and Doppler Data of Duplex Ultrasonography

Scan-head design
    Transmitting ultrasound frequency
    Ultrasound beam pattern and focusing
    Beam steering instrumentation
Doppler ultrasound system
    Time of image acquisition—frame rate
    Sample volume size
    Pulse repetition frequency
Frequency analyzer
    Method of velocity spectrum analysis—fast Fourier
    transform
    Characteristic frequency and spectral width
Display devices
    Real-time imaging and velocity spectral display
    Compensation for aliasing
    Doppler sample volume/angle superimposed on B-mode image
    Color power angiography

Table 3 Ultrasound Frequency for the Strongest Doppler Signal Relative to Vessel Depth and Type of Overlying Tissue

	Ultrasound Frequency (MHz)			
Depth (cm)	Blood (0.18)[a]	Fat (0.63)	Muscle (1.2)	Bone (20)
0.5	97	28	5.0	0.9
2.0	24	7	7.0	0.2
5.0	10	3	0.5	0.1
8.0	6	2	0.3	—
15.0	3	1	0.5	—

[a] All values for attenuation expressed as dB/cm/MHz.
Source: Modified from Ref. (26).

subclavian artery is an example of a refractive distortion caused by reflection of ultrasound from the pleura. Duplications appear in both B-mode and color images, and spectral waveforms can be obtained from both images. The only defense against misdiagnosis is a knowledge of anatomy and anatomical anomalies and the concept of refractive distortion.

Ultrasound beam steering can also introduce error measurement of blood-flow velocity. An experimental study using a velocity-calibrated string phantom demonstrated significant overestimation of recorded velocity when a multielement scan head was used in steered versus unsteered modes (4). Differences in the range of 20–50% were recorded when end elements of the scan head were used to record the Doppler signal. Errors of this magnitude are worrisome, since measurements of peak systolic and end-diastolic velocity are used clinically to recommend intervention for internal carotid artery or vein bypass graft stenosis. The reasons for velocity overestimation are complex and related to characteristics of the ultrasound system, including transducer beam width, aperture size, transmitting frequency, and angle of Doppler beam insonation. Manufacturers should be encouraged to include velocity calibration in routine instrument maintenance using test phantoms. In clinical situations where peak velocity measurements approach thresholds levels, a linear-array scan head should be used in the steered configuration with the Doppler cursor positioned at the end of the transducer array, so that pulse Doppler signal recording will be at the lowest angle of incidence to the axis of flow. Another strategy is to repeat the study using a phased-array transducer and compare the values to those obtained with the linear-array transducer.

Duplex ultrasound systems continue to undergo rapid evolution in terms of image resolution, color Doppler imaging, cost, and size. Some instruments provide velocity measurements from peripheral arteries without any assumption about the Doppler examination angle (5). When color-flow imaging was introduced, it was hoped that diagnostic accuracy would improve. A comparison between color Doppler velocity and spectral waveform velocity demonstrates that values can differ due to angle adjustments or differences in signal processing. The definition of velocity is obscure, since duplex instrumentation records blood cell movement from a volume or voxel and the velocity components displayed in the spectral display represent amplitude of multiple velocity vectors. A reproducible value can be obtained only when a consistent examination angle is used. This is important clinically for the diagnosis of disease progression. Serial duplex examinations should be performed with the same instrument and Doppler signals recorded at the same Doppler angle from an identical image as that acquired in the prior study. Because of the confusion produced by real-time color imaging and color map aliasing, some instruments provide a feature called "color power angiography," which shows pixels of blood motion in color without showing direction. The resultant image permits the selection of pulsed Doppler recording sites at and downstream from the location of maximum luminal stenosis. This minimizes the likelihood that regions of slow blood flow or vessel segments insonated at high (80 -to 90-degree) Doppler beam angles will be coded as showing no flow. When regions of no flow are identified, it is essential to scan from at least two lines of sight to improve the angle at which scan lines intersect with blood flow and thereby increase the likelihood of color-coding blood flow if present. As a rule, if the tissue (i.e., blood) velocity is less than 1 cm/s, the velocity is considered to be zero and color is not shown. If a wall filter is activated, velocities below about 10 cm/s are not shown.

In "real-time" color Doppler ultrasound, the image is not formed instantly but processed from the Doppler data from left to right over 30–50 ms. This produces a time distortion in all color-flow images. The speed of acquisition is approximately 150 cm/s which is comparable to speeds in the vascular system: wall motion <1 cm/s, average arterial blood velocity = 30 cm/s, pulse propagation speed = 1000 cm/s. Careful inspection of a single color-flow image demonstrates that the speed of Doppler acquisition is slower than the pulse propagation speed, resulting in a "systolic velocity bolus" approximately 2 cm long. Thus, each color image frame depicts velocity data at a specific time during the pulse cycle that is often different from that of the velocity spectra displayed below. The correct representation of blood-flow patterns at an arterial stenosis cannot be depicted in a single color-flow image.

B. Examination Technique

Obtaining high-quality noninvasive vascular data suitable for interpretation requires skill, experience, and knowledge of vascular anatomy and hemodynamics. Lack of expertise on the part of the examiner and adherence to the testing protocol are two important causes of measurement error and variability. Peripheral arterial and venous Doppler studies require the examiner to prepare the patient properly, manipulate the probe with care, and develop a standard testing protocol with examination of both extremities for comparison. Although indirect hemodynamic tests, such as segmental pressure measurement with Doppler waveform analysis and pulse volume recording, are less subject to examiner error, a number of pitfalls must be avoided (Table 4). When hemodynamic data are recorded from the arterial or venous circulation, the patient should be rested before examination and positioned appropriately for the testing method and indication for testing. To avoid false-positive findings with indirect hemodynamic testing, it is recommended that when abnormal values are obtained, the examination be repeated several times.

Duplex ultrasonography requires considerable learned expertise in ultrasound physics, vascular anatomy, and velocity spectral recording. To achieve a high level of correlation with contrast arteriography, the gold standard, a variety of pitfalls must be avoided (Table 5). The two most prominent problems are (a) assignment of the Doppler examination angle and (b) aliasing. An understanding of these two concepts is essential, particularly during the examination of tortuous or kinked arterial segments. In color Doppler instruments, color-coding of flow is based on the direction and velocity of blood flow. Since vascular anatomy is complex, with curves, branching, and dilatations, attention to the angle of insonation with the vessel is critical for assessing patency, directionality, and flow-pattern

Table 4 Testing Errors and Limitations of Segmental Pressure Measurements

Causes of erroneously high systolic pressure measurement
  Medial sclerosis—calcified arteries
  Hypertension
  Edema
  Narrow cuff width relative to limb girth
Causes of erroneously low systolic pressure meassurement
  Measurement after exercise or smoking
  Low ambient temperature
  Congestive heart failure
  Inadequate resting period
  Rapid (>5 mmHg/s) cuff deflation
  Unrecognized subclavian artery stenosis or occlusion

characteristics. The vascular group at the University of Washington has recommended that an examination angle of 60 degrees be used for all studies and remain constant for serial studies of the same artery. This is possible with current duplex ultrasound systems, which allow electronic steering of the color image, pulsed Doppler beam, or both. The percentage change in velocity relative to a velocity measured at 60 degrees increases dramatically at insonation angles greater than 70 degrees (Fig. 1). In the range of 30–60 degrees, an angle assignment error of $\pm$ 5 degrees will results in a 10–20% error in calculated velocity. By contrast, at an angle of 70 degrees or greater, the error in calculated velocity will be approximately 25%; but it will exceed 100% at an angle of 80 degrees. Thus, velocity spectra recorded at high (>65 degrees) insonation angles cannot be used to calculate peak systolic or end-diastolic velocity waveform values and thereby to classify stenosis severity or measure volume flow. As the angle of insonation decreases toward zero, the Doppler frequency shift will increase. When the detected frequency shift exceeds one-half the pulse repetition frequency (PRF), known as the Nyquist limit of the instrument, aliasing occurs. Aliasing in color Doppler results in improper color assignment of both direction and amplitude data, with the resulting flow pattern erroneously interpreted as abnormal or turbulent flow. Aliasing is easily recognized during pulsed Doppler spectral analysis; the artifact can be decreased or eliminated by increasing the angle of insonation or PRF of the instrument or by changing the scan plane of the transducer to decrease the depth of imaging. Accurate

Table 5 Potential Pitfalls of Color Duplex Ultrasonography

Vessel misidentification
Improper Doppler angle assignment
Aliasing
Incorrect color gain settings
Calcified vessel wall producing acoustic shadowing
Vessel tortuousity
Tandem occlusive lesions
Incorrect sample volume placement
Improper scanning technique
Overinterpretation of color-flow image

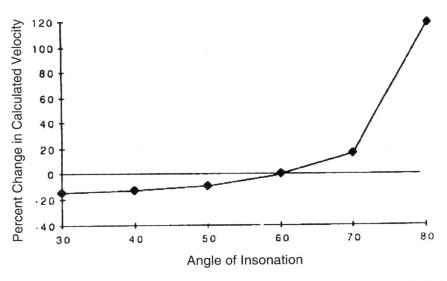

Figure 1   Percentage change in calculated velocity relative to duplex-derived velocity calculated at a 60-degree angle of insonation.

color duplex imaging compels the examiner to be vigilant at keeping a 60-degree or less angle between vessels walls (the axis of blood flow) and the transducer scan lines. Reports that have analyzed the variability of duplex-acquired velocity measurements have found variance to be within clinically acceptable levels and to be caused primarily by problems with the examination technique (failure to record the Doppler signal downstream from a stenosis, vessel tortousity precluding reproducible angle assignment) rather than inaccurate measurement of waveform parameters or changes in patient hemodynamics (6,7).

III.   INTERPRETATIVE AND STATISTICAL PITFALLS

Noninvasive vascular diagnostic testing is subject to interpretative errors independent of problems related to the instrumentation or examination technique. Indirect physiological testing and duplex ultrasonography can yield false-positive results because of anatomical variation, multilevel or bilateral disease, or concomitant medical conditions (congestive heart failure, hypertension, hypotension, vasospasm) that alter arterial flow. Elevation of segmental pressure measurements caused by heavily calcified vessels that cannot be compressed with cuff inflation is a common interpretative pitfall. Artery wall calcification, in the media or an atherosclerotic plaque, also severely attenuates ultrasound transmission and leads to blind areas (acoustic shadowing) in the B-mode image, rendering studies uninterpretable or impairing the ability to accurately identify the site of maximum stenosis. Acoustic shadowing is common in complex atherosclerotic plaques and is the primary reason why direct measurement of arterial luminal reduction is inaccurate for >50% diameter-reduction stenosis (8,9). The incorporation of sensitive Doppler flow-sensing capability, including color power angiography, in modern ultrasound systems decreases the likelihood of interpretating a high-grade stenosis with plaque calcification as a total occlusion.

An abnormal hemodynamic state that increases basal flow is another interpretative error associated with overestimation of stenosis severity. In patients with severe carotid stenosis or internal carotid occlusion, compensatory collateral flow can be present in the contralateral internal carotid artery (ICA) if the circle of Willis is intact and blood flow is provided to both cerebral hemispheres. This condition will result in overestimation of ICA stenosis, since diagnostic criteria depend on the measured levels of peak systolic and end-diastolic velocity (10,11).

This effect is most evident in the misclassification of the 40–60% stenosis category to a more severe and thus clinically important disease category. Similarly, the severity of peripheral arterial or infrainguinal graft stenosis may be overclassified if an arteriovenous fistula or postrevascularization hyperemic state is present downstream.

The interpretation of noninvasive vascular testing is complicated by the absence of uniform diagnostic criteria. Various criteria have been published for the grading of carotid and peripheral arterial stenosis. In general, it is recommended that an individual vascular laboratory initially utilize "published" criteria appropriate for their instrumentation and examination protocol, and then validate these criteria by comparison with angiography. Medical Directors of noninvasive vascular laboratories are responsible for ensuring "quality testing," which includes implementation of an independent, blinded correlation of test interpretation with a gold standard. Such a review process should expose not only pitfalls of testing related to inadequate diagnostic criteria but also problems related to the precise of the instrumentation and technologist performance. Suggested standards for the reporting noninvasive vascular testing have been developed by the national vascular surgery societies.

Angiography and venography have been considered the reference standard for comparison of noninvasive vascular testing. But these gold standards are also associated with significant inter-and intraobserver interpretation variability. Investigators have shown that the agreement between duplex ultrasound and angiography for both carotid and peripheral arterial disease classification has a variability similar to the agreement of two radiologists reading the same angiograms (sensitivity 87%, specificity 94%) (12,13). The reliability of the gold standard remains an unresolved problem in defining the accuracy of noninvasive testing, especially duplex ultrasonography. For selected clinical applications, such as the diagnosis of acute deep venous thrombosis (DVT), the accuracy of duplex ultrasound is considered to be superior to that of contrast imaging studies. The inter-and intraobserver variability of duplex studies can be minimized by adherence to a rigid testing protocol and the use of diagnostic criteria based on nonsubjective data acquisition (6). As in the case of other imaging studies, duplex classification of disease severity into minimal or moderate categories accounts for the majority of variability in interpretation.

IV. PERIPHERAL ARTERIAL TESTING

Testing for peripheral artery disease is used to detect, identify the extent, and grade the severity of obstructive and aneurysmal disease. Measurement of systolic pressure at multiple levels in combination with pulse (Doppler pulse volume recording) waveform analysis is an essential component of upper and lower limb arterial testing. Pressure measurements establish the presence and severity of arterial occlusive disease and, in conjunction with exercise testing, the diagnosis of intermittent claudication can thus be accurately determined. Arterial wall calcification, obesity, and limb edema are important factors limiting the diagnostic accuracy of peripheral arterial testing by contributing to cuff artifact or impairing ultrasound imaging of the arteries. Multilevel disease—which is commonplace in patients with symptomatic lower limb ischemia—also lessens the diagnostic accuracy of segmental pressure measurements for disease localization (aortoiliac, femoropopliteal, popliteal-tibial), and duplex mapping of disease in specific arteries (iliac, common femoral, superficial femoral, popliteal, tibial). The presence of adjacent stenosis or occlusion reduces the diagnostic accuracy of duplex scanning in the aortoiliac segment from >90 to 63% and in the superficial femoral artery from 93 to 83% (14).

An important clinical limitation of indirect physiological testing is that it provides no information as to the morphology (stenosis versus occlusion) of the occlusive process. This characteristic limits its usefulness for preintervention planning (bypass versus angioplasty) and postoperative surveillance following intervention to detect developing stenosis. The diagnostic accuracy of segmental pressure measurements to detect any arterial segment as abnormal is high (87%), with a positive predictive value of 96%, but these values are diminished in the presence of diabetes (15).

Color duplex ultrasonography can be used to image the entire lower limb arterial tree from the pararenal aorta to the pedal arteries; discriminating between occluded, stenotic, and nonstenotic arterial segments (16). Mapping of the arterial tree permits patient counseling regarding both diagnosis and the nature of intervention required to correct vascular problem [percutaneous transluminal angioplasty (PTA), direct surgery], or whether disease severity and extent dictates the need for a femoropopliteal or an infrageniculate bypass. In general, when duplex scanning identifies single-level long-segment occlusion or focal high-grade stenosis not amenable to PTA, arterial surgery can be performed without angiography. The accuracy in predicting intervention by endovascular or "open" surgical bypass exceeds 90% and, more importantly, PTA or bypass patency is not reduced compared to patients evaluated by contrast angiography (17–20). In cases of severe multilevel disease, particularly with involvement of the infrageniculate arteries, duplex scanning is plagued by several pitfalls that impair obtaining an accurate, detailed anatomical and hemodynamic definition of the arterial trees, including artifacts produced by calcific disease, poor imaging of the tibioperoneal trunk, and examiners with insufficient experience to perform arterial mapping studies.

V. CEREBROVASCULAR TESTING

Evaluation of cerebrovascular—i.e., extracranial carotid/vertebral and subclavian arteries—disease differs from peripheral arterial testing in that detection of lesions with embolic potential, in addition to pressure-and flow-reducing lesions, must be identified. Duplex ultrasonography is required to image, detect, and grade obstructive or aneurysmal lesions. The diagnostic accuracy of cerebrovascular testing is high (approximately 90%), with positive predictive values in excess of 90–95% for the detection of >50% and >70% diameter reduction ICA stenosis. Negative predictive values exceed 95% for all categories of stenosis and the diagnosis of ICA occlusion. The clinical confidence and experience with carotid duplex scanning is such that carotid endarterectomy based on ultrasound studies alone is common (60–90% of procedures) in both community and academic vascular surgery practices (20,21). For symptomatic patients, lesions with velocity spectra of a >50% stenosis are clinically important. In asymptomatic patients, only a high-grade ICA stenosis increases the risk of stroke. Appropriate values of peak systolic and end-diastolic velocity should be used. It is recommended that criteria that correlate with a positive predictive value of 95% or greater be used to recommend carotid endarterectomy in asymptomatic patients (22). Acoustic shadowing, slow flow in the distal ICA, vessel tortuosity, and compensatory collateral flow are the major diagnostic pitfalls. In general, carotid duplex testing tends to overclassify the severity of stenosis when correlated with blinded angiographic grading of ICA stenosis.

VI. PERIPHERAL VENOUS TESTING

Duplex ultrasonography is the recommended test for the diagnosis of acute lower and upper limb DVT. Diagnostic accuracy exceeds 95% with specificity approaching 100% when an examination of technical adequacy is achieved (23,24). The addition of color Doppler has enabled technologists to perform a more complete and rapid assessment of above-and below-knee veins. Although imaging of vein segments transversely and then applying pressure to coapt anterior and posterior walls is the best evidence of normal, thrombus-free vein, pulsed Doppler waveform analysis is also important to confirm flow phasicity with respiration and maneuvers to augment flow. Imaging permits diagnosis of thrombus in duplicated venous segments as well as nonoccluding thrombus. Duplex ultrasound has replaced both contrast venography and physiological testing for screening symptomatic and asymptomatic patients for DVT. Air and photoplethysmographic techniques are used primarily for the hemodynamic evaluation of chronic venous insufficiency to grade the severity of venous obstruction (impaired venous outflow) or venous reflux (short venous refilling time, ambulatory venous hypertension).

As in other areas of vascular testing, venous duplex testing is dependent on examiner experience and the technical quality of the examination. Erroneous or equivocal studies can be minimized by meticulous examination of the infrapopliteal vein, recognition of the segmental incompressibility of the superficial femoral vein within the adductor canal as a normal finding, and better estimation of the age of the thrombotic process (25). An intraluminal filling defect, a dilated vein, impaired flow, and homogenous echogencity of the thrombus are important features of acute DVT. Chronic DVT demonstrates differences in compressibility and thrombus imaging (Table 6). Obesity, limb edema, anatomically deep vascular structures, small vein caliber, thrombus outside the scan field, and bowel gas impairing imaging of the vena cava and iliac veins are other factors that limit the diagnostic accuracy of venous duplex studies. When an equivocal study is encountered, repeat scanning in 1–2 days is recommended. This approach has been demonstrated to be safe. The development of fatal pulmonary embolus is rare, but proximal DVT developed in 2–5% of patients based on serial examinations. In some patients, especially if central (vena cava,

Table 6 Differences in Duplex Ultrasound Criteria Between Acute and Chronic Deep Venous Thrombosis (DVT)

Characteristic	Acute DVT	Chronic DVT
Compressibility	Compress to medium probe pressure	None
Echogenicity	Homogenous	Heterogenous
Surface features	Smooth	Irregular
Attachment	Free-floating	Firm
Vein caliber	Dilated	Normal or contracted
Venous flow	Low, continuous	Phasic with collaterals imaged

iliac, subclavian, brachiocephalic) venous thrombosis is suspected, venography should be performed.

VII. GOALS OF VASCULAR TESTING

The application of noninvasive testing methods, especially duplex ultrasound, permits detection of the clinical spectrum of vascular disorders involving the arterial and venous systems. Although the duplex instrumentation in the various clinical applications is similar, testing protocols and diagnostic criteria should be tailored to provide measurements that characterize the vascular condition in terms of location, extent, severity, and morphology. An important pitfall of vascular testing is the failure to consider the clinical indication for the study. Interpretation of finings should be relevant to the individual patient. For example, an abnormal carotid duplex study in an asymptomatic patient should focus primarily on whether or not a high-grade stenosis has been identified. Plaque surface features and composition suggesting embolic potential are more relevant in an examination of a symptomatic patient. If intervention is based solely on duplex findings, threshold criteria with a positive predictive value in excess of 90% should be used.

Decisions regarding extent of testing for arterial and venous disorders are complex. The type of information required can vary depending on the need to establish only a diagnosis versus determining a treatment plan or assessing the result of intervention or diagnosing disease progression. Regardless of the indication for testing, the precision and reproducibility of measurements are important. Avoidance of the known pitfalls of noninvasive vascular instrumentation, testing protocols, and interpretation results in improved diagnostic accuracy and patient care.

REFERENCES

1. Sumner DS. Evaluation of noninvasive testing procedures. Data analysis and interpretation. In: Berstein EF, ed. Noninvasive Diagnostic Techniques in Vascular Disease. 3d ed. St Louis: Mosby, 1985:861–889.
2. Johnston KW, Hosang MY, Andrews DF. Reproducibility of noninvasive vascular laboratory measurement of the peripheral circulation. J Vasc Surg 1987; 6:147–151.
3. Kirkendall WM, Burton AC, Epstein FH, et al. Recommendations for human blood pressure determination by sphygmomanometers: report of a subcommittee of the postgraduate education committee, American Heart Association. Circulation 1978; 36:980–988.
4. Daigle RJ, Stavros AT, Lee RM. Overestimation of velocity and frequency values by multi-element linear array Doppler. J Vasc Technol 1990; 14:206–213.
5. Beach KW, Dunmire B, Overbeck JR, et al. Vector Doppler systems for arterial studies. J Vasc Invest 1996; 2:155–165.
6. Kohler T, Langlois Y, Roederer GO, et al. Sources of variability in carotid duplex examination— A prospective study. Ultrasound Med Biol 1985; 11:571–576.
7. Rizzo RJ, Sandager G, Astleford P, et al. Mesenteric flow velocity variations as a function of angle of insonation. J Vasc Surg 1990; 11:694–699.
8. Comerota AJ, Cranley JJ, Katz ML, et al. Real-time B-mode carotid imaging: a three year multicenter experience. J Vasc Surg 1984; 1:84–95.
9. Erickson SJ, Mewissen MW, Foley WD, et al. Stenosis of the internal carotid artery: assessment using color Doppler imaging compared with angiography. Am J Radiol 1989; 152:1299–1305.
10. Spadone DP, Barkmeier LD, Hodgson KJ, et al. Contralateral internal carotid artery stenosis

or occlusion: pitfall of correct ipsilateral classification—A study performed with color flow imaging. J Vasc Surg 1990; 11:642–649.

11. Fujitani RM, Mill JL, Wang LM, et al. The effect of unilateral internal carotid arterial occlusion upon contralateral duplex study: Criteria for accurate interpretation. J Vasc Surg 1992; 16:459–468.

12. Chikos PM, Fisher LD, Hirsh JA, et al. Observer variability in evaluating extracranial carotid artery stenosis. Stroke 1983; 14:885–889.

13. Jager KA, Phillips DJ, Martin RRL, et al. Noninvasive mapping of lower limb arterial lesions. Ultrasound Med Biol 1985; 11:515–520.

14. Allard I, Cloutier G, Durand LG, et al. Limitations of ultrasonic duplex scanning for diagnosing lower limb arterial stenosis in the presence of adjacent segment disease. J Vasc Surg 1994; 19:650–657.

15. AbuRahma AF, Khan S, Robinson PA. Selective use of segmental Doppler pressures and color duplex imaging in the localization of arterial occlusive disease of the lower extremities. Surgery 1995; 118:496–503.

16. Wain RA, Berdejo GL, Delvalle WN, et al. Can duplex scan arterial mapping replace contrast arteriography as the test of choice before infrainguinal revascularization. J Vasc Surg 1999; 29:100.

17. Ligush J Jr, Reavis SW, Preisser JS, Hansen KJ. Duplex ultrasound scanning defines operative strategies for patients with limb-threatening ischemia. J Vasc Surg 1998; 28:482–490.

18. Ascher E, Mazzariol F, Hingorani A, et al. The use of duplex ultrasound arterial mapping as an alternative for primary and secondary infrapopliteal bypasses. Am J Surg 1999; 178:162.

19. Mazzariol F, Ascher E, Hingorani A, Gunduz Y, Yorkovich W, Salles-Cunha S. Lower-extremity revascularisation without preoperative contrast arteriography in 185 cases: lessons learned with duplex ultrasound arterial mapping. Eur J Vasc Endovasc Surg 2000; 19:509–515.

20. Proia RR, Walsh D, Nelson PR, et al. Early results of infragenicular reconstruction based solely on duplex arteriography. J Vasc Surg 2001; 33:1165.

21. Dawson DL, Zierler RE, Strandness DE Jr, et al. The role of duplex scanning and arteriography before carotid endarterectomy: a prospective study. J Vasc Surg 1993; 18:673–683.

22. Samson RH, Bandyk DF, Showalter, Yunis J. Carotid endarterectomy based on duplex ultrasonography: a safe approach associated with long-term stroke prevention. Vasc Surg 2000; 34:125–136.

23. Lensing AWA, Prandoni P, Brandjes D. Detection of DVT by real-time B-mode ultrasonography. N Engl J Med 1989; 320:342–345.

24. Rose SC, Zwiebel WJ, Nelson BD, et al. Sympotmatic lower extremity deep venous thrombosis: accuracy, limitations, and role of color duplex flow imaging in diagnosis. Radiology 1990; 175:639–644.

25. Wright DJ, Shepard AD, McPharlin M, Ernst CB. Pitfalls in lower extremity venous duplex scanning. J Vasc Surg 1990; 11:675–679.

26. Beach KW. Physics and instrumentation for ultrasonic duplex scanning. In: Strandness DE Jr, ed. Duplex Scanning in Vascular Disorders. NewYork: Raven Press, 1990:196–227.

2

Cardiopulmonary Complications Related to Vascular Surgery

W. Darrin Clouse*

Massachusetts General Hospital and Harvard Medical School, Boston, Massachusetts, and F. Edward Hébert School of Medicine, Uniformed Services University of the Health Sciences, Bethesda, Maryland, U.S.A.

David C. Brewster

Massachusetts General Hospital and Harvard Medical School, Boston, Massachusetts, U.S.A.

I. INTRODUCTION

In addition to having systemic atherosclerosis, patients undergoing vascular surgery are also commonly advanced in age, afflicted with chronic obstructive pulmonary disease (COPD), showing effects of tobacco abuse, and suffering from other medical comorbidities. Accordingly, cardiopulmonary complications are the most frequent perioperative problem facing this patient population. As with any complication, evaluating and intervening in an attempt to avoid potential problems is preferred to attending them after they occur. Hence, a considerable amount of investigation has been performed in an effort to better define, profile, and preemptively address those at high risk for cardiopulmonary difficulties after vascular surgery. Obviously, this strategy is an attempt to minimize the short- and long-term morbidity and mortality from cardiopulmonary disease experienced by this population. Yet it remains difficult to clearly define specifics regarding the risks and benefits of preoperative evaluation; the ability to approach this analysis sensibly is one of the most important aspects in the management of the vascular surgical patient.

* *Current affiliation*: Wilford Hall Medical Center, Lackland Air Force Base, Texas, U.S.A.

15

II. CARDIAC COMPLICATIONS

A. Coronary Artery Disease in Peripheral Vascular Patients

Some amount of coronary artery disease (CAD) is present in nearly all vascular surgery patients due to the systemic nature of atherosclerosis. In a sentinel report from the Cleveland Clinic, Hertzer and colleagues performed coronary angiography in 1000 consecutive patients being evaluated for peripheral vascular surgery (1). Coronary artery disease, to varying degrees, was present in 92%. Moreover, 25% had severe, correctable CAD and almost 20% suffered from three-vessel coronary atherosclerosis. The severity of CAD appeared to be independent of vascular disease distribution, as CAD was severe in 36% of those with abdominal aortic aneurysm (AAA), 28% of those with lower extremity ischemia, and 32% of patients with cerebrovascular disease. Further, contemporary series reveal clinical evidence of CAD in 30–50% of patients undergoing various peripheral vascular procedures (2–15).

Not surprisingly, cardiac morbidity [usually defined as myocardial infarction, unstable angina, congestive heart failure (CHF), dysrhythmia, and cardiac death] is among the leading causes of perioperative morbidity and mortality in those undergoing peripheral vascular operation. Vascular patients are apparently at highest risk for postoperative cardiac events. Lee and colleagues, in evaluating 4315 patients undergoing noncardiac surgery, found that AAA repair and other peripheral vascular operations had a 3.6 and 3.9 relative risk, respectively, for cardiac events compared to other types of procedures (16). Acute myocardial infarction (AMI) was responsible for the majority of these events and is the leading postoperative cardiac event in most series. Although the pathophysiology of perioperative AMI is complex, numerous factors are likely involved. Both surgery and anesthesia initiate processes that place added stress on the myocardium. Catechol release, increased myocardial sensitivity to catechols, fluid shifts, blood pressure fluctuations, alterations in oxygen delivery, transient hypercoagulability, and tachycardia all may compromise the coronary circulation's ability to supply oxygen postoperatively.

Recent studies retrospectively delineating the incidence of postoperative AMI in vascular patients reveal roughly a 1–7% chance of infarction in those having operations for aneurysm, cerebrovascular disease, lower extremity ischemia, or other major peripheral vascular disease (Table 1). But when studied prospectively with aggressive diagnostic physiological parameters, AMI may occur in as many as 15% of patients (17). Several factors could explain this disparity. Postoperative myocardial ischemia is commonly silent, can occur any time during the postprocedural course, and is not uncommon in those without preoperative evidence of CAD. Illustrating this last point, in Hertzer's angiographic evaluation of 1000 vascular patients, 15% of those without clinical evidence of CAD had severe disease and 22% had advanced disease (1). Therefore, coronary disease is prevalent in this population even without clinical indicators. Silent ischemia is a harbinger of myocardial infarction and cardiac morbidity, and unexplained persistent tachycardia may be the only suggestion of ischemia postoperatively. Using perioperative ambulatory electrocardiographic (ECG) monitoring, Pasternak and coworkers reported that silent myocardial ischemia occurred in some 60% of 200 vascular surgery patients, and both the duration and number of ischemic episodes were significant predictors of postoperative AMI, which occurred in 4.5% (18). Even more disturbing, Krupski et al. documented postoperative ischemic ECG changes in 57% of infrainguinal reconstructions and 31% of aortic operations, with a staggering 98% being silent (15). Others have reported similarly large proportions of vascular patients experiencing silent postoperative ischemia (19–21). AMI has

Table 1 Postoperative Myocardial Infarction (MI) Rate in Contemporary Vascular Surgery Reports

Report[a]	Year	Number of patients/operations	MI (%)
Aortic surgery			
Cambria et al. (TAA) (106)	2002	337	3.9
Berry et al. (AAA) (128)	2001	856	1.3
Romero et al. (EAAA) (107)	2001	173	4.6
Hovsepian et al. (EAAA) (108)	2001	144	2.8
Becker et al. (EAAA) (109)	2001	305	0.6
Ponovost et al. (AAR) (110)	2001	2,987	3.3
Axelrod et al. (AAA) (111)	2001	1,001	3.1
Martin et al. (SR/TAAIII/IV) (112)	2000	165	5.0
Pearce et al. (AAA) (113)	1999	13,415	1.8
Carotid surgery			
Sternbach et al. (114)	2002	550	1.1
Azia et al. (6)	2001	123	1.6
AbuRhama et al. (115)	2001	389	0.3
James et al. (116)	2001	324	0.9
Hamdan et al. (117)	1999	1,001	0.5
Pearce et al. (113)	1999	45,744	0.8
Cao et al. (118)	1998	1,353	0.4
Infrainguinal surgery			
Conte et al. (all indications) (119)	2001	1,642	3.0
Kalra et al. (pedal bypass) (120)	2001	280	6.4
Faries et al. (all indications) (121)	2000	740	1.5
Nicoloff et al. (limb salvage) (122)	1998	112	9.0
Matsuura et al. (elective) (123)	1997	205	3.4
Major vascular surgery (procedures combined)			
Boersma (44)	2001	1,351	3.3
Landesberg et al. (23)	2001	185	6.5
Sprung et al. (3)	2000	6,948	1.5
Van Damme et al. (9)	1997	142	2.1
Landsberg et al. (35)	1997	405	4.7
Mamode et al. (22)	1996	204	6.9

[a] AAA = abdominal aortic aneurysm; AAR = abdominal aortic reconstruction (i.e., both aneurysm and occlusive disease); EAAA = endovascular abdominal aortic aneurysm repair; SR = suprarenal aortic aneurysm; TAA = thoracoabdominal aneurysm.

been estimated to be silent in nearly one-third of patients experiencing infarction after undergoing vascular surgery (13,22). A recent prospective evaluation by Landesberg et al. studied 185 vascular patients for ischemia and infarction with continuous postoperative ECG monitoring for 48–72 h and daily cardiac enzyme panels (23). Those with recent MI or unstable angina were excluded. Myocardial ischemia developed in 38 (20.5%) patients, with AMI occurring in 12 (6.5%). Ischemia was silent in over 80%, and in 42% of those with AMI.

Postoperative silent myocardial ischemia in noncardiac surgery has also recently been evaluated by Swear and colleagues and Higham et al. (20,21). Results were similar, with 40% of vascular patients having silent ischemia postoperatively; those going through vascular surgery were at highest risk for its development. It is not surprising that myocardial ischemia is silent in these patients, as it may be confounded by incisional pain and drug effects. The proper recognition of and intervention in postoperative cardiac events in terms of timing is another problem. Krupski and others have noted that a significant proportion of cardiac events occur 3 or more days after vascular surgery, when patients are usually not monitored or being routinely tested for laboratory evidence of myocardial ischemia (3,15,22,24,25). These several factors make it difficult to consistently identify or prepare for cardiac morbidity after vascular surgery.

Cardiac death is the most common cause of perioperative mortality in vascular surgery. As mentioned, AMI accounts for the bulk of these events. It has been projected that up to 40% of postvascular surgery MIs result in death (26). L'Italien reported on 547 consecutive patients referred for coronary evaluation prior to vascular surgery and found that 33% of postoperative AMI resulted in mortality (10). During the early 1980s, several reports from Hertzer's group at the Cleveland Clinic reported that half of their postoperative deaths resulted from AMI in the vascular population (27–29). Sprung et al. recently reviewed almost 7000 consecutive cases from the Cleveland Clinic vascular registry and found postoperative AMI occurred in an enviable 1.5%, with 21% dying as a result (3). Also, cardiac death is the leading reason for late demise in those with peripheral vascular disease. Regardless of required procedure, authors have repeatedly implicated cardiac death as the leading source of late mortality after vascular surgery (10,14). Therefore it is clear that cardiac intervention could not only potentially lessen morbidity surrounding these operations but also perhaps improve long-term survival.

B. Clinical Risk Assessment

Because vascular patients are at an increased perioperative cardiac risk, any preoperatively identified indicators of enhanced vulnerability to events may help in selecting patients for further cardiac evaluation. Several studies have identified physical findings or historical factors associated with increased cardiac risk in those undergoing surgery and have combined these markers into indices designed to effectively quantitate risk. While some large series have evaluated clinical predictors of cardiac events in all noncardiac surgical patients, others have focused on those undergoing vascular surgery (Table 2). Based on these studies, several clinical criteria have been identified as independently important in the development of postoperative cardiac complications. To varying degrees these have included age >70 years, angina, prior myocardial infarction, significant arrhythmias, severe valvular disease, CHF, ECG abnormalities, prior stroke, diabetes mellitus, renal insufficiency and high risk (i.e., abdominal, thoracic, vascular, and emergent) surgery.

Recognizing a need for refinement of the factors predicting cardiac morbidity, the American College of Cardiology and the American Heart Association (ACC/AHA) Task Force on Practice Guidelines has categorized these variables into major, intermediate, and minor clinical predictors of perioperative cardiac risk (Table 3) (30,31). The surgical procedures were stratified into those having high, intermediate, and low cardiac risk. Aortic and peripheral vascular surgical procedures are considered high-risk procedures, while carotid endarterectomy is deemed intermediate in risk. Further, the task force described a historical estimation of functional capacity based upon metabolic equivalents (METs), where 1 MET

Table 2 Clinical Risk Predictors for Adverse Postoperative Cardiac Events[a]

Report	Year	Independent predictors
Noncardiac surgery		
Goldman et al. (99)	1977	Age >70, MI in previous 6 months
		S$_3$ gallop or JVD, aortic stenosis
		Rhythm other than sinus or PAC, >5 PVC/min,
		Poor general medical status (PaO$_2$ <60 or
		PCO$_2$ >50, K<3.0 or HCO$_3$ <20, BUN >50 or Cr
		>3.0, elevated SGOT)
		Intraperitoneal or intrathoracic or aortic or
		emergency operation
Detsky et al. (101)	1986	Age >70, any prior MI, angina pectoris
		Pulmonary edema, critical aortic stenosis
		Rhythm other than sinus, >5 PVC/min
		Poor general medical status (PaO$_2$ <60 or
		PCO$_2$ >50, K <3.0 or HCO$_3$ <20, BUN >50 or Cr
		>3.0, elevated SGOT)
		Emergency surgery
Lee et al. (16)	1999	Ischemic heart disease
		History of CHF
		History of CVD
		Insulin-dependent diabetes mellitus
		Preoperative serum creatinine >2.0
		High-risk surgery
Vascular surgery		
Eagle et al. (52)	1987	Age >70
		Q waves on ECG
		History of angina pectoris
		History of ventricular ectopy requiring therapy
		Diabetes mellitus requiring therapy
Sprung et al. (3)	2000	Valvular heart disease (aortic or mitral)
		Coronary artery disease
		History of CHF
		Operative transfusion
		Prior CABG (protective)
Boersma et al. (44)	2001	History of CVD
		History of CHF
		Prior MI
		Current or prior angina pectoris
		Age >70
		Beta-blocker therapy (protective)

[a] BUN = blood urea nitrogen; CABG = coronary artery bypass grafting; CHF = congestive heart failure; CVD = cerebrovascular disease; HCO$_3$ = serum bicarbonate; JVD = jugular venous distention; K = serum potassium; MI = myocardial infarction; PAC = premature atrial contraction; PVC = premature ventricular contraction; PaO$_2$ = arterial oxygen tension; PaCO$_2$ = arterial carbon dioxide tension; SGOT = serum glutamic oxaloacetate transaminase.

Table 3 Clinical Risk Factors for Adverse Postoperative Cardiac Event

Major
    Unstable coronary syndromes
        Acute or recent myocardial infarction with clinical symptoms or
            noninvasive study evidence of ischemic risk
        Unstable or severe angina pectoris
    Decompensated heart failure
    Significant arrhythmias
        High-grade atrioventricular block
        Symptomatic ventricular arrhythmias with underlying heart disease
        Supraventricular arrhythmias with uncontrolled ventricular rate
Intermediate
    Mild angina pectoris
    Previous myocardial infarction by history or Q waves
    Compensated or previous heart failure
    Diabetes mellitus
    Renal insufficiency
Minor
    Advanced age
    Abnormal ECG
        Left ventricular hypertrophy
        Left bundle branch block
        ST-T abnormalities
    Rhythm other than sinus
    Low functional capacity
    Stroke history
    Uncontrolled hypertension

Sources: Refs. 30 and 31.

represents the oxygen consumption of a 40-year-old man in a resting state. Using these scales, an algorithmic approach to preoperative cardiac risk assessment was then presented (30,31). This algorithm delineated four specific clinical scenarios:

1. Patients who need emergency surgery, have undergone coronary revascularization within 5 years without recurrent signs and symptoms of CAD, or have had a recent favorable coronary evaluation without clinical changes should go directly for operation.

2. Those with major clinical predictors should have elective surgery canceled and coronary artery evaluation and intervention as necessary.

3. Those with intermediate clinical predictors and poor functional capacity (<4 METs) should have noninvasive coronary evaluation, while those with moderate or excellent functional capacity (>4 METs) should undergo noninvasive study when the proposed procedure is high risk in nature. When the procedure is intermediate or low in risk, the patient should proceed to surgery.

4. In those with minor or no clinical CAD predictors and poor functional capacity (<4 METs) who are to undergo a high-risk operation, noninvasive coronary evaluation is recommended. Those with moderate or excellent functional capacity (>4

METs) or those with poor capacity who are to undergo intermediate- or low-risk procedures should proceed to operation.

If evidence of coronary ischemia is found on noninvasive testing, cardiology referral should take place, with further coronary artery evaluation and revascularization when indicated or, in those found to have less extensive disease, risk-factor modification prior to operation.

Within this schema, vascular surgery patients are frequently within the category of those requiring noninvasive evaluation. A recent retrospective evaluation of the ACC/AHA guidelines in 133 consecutive patients undergoing aortic surgery was performed by Samain and coworkers (5). All had routine cardiac evaluation prior to surgery. Following the algorithm, 60 patients (45%) required noninvasive testing and the algorithm classified all those with postoperative events as being at high risk. The authors concluded that the ACC/AHA guidelines were valid in patients undergoing major vascular surgery. These recommendations appear to have helped to streamline thinking about cardiac clinical risk assessment prior to vascular surgery. However, while the use of clinical risk factors alone does not provide complete postoperative cardiac prognosis, it allows surgeons to identify those at increased risk who need further evaluation or procedure modification and those who may proceed to surgery knowing that their risk, although not absent, is minimal.

C. Adjunctive Screening Methods for Cardiac Risk Stratification

Once the need for further preoperative cardiac evaluation beyond clinical assessment is deemed necessary, another decision must be made on how best to accomplish this task. While coronary angiography is appropriate in those patients with unstable angina, recent myocardial infarction, decompensating CHF, and new arrhythmias, it is invasive, with complications of its own, and provides only anatomical information. Thus, no functional information is obtained and its predictive value is limited. Its principal use in preoperative risk stratification is after noninvasive studies have determined the patient to be at high risk for cardiac events and shown that catheterization may provide therapeutic benefit. Thus, the use of routine coronary angiography to stratify vascular patients is historical. A variety of noninvasive techniques have been developed that provide functional and/or metabolic definition of the myocardium.

Exercise-stress ECG testing was the earliest method used to investigate CAD severity. It is valuable in that this test provides data on functional workload capacity in addition to identifying major CAD presence. Significant induced ischemia at low-level exercise is clearly predictive of postoperative cardiac events, with negative predictive values of over 90% (30,32). However, because of age, deconditioning, severe claudication, ischemic ulcerations, prior amputation, stroke, severe lung disease, arthritis, or other infirmities, peripheral vascular surgery patients are frequently incapable of adequate exercise to achieve the necessary 75–85% of the maximal predicted heart rate required for proper testing. Submaximal testing may decrease sensitivity in this population with a high prevalence of CAD and silent ischemia; because this is also the surgical population at highest risk of cardiac events, ECG stress testing plays a limited role in noninvasive evaluation. Ambulatory ECG (Holter) monitoring with evidence of myocardial ischemia and left ventricular hypertrophy has also been shown by some to correlate with postoperative cardiac events (18,19,33–35). One prospective study, however, has shown that evidence of myocardial ischemia on preoperative Holter monitoring did not predict postoperative AMI (36). Again, however, this method is limited for several reasons. First, there is no protocol to standardize results using this method. Second, baseline ECG characteristics obviate the ability to critically interpret ST segments in a significant proportion of vascular patients. And last, while positive results may identify patients at increased perioperative cardiac risk, prognostic stratification parameters are lacking, and how to manage those with positive findings remains unclear.

Radionuclide ventriculography [gated blood pool scan, multiple gated acquisition (MUGA) scan] is a noninvasive technique that provides for assessment of left ventricular function and wall motion. Most studies have shown an increase in postoperative cardiac events with a left ventricular ejection fraction (LVEF) less than normal (55%), and the risk appears to be higher with LVEF less than 35% (17,37–39). Franco and colleagues, however, suggested that resting radionuclide ventriculography did not contribute insight into postoperative cardiac events (40). Exercise testing may be added to enhance functional changes in LVEF and wall motion indicative of CAD that is limiting myocardial perfusion, and positive findings with this method correlate well with postoperative cardiac risk (41). However, the development of echocardiography, which assesses both LVEF and wall motion without the need for radioactive material—as well as improvements in myocardial scintigraphy including newer tracer agents that allow both evaluation of ventricular function as well as myocardial perfusion—has diminished enthusiasm to utilize this technique for cardiac risk stratification (42).

Two techniques to noninvasively evaluate CAD in those with inadequate functional capacity to undergo proper exercise testing have been devised. The newest method of noninvasive cardiac testing is dobutamine stress echocardiography (DSE), which allows stress evaluation of the myocardium without exercise. Dobutamine is a beta$_1$ receptor–selective agonist that increases heart rate and contractility and thus myocardial oxygen consumption. When dobutamine is given in conjunction with echocardiography before and after administration, differences in left ventricular function and wall motion are detected. These findings suggest unmasking of flow-limiting CAD with resultant myocardial dysfunction. Positive ischemic endpoints are noted as new or worsening wall motion abnormalities (NWMA) and the myocardium defined in segments. Although DSE has not been as extensively studied as myocardial scintigraphy, its utility as an adjunct to cardiac risk assessment is being defined. Indeed, the existence of wall motion abnormalities at rest correlates with postoperative events in vascular patients (43,44). The positive predictive value of stress-induced ischemia using DSE appears to be 10–40% and the negative predictive value without NWMA 95–100% (9,30,43–45). Two studies have used DSE to report stratification schemes for those requiring noninvasive testing. Poldermans and colleagues studied 300 vascular surgery patients by clinical risk assessment using Detsky and Eagle criteria and DSE (43). All patients who suffered a postoperative cardiac event had a positive DSE. Thus, the negative predictive value was 100% and the positive predictive value 38%. Further, the authors found that the lower the heart rate at the time of NWMA onset, the greater the risk of a postoperative event. Recently, Boersma et al. evaluated 1351 consecutive major vascular surgery patients (44). DSE was performed in 1079 patients and a positive DSE was independently associated with adverse cardiac events. Also, those with NWMA in five or more segments had a four- to sixfold increase in events compared to those with one to four segments affected. By incorporating the Lee clinical risk index, the authors found that in those with fewer than three risk factors, the adverse cardiac event rate was 2%, and DSE added little to the patient's risk stratification. In those with more than three factors, DSE was predictive of adverse cardiac events, as the event rate was 4.6% in those with no NWMA, 13% in those with one to four affected, segments and 35% when five or more segments became ischemic. The protective effect of beta blockade in vascular patients was impressive in this series as well and is discussed below. The major criticism of DSE as a method of noninvasive evaluation is a lack of standardized protocols and criteria to describe positive tests and the subjective nature of NWMA. Also, problems with dobutamine administration—such as arrhythmias, myocardial infarction, angina, hypotension and drug reactions—may occur. However, at present, this appears to be a useful technique in the risk stratification of vascular patients.

The second and most studied method of noninvasive cardiac evaluation in vascular patients unable to exercise is dipyridamole-thallium scintigraphy. This method was first applied to risk assessment prior to vascular surgery by Boucher in 1985, and we have used it extensively at the Massachusetts General Hospital (46). The nuclear imaging technology has continued to improve and newer radiotracers based on technitium 99m (^{99m}Tc), with shorter half-lives, allow both assessment of ventricular function as well as myocardial viability imaging (42). Dipyridamole administered intravenously inhibits the natural transport processes of adenosine, a potent coronary vasodilator, causing increased levels. This results in coronary vasodilatation with increased flow in those coronary arteries without significant disease, while arteries with significant atherosclerotic disease fail to dilate. Flow is preferential to myocardial segments supplied by normal arteries, with hypoperfusion in the distribution of severely disease coronary arteries. Adenosine itself is now also used to precipitate pharmacologically induced coronary vasodilatation, and the use of dobutamine-induced stress for scintigraphy has also been reported (9,42). Thallium 201 (^{201}Th) and the newer ^{99m}Tc- labeled tracers enter myocardial cells in proportion to blood flow; thus they enter viable areas. The myocardium normally has homogeneous radiotracer uptake unless there are regions of hypoperfusion.

The current myocardial scintigraphy technique used for cardiac risk assessment prior to vascular surgery at the Massachusetts General Hospital is described in Figure 1. Intravenous adenosine is used for pharmacological stress and ^{99m}Tc sestamibi (mibi) is the currently used radiotracer. Imaging occurs with the use of stress single-photon-emission computed tomography (SPECT). Initial resting scans are obtained 30–45 min after radiotracer injection (10 mCi ^{99m}Tc mibi). Then the stress sequence begins with low-level exercise and adenosine infusion (140 ug/kg/min). The radiotracer (30 mCi ^{99m}Tc mibi) is again injected 2 min after the adenosine is started. Once the stress sequence is complete, repeat images are obtained 45 min after tracer injection, using ECG gating to provide LVEF data. Normally perfused myocardium quickly absorbs the radiotracer and is visualized on both resting and stress images. Viable ischemic myocardium, beyond a fixed coronary artery stenosis that cannot dilate, takes up the radiotracer at a reduced rate and is seen only in the resting baseline images (Fig. 2). Hence, any areas of hypoperfusion appear as decreased radiotracer uptake or "cold spots" on the stress scans. If these initially underperfused areas show more homogeneous uptake of the radiotracer on the resting baseline images, this is referred to as "fill in" or redistribution (Fig. 3) (46). A scan is considered positive if regions of redistribution are confirmed. These areas represent regions of ischemic but viable myocardium at risk for perioperative ischemia or infarction. Regions of persistent decreased uptake represent nonviable myocardium from previous infarction (i.e., "scarred") and are considered not to be at risk for further events. Such a scan is not considered positive (47). The sensitivity of scintigraphy may be enhanced by low-level exercise; we use low stress treadmill walking for this purpose. If patients experience any adverse reactions to dipyridamole or adenosine (i.e., flushing, wheezing, dizziness, angina, arrhythmias, and hypotension), the infusion is stopped. Aminophylline may need to be

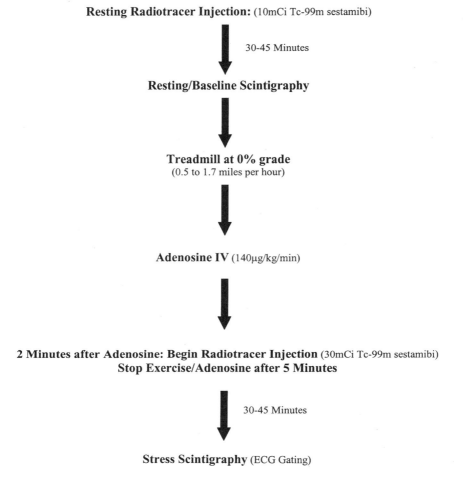

Resting Radiotracer Injection: (10mCi Tc-99m sestamibi)

30-45 Minutes

Resting/Baseline Scintigraphy

Treadmill at 0% grade
(0.5 to 1.7 miles per hour)

Adenosine IV (140μg/kg/min)

2 Minutes after Adenosine: Begin Radiotracer Injection (30mCi Tc-99m sestamibi)
Stop Exercise/Adenosine after 5 Minutes

30-45 Minutes

Stress Scintigraphy (ECG Gating)

Figure 1 Our current myocardial scintigraphy protocol for cardiac risk stratification screening prior to vascular surgery.

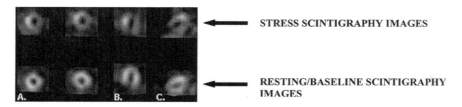

STRESS SCINTIGRAPHY IMAGES

RESTING/BASELINE SCINTIGRAPHY
IMAGES

Figure 2 Myocardial scintigraphy images using the radiotracer technetium-99m sestamibi showing apical (A) inferior (B) and lateral (C) "redistribution" consistent with viable ischemic myocardium at risk.

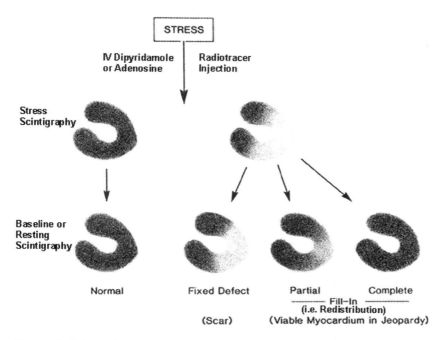

Figure 3 Schematic representation of possible myocardial scintigraphy results. Normal stress and resting myocardial scintigraphy showing homogenous uptake of radiotracer during both stress and rest. Stress scintigraphy images obtained after pharmacological coronary vasodilation revealing poor radiotracer uptake in a myocardial distribution may persist at rest as a fixed defect suggesting scar, or resting images may partially or completely "fill in" the defect, suggesting viable myocardium at risk.

used to compete for adenosine receptors. Patients taking methylxanthines must obviously discontinue these prior to undergoing this test.

Stress scintigraphy has been widely evaluated in vascular patients in an attempt to identify those at highest risk of cardiac complications. L'Italien found that in 547 consecutive patients referred for dipyridamole-thallium scanning prior to aortic, infrainguinal, or carotid surgery, redistribution on scanning was the most significant predictor of postoperative MI. Those with a positive test were over 3 1/2 times more likely to experience infarct (10). The significance of redistribution on scintigraphy has also been suggested predictive of postoperative cardiac events by others (10,11,48–51). Eagle et al. reported that the predictive value of dipyridamole-thallium redistribution could be significantly increased by combining scan results with clinical criteria (52). This landmark study categorized patients into three risk groups based on the presence of these clinical factors. Low-risk patients were those with no clinical markers. One or two factors placed the patient in the intermediate-risk group, and three or more markers defined the high-risk group (Fig. 4). The risk of untoward postoperative cardiac ischemic events was small in the low-risk group (3% events, no deaths); scintigraphy is not warranted in these patients. The event rate in the high-risk group was so high (50%) that scan results would not improve the risk prediction or alter preoperative workup or perioperative management. Consideration of a more extensive coronary artery evaluation (i.e., catheterization) and intervention as well as alternative surgical approaches

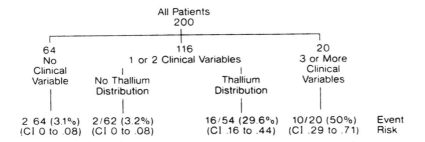

* Q wave on electrocardiogram, age > 70 yrs, history of angina,
history of ventricular ectopic activity requiring treatment, and
diabetes mellitus requiring treatment.

Figure 4 Selective cardiac screening efficacy using clinical predictors and myocardial scintigraphy to identify patients at increased risk for adverse cardiac events after vascular surgery. *Event* refers to postoperative cardiac ischemic events, including unstable angina, ischemic pulmonary edema, myocardial infarction, or cardiac death. CI = 95% confidence interval. (From Ref. 52.)

or cancellation would be more productive. However, in the moderate-risk patients, stress-thallium scintigraphy was extremely helpful, as those with normal perfusion had a post-operative event rate (3%) equating that of the low-risk cohort, whereas redistribution indicated a 30% risk and suggested that a more detailed CAD assessment was prudent. Using this strategy, the test's sensitivity and specificity for identifying postoperative adverse cardiac events were 83% and 66%, respectively, with a positive predictive value of 30% and a negative predictive value of 96%. The authors concluded that the method's ability to stratify patients was enhanced by combining clinical risk factors with selective myocardial scintigraphy and that it could effectively limit the number of patients requiring extensive coronary evaluation (52). Also, Levinson and colleagues have reported that quantification of redistribution by ischemic segments, number of positive views, and number of coronary territories affected further identifies those at highest risk for postoperative cardiac events after vascular surgery (Table 4) (53). Others have also found quantitative interpre-

Table 4 Maximizing Myocardial Scintigraphy Interpretation

Variables	Probability of cardiac event
Ischemic segments	
<3	12% ($p=0.03$)
>4	38%
Number of views with ischemia	
<1	0% ($p=0.005$)
>2	36%
Number of coronary territories with ischemia	
<3	13% ($p=0.007$)
>4	43%

Source: Ref. 53.

tation of redistribution to improve the positive predictive value of myocardial scintigraphy (54,55).

However, there is no consensus regarding the use of myocardial scintigraphy for the purpose of preoperative cardiac risk stratification and predicting cardiac morbidity and mortality in vascular surgery patients. Several authors have suggested that routine stress cardiac scintigraphy before vascular surgery is not helpful in predicting events (56–59). Baron, et al. evaluated the usefulness of dipyridamole-thallium and LVEF in 513 consecutive patients who were to undergo elective abdominal aortic surgery (60). Those with clear indications for coronary catheterization as well as those with incomplete clinical or imaging data were excluded. In all, 457 patients were analyzed and the authors found no correlation between preoperative redistribution and postoperative events. Most recently, in a blinded, prospective study, de Virgilio and coworkers concluded that no association existed between redistribution and postoperative cardiac events in 80 patients with at least one Eagle risk factor (2). They reported a sensitivity and specificity of 44% and 65%, respectively, with positive and negative predictive values of 14% and 90% in their selective cohort.

At present, there is no clearly superior method of noninvasive evaluation for cardiac stratification prior to vascular surgery. While exercise stress ECG is a powerful tool to evaluate CAD, patients afflicted with peripheral vascular disease are, for the most part, unable to undergo meaningful exercise stress testing for health related reasons. Also, a significant proportion have baseline ECG abnormalities. Pharmacological stress testing with dipyridamole, adenosine, or dobutamine is, therefore, useful to instigate myocardial stress in these patients. Stress imaging by either DSE or myocardial scintigraphy appears to help further define risks in those requiring noninvasive cardiac evaluation; these are the most often used techniques in this population. Current reviews reveal a negative predictive value of these noninvasive methods of roughly 98% (42). Further, there is evidence that both myocardial scintigraphy and DSE provide long-term coronary artery prognostic information in vascular patients (10,59,61–63). Even though their use in preoperative stratification is still hotly debated, their strongest use may be in identifying those at highest risk for long-term CAD events and in reducing late cardiac morbidity and mortality.

D. Risk Stratification Postures for Cardiac Assessment Prior to Vascular Surgery

Albeit clinical variables important to the development of postoperative cardiac complications are widely recognized and critical evaluation to find the elusive perfect noninvasive technique is ongoing, what remains critical to vascular surgeons when their patients are found to be at increased cardiac risk is what can be done to improve their patients' course and long-term health. A lowering of postoperative cardiac morbidity and mortality by aggressive preoperative evaluation for CAD and revascularization within this population remains, at present, unproven, and several general postures toward cardiac risk stratification have evolved.

First, an aggressive stance may be taken that all patients who are to have a major vascular surgical procedure should be critically evaluated and treated for the presence of significant CAD in the hopes of both reducing perioperative morbidity and improving long-term survival. The cornerstone of this approach is the hypothesis that coronary revascularization improves postoperative outcomes after vascular surgery. The literature over the last three decades has delineated a potential benefit, both perioperatively and in the long term, in those who undergo coronary artery bypass grafting (CABG) prior to noncardiac surgery. This was evident from the Coronary Artery Surgery Study (CASS), when Eagle et al. reported on nearly 3400 patients undergoing various noncardiac procedures. Previous CABG was independently protective in those undergoing high-risk surgery and the protective effect was present for up to 6 years after coronary revascularization (64). Hertzer and colleagues studied over 1000 vascular patients and found those identified preoperatively with significant surgically reconstructable CAD who underwent CABG had fewer postoperative cardiac complications after vascular surgery than those who did not. Further, the long-term (5-year) survival in those who had coronary revascularization was significantly enhanced (75%) compared to those without CABG (29%) (1,65,66). This result has been echoed by several authors (67,68). Sprung and associates reviewed the recent Cleveland Clinic experience with postoperative myocardial infarction in nearly 7000 vascular surgical patients (3). While they did not find CABG protective for the occurrence of AMI, they did find it to be protective against cardiac death. Those with prior coronary grafting experienced a 79% reduction (27.9 vs. 7.7%; $p = 0.01$) in postoperative death due to cardiac causes.

Fewer reports have studied the effects of preoperative percutaneous coronary revascularization on perioperative outcomes. Several small studies have implicated a protective effect of percutaneous transluminal coronary angioplasty (PTCA) prior to noncardiac surgery (69,70). One study by Elmore and colleagues from the Mayo Clinic evaluated 84 patients who underwent CABG and 14 with PTCA before AAA repair (71). They found that both groups had similar postoperative cardiac event rates and 3-year survival. The PTCA cohort was able to undergo AAA repair a mean of 10 days after coronary revascularization, while those undergoing CABG had to wait 68 days. However, the PTCA group had significantly more late cardiac events (57 vs. 27%; $p = 0.002$). Gottlieb and coworkers analyzed 194 patients who had PTCA within 18 months before undergoing vascular surgery (72). Three-quarters of these patients underwent PTCA within 50 days of surgery and the postoperative MI rate and occurrence of CHF were both an excellent 0.5%, suggesting a beneficial effect to preoperative percutaneous revascularization. Recently, the Bypass vs. Angioplasty Revascularization Investigation (BARI) reported its results in patients undergoing noncardiac surgery believed to require preoperative coronary revascularization (73). Patients were randomly assigned to undergo CABG or PTCA prior to surgery. The perioperative cardiac morbidity and mortality were no different between groups; however, only 11% of the procedures were vascular and only one-third were high risk in nature. Although small in number and biased by nonvascular operations, data suggest that PTCA may provide similar perioperative cardiac protection compared to CABG in vascular surgery patients with CAD appropriate for percutaneous intervention.

Not all reports conclude a salutary effect of coronary revascularization on cardiac events after vascular surgery (49). Mason and colleagues developed models evaluating the effect of preoperative coronary angiography and revascularization on perioperative vascular surgery results (74). Only when the vascular operative mortality was substantial (greater than 5%) and the risks of coronary revascularization low did a mortality benefit occur. This benefit was small (less than 1%), however, and was only present when those with unreconstructable CAD had their vascular surgery canceled. In all models performed, patients with preoperative coronary angiography and revascularization had more perioperative morbidity. Moreover, this strategy doubled the cost of patient care, but long-term consequences were not addressed. Massie and associates compared 70 vascular patients who underwent coronary angiography due to redistribution on myocardial scintigraphy with 70 matched controls (75). Coronary revascularization was required in 25 of the 70 angiography patients. Although fewer postoperative cardiac events occurred in the angiography/revascularization cohort, complications secondary to the invasive coronary evaluation led to no difference in perioperative outcome between groups. Also, the invasively studied/revascularized patients had significantly fewer long-term cardiac events, but long-term survival was similar. The authors concluded that in vascular surgery patients with abnormal myocardial scintigraphy, coronary angiography and revascularization did not improve overall outcomes. The above studies suggest that the additive morbidity and mortality of invasive coronary evaluation and revasculariztion prior to vascular surgery may offset any benefit. Thus, currently, there is no consensus regarding the efficacy of coronary revascularization prior to vascular surgery in preventing postoperative cardiac events. To assist in answering questions surrounding this controversy, the Coronary Artery Revascularization Prophylaxis for Elective Vascular Surgery Study (CARP) is ongoing and should shed light on how best to approach coronary revascularization perioperatively in vascular patients with significant CAD (76).

The lack of clear evidence supporting a protective effect of preoperative coronary revascularization on postoperative adverse cardiac events has generated another outlook on risk stratification. This posture toward preoperative cardiac risk assessment is a minimalist approach. Taylor et al. prospectively evaluated 491 vascular surgery patients through 534 procedures during a 1-year period (13). The authors were unconvinced that preoperative cardiac risk screening prior to vascular surgery was efficacious and wanted to study the outcome with limited use of preoperative testing. Only when clinical evidence suggested severe CAD did evaluation beyond history, physical examination and resting ECG take place. In 31 (5.8%) patients, further testing was performed. The overall AMI rate was an enviable 3.9% and no differences in event rates were found between patients with or without clinical evidence of CAD or those undergoing detailed cardiac evaluation. Taylor and colleagues concluded that preoperative cardiac evaluation in vascular patients should be limited to those with severe symptomatic disease. This minimalist approach has recently been advocated in several communications by de Virgilio and coworkers. Their work has described no association between dipyridamole myocardial scintigraphy results and post-vascular surgery events even in the intermediate-risk category (2,7). They conclude that, as in selective stratification, those with no clinical risk factors should proceed to surgery and those with major clinical risk factors continue with extensive coronary evaluation. However, in the intermediate-risk category, they propose proceeding to surgery under beta blockade (77,78). Others have found no overall event reduction with preoperative cardiac evaluation (58,75). Further, these groups argue that the complications of noninvasive testing proceeding to invasive coronary evaluation and therapy are additive, and even if they actually decrease the operative cardiac morbidity and mortality after vascular surgery, the complications due to the other prevascular procedures at least offset the gain (79). Also, they suggest that more money is spent per person undergoing extensive coronary evaluation for no apparent overall benefit (74).

As the benefits of aggressive evaluation for CAD before vascular operation in all patients remains questioned, and due to concern regarding the high CAD incidence in these individuals, another position regarding preoperative stratification has developed. This method is referred to as selective screening for coronary disease. The basis for this approach lies in the use of clinical factors and noninvasive testing to identify those patients at increased cardiac risk and to intervene in them in some fashion to reduce risk. Thereby the cost, predictive value, and benefits of preoperative coronary studies may be enhanced. As mentioned above, dipyridamole-thallium scintigraphy was used by Eagle and colleagues after clinically scoring 200 patients who were to undergo vascular surgery (Fig. 4) (52). Those with no clinical variables had a low (3%) cardiac event rate and those with three or more clinical variables had a high risk for events (50%). The intermediate-risk group, however, was further stratified by the use of myocardial scintigraphy. If redistribution was present on scanning, 30% of patients suffered a postoperative adverse cardiac event, while those with no redistribution had just as low a risk as those with no clinical risk factors (3%). This study initiated the idea of selective screening, as it proved that higher-risk patients could be identified and therapies initiated in an attempt to reduce risk and that routine study of patients at clinically low risk is not justified. This selective scheme using clinical and scintigraphy data was subsequently validated by L'Italien and colleagues in 1081 vascular surgery patients (11). The ability to select patients at higher cardiac risk was also noted by van Damme et al. (9). They extensively studied 156 consecutive patients scheduled for major vascular surgery. After clinical evaluation and noninvasive testing, 142 remained as 11 proceeded to coronary angiography and 3 more had incomplete data. In those without clinical evidence of CAD, the postoperative cardiac event rate was 0–3% regardless of dobutamine stress test results. In those with clinically evident CAD and positive dobutamine stress myocardial scintigraphy, the event rate was 25%; in those with positive dobutamine stress echocardiography, it was 18%. However, if scintigraphy or DSE was negative, the rates were reduced to 1.8 and 4%, respectively. The ability to reduce risk therapeutically within a noninvasively selected stratification category was recently reported by Boersma and coworkers (44). Using DSE, the authors found that in those with Lee cardiac risk indices of 3 or greater and NWMA in one to four segments, those taking beta blockers had a 92% risk reduction compared to those without beta blockade. Patients with five or more segments having NWMA were unaffected by beta blockade, as postoperative event rates were 33 and 36% in those not taking and taking beta blockers, respectively.

Thus, noninvasive evaluation in conjunction with clinical risk stratification may be used to identify patients who are at highest risk for postoperative cardiac events and lead to more aggressive therapeutic strategies for CAD in this group. Further, an intermediate-risk group may be identified, within which proceeding to vascular surgery with risk-reducing methods, such as beta blockade, is reasonable. Selective stratification is our preferred posture toward cardiac risk evaluation, given the experience of the Massachusetts General Hospital with the use of stress myocardial scintigraphy. Our current selective process incorporating clinical scoring with functional capacity along with noninvasive evaluation (i.e., myocardial scintigraphy) is represented in Table 5. We believe that it optimizes the predictive value and cost-effectiveness of noninvasive testing, identifies patients in whom vascular surgical plans should be altered or canceled when feasible, adequately selects patients who need further coronary evaluation, and may justifiably identify patients who can proceed to vascular surgery with risk-reducing strategies.

The multitude of data in the literature supporting several approaches to preoperative cardiac screening and stratification have made this a difficult arena in which to clearly prove the best methodology to practice. However, as mentioned, the Prophylactic Coronary Artery Revascularization for Elective Vascular Surgery (CARP) trial is a prospective, randomized trial of coronary revascularization (either CABG or PTCA based upon patient anatomy) versus no revascularization in intermediate-risk patients who have significant clinical risk and/or positive noninvasive testing (76). This trial should help answer questions regarding the benefits and proper extent of cardiac evaluation in intermediate-risk patients,

Table 5 Selective Approach to Cardiac Stratification

Operative risk	Clinical risk predictors	Functional capacity	Approach
		(Poor <4 MET[a])	
Emergent case			
Coronary revascularization ≤5 years without symptoms			Operation
Recent favorable coronary evaluation			
High risk (i.e., AAA)	Major	Any	Coronary evaluation (cardiology)
	Intermediate	Any	Noninvasive testing[b]
	Minor/none	Good	Operation
		Poor	Noninvasive testing[b]
Intermediate risk (e.g., CEA)	Major	Any	Coronary evaluation (cardiology)
	Intermediate	Good	Operation
		Poor	Noninvasive testing[b]
	Minor/none	Any	Operation
Low risk (e.g., amputation)	Major	Any	Coronary evaluation (cardiology)
	Intermediate	Good	Operation
		Poor	Noninvasive testing[b]
	Minor/none	Any	Operation

[a] MET = metabolic equivalent = oxygen consumption of 40 year-old male at rest.
[b] Noninvasive testing = our preference is myocardial scintigraphy.

the ability of coronary revascularization to protect against postoperative events, and the comparability of CABG and PTCA prior to vascular surgery.

E. Risk-Reduction Techniques

1. Beta Blockade and Medical Therapies

Although the use and impact of coronary revascularization on cardiac outcome in vascular surgery patients remains unclear, several other modes of risk reduction are employed. Use of beta blockade to reduce the risk of postoperative cardiac events has been intensively studied over the last several years. Mangano et al. studied 200 noncardiac surgery patients who had clinical evidence of CAD and/or at least two risk factors for CAD (80,81). The majority of enrolled patients were undergoing major vascular surgery. The investigators performed a randomized, double-blinded trial of atenolol versus placebo before induction of anesthesia and continuing through hospitalization; cardiac morbidity and mortality were evaluated over the ensuing 2 years. Interestingly, patients administered atenolol perioperatively had significantly lower long-term mortality and overall cardiac morbidity than those taking placebo (80). During the postoperative period, no differences in myocardial infarction or cardiac death were evident; however, the atenolol group had significantly less myocardial ischemia detected on continuous ECG monitoring (81). Subsequently, Poldermans and colleagues evaluated intermediate-risk vascular surgery patients (at least one clinical risk variable) who were not previously on beta blockers (82). All patients underwent DSE, and those with extensive NWMA were excluded. The remaining 112 patients were randomized to the addition of beta blockade or standard perioperative care. Bisoprolol was started 1 week before vascular surgery and titrated to keep the heart rate at 60; it was then continued for 30 days afterward. Cardiac death and nonfatal AMI were significantly reduced (91% risk reduction) in the postoperative period in the patients taking beta blockers. Bisoprolol was continued in the treatment-arm patients postoperatively, and these authors have recently reported the long-term effects of beta blockade in this cohort (83). They found that the protective effect of beta blockade was persistent, as cardiac death and nonfatal myocardial infarction rates remained significantly less in the treated group over the next 2 years.

Recently, this same group reported on their overall experience in screening 1351 patients for the above study, and they evaluated the utility of clinical scoring and DSE for screening and the effects of beta blockade in select groups (44). The authors found the use of clinical risk scoring (Lee's revised risk index) useful for identification, DSE valuable for patient stratification, and the use of perioperative beta blockade to be protective for specific patients. Regarding those either taking beta blockers before evaluation or placed on them as part of the study protocol, event rates were reduced as clinical risk scoring increased. Specifically, in those with no clinical risk factors not taking beta blockers, the cardiac event rate was 1.2%, while no patient taking beta blockers suffered a postoperative event. Patients with one to three risk factors not taking beta blockers suffered a 9% postoperative cardiac event rate, versus 3% in those on the medication. Patients not on beta blockers with more than three clinical risk variables and a normal DSE had a 5.8% adverse cardiac event rate; this was reduced to 2% for those on beta blockers. In those with one to four NWMA, the risk of event was reduced 92% by beta blocker usage (33 vs. 2.8%). This reduction led to a rate approaching that of those patients with no clinical risk factors or NWMA. In the group of vascular patients with five or more NWMA, beta blockers made no difference in adverse cardiac outcome, as both groups had unacceptably high event rates (33 vs. 36%). Although the proper dosage and timing of administration are not clearly defined, these newer data suggest that vascular surgery patients with known or clinical evidence of CAD and those with risk factors for CAD should be on perioperative beta blockade for the purpose of reducing risk of cardiac complications.

Several other medications—such as nitroglycerin, calcium channel blockers, and alpha$_2$ adrenergic agonists—have been used perioperatively in an attempt to reduce cardiac risk in vascular and noncardiac surgery patients (24,84,85). Currently, these studies have not been conclusive enough to make specific recommendations regarding their use in this capacity. Also of special mention is analgesia selection postoperatively. While considerable benefits to the use of epidural analgesia in patients at risk for cardiac events after surgery have been proposed, these benefits remain largely unproven. A stimulating metaanalysis combining studies wherein randomized epidural use was continued for 24 h or more after surgery has recently been performed (86). All but one small study consisted of vascular surgery patients, and a combined total of nearly 1200 patients were included. Although in-hospital deaths were similar among epidural versus no epidural patients, the postoperative myocardial infarction rate (6.3% overall) was significantly reduced by the use of epidural analgesia (minus 3.8%; $p = 0.05$). Further, this reduction was more pronounced (minus 5.3%) with the use of thoracic epidural analgesia. Thus, it appears that the use of postoperative epidural analgesia may reduce the risk of postoperative AMI in vascular surgery patients.

2. Monitoring

Initial reports on pulmonary artery catheter (PAC) use to aid in the management of vascular surgery patients to prevent adverse cardiac events were encouraging (87). However, over the last several decades a modest body of literature has developed evaluating the morbidity and mortality effects of such PAC use (88–90). In general, these studies have found no reduction in perioperative cardiac events. A randomized, prospective trial by Valentine and coworkers found no difference in overall or cardiac complications based on PAC use in aortic surgery patients (91). Those with recent AMI, severe valvular disease, or unstable coronary syndromes were excluded. Patients with PAC placement were preoperatively "optimized" by Starling curve performance. Intriguingly, those with PAC use had significantly more cardiopulmonary intraoperative complications and received more intravenous fluid. The authors recommended continuing use of central venous access during aortic surgery, however, for contingency purposes and to expedite PAC placement in those with situations where it is deemed necessary. These findings were reinforced by Ziegler et al (4), who performed a randomized, prospective trial of preoperative hemodynamic "optimization" using the PAC to achieve central venous oxygen saturations of greater than 65%. The control group had PAC placement without therapy to achieve "optimization." No differences in cardiovascular complications were found between groups, suggesting that the use of PAC did not reduce complications. A recent strict metaanalysis of the prospective, randomized studies of PAC use in moderate-risk vascular surgery patients by Barone et al indicated no difference in postoperative mortality or morbidity based on management with a PAC (92). We concur that in the patient with moderate cardiac risk undergoing major vascular surgery the use of a PAC generally does not improve postoperative cardiac outcome and is not indicated. While not clearly delineated, these catheters may still have a place in high-risk patients and in select patients with cardiac complications after vascular surgery.

The use of transesophageal echocardiography (TEE) intraoperatively to direct fluid management and pharmacological modification of cardiac function during vascular surgery has been described (93). Given the excellent quality of today's echocardiography and Doppler measurement capabilities, this seemingly could improve or add to patient management and perhaps reduce events in this patient population. Further, TEE is considered to detect myocardial dysfunction not observed by standard monitoring techniques (94). Studies have suggested some degree of therapeutic usefulness in vascular and noncardiac surgery (95–98). However, prospective data supporting and defining the use of TEE are lacking (31). Currently, it seems prudent to consider its use in high-risk patients, such as those with valvular disease, congestive heart failure, or recent AMI requiring vascular surgery.

F. Valvular Disease

As congestive heart failure (CHF) and left-sided valvular lesions have been shown to be independent predictors of adverse cardiac events after surgery in several analyses, the impact valvular lesions may have on a vascular patient's course are significant. Goldman and associates reported a 20% incidence of postoperative CHF in patients with valvular disease (99,100). Stenotic lesions are particularly concerning, as they have been implicated in increasing postoperative mortality to the range of 10–20% as well as perioperative CHF and shock (31,99–102). And while a few small studies have suggested that recent advances in anesthetic technique may have attenuated some of the risk in asymptomatic patients, severe and symptomatic aortic and mitral stenosis should be evaluated and repaired, either by valvulotomy or replacement, prior to major surgery (31,103,104). Patients with stenotic valvular lesions should be well hydrated, and both tachycardia and afterload reduction should be avoided. Aortic or mitral regurgitation is, on the whole, better tolerated than stenotic lesions. When left ventricular function is normal, noncardiac surgery may be entertained with vigilant medical control and monitoring. However, symptomatic regurgitation should also undergo critical preoperative evaluation, as patients with reduced ventricular function or multiple lesions may well be served by addressing these before surgery. Proper fluid balance, afterload reduction, and postoperative diuresis are critical in these patients. In patients with valvular disease, perioperative use of a PAC should be strongly considered to aid in the above endeavors. Bacterial endocarditis prophylaxis should be adhered to according to the AHA guidelines whenever patients with valvular disease are being operated on (105).

III. PULMONARY COMPLICATIONS

A. Importance in Peripheral Vascular Patients

Pulmonary complications are a significant cause of morbidity after vascular surgery. While not as extensively studied as cardiac complications, postoperative respiratory issues are common and cause significant prolongation of intensive care unit (ICU) and hospital stay (124,125). The impact pulmonary issues may have is not surprising. Advancing age, tobacco abuse associated with chronic obstructive pulmonary disease (COPD), and other comorbid states frequently accompany peripheral vascular disease. Vascular operations may also be extensive, involving the thoracic and abdominal cavities and leading to inhibition of the patient's ability to breathe fully. The incidence of pulmonary complications after vascular surgery is dependent on how they are defined and the vascular surgery performed. Aortic operations carry a more significant risk than those for peripheral occlusive disease or carotid artery disease (126). Reported rates vary from as high as 40% for thoracoabdominal aneurysm repair to the 1–2% range for carotid endarterectomy (126–128). Typical respiratory complications that may occur include prolonged mechanical ventilation, need for reintubation, respiratory failure, pneumonia, symptomatic pleural effusion, atelectasis/collapse, and the acute respiratory distress syndrome (ARDS). Although the specifics of these entities are beyond the scope of this chapter, great advances have been made in the diagnosis and treatment of postoperative pneumonia and ARDS. These issues are critically reviewed elsewhere (129–131). Our focus is on the identification of those at risk for these complications and on a review of risk assessment and risk-reducing strategies.

B. Clinical Risk Assessment

Albeit perhaps not as extensive as the evaluation of clinical risk factors for cardiac complications, studies have evaluated preoperative clinical variables attempting to identify those at highest risk for pulmonary complications after vascular and noncardiac surgery. Important factors generally implicated are increasing age, smoking, COPD, chronic cough with changes in sputum character and amount, general functional status [both American Society of Anesthesiologists (ASA) and Goldman cardiac risk criteria], obesity, type and length of surgery, anesthesia used, and spirometric findings. These variables can be organized into patient- and procedure-specific items. The data behind the assertion of these risk factors have recently been reviewed (132). Many of these evaluations have been performed in noncardiac abdominal surgery patients (124,133–135).

Four studies have been performed in patients undergoing aortic aneurysm surgery. Money and coworkers studied factors predictive of postoperative respiratory failure in 100 consecutive thoracoabdominal aneurysm (TAA) resections (136). Increasing age, aneurysm extent, amount of intraoperative blood transfusion, postoperative renal insufficiency, and pneumonia were found to be independent correlates of respiratory failure. A similar report by Svensson et al., in 1400 TAA patients, found that 112 (8%) had postoperative respiratory failure, with COPD, smoking, complications in other organ systems (cardiac and renal) and spirometric evaluation, specifically the mid-expiratory flow (FEF_{25}), being predictive (137). More recently, advanced age, smoking, aortic cross-clamp time, operative transfusion, and diaphragmatic division were found to be independent predictors of prolonged ventilation after 387 TAA or thoracic aneurysm repairs by Engle and colleagues (138). Age, obesity, and spirometric findings were also found to be important risk factors for pulmonary complications by Calligaro and associates in elective abdominal aortic reconstruction (139).

Recently, the National Veterans Administration Surgical Quality Improvement Program reported a clinical risk index predicting respiratory failure after noncardiac surgery (140). Nearly 100,000 male patients were studied after model development, and postoperative respiratory failure developed in 2746 (3.4%). Only clinical variables were considered. No objective preoperative testing data were included. Independently predictive factors included type of surgery, serum albumin, blood urea nitrogen levels, independent versus dependent functional status, COPD, and age. These critical factors were score-weighted and a risk index developed (Table 6). The index is based upon point totals and its categorization is presented in Table 7 and correlates with increasing risk of postoperative respiratory failure. Of note, patients undergoing AAA repair and peripheral vascular procedures were 14 times and 4 times more likely, respectively, to develop respiratory failure. In fact, AAA repair was the operative procedure at highest risk. The authors suggested this risk index be used to identify patients at increased risk for postoperative pul-

Table 6 Preoperative Clinical Predictors of Postoperative Respiratory Failure with Respiratory Failure Index[a]

Variable	Odds ratio (95% CI)	Point value
Type of surgery		
Abdominal aortic aneurysm	14.3 (12.0–16.9)	27
Thoracic	8.14 (7.17–9.25)	21
Peripheral vascular, upper abdominal, or neurosurgery	4.21 (3.80–4.67)	14
Neck	3.10 (2.40–4.01)	11
Emergency surgery	3.12 (2.83–3.43)	11
Albumin (<30 g/dL)	2.53 (2.28–2.80)	9
Blood urea nitrogen (>30 mg/dL)	2.29 (2.04–2.56)	8
Partially or fully dependent living status	1.92 (1.74–2.11)	7
History of chronic obstructive pulmonary disease	1.81 (1.66–1.98)	6
Age (years)		
≥70	1.91 (1.71–2.13)	6
60–69	1.51 (1.36–1.69)	4

[a]Respiratory failure defined as mechanical ventilation for more than 48 h or reintubation after extubation.
Source: Ref. 140.

Table 7   Respiratory Failure Index[a]

Point total	Predicted probability[b] of respiratory failure
<10	0.5%
11–19	2.2%
20–27	5.0%
28–40	11.6%
>40	30.5%

[a] Respiratory failure defined as mechanical ventilation for more than 48 h or reintubation after extubation.
[b] Prediction based on model development with cohort confirmation.
Source: Ref 140.

monary insufficiency who may benefit from further objective pulmonary testing prior to operation.

C. Preoperative Evaluation

A detailed history and physical examination are invaluable in identifying patients with significant pulmonary disease. Physical examination should detect hypoventilation in weak or debilitated patients, and wheezing, rhonchi, prolonged expiration, and poor air movement in those with COPD. Lung examination abnormalities clearly increase the risk of adverse pulmonary events after operation (124). Although the degree of dyspnea on exertion may be an indicator of significant pulmonary insufficiency, many vascular patients lead sedentary lives, and the historical information given is of limited value. Obviously, as indicated above, obtaining a smoking history is of critical value. The nature and quantity of sputum production may provide insight into chronicity of disease and underlying infection. Recent studies have found sputum production and chronic cough prior to noncardiac surgery to be independent correlates with pulmonary complications (133,135). Preoperative (or recent) anteroposterior and lateral chest x-ray is indicated in those over 40 years of age with a history of or examination evidence of cardiopulmonary disease, smoking history or active symptoms. Ostensibly, based on these criteria, chest x-ray should be routine for nearly all vascular surgery patients.

Once a patient has been deemed at risk for pulmonary complications after vascular surgery by clinical and physical stratification, further pulmonary function testing (PFT) and arterial blood gas (ABG) evaluation is indicated. Pulmonary function testing provides both volume (Fig. 5) and flow information implicating type and extent of lung disease present, while room-air ABG analysis indicates the degree of current compensation. Most evidence suggests association between PFT abnormalities—specifically flow variables such as FEV_1 and FEF_{25}—and elevated Pa_{CO2} levels and the development of postoperative pulmonary complications (Table 8) (126,132,137,141). This is not universal in the literature, however, and although there are no agreed upon criteria whereby pulmonary function is in and of itself prohibitive for operation, they may aid in identifying those with such severe disease that it is prudent to alter the operation or anesthesia, cancel elective surgery, or aggressively use risk-reduction strategies perioperatively (132).

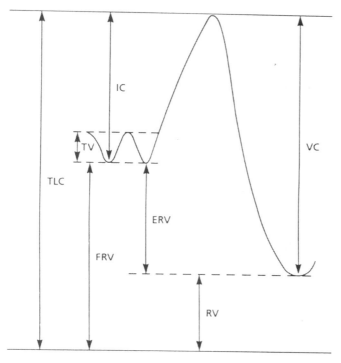

Figure 5 Spirometric lung volumes obtained during pulmonary function testing (PFT). TLC = total lung capacity; TV = tidal volume; FRV = functional residual volume; IC = inspiratory capacity; ERV = expiratory reserve volume; RV = residual volume; VC = vital capacity.

D. Risk Reduction

Vascular surgery procedures on the thoracic and abdominal aorta require thoracotomy or laparotomy incisions. These incisions alter chest wall, diaphragmatic, and lung function. Postoperative incisional pain causes splinting and decreases both tidal volume and functional residual capacity (142). This pain also prevents the patients from coughing effectively. The cumulative effects of these mechanical problems is closure of small airways (microatelectasis) due to decreased volumes and bronchial occlusion and regional atelec-

Table 8 Preoperative Pulmonary Function Assessment

	Normal	High Risk
Vital capacity	30–50 mL/kg; >80% predicted	<30–50%
Forced expiratory volume, 1 s (FEV_1)	>80% predicted	<40–50%
Maximal midexpiratory flow ($FEF_{25\%-75\%}$)	150–200 L/min; >80% predicted	<35–50%
Maximal voluntary ventilation	150–500 L/min; >80% predicted	<35–50%
Pa_{O_2}, room air	85 ± 5 mmHg	<50–55 mmHg
Pa_{CO_2}, room air	40 ± 4 mmHg	>45–55 mmHg

Souce: Ref. 159.

tasis (macroatelectasis) from poor pulmonary toilet (132,143,144). While enthusiasm for retroperitoneal approaches for abdominal aortic surgery as opposed to transperitoneal operations has been purported to reduce pulmonary complications this remains unproven; our own prospective, randomized study revealed no benefit (145,146). Those identified by clinical and objective data to be at highest risk for postoperative pulmonary complications should be strongly considered for endovascular or extra-anatomic revascularization to reduce this potential.

Methods to expand the lungs and prevent this micro- and macrocollapse are proven and easily accomplished. Two maneuvers with equal efficacy are deep-breathing exercises and incentive spirometry (147–149). The greatest benefit by these modalities is achieved by preoperative education and training prior to surgery (147,150). When patients are unable to utilize these methods adequately after vascular surgery, intermittent positive-pressure breathing (IPPB) or continuous positive airway pressure (CPAP) are beneficial, as they are not dependent upon patient effort. However, complications occur more frequently, and these measures are more expensive than patient-driven modalities such as incentive spirometry (144,147,151). Chest physiotherapy and nasotracheal suctioning may be indicated for those with substantial atelectasis or preexisting lung disease causing problems with the clearance of secretions (144).

Beside preoperative education and training regarding lung-expansion techniques, other preoperative strategies to reduce risk include smoking cessation at least 8 weeks before surgery, optimization of respiratory flow dynamics in those with obstructive disease, and treatment of any present respiratory infection well in advance of surgery. The impact that cigarette smoking has on postoperative pulmonary complications was recently reiterated by Bluman and associates (135). Patients undergoing noncardiac surgery who were smoking at the time of operation were over five times more likely to have lung-related complications compared to patients who had never smoked. Intriguing was the fact that among smokers, those who reduced or quit smoking within 1 month of surgery were at significantly higher risk of pulmonary complications than those who did not. Warner et al. studied patients undergoing CABG and found that those patients who quit smoking within 2 months of surgery had more pulmonary complications than those who quit at least 2 months before surgery (152). While unexplained at present, these data suggest that, when possible, smoking cessation should be strongly encouraged to occur at least 8 weeks before a planned operation. Patients with obstructive lung disease are at increased risk for lung-related complications postoperatively. When patients remain symptomatic prior to vascular surgery, pulmonary medical consultation is wise. Ipratropium, beta agonists, and methylxanthines should be added to the therapy regimen serially so as to maximize flow and the clearance of secretions (132). When patients remain symptomatic despite aggressive, escalating therapy, corticosteroids for 14 days may be initiated with minimal sequelae (153). Although there is no place for antibiotics for preoperative "preparation," treatment of respiratory tract infection should be completed with clear resolution prior to entertaining operation.

The conduct and effects of anesthesia have a profound influence on ventilatory mechanics and pulmonary function postoperatively. General anesthesia alters the mechanical properties of the chest wall and lung. The required positive-pressure circuit leads to atelectasis in the dependent areas, with decreased compliance. Inhalation anesthetics cause respiratory muscle dysfunction and incoordination, thus contributing to this phenomenon (143). Pulmonary problems have been identified in those under neuromuscular blockade with pancuronium as opposed to the shorter-acting agents (154). This effect is related to the longer duration of action of pancuronium, thus leading to longer durations of neuromuscular blockade and hypoventilation. To this end, Mitchell and coworkers found the duration of anesthesia to be an independent predictor of pulmonary complications after elective surgery (133). The use of neuroaxial blockade (epidural/spinal) techniques, either as "stand alone" anesthetic methods or in conjunction with general anesthesia, has proven helpful in reducing postoperative pulmonary complications (132,134,143,155–158). These strategies allow for excellent postoperative analgesia as well and reducing the medications depressing respiratory function, such as systemic opioids, required both during operation and postoperatively. This currently allows extubation in the operating room in over 90% of our patients undergoing major aortic operations.

IV. CONCLUSION

The typical vascular surgery patient presents with systemic atherosclerosis, which includes CAD to varying degrees as well as pulmonary disease such as COPD due to smoking. This patient population is at highest risk for postoperative cardiac and pulmonary morbidity and mortality. A dedicated approach to the preoperative identification, evaluation, and stratification of patients with regard to cardiopulmonary risk helps to maximize benefit when these patients undergo vascular procedures. Further, long-term outcomes beyond the procedure at hand are also affected. Preoperative preparation, intraoperative techniques, alternative surgical approaches, and postoperative care may all play a role in addressing cardiopulmonary problems in this population, and the ability to approach these topics sensibly is one of the most important in vascular surgery.

REFERENCES

1. Hertzer NR, Beven EG, Young JR, O'Hara PJ, Ruschhaupt WF III, Graor RA, DeWolfe VG, Maljoved LC. Coronary artery disease in peripheral vascular patients: A classification of 1000 coronary angiograms and results of surgical management. Ann Surg 1984; 199:223–233.
2. de Virgilio C, Toosie K, Ephraim L, Elbassir M, Donayre C, Baker D, Narahara K, Mishkin F, Lewis RJ, Chang C, White R, Mody FV. Dipyridamole-thallium/sestamibi before vascular surgery: A prospective blinded study in moderate-risk patients. J Vasc Surg 2000; 32:77–89.
3. Sprung J, Abdelmalak B, Gottlieb A, Mayhew C, Hammel J, Levy PJ, O'Hara PJ, Hertzer NR. Analysis of risk factors for myocardial infarction and cardiac mortality and after major vascular surgery. Anesthesiology 2000; 93:129–140.
4. Ziegler DW, Wright JG, Choban PS, Flancbaum L. A prospective randomized trial of preoperative "optimization" of cardiac function in patients undergoing elective peripheral vascular surgery. Surgery 1997; 122:584–592.
5. Samain E, Farah E, Leseche G, Marty J. Guidelines for perioperative cardiac evaluation from the American College of Cardiology/American Heart Association task force are effective for stratifying cardiac risk before aortic surgery. J Vasc Surg 2000; 31:91–99.
6. Aziz I, Lewis JR, Baker JD, de Virgilio C. Cardiac morbidity and mortality following carotid endarterectomy: The importance of diabetes and multiple eagle risk factors. Ann Vasc Surg. 2001; 15:243–246.
7. de Virgilio C, Wall DB, Ephraim L, Toosie K, Donayre C, White R, Elbassir M. An abnormal dipyridamole thallium/sestamibi fails to predict long-term cardiac events in vascular surgery patients. Ann Vasc Surg 2001; 15:267–271.
8. de Virgilio C, Toosie K, Lewis RJ, Stabile BE, Baker JD, White R, Donayre CE, Ephraim L. Cardiac morbidity and operative mortality following lower-extremity amputation: The significance of multiple Eagle criteria. Ann Vasc Surg 1999; 13:204–208.

9. van Damme H, Pierard L, Gillain D, Benoit T, Rigo P, Limet R. Cardiac risk assessment before vascular surgery: A prospective study comparing clinical evaluation, dobutamine stress echocardiography, and dobutamine Tc-99m sestamibi tomoscintigraphy. Cardiovasc Surg 1997; 5:54–64.

10. L'Italien GJ, Cambria RP, Cutler BS, Leppo JA, Paul SD, Brewster DC, Hendel RC, Abbott WM, Eagle KA. Comparative early and late morbidity among patients requiring different vascular surgery procedures. J Vasc Surg 1995; 21:935–944.

11. L'Italien GJ, Paul SD, Hendel RC, Leppo JA, Cohen MC, Fleisher LA, Brown KA, Zarich SW, Cambria RP, Cutler BS, Eagle KA. Development and validation of a Bayesian model for perioperative cardiac risk assessment in a cohort of 1,081 vascular surgical candidates. J Am Coll Cardiol 1996; 27:779–786.

12. de Virgilio C, Bui H, Donayre C, Ephraim L, Lewis RJ, Elbassir M, Stabile BE, White RE. Endovascular vs. open abdominal aortic aneurysm repair. Arch Surg 1999; 134:947–951.

13. Taylor LM, Yeager RA, Moneta GL, McConnell DB, Porter JM. The incidence of perioperative myocardial infarction in general vascular surgery. J Vasc Surg 1991; 15:52–61.

14. Krupski WC, Layug EL, Reilly LM, Rapp JH, Mangano DT. Comparison of cardiac morbidity rates between aortic and infrainguinal operations: Two-year follow-up. J Vasc Surg 1993; 18:609–617.

15. Krupski WC, Layug EL, Reilly LM, Rapp JH, Mangano DT. Comparison of cardiac morbidity rates between aortic and infrainguinal operations. J Vasc Surg 1992; 15:354–365.

16. Lee TH, Marcantonio ER, Mangione CM, Thomas EJ, Polanczyk CA, Cook EF, Surgarbaker DJ, Donaldson MC, Poss R, Ho KKL, Ludwig LE, Pedan A, Goldman L. Derivation and prospective validation of a simple index for prediction of cardiac risk of major noncardiac surgery. Circulation 1999; 100:1043–1049.

17. Yeager RA. Basic data related to cardiac testing and cardiac risk associated with vascular surgery. Ann Vasc Surg 1990; 4:193–197.

18. Pasternak PF, Grossi EA, Baumann G, Riles TS, Lamparello PJ, Giangola G, Primis LK, Mintzer R, Imparato AM. The value of silent myocardial ischemia monitoring in the prediction of perioperative myocardial infarction in patients undergoing peripheral vascular surgery. J Vasc Surg 1989; 10:617–625.

19. Mangano DT, Hollenberg M, Fegert G, Meyer LM, London MJ, Tubau JF, Krupski WC. Perioperative myocardial ischemia in patients undergoing noncardiac surgery: I. Incidence and severity during the 4 day perioperative period. J Am Coll Cardiol 1991; 17:843–850.

20. Sear JW, Foex P, Howell SJ. Effect of chronic intercurrent medication with β-adrenoceptor blockade on postoperative silent myocardial ishemia. Br J Anaesth 2000; 84:311–315.

21. Higham H, Sear JW, Neill F, Sear YH, Foex P. Peri-operative silent myocardial ischaemia and long-term adverse outcomes in non-cardiac surgical patients. Anaesthesia 2001; 56:630–637.

22. Mamode N, Scott RN, McLaughlin SC, McLelland A, Pollock JG. Perioperative myocardial infarction in peripheral vascular surgery. Br Med J 1996; 312:1396–1397.

23. Landesberg G, Mosseri M, Zahger D, Wolf Y, Perouansky M, Anner H, Drenger B, Hasin Y, Berlatzky Y, Weissman C. Myocardial infarction after vascular surgery: The role of prolonged, stress-induced, ST-depression-type ischemia. J Am Coll Cardiol 2001; 37:1839–1845.

24. Oliver MF, Goldman L, Julian DG, Holme I. The effect of mivazerol on perioperative cardiac complications during non-cardiac surgery in patients with coronary artery disease: The European Mivazerol Trial (EMIT). Anesthesiology 1999; 91:951–961.

25. Mangano DT, Wong MG, London MJ, Tubau JF, Rapp JA. Perioperative myocardial ischemia in patients undergoing noncardiac surgery: II. Incidence and severity during the 1st week after surgery. J Am Coll Cardiol 1991; 17:851–857.

26. Mangano DT. Perioperative cardiac morbidity. Anesthesiology 1990; 72:153–184.

27. Hertzer NR, Avellone JC, Farrell CJ, Plecha FR, Rhodes RS, Sharp WV, Wright GF. The risk of vascular surgery in a metropolitan community with observations on surgeon experience and hospital size. J Vasc Surg 1984; 1:13–21.

28. Hertzer NR. Fatal myocardial infarction following lower extremity revascularization. Ann Surg 1981; 193:492–498.

29. Hertzer NR. Fatal myocardial infarction following abdominal aortic aneurysm resection. Ann Surg 1980; 192:667–673.

30. Eagle KA, Brundage BH, Chaitman BR, Ewy GA, Fleisher LA, Hertzer NR, Leppo JA, Ryan T, Schlant RC, Spencer WH III, Spittell JA Jr, Twiss RD. Guidelines for perioperative cardiovascular evaluation for noncardiac surgery: Report of the American College of Cardiology/American Heart Association Task Force on Practice Guidelines (Committee on Perioperative Cardiovascular Evaluation for Noncardiac Surgery). Circulation 1996; 93:1278–1317.

31. Eagle KA, Berger PB, Calkins H, Chaitman BR, Ewy GA, Fleischmann KE, Fleisher LA, Froehlich JB, Gusberg RJ, Leppo JA, Ryan T, Schlant RC, Winters WL Jr, ACC/AHA Guidelines update for perioperative cardiovascular evaluation for noncardiac surgery-executive summary: A report of the American College of Cardiology/American Heart Association Task Force on Practice Guidelines (Committee to update the 1996 guidelines n perioperative cardiovascular evaluation for noncardiac surgery). Circulation 2002; 105:2157–1267.

32. Cutler BS, Wheeler HB, Paraskos JA, Cardullo PA. Applicability and interpretation of electrocardiographic stress testing in patients with peripheral vascular disease. Am J Surg 1981; 141:501–506.

33. Raby KE, Goldman L, Creager MA, Cook EF, Weisberg MC, Whittemore AD, Selwyn AP. Correlation between preoperative ischemia and major cardiac events after peripheral vascular surgery. N Engl J Med 1989; 321:1296–1300.

34. Mangano DT, Hollenberg M, Fegert G, Meyer ML, London MJ, Tubau JF, Krupski WC. Perioperative myocardial ischemia in patients undergoing noncardiac surgery: I. Incidence and severity during the 4 day perioperative period. The Study of the Perioperative Ischemia (SPI) Research Group. J Am Coll Cardiol 1991; 17:851–857.

35. Landesberg G, Einav S, Christopherson R, Beattie C, Berlatzky Y, Rosenfeld B, Eidelman LA, Norris E, Anner H, Mosseri M, Cotev S, Luria MH. Perioperative ischemia and cardiac complications in major vascular surgery: Importance of the preoperative twelve-lead electrocardiogram. J Vasc Surg 1997; 26:570–578.

36. Kirwin JD, Ascer E, Gennana M, Mohan C, Jonas S, Yorkovich W, Matano R. Silent myocardial ischemia is not predictive of myocardial function in peripheral vascular surgery patients. Ann Vasc Surg 1993; 7:27–32.

37. Pasternack PF, Imparato AM, Bear G, Riles TS, Baumann FG, Benjamin D, Sanger J, Kramer E, Wood RP. The value of radionuclide angiography as a predictor of perioperative myocardial infarction in patients undergoing abdominal aortic aneurysm resection. J Vasc Surg 1984; 1:320–325.

38. Kazmers A, Cerquieira MD, Zierler RE. The role of preoperative radionuclide left ventricular ejection fraction for risk assessment in carotid surgery. Arch Surg 1988; 123:416–419.

39. Kazmers A, Cerquieira MD, Zierler RE. The role of preoperative radionuclide ejection fraction in direct abdominal aortic aneurysm repair. J Vasc Surg 1988; 8:128–136.

40. Franco CD, Goldsmith J, Veith FJ, Ascer E, Wengerter KR, Calligaro KD, Gupta SK. Resting gated pool ejection fraction: A poor predictor of perioperative myocardial infarction in patients undergoing vascular surgery for infrainguinal bypass grafting. J Vasc Surg 1989; 10:656–661.

41. Beller GA, Gibson RS. Sensitivity, specificity, and prognostic significance of noninvasive testing for occult or known coronary artery disease. Prog Cardiovasc Dis 1987; 29:241–270.

42. Lee TH, Boucher CA. Noninvasive tests in patients with stable coronary artery disease. N Engl J Med 2001; 344:1840–1845.

43. Poldermans D, Arnese M, Fioretti PM, Salustri A, Boersma E, Thomson IR, Roelandt JRTC, van Urk H. Improved cardiac risk stratification in major vascular surgery with dobutamine-atropine stress echocardiography. J Am Coll Cardiol 1995; 26:648–653.

44. Boersma E, Poldermans D, Bax JJ, Steyerberg EW, Thomson IR, Banga JD, Van de ven LLM, van Urk H, Roelandt JRTC. Predictors of cardiac events after major vascular surgery: Role of clinical characteristics, dobutamine echocardiography, and β-blocker therapy. JAMA 2001; 285:1865–1873.

45. Shaw LL, Eagle KA, Gersh BJ, Miller DD. Meta-analysis of intravenous dipyridamole-thallium-201 imaging (1985–1994) and Dobutamine echocardiography (1991–1994) for risk stratification before vascular surgery. J Am Coll Cardiol 1996; 27:787–798.

46. Boucher CA, Brewster DC, Darling RC, Okada RD, Strauss HW, Pohost GM. Determination of cardiac risk by dipyridamole-thallium imaging before peripheral vascular surgery. N Engl J Med 1985; 312:389–394.

47. Eagle KA, Strauss HW, Boucher CA. Dipyridamole myocardial perfusion imaging for coronary heart disease. Am J Cardiac Imaging 1988; 2:230–292.

48. Vanzetto G, Machecourt J, Blendea D, Fagret D, Borrel E, LucMagne J, Gattaz F, Guidicelli H. Additive value of thallium single-photon emission computed tomography myocardial imaging for prediction of perioperative events in clinically selected high cardiac risk patients having abdominal aortic surgery. Am J Cardiol 1996; 77:143–148.

49. Cutler BS, Leppo JA. Dipyridamole thallium 201 scintigraphy to detect coronary artery disease before abdominal aortic surgery. J Vasc Surg 1987; 5:91–100.

50. Eagle KA, Singer DE, Bewster DC, Darling RC, Mulley AG, Boucher CA. Dipyridamole-thallium scanning in patients undergoing vascular surgery: Optimizing preoperative evaluation of cardiac risk. JAMA 1987; 257:2185–2189.

51. Brewster DC, Okada RD, Strauss HW, Abbott WM, Darling RC, Boucher CA. Selection of patients for preoperative coronary angiography: Use of dipyridamole-stress thallium myocardial imaging. J Vasc Surg 1985; 2:504–509.

52. Eagle KA, Coley CM, Newell JB, Brewster DC, Darling RC, Strauss HW, Guiney TE, Boucher CA. Combining clinical and thallium data optimizes preoperative assessment of cardiac risk before major vascular surgery. Ann Intern Med 1989; 110:859–866.

53. Levinson JR, Boucher CA, Coley CM, Guiney TE, Strauss HW, Eagle KA. Usefulness of semiquantitative analysis of dipyridamole-thallium-201 redistribution for improving risk stratification before vascular surgery. Am J Cardiol 1990; 66:406–410.

54. Hendel RC, Whitfield SS, Villegas BJ, Cutler BS, Leppo JA. Prediction of late cardiac events by dipyridamole thallium imaging in patients undergoing elective vascular surgery. Am J Cardiol 1992; 70:1243–1249.

55. Lette J, Waters D, Cerino M, Picard M, Champagne P, Lapointe J. Preoperative coronary artery disease risk stratification based on dipyridamole imaging and a simple three-step, three-segment model for patients undergoing noncardiac vascular surgery or major general surgery. Am J Cardiol 1992; 69:1553–1558.

56. Mangano DT, London MJ, Tubau JF, Browner WS, Hollenberg M, Krupski W, Layug EL, Massie B. Diypridamole thallium-201 scinitgraphy as a preoperative screening test: A reexamination of its predictive potential. Circulation 1991; 84:493–502.

57. Schueppert MT, Kresowik TF, Corry DC, Jacobovicz C, Mohan CR, Slaymaker E, Hoballah JJ, Sharp WJ, Grover-McKay M, Corson JD. Selection of patients for cardiac evaluation before peripheral vascular operations. J Vasc Surg 1996; 23:802–809.

58. Seeger J, Rosenthal G, Self S, Flynn TC, Limacher MC, Harward TR. Does routine stress-thallium cardiac screening reduce postoperative cardiac complications? Ann Surg 1994; 6: 654–663.

59. Stratmann H, Younis L, Wittry M, Amato M, Miller DD. Diypridamole technetium-99m sestamibi myocardial tomography in patients evaluated for elective vascular surgery: Prognostic value for perioperative and late cardiac events. Am Heart J 1995; 131:923–929.

60. Baron JF, Mundler O, Bertrand M, Vicaut E, Barre E, Godet G, Samama M, Coriat P, Kieffer E, Viars P. Dipyridamole-thallium scintigraphy and gated radionuclide angiography to assess cardiac risk before abdominal aortic surgery. N Engl J Med 1994; 330:663–669.

61. Poldermans D, Mariarosaria A, Fioretti PM, Boersma E, Thomson IR, Rambaldi R, van Urk H. Sustained prognostic value of dobutamine stress echocardiography for late cardiac events after major noncardiac vascular surgery. Circulation 1997; 95:53–58.

62. Cohen MC, Curran PJ, L'Italien, Mittleman MA, Zarich SW. Long-term prognostic value of preoperative dipyridamole thallium imaging and clinical indexes in patients with diabetes mellitus undergoing peripheral vascular surgery. Am J Cardiol 1999; 83:1038–1042.

63. Fleisher LA, Eagle KA, Shaffer T, Anderson GF. Perioperative and long-term mortality rates after major vascular surgery: The relationship to preoperative testing in the medicare population. Anesth Analg 1999; 89:849–855.

64. Eagle KA, Rihal CS, Mickel MC, Holmes DR, Foster ED, Gersh BJ. Cardiac risk of noncardiac surgery: Influence of coronary disease and type of surgery in 3368 operations. Circulation 1997; 96:1882–1997.

65. Hertzer NR. The natural history of peripheral vascular disease: Implications for its management. Circulation 1983; 83(S1):1–12.

66. Hertzer NR, Young J, Beven E, O'Hara PJ, Graor RA, Ruschhaupt WF, Maljovec LC. Late results of coronary bypass in patients with peripheral vascular disease: II. Five-year survival according to sex, hypertension, and diabetes. Cleve Clin J Med 1987; 54:15–23.

67. Rihal CS, Eagle KA, Mickel MC, Foster ED, Sopko G, Gersh BJ. Surgical therapy for coronary artery disease among patients with combined coronary artery and peripheral vascular disease. Circulation 1995; 91:46–53.

68. Toal K, Jacocks M, Elkins R. Preoperative coronary artery bypass grafting in patients undergoing abdominal aortic reconstruction. Am J Surg 1984; 148:825–829.

69. Huber KC, Evans MA, Bresnahan JF, Gibbons RJ, Holmes DR Jr. Outcome of noncardiac operations in patients with severe coronary artery disease successfully treated preoperatively with coronary angioplasty. Mayo Clin Proc 1992; 67:15–21.

70. Posner KL, van Norman G, Chan V. Adverse cardiac outcomes after noncardiac surgery in patients with prior percutaneous transluminal coronary angioplasty. Anesth Analg 1999; 89:553–560.

71. Elmore JR, Hallett JW Jr, Gibbons RJ, Naessens JM, Bower TC, Cherry KJ, Gloviczki P, Pairoleiro PC. Myocardial revascularization before abdominal aortic aneurysmorrhaphy: Effect of coronary angioplasty. Mayo Clin Proc 1993; 68:637–641.

72. Gottlieb A, Banoub M, Sprung J, Levy PJ, Beven M, Mascha EJ. Perioperative cardiovascular morbidity in patients with coronary artery disease undergoing vascular surgery after percutanous transluminal coronary angioplasty. J Cardiothorac Vasc Anesth 1998; 12:501–506.

73. Hassan SA, Hlatky MA, Boothroyd DB, Winston C, Mark DB, Brooks MM, Eagle KA. Outcomes of noncardiac surgery after coronary bypass surgery or coronary angioplasty in the bypass angioplasty revascularization investigation (BARI). Am J Med 2001; 110:260–266.

74. Mason JJ, Owens DK, Harris RA, Cooke JP, Hlatky MA. The role of coronary angiography and coronary revascularization before noncardiac vascular surgery. JAMA 1995; 273:1919–1925.

75. Massie MT, Rohrer MJ, Leppo JA, Cuter BS. Is coronary angiography necessary for vascular surgery patients who have positive results of dipyridamole thallium scans? J Vasc Surg 1997; 25:975–983.

76. McFalls EO, Ward HB, Krupski WC, Goldman S, Littooy F, Eagle K, Nyman JA, Moritz T, McNabb S, Henderson WG. Prophylactic coronary artery revascularization for elective vascular surgery: Study design. Control Clin Trials 1999; 20:297–308.

77. Bui H, de Virgilio C. Preoperative evaluation and interventions before aortic surgery: Are they justified? Perspect Vasc Surg 2000; 12:25–54.

78. Romero L, de Virgilio C. Preoperative cardiac risk assessment: An updated approach. Arch Surg 2001; 136:1370–1376.

79. Krupski WC, Nehler MR, Whitehill TA, Lawson RC, Strecker PK, Hiatt WR. Negative impact of cardiac evaluation before vascular surgery. Vasc Med 2000; 5:3–9.

80. Mangano DT, Layug EL, Wallace A, Tateo I. Effect of atenolol on mortality and cardio-vascular morbidity after noncardiac surgery. N Engl J Med 1996; 335:1713–1720.

81. Wallace A, Layug B, Tateo I, Li J, Hollenberg M, Browner W, Miller D, Mangano DT. Prophylactic atenolol reduces postoperative myocardial ischemia. Anesthesiology 1998; 88: 7–17.

82. Poldermans D, Boersma E, Bax JJ, Thomson IR, van de Ven LLM, Blankensteijn JD, Baars HF, Yo T, Trocino G, Vigna C, Roelandt JRTC, van Urk H. The effect of bisoprolol on perioperative mortality and myocardial infarction in high-risk patients undergoing vascular surgery. N Engl J Med 1999; 341:1789–1794.

83. Poldermans D, Boersma E, Baxx JJ, Thomson IR, Paelinck B, van de Ven LLM, Scheffer MG, Trocino G, Vigna C, Baars HF, van Urk H, Roelandt JRTC. Bisoprolol reduces cardiac death and myocardial infarction in high-risk patients as long as 2 years after successful major vascular surgery. Eur Heart J 2001; 22:1353–1358.

84. Dodds TM, Stone JG, Coromilas J, Weinberger M, Levy DG. Prophylactic nitroglycerine infusion during noncardiac surgery does not reduce perioperative ischemia. Anesth Analg 1993; 76:705–713.

85. Godet G, Coriat P, Baron JF, Bertrand M, Diquet B, Sebag C, Viars P. Prevention of intraoperative myocardial ischemia during noncardiac surgery with intravenous diltiazem: A randomized trial versus placebo. Anesthesiology 1987; 66:241–245.

86. Beattie WS, Badner NH, Choi P. Epidural analgesia reduces postoperative myocardial infarction: A meta-analysis. Anesth Analg 2001; 93:853–858.

87. Whittemore AD, Clowes AW, Hechtman HB, Mannick JA. Aortic aneurysm repair: Reduced operative mortality associated with maintenance of optimal cardiac performance. Ann Surg 1980; 192:414–421.

88. Berlauk JF, Abrams JH, Gilmour IJ, O'Connor SR, Knighton DR, Cerra FB. Preoperative optimization of cardiovascular hemodynamics improves outcome in peripheral vascular surgery. Ann Surg 1991; 214:290–299.

89. Bender JS, Smith-Meek MA, Jones CE. Routine pulmonary artery catheterization does not reduce morbidity and mortality of elective vascular surgery. Ann Surg 1997; 226:229–237.

90. Isaacson IJ, Lowdon JD, Berry AJ, Smith RB III, Knos GB, Weitz FI, Ryan K. The value of pulmonary artery and central venous monitoring in patients undergoing abdominal aortic reconstructive surgery: A comparative study of two selected, randomized groups. J Vasc Surg 1990; 12:754–760.

91. Valentine RJ, Duke ML, Inman MH, Grayburn PA, Hagino RT, Kakish HB, Clagett GP. Effectiveness of pulmonary artery catheters in aortic surgery: A randomized trial. J Vasc Surg 1998; 27:203–212.

92. Barone JE, Tucker JB, Rassias D, Corvo PR. Routine perioperative pulmonary artery catheterization has no effect on rate of complications in vascular surgery: A meta-analysis. Am Surg 2001; 67:674–679.

93. Gewertz BL, Kremser PC, Zarins CK, Smith JS, Ellis JE, Feinstein SB, Roizen MF. Transesophageal echocardiographic monitoring of myocardial ischemia during vascular surgery. J Vasc Surg 1987; 5:607–613.

94. Smith JS, Cahalan MK, Benefiel DJ, Byrd BF, Lurz FW, Shapiro WA, Roizen MF, Bouchard A, Schiller NB. Intraoperative detection of myocardial ischemia in high-risk patients: Elec-trocardiography versus two-dimensional transesophageal echocardiography. Circulation 1985; 72:1015–1021.

95. Eisenberg MJ, London MJ, Leung JM, Browner WS, Hollenberg M, Tubau JF, Tateo IM, Schiller NB, Mangano DT. Monitoring for myocardial ischemia during noncardiac surgery. A technology assessment of transesophageal echocardiography and 12-lead electrocardiography. The Study of Perioperative Ischemia Research Group. JAMA 1992; 268:210–216.

96. Iafrati MD, Gordon G, Staples MH, Mackey WC, Belkin M, Diehl J, Schwartz S, Payne D, O'Donnell TF. Transesophageal echocardiography for hemodynamic management of thoraco-abdominal aneurysm repair. Am J Surg 1993; 166:179–185.

97. Suriani RJ, Neustein S, Shore-Lesserson L, Konstadt S. Intraoperative transesophageal echocardiography during noncardiac surgery. J Cardiothorac Vasc Anesth 1998; 12:274–280.

98. Schmidlin D, Bettex D, Bernard E, Germann R, Tornic M, Jenni R, Schmid ER. Transo-esophageal echocardiography in cardiac and vascular surgery: Implications and observer var-iablility. Br J Anesth 2001; 86:497–505.

99. Goldman L, Caldera DL, Nussbaum SR, Southwick FS, Drogstad D, Murray B, Burke DS, O'Malley TA, Goroll AH, Caplan CH, Nolan J, Carabello B, Slater EE. Multifactorial index of cardiac risk in noncardiac surgical procedures. N Engl J Med 1977; 297:845–850.

100. Goldman L. Cardiac risks and complications of noncardiac surgery. Ann Intern Med 1983; 98:504–513.

101. Detsky AS, Abrams HB, Forbath N, Scott JG, Hilliard JR. Cardiac assessment for patients undergoing noncardiac surgery: A multifactorial risk index. Arch Intern Med 1986; 146:2131–2134.

102. Detsky AS, Abrams HB, McLaughlin JR, Drucker DJ, Sasson Z, Johnston N, Scott JG, Forbath N, Hilliard JR. Predicting cardiac complications in patients undergoing noncardiac surgery. J Gen Intern Med 1986; 1:211–219.

103. Raymer K, Yang H. Patients with aortic stenosis: Cardiac complications in non-cardiac surgery. Can J Anesth 1998; 45:855–859.

104. Torsher LC, Shub C, Rettke SR, Brown DL. Risk of patients with severe aortic stenosis undergoing noncardiac surgery. Am J Cardiol 1998; 81:448–452.

105. Dajani AS, Taubert KA, Wilson W, Bolger AF, Bayer A, Ferrieri P, Gewitz MH, Shulman ST, Nouri S, Newburger JW, Hutto C, Pallasch TJ, Gage TW, Levison ME, Peter G, Zuccaro G Jr. Prevention of bacterial endocarditis: Recommendations by the American Heart Asso-ciation. JAMA 1997; 277:1794–1801.

106. Cambria RP, Clouse WD, Davison JK, Dunn PF, Corey M, Dorer DJ. Thoracoabdominal aneurysm repair: Results with 337 operations performed over a 15-year interval. Ann Surg 2002; 216:471–479.

107. Romero L, de Virgilio C, Donayre C, Stabile BE, Lewis RJ, Narahara K, Lippmann M, White R, Chang C. Trends in cardiac morbidity and mortality after endoluminal abdominal aortic aneurysm repair. Arch Surg 2001; 136:996–1000.

108. Hovsepian DM, Hein AN, Pilgram TK, Cohen DT, Kim HS, Sanchez LA, Rubin BG, Picus D, Sicard GA. Endovascular abdominal aortic aneurysm repair in 144 patients: Correlation of aneurysm size, proximal aortic neck length, and procedure-related complications. J Vasc Intervent Radiol 2001; 12:1373–1382.

109. Becker GJ, Kovacs M, Mathison MN, Katzen BT, Benenati JF, Zemel G, Powell A, Almeida JI, Alvarez J Jr. Coello AA, Ingegno MD, Kanter SR, Katzman HE, Puente OA, Reiss IM, Rua I, Gordon R, Baquero J. Risk stratification and outcomes of transluminal endografting for abdominal aortic aneurysm: 7-year experience and long-term follow-up. J Vasc Intervent Radiol 2001; 12:1033–1046.

110. Pronovost P, Garrett E, Dorman T, Jenckes M, Webb TH III, Breslow M, Rosenfeld B, Bass E. Variations in complication rates and opportunities for improvement in quality of care for patients having abdominal aortic surgery. Langenbeck's Arch Surg 2001; 386:249–256.

111. Axelrod DA, Henke PK, Wakefield TW, Stanley JC, Jacobs LA, Graham LM, Greenfield LJ, Upchurch GR. Impact of chronic obstructive pulmonary disease on elective and emergency abdominal aortic aneurysm repair. J Vasc Surg 2001; 33:72–76.

112. Martin GH, O'Hara PJ, Hertzer NR, Mascha EJ, Krajewski LP, Beven EG, Clair DG, Ouriel K. Surgical repair of aneurysms involving the suprarenal, visceral, and lower thoracic aortic segments: Early results and late outcome. J Vasc Surg 2000; 31:851–862.

113. Pearce WH, Parker MA, Feinglass J, Ujiki M, Manheim LM. The importance of surgeon

volume and training in outcomes for vascular surgical procedures. J Vasc Surg 1999; 29:768–778.

114. Sternbach Y, Illig KA, Zhang R, Shortell CK, Rhodes JM, Davies MG, Lyden SP, Green RM. Hemodynamic benefits of regional anesthesia for carotid endarterectomy. J Vasc Surg 2002; 35:333–339.

115. AbuRhama AF, Jennings TG, Wulu JT, Tarakji L, Robinson PA. Redo carotid endarterectomy versus primary carotid endarterectomy. Stroke 2001; 32:2787–2792.

116. James DC, Hughes JD, Mills JL, Westerband A. The influence of gender on complications of carotid endarterectomy. Am J Surg 2001; 182:654–657.

117. Hamdan AD, Pomposelli FB, Gibbons GW, Campbell DR, LoGerfo FW. Perioperative strokes after 1001 consecutive carotid endarterectomy procedures without an electroencephalogram. Arch Surg 1999; 134:412–415.

118. Cao P, Giordano G, De Rango P, Zannetti S, Chiesa R, Coppi G, Palombo D, Spartera C, Stancanelli V, Vecchiati E. A randomized study on eversion versus standard carotid endarterectomy: Study design and preliminary results: The EVEREST Trial. J Vasc Surg 1998; 27:595–605.

119. Conte MS, Belkin M, Upchurch GR, Mannick JA, Whittemore AD, Donaldson MC. Impact of increasing comorbidity on infrainguinal reconstruction: A 20-year perspective. Ann Surg 2001; 233:445–452.

120. Kalra M, Gloviczki P, Bower TC, Panneton JM, Harmsen WS, Jenkins GD, Stanson AW, Toomey BJ, Canton LG. Limb salvage after successful pedal bypass grafting is associated with improved long-term survival. J Vasc Surg 2001; 33:6–16.

121. Faries PL, LoGerfo FW, Arora S, Hook S, Pulling MC, Akbari CM, Campbell DR, Pomposelli FB. A comparative study of alternative conduits for lower extremity revascularization: All-autogenous conduit versus prosthetic grafts. J Vasc Surg 2000; 32: 1080–1090.

122. Nicoloff AD, Taylor LM, McLafferty RB, Moneta GL, Porter JM. Patient recovery after infrainguinal bypass grafting for limb salvage. J Vasc Surg 1998; 27:256–266.

123. Matsuura JH, Sobel M, Wong J, Dattilo JB, Poletti LF, Makhoul RG, Posner MP, Lee HM. The limits of generalized cardiac screening tests for predicting cardiac complications after infrainguinal arterial reconstruction. Ann Vasc Surg 1997; 11:620–625.

124. Lawrence VA, Dhanda R, Hilsenbeck SG, Page CP. Risk of pulmonary complications after elective abdominal surgery. Chest 1996; 110:744–750.

125. Kazmers A, Jacobs L, Perkins A. The impact of complications after vascular surgery in Veterans Affairs medical centers. J Surg Res 1997; 67:62–66.

126. Kispert JF, Kazmers A, Roitman L. Preoperative spirometry predicts perioperative pulmonary complications after major vascular surgery. Am Surg 1992; 8:491–495.

127. Rectenwald JE, Huber TS, Martin TD, Ozaki K, Devidas M, Wellborn MB, Seeger JM. Functional outcome after thoracoabdominal aortic aneurysm repair. J Vasc Surg 2002; 35:640–647.

128. Berry AJ, Smith RB III, Weintraub WS, Chaikof EL, Dodson TF, Lumsden AB, Salam AA, Weiss V, Konigsberg S. Age versus comborbidities as risk factors for complications after elective abdominal aortic reconstructive surgery. J Vasc Surg 2001; 33:345–352.

129. Rowe S, Cheadle WG. Complications of nosocomial pneumonia in the surgical patient. Am J Surg 2000; 179(suppl 2A):63S–68S.

130. Croce MA. Diagnosis of acute respiratory distress syndrome and differentiation from ventilator-associated pneumonia. Am J Surg 2000; 179(suppl 2A):26S–30S.

131. Meade MO, Herridge MS. An evidence-based approach to acute respiratory distress syndrome. Respir Care 2001; 46:1368–1376.

132. Smetana GW. Preoperative pulmonary evaluation. N Engl J Med 1999; 340:937–944.

133. Mitchell CK, Smoger SH, Pfeifer MP, Vogel RL, Pandit MK, Donnelly PJ, Garrison RN, Rothschild MA. Multivariate analysis of factors associated with postoperative pulmonary complications following general elective surgery. Arch Surg 1998; 133:194–198.

134. Brooks-Brunn JA. Predictors of postoperative pulmonary complications following abdominal surgery. Chest 1997; 111:564–571.

135. Bluman LG, Mosca L, Newman N, Simon DG. Preoperative smoking habits and postoperative pulmonary complications. Chest 1998; 113:883–889.

136. Money SR, Rice K, Crockett D, Becker M, Abdoh A, Wisselink W, Kazmier F, Hollier LH. Risk of respiratory failure after repair of thoracoabdominal aortic aneurysm. Am J Surg 1994; 168:152–155.

137. Svensson LG, Hess KR, Coselli JS, Safi HJ, Crawford ES. A prospective study of respiratory failure after high-risk surgery on the thoracoabdominal aorta. J Vasc Surg 1991; 14:271–282.

138. Engle J, Safi HJ, Miller CC III, Campbell MP, Harlin SA, Letsou GV, Lloyd KS, Root DB. The impact of diaphragm management on prolonged ventilator support after thoraco-abdominal aortic repair. J Vasc Surg 1999; 29:150–156.

139. Calligaro KD, Azurin DJ, Dougherty MJ, Dandora R, Bajgier SM, Simper S, Savarese RP, Raviola A, DeLaurentis DA. Pulmonary risk factors of elective abdominal aortic surgery. J Vasc Surg 1993; 18:914–921.

140. Arozullah AM, Daley J, Henderson WG, Khuri SF. Multifactorial risk index for predicting postoperative respiratory failure in men after major noncardiac surgery. Ann Surg 2000; 232: 242–253.

141. Kroenke K, Lawrence VA, Theroux JF, Tuley MR, Hilsenbeck S. Postoperative complications after thoracic and major abdominal surgery in patients with and without obstructive lung disease. Chest 1993; 104:1445–1451.

142. Meyers JR, Lembeck L, O'Kane H, Baue AE. Changes in functional residual capacity of the lung after operation. Arch Surg 1975; 110:576–583.

143. Warner DO. Preventing postoperative pulmonary complications: The role of the anesthesiologist. Anesthesiology 2000; 92:1467–1472.

144. Brooks-Brunn JA. Postoperative atelectasis and pneumonia. Heart Lung 1995; 24:94–115.

145. Cambria RP, Brewster DC, Abbott WM, Freehan M, Megerman J, LaMuraglia G, Wilson R, Wilson D, Teplick R, Davison JK. Transperitoneal versus retroperitoneal approach for aortic reconstruction: A randomized, prospective study. J Vasc Surg 1990; 11:314–325.

146. Sicard GA. Surgical techniques for repair of abdominal aortic aneurysms. In: Gewertz BL Schwartz LB, eds. Surgery of the Aorta and Its Branches. Philadelphia: Saunders 2000:124–175.

147. Celli BR, Rodriguez KS, Snider GL. A controlled trial of intermittent positive pressure breathing, incentive spirometry, and deep breathing exercises in preventing pulmonary complications after abdominal surgery. Am Rev Respir Dis 1984; 130:12–15.

148. Chumillas S, Ponce JL, Delgado F, Viciano V, Mateu M. Prevention of postoperative pulmonary complications through respiratory rehabilitation: A controlled clinical study. Arch Phys Med Rehabil 1998; 79:5–9.

149. Thomas JA, McIntosh JM. Are incentive spirometry, intermittent positive pressure breathing and deep breathing exercises effective in the prevention of postoperative pulmonary complications after upper abdominal surgery? A systematic overview and meta-analysis. Phys Ther 1994; 74:3–16.

150. Castillo R, Haas A. Chest physical therapy: Comparative efficacy of preoperative and postoperative in the elderly. Arch Phys Med Rehabil 1985; 66:376–379.

151. Stock MC, Downs JB, Gauer PK, Alster JM, Imrey PB. Prevention of postoperative pulmonary complications with CPAP, incentive spirometry, and conservative therapy. Chest 1985; 87:151–157.

152. Warner MA, Offord KP, Warner ME, Lennon RL, Conover MA, Jansson-Schumacher U. Role of preoperative cessation of smoking and other factors in postoperative pulmonary complications: A blinded, prospective study of coronary artery bypass patients. Mayo Clin Proc 1989; 64:609–616.

153. Kabalin CS, Yarnold PR, Grammer LC. Low complication rate of corticosteroid-treated asthmatics undergoing surgical procedures. Arch Intern Med 1995; 155:1379–1384.

154. Berg H, Roed J, Viby-Mogensen J, Mortensen CR, Engbaek J, Skovgaard LT, Krintel JJ. Residual neuromuscular block is a risk factor for postoperative pulmonary complications: A prospective, randomised, and blinded study of postoperative pulmonary complications after atracurium, vecuronium, and pancuronium. Acta Anaesthesiol Scand 1997; 41:1095–1103.

155. Her C, Kizelshteyn G, Walker V, Hayes D, Lees DE. Combined epidural and general anesthesia for abdominal aortic surgery. J Cardiothorac Anesth 1990; 4:552–557.

156. Kehlet H, Holte K. Effect of postoperative analgesia on surgical outcome. Br J Anaesth 2001; 87:62–72.

157. Rodgers A, Walker N, Schug S, Kehlet H, van Zundert A, Sage D, Futter M, Saville G, Clark T, MacMahon S. Reduction of postoperative mortality and morbidity with epidural or spinal anaesthesia: Results from overview of randomised trials. Br Med J 2000; 321:1–12.

158. Ballantyne JC, Carr DB, de Ferranti S, Suarez T, Lau J, Chalmers TC, Angelillo A, Mosteller F. The comparative effects of postoperative analgesic therapies on pulmonary outcome: Cumulative meta-analysis of randomized, controlled trials. Anesth Analg 1998; 86:598–612.

159. Wakefield TW, Stanley JC. Cardiopulmonary assessment for major vascular reconstructive procedures. In: Haimovici H, ed. Vascular Surgery. 4th ed. Cambridge, MA: Blackwell Science 1996:209–221.

3

Renal Failure and Fluid Shifts Following Vascular Surgery

Gregory S. Cherr

State University of New York at Buffalo, Buffalo, New York, U.S.A.

Kimberley J. Hansen

Wake Forest University School of Medicine, Winston-Salem, North Carolina, U.S.A.

The morbidity and mortality of acute renal failure (ARF) after vascular surgery was recognized in the earliest series describing aortic reconstruction (1–3). With better understanding of perioperative fluid shifts, the incidence of renal dysfunction has subsequently fallen, but ARF remains a frequent complication after vascular surgery (4–15). Because of the limited ability to alter the course of established ARF and the high mortality associated with ARF after vascular surgery, it is imperative that the vascular surgeon take measures to prevent this complication.

Articles describing ARF use varying terminology and lack concise reporting standards. Consequently, review of the topic is potentially confusing and direct comparisons between studies are difficult (5,16). For the sake of clarity, in this review the term *acute renal failure* is used to describe an abrupt rise in serum creatinine and/or blood urea nitrogen (BUN) with or without oliguria (urine output <400 mL/day). Because patients with ARF do not necessarily require renal replacement therapy, the distinction between ARF and renal replacement therapy is noted. Following a brief description of normal renal physiology, the causes of ARF are reviewed. From this reference point, the diagnosis, management, and potential preventive strategies of ARF associated with vascular surgery are discussed. Because ARF occurs more commonly after aortic reconstruction and has been well described in this patient population, particular emphasis is placed on the management of these patients.

I. THE INCIDENCE OF ACUTE RENAL FAILURE ASSOCIATED WITH VASCULAR SURGERY

Because ARF is an unusual complication of infrainguinal or cerebrovascular reconstruction, it has not been well described in the literature. Acute renal failure in these popu-

Table 1 The Incidence of Acute Renal Failure and Renal Replacement Therapy After Aortic Surgery

Procedure	ARF (%)	Mortality with ARF (%)	RRT (%)	Mortality with RRT (%)
Infrarenal AAA (6)			CrCl>45: 0	0.6
			CrCl<45: 7.0	45.5
Infrarenal AAA (7)	13.9		1.8	
Suprarenal AAA (7)	38.5		2.6	
TAA (9)		16.0	11.9	41.0
Ruptured TAA (9)			22.2	
TAA (10)	15.9		13.0	20.5 (comb)
TAA (11)	17.3	38.0	8.0	56.0
TAA (12)	15.0		2.5	49.0 (comb)
Ruptured AAA (13)	27.7	65.8	6.3	85.7
Ruptured AAA (14)	29.0			
Ruptured AAA (15)	11.4		18.1	65.0 (comb)

Abbreviations: ARF, acute renal failure; RRT, renal replacement therapy; AAA, abdominal aortic aneurysm; CrCl, creatinine clearance (mL/min); TAA, thoracoabdominal aneurysm; comb, combined mortality for ARF and RRT.

lations is likely related to preexisting renal dysfunction and/or contrast nephrotoxicity. However, ARF following aortic surgery is a relatively common complication associated with high mortality (Table 1). Although it is reported to have an incidence ranging from 0–13.9% after elective infrarenal aortic repair (4–8), the occurrence of ARF increases with the addition of inciting factors such as urgent or emergency operation, proximal aortic repair, preoperative renal dysfunction, adverse intraoperative and postoperative events, and medical comorbidity (such as diabetes or coronary artery or liver disease) (7,9,13,17). The incidence of ARF following repair of ruptured abdominal aortic aneurysm (AAA) ranges from 20 to 29% (13,14,18) and has not changed appreciably in the past 25 years (19–22). Moreover, the mortality of ARF requiring renal replacement therapy after repair of intact or ruptured AAA is 58–86% and likely represents the mortality risk associated with ARF as part of multisystem organ dysfunction (13,23–25).

II. NORMAL RENAL FUNCTION

While a complete discussion of normal renal physiology is beyond the scope of this chapter, a basic understanding of intrarenal and excretory renal function is necessary to understand abnormal renal function complicating the evaluation and management of vascular disorders.

The kidney serves as the dominant site for maintenance of normal intravascular volume and composition. Under normovolemic, unstressed conditions, the kidneys receive approximately 25% of the cardiac output. Based on a cardiac output of 5 L/min, the kidneys will receive approximately 900 L/day of plasma flow. Given the fact that the glomeruli filter 20% of the renal plasma flow and that the normal 24-h urinary output for a 70-kg man is less than 1.8 L, the kidneys' tubular system must reabsorb more than 99% of the 180 L/day of filtered plasma to maintain homeostasis. Moreover, the initial composition of the ultrafiltrate is the electrolyte and solute concentration of plasma. Therefore, electrolytes and other solutes such as glucose must also be almost totally reabsorbed (26).

Reabsorption of electrolytes from the tubular fluid occurs both by active transport and by passive back-diffusion. The sodium ion is reabsorbed in the early proximal tubule by its cotransportation with organic solutes, bicarbonate, and divalent cations through an active transport mechanism. Similarly, sodium is actively transported in the late proximal tubule in combination with chloride transport. Since water freely follows this movement of solutes and ions, the tubular fluid is iso-osmotic to plasma as it enters the loop of Henle (26).

Depending on their location, the tubular cells of the loop of Henle vary in their permeability. This variable permeability establishes a hypotonic tubular fluid and medullary osmotic gradient. Whereas the descending loop of Henle is permeable to water but relatively impermeable to sodium and chloride, the ascending loop of Henle is impermeable to water but actively transports the chloride ion, with sodium passively following. The resulting countercurrent mechanism produces a medullary osmotic gradient that regulates urine osmolarity from 50 to 1200 mOsm. Distal tubular reabsorption of sodium is also active. In the distal tubule and the proximal collecting ducts, sodium is actively and almost completely reabsorbed under the control of aldosterone. Of the approximately 25,000 mEq of sodium filtered daily, only 50 to 200 mEq is ultimately excreted (less than 1%) (26).

Filtered potassium is almost totally reabsorbed in the proximal tubule and the loop of Henle. Influenced by the electrochemical gradient and the intracellular concentration of potassium, however, potassium is also passively secreted by the distal tubules and early collecting ducts into the tubular lumen. Essentially all of the potassium in the urine is transported there through this process (26,27).

A. Neuroendocrine Modulators of Renal Function

Intravascular volume is regulated primarily by a series of stretch or baroreceptors located in the arterial tree and the atria. Since these receptors not only sense pressure or volume changes (atrial receptors) but also monitor the rates of change during the cardiac cycle, they govern the effective circulating volume. Factors that decrease cardiac performance will alter the intravascular volume perceived by these receptors and thereby also alter the renal function to retain water and increase the effective circulating volume. Similarly, when the concentration of circulating plasma proteins is reduced, there is a net diffusion of intravascular water into the extravascular space secondary to the decreased intravascular oncotic pressure. This net decrease in circulating volume is sensed by these same receptors, and neuroendocrine regulators of urinary output inhibit excretion of water to correct the volume deficiency.

When the baroreceptors perceive a reduction in circulating volume, their afferent signals are reduced, which decreases their tonic inhibition over the neuroendocrine system. This leads to increased secretion of vasopressin, beta endorphins, growth hormone, and adrenocorticotropic hormone through the central nervous system (CNS) and to an increase in release of epinephrine from the adrenal medulla. Within the kidneys, at the level of the nephron, baroreceptors within the macula densa cells of the juxtaglomerular apparatus perceive a decrease in intravascular pressure or plasma ion concentration and stimulate juxtaglomerular cells to release renin. Renin, in turn, stimulates the production of angiotensin I from angiotensinogen, which ultimately forms angiotensin II. Angiotensin II functions to raise blood pressure by direct vasoconstriction and, through its stimulation of aldosterone, indirectly functions to increase circulating plasma volume.

The primary hormonal regulators of fluid and electrolyte balance are aldosterone, cortisol, vasopressin, and angiotensin. However, the interactions between insulin, epinephrine, plasma glucose concentration, acid-base balance of the plasma, and other factors play a vital role in modulating the release of these hormones and directly affect the renal tubular management of water and the respective filtered solutes (26,27). Here, discussion of these interactions and impact on renal function and fluid shifts is limited to the effects of major vascular surgery.

III. FLUID SHIFTS ASSOCIATED WITH VASCULAR SURGERY

Because of the fluid shifts associated with vascular surgery, inappropriate fluid and electrolyte administration after vascular reconstruction will place the patient at risk for ARF. Causes of fluid shifts include tissue trauma from operative dissection, hemodynamic response to arterial clamping, and operative blood loss. Due to the importance and predictability of these fluid shifts after vascular surgery, this physiology is briefly reviewed.

Movement of water and solutes from the intravascular to the extravascular, extracellular space normally takes place at the precapillary level due to increased hydrostatic pressure. The reentry of fluid into the intravascular space in the distal capillaries results from the oncotic pressure gradient of intravascular proteins (predominantly albumin). Operative dissection and disruption of lymphatic channels combined with inflammatory mediators causing alterations in tissue perfusion result in increased capillary membrane permeability to albumin (28). Reduced plasma albumin concentration leads to decreased water reabsorption into the intravascular space. The resulting decreased intravascular volume causes activation of neuroendocrine mechanisms that decrease renal excretion of sodium and free water (29). In addition, ischemia-reperfusion and/or shock secondary to blood loss causes changes in the cellular transmembrane potential with movement of sodium and water into the intracellular space from the extracellular space (30). The normal response to decreased intravascular volume is mobilization of extracellular fluid. Because of its increased oncotic pressure after vascular surgery, the extracellular fluid is less available for expansion of the intravascular space. Finally, anesthesia may cause decreased renal blood flow through reductions in effective blood volume and reduced mean arterial pressure (16). The net result of these mechanisms is the potential for renal hypoperfusion and ARF.

Because of the presence of fluid shifts and intravascular hypovolemia after vascular surgery, determination of intravascular volume and serum electrolytes plays a vital role in preventing dysfunction of the kidneys. Isotonic crystalloid is used for fluid resuscitation during and after vascular surgery with blood transfusions reserved for significant reductions of hemoglobin. However, routine albumin resuscitation in the postoperative period does not appear beneficial after aortic reconstruction (31). Finally, time to mobilization of the sequestered third-space fluid is variable, usually ranging from 2 to 5 days, depending on the magnitude of perioperative stress, cardiac performance, and intravascular oncotic pressure. If not managed with appropriate reduction in intravenous fluid administration (and occasionally the addition of diuretic therapy), reabsorption of extracellular fluid can lead to intravascular volume overload and acute congestive heart failure.

IV. CATEGORIES OF RENAL DYSFUNCTION

Potential causes of renal dysfunction are summarized in Table 2.

A. Prerenal Dysfunction

Prerenal causes are the most frequent source of ARF in the postoperative period. Renal failure from a prerenal cause is usually the result of a contracted intravascular volume

Table 2 Potential Causes of Acute Renal Dysfunction in the Patient Undergoing Vascular Reconstruction

Prerenal	Parenchymal	Postrenal
Low cardiac output/cardiogenic shock	Nephrotoxic drugs	Catheter kinking
Increased vascular space	Acute tubular necrosis	Catheter clot
Septic shock	Radiological contrast	Bladder clot
Hypovolemia	Myoglobinuria	Ureteral obstruction
Blood loss	Other causes	Renal pelvic obstruction
Dehydration		
Third-space sequestration		

resulting from inadequate replacement of intraoperative or postoperative fluid losses. Less commonly, it is caused by a reduction in cardiac performance triggering neurohormonal mechanisms that lead to increased reabsorption of sodium and water. In their pure forms, these two causes of reduced renal function are clinically distinguishable. While hypovolemia is associated with flat neck veins, dry mucous membranes, and reduced pulmonary artery wedge and end-diastolic pressures, renal dysfunction from poor cardiac performance is manifest by distended neck veins, clinical fluid overload, and elevated pulmonary artery wedge pressure. Patients with hypovolemia are resuscitated with isotonic crystalloid (and blood or blood products as needed), while those with ARF of cardiogenic origin require improvement in myocardial performance (with afterload-reducing agents and/or inotropic agents) and reduction of left ventricular preload (with diuretic and/or nitrate therapy).

Since the patient undergoing vascular surgery frequently has associated coronary artery disease and impaired left ventricular systolic and diastolic function (3,33), distinction between hypovolemic and cardiogenic ARF can be difficult. Preexisting heart disease may raise the baseline total body volume with associated higher central filling pressures. In patients with diastolic dysfunction, normal or low-normal filling pressures may actually reflect relative hypovolemia. In this clinical situation, the authors maintain a constant infusion of both afterload-reducing and inotropic agents and cautiously administer small boluses of isotonic crystalloid while monitoring cardiac output, pulmonary artery wedge pressure, and right ventricular end-diastolic volume. If urinary response is negligible once filling pressures begin to rise, diuretic therapy may be required. The frequent presence of left ventricular dysfunction in patients undergoing vascular reconstruction requires that measures of cardiac function and filling pressures be established before starting diuretic or inotropic therapy (32,33).

B. Postrenal Dysfunction

Postrenal dysfunction (obstruction of flow from the kidney) is an uncommon cause of renal dysfunction after vascular surgery. The obstruction is usually at the level of the urethra or urinary catheter and rarely at the ureters. Hematuria or traumatic catheter insertion may lead to clot formation, catheter obstruction, and obstructive uropathy. For this reason, an abrupt decline in urine output should prompt maneuvers—such as catheter irrigation or replacement—to exclude mechanical causes. Urethral strictures, clots, or other abnormalities during catheter insertion should be noted.

Ureteral or renal pelvic obstruction should be considered after other causes of postrenal dysfunction have been excluded. Causes include kidney stones, iatrogenic injury, extrinsic compression of the ureter by a graft limb, or fibrotic reaction to surgery. Preliminary diagnosis is suggested by renal ultrasound or renogram and confirmed by retrograde urography. Delayed diagnosis and treatment reduces the chance of recovery of renal function, so that prompt recognition of the pathology is paramount (34). Therapy may require the placement of ureteral stents or percutaneous nephrostomy (16,35).

Acute urinary retention leading to obstructive uropathy may complicate the removal of a bladder catheter. Patients at risk include those with prostatic hypertrophy or epidural catheters for pain control. To avoid urinary retention, we generally allow 6–12 h time to elapse after epidural analgesia is discontinued prior to removal of urinary catheters.

C. Renal Parenchymal Dysfunction

Parenchymal causes of ARF are diverse and pose the greatest risk for permanent damage to the kidney. Potential sites of parenchymal injury include the renal tubule, vessels, or glomerulus (16). Parenchymal dysfunction caused by injury of the renal tubules mediated by ischemia or toxins is most relevant to the patient undergoing vascular surgery. Common causes of renal ischemia after vascular surgery include suprarenal aortic cross-clamping and systemic inflammatory response associated with multisystem organ dysfunction, hypovolemia, shock, or atheroembolism. Prerenal and parenchymal dysfunction are linked when severe reductions in renal blood flow causes ischemic injury to the tubular cells (16). Causes of toxic injury associated with vascular reconstruction include aminoglycoside therapy, myoglobinuria, and radiological contrast. Other causes of parenchymal dysfunction (such as acute interstitial nephritis and glomerulonephritis) are uncommon after vascular surgery and are not further discussed in this chapter (16).

1. Acute Ischemic Injury

The pathophysiology of acute ischemic injury is likely twofold. First, as a consequence of the magnitude and duration of ischemia, tubular cell swelling occurs following reperfusion. This may cause tubular obstruction and reduction of glomerular filtration. Second, ischemia may cause tubular cell necrosis, apoptosis, or loss of basement membrane attachment (from interstitial edema during reperfusion), with sloughing of cells into the tubule. The medullary thick ascending loop of Henle and the pars recta of the proximal tubule are the segments of the tubular epithelium most sensitive to ischemia. Following loss of the tubular cell, a back leak of glomerular filtrate into the renal parenchyma then develops (36–38).

Aortic repair requiring a suprarenal cross clamp poses a significant risk for renal ischemia. The risk is greater for repair of thoracoabdominal aneurysm (TAA), where longer periods of renal ischemia can be anticipated. Rates of ARF as high as 17% are reported in larger series for elective repair of TAA (10–12). Predictors of renal dysfunction included preoperative creatinine >1.5 mg/dL and cross-clamp time >100 min. These results were similar to those from series in which partial left heart bypass and distal aortic perfusion were utilized (39). Recovery of renal function after suprarenal cross-clamping relates to preexisting renal dysfunction, patient age, and the duration of renal ischemia (cross-clamp time) (7,9,11,14,40).

Vascular surgery complicated by sepsis, myocardial dysfunction, or reperfusion injury may cause renal ischemia leading to ARF. When it is part of the systemic inflammatory response syndrome, ARF may be mediated by increases in proinflammatory mediators such as endotoxin, tumor necrosis factor, interleukin (IL)-1, IL-6, IL-8, prostaglandins, or leukotrienes (41). Recovery of renal function is dependent upon maintenance of adequate renal perfusion and requires prompt elimination of the septic focus and improvement in left ventricular performance. Hypotension from blood loss, myocardial dysfunction, or sepsis can also diminish renal blood flow and incite acute ischemic injury (6,12,42).

Atheroembolism is an underrecognized cause of ARF. Embolization of atheromatous debris from diseased segments of the pararenal aorta may complicate suprarenal cross-clamping or dissection of the aorta. Likewise, catheter manipulation during aortography may cause atheroembolization. These patients may also develop concomitant peripheral ischemia from atheroembolization to the lower extremities. The presence of serum eosino-philia and urine eosinophils may aid in the diagnosis (43). Acute renal failure from athero-embolism is usually progressive and may be fatal.

2. Toxic Injury

Aminoglycosides appear to exert their renal toxicity at the tubular cell and cause impair-ment of renal function in up to 20% of patients (44,45). Risk factors which can contribute to nephrotoxicity with aminoglycoside use include high dosage or prolonged course of an aminoglycoside, preexisting renal insufficiency, advanced age, extracellular volume deple-tion with concomitant renal ischemia, or use of other nephrotoxins (44,45). Once-daily dosing regimens for aminoglycosides are less costly and more convenient but do not appear to reduce the risk of nephrotoxicity (46). A prudent approach would be to avoid aminoglycoside therapy when possible.

Myoglobinuria is an important cause of ARF in patients undergoing vascular reconstruction after a period of prolonged muscle ischemia. Myoglobin, released from ischemic muscle, is freely filtered by the glomerulus and is thought to cause ARF through direct tubular cell injury caused by myoglobin degradation products, precipitation within the tubule, or abnormal renal blood flow (47–49). Myoglobinuria is suggested when the urine is dipstick-positive for blood but no red cells are present on microscopic analysis. Once diagnosed, myoglobinuria-induced injury to the kidney may be ameliorated by alkalinizing the urine with sodium bicarbonate and maximizing urine output with crystalloid infusion and mannitol administration (50).

Contrast agents used during angiography are a common cause of ARF. These agents cause both direct tubular cell injury (51) and transient hypoperfusion of the kidneys (52). The ionization and high osmolarity of contrast agents may contribute to their nephrotox-icity. Conventional (ionic) contrast agents contain iodine, which absorbs x-ray photons and thus allows visualization of the vasculature. Nonionic contrast agents provide comparable absorption of x-ray photons yet are significantly less charged than traditional agents. In comparing ionic and nonionic contrast agents, the rate of severe nephrotoxicity is found to be similar for patients with normal renal function. Consequently, the lower cost of ionic agents makes them preferable in this patient population (53). However, in patients with preexisting renal dysfunction, nonionic contrast agents may reduce the risk of nephrotoxicity (54). In most patients with contrast-induced ARF, serum creatinine levels peak in 4–5 days and return to their baseline level within 2 weeks (55–57).

Risk factors for contrast-induced nephrotoxicity as determined by metanalysis of prospective clinical trials include preexisting renal insufficiency, diabetes, heart failure, and dose of contrast used (58). In patients with normal renal function, the incidence of contrast nephropathy is <10%, but it increases with the addition of the previously mentioned risk factors (53,54,59). The risk of nephrotoxicity may increase exponentially for patients with a serum creatinine >1.2 mg/dL (57). For diabetic patients with normal renal function [as indicated by a normal estimated glomerular filtration rate (EGFR)], the risk of contrast-induced nephrotoxicity is similar to that for nondiabetics (54,59,60). However, the combination of diabetes and renal insufficiency increases the risk of contrast nephrotoxicity to at least twice that expected for renal insufficiency alone (54,60,61). Among patients commonly submitted to vascular surgery, diabetics with renal insufficiency appear to be at greatest risk for ARF after angiography (62).

V. STRATEGIES TO PROTECT RENAL FUNCTION

Strategies to protect renal function are summarized in Table 3.

A. Preoperative Measures

Measures to protect renal function are begun in the preoperative period. The first goal is to identify patients at increased risk for perioperative ARF. Excretory renal function should be determined in every patient undergoing vascular surgery. The best overall estimate of renal function is glomerular filtration rate. Direct measurement of glomerular filtration rate, although preferred, is rarely performed in our clinical practice. Instead, EGFR is determined using creatinine clearance calculated from measured serum creatinine (63). Using EGFR, patients with preexisting renal dysfunction are identified and presumed to be at increased risk for perioperative ARF. Elevated preoperative creatinine and associated decreased EGFR are the most consistent predictors of ARF for patients submitted to aortic reconstruction (4,7,9–15,40). Other risk factors for postoperative ARF include increased age, poor cardiac function, diabetes, and renovascular disease (5,7,9).

Before vascular repair, the greatest risk of renal dysfunction occurs during angiography. Strategies to minimize the effects of contrast-induced renal injury are controversial and lack controlled studies to confirm their efficacy. Two easily modified risk factors for contrast-induced nephrotoxicity are hypovolemia and volume of contrast agent used. Intravenous crystalloid is started before angiography and urine output is used as a measure of the adequacy of hydration. In patients with renal insufficiency undergoing coronary angiography, hydration with 0.45% saline plus mannitol or furosemide has demonstrated a greater risk of nephrotoxicity than 0.45% saline alone (61). Similarly, renal dose dopamine (0.5–2.5 (μg/kg/min) does not appear to offer further advantages over

Table 3 Summary of Measures Taken to Prevent Acute Renal Dysfunction During Vascular Reconstruction

Preoperative	Intraoperative
Identify pts at risk ($\downarrow$EGFR)	Minimize renal ischemia time
Angiography	Aortic cross-clamping
Preangiogram hydration	Heparin
Minimize contrast use	Mannitol
Acetylcysteine?	Maintenance of euvolemia
Hold ACE inhibitors, loop diuretics,	Bladder catheter
AT II receptor inhibitors	Pulmonary artery catheter
Preoperative hydration	Avoid atheroembolism

Abbreviations: pts, patients; EGFR, estimated glomerular filtration rate; ACE, angiotensin-converting enzyme; AT II, angiotensin II.

crystalloid therapy (64,65). In our practice, patients at increased risk for nephrotoxicity are routinely admitted for intravenous hydration prior to angiography (1.5 mL/kg/h for 12 h). Immediately before angiography, the patient usually receives a bolus of intravenous fluid (3 to 5 mL/kg). Finally, intravenous hydration is continued for 4–6 h after completion of the study.

Because no definitive limit on the "safe" amount of contrast agent exists, minimal contrast doses should be used. Even small doses (30 mL) of contrast may induce dialysis-dependent ARF in patients with extreme renal insufficiency (EGFR ≤15 mL/min). Conversely, 300 mL of contrast material has been safely administered to patients at low risk for nephrotoxicity (66). The authors' practice is to limit the quantity of nonionized contrast agent to less than 50 mL in patients with renal insufficiency (EGFR <30 mL/min). If additional contrast is required, further imaging is postponed to allow for recovery of renal function.

Adjuncts or alternatives to conventional angiography are appropriate in many instances. Digital subtraction techniques may be useful in limiting the quantity of contrast material required. Carbon dioxide gas can be used for angiography with minimal renal risk (67,68). Because it offers limited detail, CO_2 angiography is often used to identify the site of disease, which is then better defined with conventional contrast agents. Other alternatives to conventional angiography that reduce or eliminate the risk of nephrotoxicity include the use of gadolinium as a contrast agent for angiography (69), magnetic resonance angiography (70), and abdominal ultrasound with visceral/renal artery duplex sonography.

By scavenging reactive oxygen species, acetylcysteine may protect against contrast-induced nephrotoxicity. Tepel and colleagues studied patients with chronic renal dysfunction who required nonionic contrast for computed tomography. They documented a significant reduction in serum creatinine with the use of oral acetylcysteine and hydration compared to placebo and hydration (71). Although further study is needed to better define the role of acetylcysteine during arteriography, we administer two oral doses of acetylcysteine (600 mg) before and after these studies in patients at high risk for contrast nephrotoxicity.

Finally, high-dose loop diuretics, angiotensin-converting enzyme (ACE) inhibitors, and angiotensin II receptor antagonists are held for at least 72 h prior to aortic reconstruction. Selective beta blockers and calcium channel blockers (i.e., nifedipine) are substituted when necessary. With this approach, we hope to optimize renal perfusion through avoidance of hypovolemia and renal vasoconstriction (72).

B. Operative Measures

Perioperative measures to protect renal function during vascular surgery are widely practiced by vascular surgeons. These include providing adequate circulating blood volume through preoperative intravenous hydration, adequately replacing lost blood volume, avoiding repetitive or prolonged renal ischemia, and optimizing myocardial performance. Additional modalities may include the use of dopamine or fenoldopam and mannitol to enhance renal perfusion (73–76). It is our belief that these preventive measures may lessen the severity and duration of ARF after vascular surgery (73,74).

Particular attention to the patient's volume status is imperative. Patients are admitted at least 12 h before operation for intravenous hydration. Without hydration, patients are frequently hypovolemic from the combined effects of bowel preparation and an overnight fast. Bladder catheters are placed to monitor urine output during and immediately after the operation. For patients requiring aortic reconstruction, we routinely use pulmonary artery catheters to help guide fluid resuscitation and monitor myocardial performance. For patients with severe systolic and/or diastolic dysfunction, transesophageal echocardiography is used intraoperatively to guide fluid and vasoactive agent management, especially during cross clamping of the aorta.

When possible, warm renal ischemia time should be limited by using efficient, meticulous surgical technique. The normally perfused kidney can tolerate 45 min of warm ischemia. For the chronically ischemic kidney, the duration of safe warm ischemic time may be longer but ultimately depends on the amount and effectiveness of collateral blood flow. Regional renal hypothermia may be a helpful adjunct for the protection of renal function during periods of ischemia. Decreases in the core temperature of the kidney significantly reduce metabolic needs and may reduce the incidence of postischemic ARF. In animal models of renal ischemia, a modest decrease in core renal temperature (35°C) had a protective effect on both renal tubular morphology and postprocedure serum creatinine levels (77). Although we frequently use cold perfusion preservation techniques during ex vivo renal artery repair, we do not routinely perfuse the in situ kidney with cold electrolyte solution during aortic reconstruction. Rather, we use topical ice slush when warm renal ischemia is likely to exceed 45 min during aortic repair.

A number of adjunctive measures may be employed at the time of aortic cross-clamping. We routinely administer heparin (1 mg/kg) and confirm systemic anticoagulation by measurement of activated clotting time. We also use mannitol in small bolus doses (12.5–25 g IV) during pararenal dissection and before and after periods of renal ischemia up to a total dose of 1 g/kg of the patient is body weight. Potential protective actions of mannitol include osmotic diuresis, decreased renovascular resistance that enhances cortical and medullary blood flow, free-radical scavenging, and increased glomerular filtration during renal hypoperfusion (50,78). When compared to saline administration before aortic cross-clamping during infrarenal AAA repair, mannitol causes a reduction in subclinical glomerular and renal tubular damage (73).

Dopamine is frequently administered during vascular surgery. "Renal dose" dopamine (0.5–3 (μg/kg/min) in healthy adults causes increased renal perfusion, glomerular filtration rate, and urine output (79). However, the effect of low-dose dopamine in patients undergoing vascular surgery is less well understood. During aortic reconstruction, dopamine administration may cause increased urine output through its inotropic effects (74,80). However, the clinical benefit of prophylactic dopamine administration in patients undergoing vascular surgery is unproved (74,81,82). Because dopamine may cause tachyarrhythmias, myocardial ischemia, pulmonary shunting, or mesenteric vasoconstriction (81–83), its routine use should be approached with caution.

Fenoldopam is a dopaminergic type 1 receptor agonist that may reduce the risk of ARF. Two dopamine receptors are found in the kidney: DA1 and DA2. Activation of the DA1 receptor causes increased glomerular filtration likely mediated by increased blood flow to the inner cortex and medulla of the kidney. Activation of the DA2 receptor causes a reduction in renal blood flow and glomerular filtration rate (84). Fenoldopam is a potent antihypertensive agent used to treat patients with severe hypertension (85). Fenoldopam significantly increases renal blood flow in healthy adults (76) and maintains kidney perfusion in animal models of radiocontrast-induced nephrotoxicity (86) and aortic cross-clamping (87). However, fenoldopam also causes significant reductions in cerebral blood flow in healthy adults (88). Although preliminary evidence indicates that fenoldopam may prevent contrast-induced nephropathy (89) and renal dysfunction after aortic surgery (75), additional investigation is needed to better elucidate the role of fenoldopam during vascular surgery.

Specific intraoperative techniques may help to prevent microembolization of atheromatous debris during juxtarenal aortic dissection and clamping. One should avoid repetitive aortic cross-clamping, as this increases the risk of atheroembolization to the renal arteries. Because the embolic potential of the debris cannot be judged definitively until after the aorta is opened, one should assume its presence. When either suprarenal or juxtarenal aortic control is required, we temporarily occlude renal artery flow immediately before the application of the aortic clamp. Although we can provide only anecdotal support for this maneuver, we believe that it has been an important adjunct in minimizing the incidence of postoperative ARF due to atheroembolization among our patients.

Atheroembolism is the likely cause of ARF in patients without prolonged renal ischemia, excessive blood loss, hypotension, or other recognized nephrotoxic insult (90). The quantity of emboli produced during manipulation of the aorta depends on the stability and amount of atheromatous debris and the operative techniques employed. The clinical impact of renal emboli depends on the amount of renal parenchyma affected and the presence of concomitant renal insults. In patients without other risk factors for ARF or preexisting renal dysfunction, large amounts of atheromatous emboli can occur without immediate impact on renal function (91). In contrast, in patients with minimal renal reserve, the added insult of minor emboli can lead to ARF. Because the prognosis for recovery of renal function after atheroembolism is poor, prevention of this complication is important.

Distal aortic perfusion may be used to maintain renal perfusion during repair of TAA. This technique is most attractive during the repair of an isolated TAA (92) or when complex disease precludes prompt completion of the proximal thoracic aortic anastamosis (93). Distal aortic perfusion may be modified with "octopus" catheters to directly perfuse the renal arteries during distal reconstruction (12). Since the routine use of distal aortic perfusion has been associated with an increased incidence of ARF despite renal and spinal cord protection in extensive (type II) TAA, we have preferred other strategies to provide renal protection (12,94).

VI. DIAGNOSIS AND TREATMENT OF RENAL DYSFUNCTION

The diagnosis of ARF is based on an acute rise in serum creatinine and BUN with or without a concomitant decrease in urine output. However, creatinine and BUN are relatively insensitive markers of excretory renal function. The glomerular filtration rate may fall by 50% before a rise in serum creatinine is noted due to the kidney's compensatory increase in creatinine excretion (95,96). Conversely, creatinine and BUN may rise without an associated decrease in glomerular filtration. Causes of isolated increased creatinine without associated renal dysfunction include increased release from muscle and decreased secretion from the proximal tubules (e.g., trimethoprim or cephalosporin therapy). Causes of rising BUN without worsening renal function include increased protein intake, infusion of amino acids, catabolism, gastrointestinal bleeding, and steroid therapy (97,98). Despite these limitations, serial determinations of serum creatinine and BUN, calculation of EGFR, and measurement of urine output are the mainstays of renal function monitoring.

An organized plan of diagnosis and treatment is important when faced with the patient with ARF after vascular surgery. The evaluation includes a thorough physical examination.

Table 4 Urinary and Blood Parameters that May Aid in the Evaluation of the Patient with Acute Renal Dysfunction

Characteristic	Prerenal dysfunction	Renal parenchymal dysfunction	Postrenal dysfunction
Urine specific gravity	>1.020	<1.020	<1.020
Urine osmolarity (mOsm/L)	>400	<400	<400
Urine/plasma (U/P) osmolarity	>1.5	~1	~1
Urine Na (mEq/L)	<20	>30	<30[a]
Fractional excretion of Na	<1%	>1%	<1%[a]
BUN:Cr	>20	<10	10–20[a]
U/P Cr	>40	<20	<20

[a] First 24 h only.

Evidence of intravascular volume depletion, hemodynamic instability, sepsis or congestive heart failure directs the differential diagnosis toward possible prerenal, renal, and postrenal causes for renal dysfunction. Prerenal causes are the most frequent source of ARF in the early postoperative period. The patient's intravascular volume status and cardiac performance should be evaluated. Patients with signs of volume depletion (flat neck veins, dry mucous membranes, and reduced filling pressures) require fluid resuscitation with isotonic crystalloid. Potassium-containing solutions and blood products are avoided until adequate renal function is confirmed. Patients with signs of inadequate cardiac performance (distended neck veins, S3 gallop, pulmonary edema, acute electrocardiographic changes, dysrhythmias, decreased cardiac output, and elevated filling pressures) require judicious inotropic support while indices of cardiac performance are measured. If correction of filling pressures or myocardial performance fails to improve urinary output, samples of urine and blood are obtained. Serum electrolytes, blood counts, and urine studies allow evaluation of other possible sources of oliguria, such as myoglobinuria. Urine studies include urinalysis, urine sodium, urea and creatinine concentrations, urine osmolality, and estimation of fractional excretion of sodium. Interpretations of these blood and urinary parameters are provided in Table 4.

VII. ESTABLISHED RENAL DYSFUNCTION AFTER VASCULAR SURGERY

Acute renal failure following vascular surgery requires multidisciplinary therapy beyond the scope of this review. Briefly, the initial goals are correction of extracellular volume deficits and optimization of cardiac performance. With restoration of intravascular volume and cardiac output, urinary output may be augmented with the addition of low-dose dopamine (0.5–3 (μg/kg/min) (99,100). The conversion of oliguric renal failure to a nonoliguric state may delay the need for renal replacement therapy and simplify fluid management. It may also be associated with fewer complications and improved survival (9,101,102), although prospective data to support this notion are lacking.

Patients with radiocontrast-induced ARF require supportive care. Renal perfusion should be optimized with fluid administration for patients with hypovolemia and diuresis of those with fluid overload. If necessary, myocardial performance can be enhanced with inotropic and/or vasodilatory agents. Further renal insults should be avoided with delay of nonurgent operations or contrast studies. Finally, nephrotoxic drugs should be avoided. Most patients' renal function will return to baseline within 2 weeks of the inciting angiogram (55–57).

As previously noted, the onset of renal failure requiring chronic replacement therapy in the postoperative period has a grave prognosis. We prefer the use of continuous venovenous hemofiltration/dialysis until the patient's hemodynamic status is stabilized. Continuous hemodialysis reduces hemodynamic instability, allows better control of fluid and metabolic status, and may affect outcome by removing deleterious cytokines (103,104). Nutritional support of the patient with ARF is important, as protein-calorie malnutrition is common in this population (105). The dosage of renally excreted medications should be adjusted appropriately. Finally, it is important to maintain a frank and realistic dialogue with the family of the patient requiring renal replacement therapy for ARF after vascular repair.

REFERENCES

1. Powers SR, Boba A, Stein A. The mechanism and prevention of distal tubular necrosis following aneurysmectomy. Surgery 1957; 42:156–162.
2. MacVaugh H, Roberts B. Results of resection of abdominal aortic aneurysm. Surg Gynecol Obstet 1961; 113:17–23.
3. Payne JH, Wood DL, Goethel JA. Oliguria and renal failure in abdominal aortic surgery. Am Surg 1963; 29:713–718.
4. Johnston KW. Multicenter prospective study of nonruptured abdominal aortic aneurysms: Part II, variables predicting morbidity and mortality. J Vasc Surg 1989; 9:437–447.
5. Novis BK, Roizen MF, Aronson S, Thisted RA. Association of preoperative risk factors with postoperative acute renal failure. Anesth Analg 1994; 78:143–149.
6. Powell RJ, Roddy SP, Meier GH, Gusberg RJ, Conte MS, Sumpio BE. Effect of renal insufficiency on outcome following infrarenal surgery. Am J Surg 1997; 174:126–130.
7. Breckwoldt WL, Mackey WC, Belkin M, O'Donnell TF. The effect of suprarenal cross-clamping on abdominal aortic aneurysm repair. Arch Surg 1992; 127:520–524.
8. Berry AJ, Smith RB, Weintraub WS, Chaikof EL, Dodson TF, Lumsden AB. Age versus comorbidities as risk factors for complications after elective aortic reconstructive surgery. J Vasc Surg 2001; 33:345–352.
9. Schepens MA, Defauw JJ, Hamerlijnck RP, Vermeulen FE. Risk assessment of acute renal failure after thoracoabdominal aortic aneurysm surgery. Ann Surg 1994; 219:400–407.
10. Svensson LG, Crawford ES, Hess KR, Coselli JS, Safe HJ. Experience with 1509 patients undergoing thoracoabdominal and aortic operations. J Vasc Surg 1993; 17:357–368.
11. Godet G, Fleron M-H, Vicaut E, Zubicki A. Risk factors for acute postoperative renal failure in thoracic or thoracoabdominal aortic surgery: A prospective study. Anesth Analg 1997; 85:1227–1232.
12. Safi HJ, Harlin SA, Miller CC, Iliopoulos DC, Joshi A, Mohasci TG, Zippel R, Letsou GV, Tabor M. Predictive factors for acute renal failure in thoracic and thoracoabdominal aortic aneurysm surgery. J Vasc Surg 1996; 24:338–344.
13. Panneton JM, Lassonde J, Laurendeau F. Ruptured abdominal aortic aneurysm: Impact of comorbidity and postoperative complications on outcome. Ann Vasc Surg 1995; 9:535–541.
14. Bauer EP, Redaelli C, von Segesser LK, Turina MI. Ruptured abdominal aortic aneurysms: Predictors for early complications and death. Surgery 1993; 114:31–35.
15. Hajarizadeh H, Rohrer MJ, Hermann JB, Cutler BS. Acute peritoneal dialysis following ruptured abdominal aortic aneurysms. Am J Surg 1995; 170:223–226.

16. Thadhani R, Pascual M, Bonventre JV. Acute renal failure. N Engl J Med 1996; 334:1448–1460.

17. Nypaver TJ, Shepard AD, Reddy DJ, Elliot JP, Smith RF, Ernst CB. Repair of pararenal abdominal aortic aneurysms. An analysis of operative management. Arch Surg 1993; 128:808–813.

18. Gordon AC, Pryn S, Collin J. Outcome of patients who required renal support after surgery for ruptured abdominal aortic aneurysm. Br J Surg 1994; 81:836–838.

19. Hicks GL, Eastland MW, DeWeese JA, Rob CG. Survival improvement following aortic aneurysm resection. Ann Surg 1975; 181:863–869.

20. McCombs PR, Roberts B. Acute renal failure following resection of abdominal aortic aneurysm. Surg Gynecol Obstet 1979; 148:175–178.

21. Gornick CC, Kjellstrand CM. Acute renal failure complicating aortic surgery. Nephron 1983; 35:145–147.

22. Fielding JL, Black J, Ashton F, Slaney G. Ruptured aortic aneurysms: postoperative complications and their aetiology. Br J Surg 1984; 71:487–491.

23. Braams R, Vossen V, Lisman BAM, Eikelboom BC. Outcome in patients requiring renal replacement therapy after surgery for ruptured and nonruptured aneurysm of the abdominal aorta. Eur J Vasc Endovasc Surg 1999; 18:323–327.

24. Chen JC, Hildebrand HD, Salvian AJ, Taylor DC, Strandberg S, Myckatyn TM, Hsiang YN. Predictors of death in nonruptured and ruptured abdominal aortic aneurysms. J Vasc Surg 1996; 24:614–620.

25. Barratt J, Parajasingam R, Sayers RD, Feehally J. Outcome of acute renal failure following surgical repair of ruptured abdominal aortic aneurysms. Eur J Vasc Endovasc Surg 2000; 20:163–168.

26. Robaczewski DL, Dean RH. Basic Science of Renovascular Hypertension. In: Sidawy AN, Sumpio BE, Depalma RG, eds. The Basic Science of Vascular Disease. Armonk, NY: Futura, 1997 pp. 691–721.

27. Valtin H. Renal function: Mechanisms preserving fluid and solute balance in health. In: Valtin H, ed. Renal Dysfunction: Mechanisms Involved in Fluid and Solute Imbalance, 3rd ed. Boston, Little Brown, 1995: pp 110–129.

28. Weissman C. Ensuring perioperative fluid homeostasis in critically ill patients. J Crit Illness 1994; 9:1077–1084.

29. Schrier RW. A unifying hypothesis of body fluid volume regulation. J R Coll Phys Lond 1992; 26:295–306.

30. Smeets HJ, Kievit J, Dulfer FT, Hermans J, Moolenaar AJ. Analysis of post-operative hypoalbuminemia: A clinical study. Int Surg 1994; 79:152–157.

31. Nielsen OM, Engell HC. Effects of maintaining normal plasma colloid osmotic pressure on renal function and excretion of sodium and water after major surgery: A randomized study. Dan Med Bull 1985; 31:182–185.

32. Hertzer NR, Beven EG, Young JR, O'Hara PJ, Rushchaupt WF, Graor RA, Dewolfe VG, Maljovec LC. Coronary artery disease in peripheral vascular patients: A classification of 1000 coronary angiograms and results of surgical management. Ann Surg 1984; 199:223–233.

33. Blombery PA, Ferguson IA, Rosengarten DS, Stuchbery KE, Miles CR, Black AJ, Pitt A, Anderson ST, Harper RW, Federman J. The role of coronary artery disease in complications of abdominal aortic aneurysm surgery. Surgery 1987; 101:150–155.

34. Shapiro SR, Bennett AH. Recovery of renal function after prolonged unilateral ureteral obstruction. J Urol 1976; 115:136–140.

35. Naude G, Bongard F. Renal failure in the vascular patient. Semin Vasc Surg 1996; 9:266–274.

36. Mason J, Joeris B, Welsch J, Kriz W. Vascular congestion in ischemic renal failure: The role of cell swelling. Miner Electrolyte Metab 1989; 15:114–124.

37. Lerman L, Textor SC. Pathophysiology of ischemic nephropathy. Urol Clin North Am 2001; 28:793–803.

38. Molitoris BA. New insights into the cell biology of ischemic acute renal failure. J Am Soc Nephrol 1991; 1:1263–1270.

39. Kashyap VS, Cambria RP, Davison JF, L'Italien GJ. Renal failure after thoracoabdominal aortic surgery. J Vasc Surg 1997; 26:949–955.

40. Crawford ES, Crawford JL, Safi HJ, Coselli JS, Hess KR, Brooks B, Norton HJ, Glaeser DH. Thoracoabdominal aortic aneurysms: preoperative and intraoperative factors determining immediate and long-term results of operations in 605 patients. J Vasc Surg 1986; 3:389–404.

41. Breen D, Bihari D. Acute renal failure as a part of multiple organ failure: The slippery slope of critical illness. Kidney Int 1998; 53:S25–S33.

42. Schepens MA, Defauw JJ, Hamerlijnck CRP, De Geest R, Vermeulen FE. Surgical treatment of thoracoabdominal aortic aneurysms by simple cross-clamping: Risk factors and late results. J Thorac Cardiovasc Surg 1994; 107:134–142.

43. Scolari F, Bracchi M, Valzorio B, Movilli E, Costantino E, Savoldi S, Zorat S, Bonardelli S, Tardanico R, Maiorca R. Cholesterol atheromatous embolism: an increasingly recognized cause of acute renal failure. Nephr Dial Trans 1996; 11:1607–1612.

44. Moore RD, Smith CR, Lipsky JJ, Mellits ED, Lietman PS. Risk factors for nephrotoxicity in patients treated with aminoglycosides. Ann Intern Med 1984; 100:352–357.

45. Boucher BA, Coffey BC, Kuhl DA, Tolley EA, Fabian TC. Algorithm for assessing renal dysfunction risk in critically ill trauma patients receiving aminoglycosides. Am J Surg 1990; 160:473–480.

46. Hatala R, Dinh T, Cook DJ. Once-daily aminoglycoside dosing in immunocompetent adults: A meta-analysis. Ann Intern Med 1996; 124:717–725.

47. Zager RA. Heme protein-ischemic interactions at the vascular, intraluminal, and renal tubular cell levels: Implications for therapy of myoglobin-induced renal injury. Renal Failure 1992; 14:341–344.

48. Zager RA. Rhabdomyolysis and myohemoglobinuric acute renal failure. Kidney Int 1996; 49: 314–326.

49. Vetterlein F, Hoffman F, Pedina J, Neckel M, Schmidt G. Disturbances in renal microcirculation induced by myoglobin and hemorrhagic hypotension in anesthetized rats. Am J Physiol 1995; 268:F839–F846.

50. Better OS, Stein JH. Early management of shock and prophylaxis of acute renal failure in traumatic rhabdomyolysis. N Engl J Med 1990; 322:825–829.

51. Donadio C, Tramonti G, Lucceshi A, Giordani R, Lucchetti A, Bianchi C. Tubular toxicity is the main renal effect of contrast media. Renal Failure 1996; 18:647–656.

52. Larson TS, Hudson K, Mertz JI, Romero JC, Knox FG. Renal vasoconstrictive responses to contrast medium. J Lab Clin Med 1983; 101:385–391.

53. Schwab SJ, Hlatky MA, Pieper KS, Davidson CJ, Morris KG, Skelton TN, Bashore TM. Contrast nephrotoxicity: a randomized controlled trial of a nonionic and an ionic radiographic contrast agent. N Engl J Med 1989; 320:149–153.

54. Rudnick MR, Goldfarb S, Wexler L, Ludbrook PA, Murphy MJ, Halpern EF, Hill JA, Winniford M, Cohen MB, VanFossen DB. Nephrotoxicity of ionic and nonionic contrast media in 1196 patients: A randomized trial. The Iohexol Cooperative Study. Kidney Int 1995; 47:254–261.

55. Berns AS. Nephrotoxicity of contrast media. Kidney Int 1989; 36:730–740.

56. Porter GA. Contrast-associated nephropathy. Am J Cardiol 1989; 64:22E–26E.

57. Wish JB, Moritz CE. Preventing radiocontrast-induced acute renal failure. J Crit Illness 1990; 5:16–25.

58. Barrett BJ. Contrast nephrotoxicity. J Am Soc Nephrol 1994; 5:125–137.

59. Davidson CJ, Hlatky M, Morris KG, Pieper K, Skelton TN, Schwab SJ, Bashore TM. Cardiovascular and renal toxicity of a non-ionic radiographic contrast agent after cardiac catheterization: A prospective trial. Ann Intern Med 1989; 110:119–124.

60. Parfrey PS, Griffiths SM, Barrett BJ, Paul MD, Genge M, Withes J, Farid N, McManamon

PJ. Contrast material-induced renal failure in patients with diabetes mellitus, renal insufficiency, or both. A prospective controlled study. N Engl J Med 1989; 320:143–149.

61. Solomon R, Werner C, Mann D, D'Elia J, Silva P. Effects of saline, mannitol and furosemide to prevent acute decreases in renal function induced by radiocontrast agents. N Engl J Med 1994; 331:1416–1420.

62. Manske CL, Sprafka JM, Strony FT, Wang Y. Contrast nephrography in azotemic diabetic patients undergoing coronary angiography. Am J Med 1990; 89:615–620.

63. Rolin HA, Hall PM, Wei R. Inaccuracy of estimated creatinine clearance for predictors of iothalamate glomerular filtration rate. Am J Kidney Dis 1984; 4:48–54.

64. Hans B, Hans SS, Mittal VK, Khan TA, Patel N, Dahn MS. Renal function to dopamine during and after arteriography in patients with chronic renal failure. Radiology 1990; 176:651–654.

65. Hall KA, Wong RW, Hunter GC, Camazine BM, Rappaport WA, Smyth SH, Bull DA, McIntyre KE, Bernhard VM, Misiorowski RL. Contrast-induced nephrotoxicity: The effects of vasodilator therapy. J Surg Res 1992; 53:317–320.

66. Cigarroa RG, Lang RA, Williams RH, Hillis LD. Dosing of contrast material to prevent contrast nephropathy in patients with renal disease. Am J Med 1989; 86:649–652.

67. Weaver FA, Pentecost MJ, Yellin AE. Carbon dioxide digital subtraction arteriography: A pilot study. Ann Vasc Surg 1990; 4:437–441.

68. Seeger JM, Self S, Harward TR, Flynn TC, Hawkins IF. Carbon dioxide gas as an arterial contrast agent. Ann Surg 1993; 217:688–697.

69. Hammer FD, Goffette PP, Malaise J, Mathurin P. Gadolinium dimeglumine: An alternative contrast agent for digital subtraction angiography. Eur Radiol 1999; 9:128–136.

70. Goyen M, Ruehm SG, Debatin JF. MR-angiography: The role of contrast agents. Eur J Radiol 2000; 34:247–256.

71. Tepel M, van der Giet M, Schwarzfeld C, Laufer U, Liermann D, Zidek W. Prevention of radiographic-contrast-agent-induced reductions in renal function by acetylcysteine. N Engl J Med 2000; 343:180–184.

72. Bonventure JV. Mechanisms of ischemic acute renal failure. Kidney Int 1993; 43:1160–1178.

73. Nicholson ML, Baker DM, Hopkinson BR, Wenham PW. Randomized control trial of the effect of mannitol on renal reperfusion injury during aortic aneurysm surgery. Br J Surg 1996; 83:1230–1233.

74. De Lasson L, Hansen HE, Juhl B, Paaske WP, Pedersen EB. A randomised, clinical study of the effect of low-dose dopamine on central and renal haemodynamics in infrarenal aortic surgery. Eur J Vasc Endovasc Surg 1995; 10:82–90.

75. Gilbert TB, Hasnain JU, Flinn WR, Lilly MP, Benjamin ME. Fenoldopam infusion associated with preserving renal function after aortic cross-clamping for aneurysm repair. J Cardiovasc Pharmacol Ther 2001; 6:31–36.

76. Mathur VS, Swan SK, Lambrecht LJ, Anjum S, Fellmann J, McGuire D, Epstein M, Luther RR. The effects of fenoldopam, a selective dopamine receptor agonist, on systemic and renal hemodynamics in normotensive subjects. Crit Care Med 1999; 27:1832–1837.

77. Pelkey TJ, Frank RS, Stanley JJ, Frank TS, Zelenock GB, D'Alecy LG. Minimal physiologic temperature variations during renal ischemia alter functional and morphologic outcome. J Vasc Surg 1992; 15:619–625.

78. Abbott WM, Austen WG. The reversal of renal cortical ischemia during aortic occlusion by mannitol. J Surg Res 1974; 16:482–489.

79. Denton MD, Chertow M, Brady HR. "Renal-dose" dopamine for the treatment of acute renal failure: Scientific rationale, experimental studies and clinical trials. Kidney Int 1996; 50:4–14.

80. Girbes AR, Lieverse AG, Smit AJ, van Veldhuisen KJ, Zwaveling JH, Miejer S, Rietsma WD. Lack of specific renal haemodynamic effects of different doses of dopamine after infrarenal aortic surgery. Br J Anaesth 1996; 77:753–757.

81. Baldwin L, Henderson A, Hickman P. Effect of postoperative low-dose dopamine on renal function after elective major vascular surgery. Ann Intern Med 1994; 120:744–747.

82. Kellum JA. The use of diuretics and dopamine in acute renal failure: A systemic review of the evidence. Crit Care 1997; 1:53–59.

83. Thompson BT, Cockrill BA. Renal-dose dopamine: a siren song? Lancet 1994; 344:7–8.

84. Kebabian JW, Calne DB. Multiple receptors for dopamine. Nature Lond 1979; 277:93–96.

85. Murphy MB, Murray C, Shorten GD. Fenoldopam: a selective peripheral dopamine-receptor agonist for the treatment of severe hypertension. N Engl J Med 2001; 345:1548–1557.

86. Bakris GL, Lass NA, Glock D. Renal hemodynamics in radiocontrast medium-induced renal dysfunction: A role for dopamine-1 receptors. Kidney Int 1999; 56:206–210.

87. Halpenny M, Markos F, Snow HM, Duggan PF, Gaffney E, O'Connell DP, Shorten GD. The effects of fenoldopam on renal blood blow and tubular function during aortic cross-clamping in anaesthetized dogs. Eur J Anaesth 2000; 17:491–498.

88. Prielipp RC, Wall MH, Groban L, Tobin JR, Fahey FH, Harkness BA, Stump DA, James RL, Cannon MA, Bennett J, Butterworth J. Reduced regional and global cerebral blood flow during fenoldopam-induced hypotension in volunteers. Anesth Analg 2001; 93:45–52.

89. Madyoon H, Croushore L, Weaver D, Mathur V. Use of fenoldopam to prevent radiocontrast nephropathy in high-risk patients. Catheter Cardiovasc Intervent 2001; 53:341–345.

90. Iliopoulos JI, Zdon MJ, Crawford BG, Pierce GE, Thomas JH, Hermreck AS. Renal micro-embolization syndrome. A cause for renal dysfunction after abdominal aortic reconstruction. Am J Surg 1983; 146:779–783.

91. Smith MC, Ghose MK, Henry AR. The clinical spectrum of renal cholesterol embolization. Am J Med 1981; 71:174–180.

92. Von Oppell U, Dunne T, DeGroot K, Zilla P. Spinal cord protection in the absence of collateral circulation: meta-analysis of mortality and paraplegia. J Card Surg 1994; 9:685–691.

93. Coselli JS. Thoracoabdominal aortic aneurysms: Experience with 372 patients. J Card Surg 1994; 9:638–647.

94. Coselli JS, LeMaire SA, Miller CC, Schmittling ZC, Koksoy C, Pagan J, Curling PE. Mortality and paraplegia after thoracoabdominal aortic aneurysm repair: A risk factor analysis. Ann Thorac Surg 2000; 69:409–414.

95. Doolan PD, Alpen EL, Theil GB. A clinical appraisal of the plasma concentration and endogenous clearance of creatinine. Am J Med 1962; 32:65–69.

96. Bennett WM, Porter GA. Endogenous creatinine clearance as a clinical measure of glomerular filtration rate. BMJ 1971; 4:84–86.

97. Berglund F, Killander J, Pompeius R. Effect of trimethoprim-sulfamethoxazole on the renal excretion of creatinine in man. J Urol 1975; 114:802–808.

98. Anderson RA. Prevention and management of acute renal failure. Hosp Pract 1993; 28:61–72.

99. Szerlip HM. Renal-dose dopamine: Fact and fiction. Ann Intern Med 1991; 115:153–154.

100. Flancbaum L, Choban PS, Dasta JF. Quantitative effects of low-dose dopamine on urine output in oliguric surgical intensive care unit patients. Crit Care Med 1994; 22:61–68.

101. Corwin HL, Bonventre JV. Factors influencing survival in acute renal failure. Semin Dial 1989; 2:220–231.

102. Lieberthal W, Levinsky NG. Treatment of acute tubular necrosis. Semin Nephrol 1990; 10:571–583.

103. Mehta RL. Therapeutic alternatives to renal replacement for critically ill patients in acute renal failure. Semin Nephrol 1994; 14:64–82.

104. Druml W. Metabolic aspects of continuous renal replacement therapies. Kidney Int 1999; 72:S56–S61.

105. Ikizler TA. Himmelfarb. Nutrition in acute renal failure patients. Adv Renal Repl Therap 1997; 4:54–63.

4

Intimal Hyperplasia: The Mechanisms and Treatment of the Response to Arterial Injury

Michael J. Englesbe and Alexander W. Clowes

University of Washington, Seattle, Washington, U.S.A.

All forms of arterial reconstruction involve vessel wall injury and repair of the injury by cells from adjacent normal tissues repair and possibly by circulating precursor cells. Intimal hyperplasia is the hallmark of this healing process, often resulting in significant luminal narrowing that predisposes the repair to failure. Since intimal hyperplasia affects 15–30% of all arterial interventions, strategies to control this injury response would have significant clinical impact (1).

This chapter reviews the biology of vessel wall healing following vascular reconstruction and the molecular mechanisms involved in smooth muscle cell (SMC) mitogenesis, migration, and extracellular matrix formation, three critical processes in intimal hyperplasia formation. Recent advances in the understanding of arterial injury response have fostered new approaches to inhibit intimal hyperplasia. (Table 1) These novel clinical approaches are discussed.

I. AUTOLOGOUS VEIN GRAFT HEALING

Vein grafts are the preferred conduits for most coronary and lower limb arterial bypasses. Nonetheless, these arterial reconstructions fail because of intimal thickening, luminal narrowing, and thrombosis. Graft failure is associated with 37–44% of aortocoronary venous bypass grafts in the 3–10 years after surgery (2,3). Without careful surveillance, patency is as low as 50% 2 years following infrainguinal bypass using saphenous vein as the conduit (4).

The causes of graft failure are categorized into three groups. In the immediate postoperative period, graft occlusion occurs because of technical issues, such as twisting or compression of the graft, poor distal arterial outflow, graft size mismatch, or flawed surgical technique. The treatment of early graft failure involves prompt revision of the

Table 1 Four General Categories of Therapeutic Approaches for Inhibiting Stenosis or Restenosis from Intimal Hyperplasia

Mechanical therapies	Cell-cycle inhibitors	Growth factor inhibitors	Antithrombotics or anticoagulants
Balloon dilatation of artery or stent Stent placement in artery or within existing stent Atherectomy	Brachytheraphy Rapamycin (sirolimus) (also inhibits migration) E2F transcription factor decoy oligonucleotides Taxol (paclitaxel) (also inhibits migration) Gene therapy-overexpression of RB, p21, gax, dominant negative mutants of *ras*, NOS	Antibodies and inhibitors of PDGFR α and β Antibody to EGFR Antibody to FGFR Antibody to TGF-β Recombinant TGF-beta RII Antibody to IGFR	Aspirin Ticlopidine Heparins

graft. From 3 months to 2 years, the graft wall thickens, or becomes "arterialized," along its entire length. In addition, focal areas of intimal thickening develop, occurring at anastomoses, valves, or vascular clamp sites. The resultant luminal stenoses reduce flow and predispose the graft to thrombosis (5–7). There is currently no good treatment for intimal hyperplastic lesions besides close graft surveillance and prompt surgical revision. The third category of graft failure occurs after 2 years because of atherosclerosis in either the graft or in the proximal or distal artery. Treatment entails aggressive risk-factor intervention, including use of lipid-lowering agents.

An understanding of the biology of vein graft healing is fundamental to developing new therapeutic approaches aimed at the prevention and regression of intimal hyperplasia. Venous endothelial and smooth muscle cells (SMC) are injured at the time of graft harvest. Techniques such as the method of vein harvesting, application of clamps, valvulotomy, ischemia, and distention of the graft variably affect the degree of injury (8,9). In addition, placement of a vein into the arterial system elicits an injury response in part due to hemodynamic stress on the vein graft wall as well as to the surgery itself (10). The medial hyperplastic response to increased wall stress is a reversible phenomenon. When flow within the graft is returned to venous levels, the response is reversed (11).

Because the time course of intimal thickening in human venous grafts is difficult to study, we must rely on animal models for a detailed description, even though these models more often provide insight into vein wall adaptation rather than pathological intimal thickening and luminal stenosis. In a rabbit model, when the external jugular vein is transposed into the carotid artery, platelets, microthrombi, and leukocytes adhere to areas of endothelial denudation (12). By 2 weeks, the areas of endothelial denudation have regenerated. Over the first 4 weeks, there is substantial intimal SMC proliferation and migration and intimal thickening begins to develop. As proliferation and migration stop, there is accumulation of extracellular matrix. In this rabbit model, graft wall thickness, circumference, and cross-sectional area reach a maximum at 12 weeks (13). Following this acute injury response, the graft continues to respond to environmental stimuli. The venous graft is a dynamic entity that adapts to changes in hemodynamic forces. The chronic response to arterialization likely mimics the arterial hypertrophic response to hypertension. Also, shear stress likely affects venous graft diameter and wall thickness.

II. PROSTHETIC GRAFT HEALING

Prosthetic grafts are preferred for large vessel replacement and when autologous conduit is inadequate. They function well when placed in vascular beds of high flow, such as in the aortobifemoral position, but are prone to failure when used in beds of relatively low flow, such as femoral-infrapopliteal bypasses (14). There are many differences between prosthetic vascular conduits and venous grafts. Prosthetic grafts are more prone to spontaneous thrombosis and infection. In animals, depending on the porosity of the vascular graft, variable amounts of endothelium line the luminal aspect of the graft. Most clinically relevant PTFE vascular grafts have low porosity (30-μm pores or smaller). In such grafts, the endothelial and SMC coverage of the luminal surface of the graft is limited to the first few centimeters of each anastomosis. It is not known why these SMCs and endothelial cells populate only the graft adjacent to the anastomosis. The central portion of the graft is covered by a pseudointima containing fibrin, platelets, and leukocytes but no endothelial cells (15). A detailed time course of graft healing in humans is not known because the tissue is inaccessible. Nonetheless, intimal thickness is likely maximal within the perianastomotic native artery and graft at approximately 12 weeks.

In contrast, polytetrafluoroethylene (PTFE) grafts with 60-μm pores demonstrate a markedly different process of graft healing. When these grafts are used in aortoiliac bypasses in baboons, a fully developed, endothelialized intima develops by 2 weeks along the entire length of the graft and continues to increase in size until 8–12 weeks (16). The SMCs and endothelial cells presumably migrate in from perigraft granulation tissue.

III. ARTERIAL HEALING FOLLOWING BALLOON ANGIOPLASTY AND STENTING

Percutaneous intravascular interventions have significant promise for patients with either coronary artery disease or peripheral vascular disease. Important limitations of balloon angioplasty are restenosis from intimal hyperplasia and pathological remodeling.

Inward or pathological remodeling is the major factor in restenosis after atherectomy and angioplasty (17,18). Animal studies suggest that adventitial cicatrization is important in inward remodeling (19,20). Time-course studies using intravascular ultrasound (IVUS) indicate that inward remodeling occurs 1–6 months following a procedure (17). Late regression of stenosis (6 months to 5 years) after angioplasty demonstrates that the ability to outwardly remodel is restored, likely from the reestablishment of an intact and functional endothelium (21). Intraluminal stent placement prevents pathological inward or outward remodeling, and luminal narrowing depends solely upon the amount of in-stent intimal hyperplasia.

The most extensively studied model for arterial healing and intimal formation after angioplasty utilizes the rat carotid balloon injury model (22) (Fig. 1). The balloon strips away the endothelial cells, stretches the underlying media, and disrupts elastin layers. Endothelial denudation alone is enough to significantly induce an intimal hyperplastic response, but the response is augmented by balloon stretch of the vessel wall (22). Immediately following injury, the exposed media is coated with platelets, which then degranulate. SMCs begin proliferating approximately 24 h after the injury. These smooth muscle cells

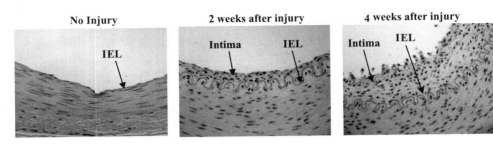

Figure 1 Balloon-injured baboon saphenous artery. (H&E staining, × 100.) Demonstrates time course of intimal growth from smooth muscle cell migration and proliferation. (IEL = internal elastic lumina.)

increase from a basal level of proliferation of 0.06% per day to 10–30% per day (23). After 4 days, SMCs migrate into the intima, continue to proliferate, and secrete substantial amounts of extracellular matrix. A steady state is reached at 12 weeks, with an intima composed of 20% cells and 80% extracellular matrix (24). Regrowth of the endothelium likely down regulates intimal SMC proliferation and migration. If the zone of injury is larger than 3 cm, endothelial repopulation of the artery never reaches the central segment of injured artery, and smooth muscle cells at the luminal surface continue to turnover (25).

Intraluminal stent placement prevents arterial recoil and pathological remodeling, reducing early (less than 6 weeks) restenosis. However, stent placement is associated with an even more vigorous intimal hyperplastic response (26), and the overall rate of late (greater than 6 weeks) stent restenosis remains approximately 15–30% in stented coronary arteries (27). With stent placement, cytokines and growth factors induce multiple signaling pathways associated with SMC migration and proliferation (28,29). Coronary stent penetration into the lipid core induces increased arterial inflammation, associated with increased neointimal growth (A. Farb, R. Virmani, personal communication). Thus, the arterial wall reacts not only to the underlying atherosclerotic process with its inflammatory components and the acute wall injury but also to the chronic inflammation induced by the foreign body.

IV. MOLECULAR MECHANISMS OF INTIMAL HYPERPLASIA

The healing of vein grafts, prosthetic grafts, balloon-dilated and stented vessels, or endarterectomized arteries is similar. There are three primary observations that apply to all forms of arterial reconstruction: (a) medial SMC proliferation is in proportion to the severity of injury, (b) all forms of injury cause endothelial denudation and accumulations of platelets in the subendothelium, and (c) serum derived from degranulated platelets and clotted blood induces SMC proliferation and migration. The best-studied model of intimal hyperplasia is the rat carotid artery response to balloon injury. An in-depth understanding of this relatively simple system of arterial injury is a critical step in developing pharmacological approaches to inhibiting the deleterious effect of intimal hyperplasia in patients.

In the rat, balloon injury leads to complete destruction of the endothelium as well as death to medial SMCs (25). The SMC response to injury and the molecules involved in the response have been categorized into four waves (25,30–32). Within the first 24 h, the first wave of injury response is initiated, which entails basic fibroblast growth factor (bFGF)-

and epidermal growth factor receptor (EGFR)- dependent medial SMC proliferation (33) (A. Chan, unpublished results). Though this first wave of SMC proliferation has no obvious relation to later SMC proliferation and migration, there is some evidence that inhibition of this initial proliferation will lead to a diminution of the eventual size of the final intimal hyperplastic lesion (34,35). The second wave involves the migration of SMCs through the internal elastic lamina into the intima, first noted at 4 days after balloon injury (25). The most important molecule in this response is thought to be platelet-derived growth factor (PDGF), specifically PDGF-BB. Rats treated with blocking antibodies to PDGF develop significantly smaller intimal lesions. These antibodies presumably inhibit migration of SMCs, because there is no reduction in mitogenesis in the media or intima (36). Similarly, infusion with PDGF-BB stimulates SMC migration and intimal thickening but has little effect on SMC proliferation (37). Whether PDGF is a significant mitogen in more complex lesion systems, such as in a human atherosclerotic vessel after angioplasty, is unclear. Transfection of PDGF-B into swine arteries causes a marked increase in replication (38). Such observations support the contention that PDGF-B may be a mitogen in in vivo systems. Matrix metalloproteinases (MMPs) are also thought to have a critical role in the migration associated with the second wave. MMPs are expressed in the intima and are required for cell movement. MMP-3 and MMP-9 are expressed following injury (39). The local overexpression of the tissue inhibitor of MMP-1 suppresses intimal thickening by inhibiting SMC migration (40).

The third wave entails the replication of intimal SMCs, which may continue for weeks to months (25). During this period, the intima overexpresses many growth factors and receptors, including PDGF-A, Ang II receptor (AT-1), and transforming growth factor (TGF-β) (41,42). In addition, insulin-like growth factor I (IGF-1) is overexpressed in the media, where there is also significant proliferation (43). The culprit molecule, blockade of which would inhibit proliferation, has not been elucidated for the third wave in rats, but there is some evidence in baboons that it is PDGF receptor (PDGFR-α and PDGFR-β) (M. Englesbe, A. Clowes, unpublished observations).

In a model of balloon arterial injury in baboons, there is a significant population of inflammatory cells within the early intima. Inflammatory mediators may significantly modulate the response to SMC to growth factors. For example, IL-1β significantly inhibits PDGF-BB–induced baboon SMC migration in an in vitro system while augmenting PDGF-BB–induced mitogenesis (G. Daum and M. Englesbe, unpublished results). In a mouse model, tumor necrosis factor alpha (TNF-α) and IL-1 modulate intimal hyperplasia induced by low shear stress (44).

The fourth wave is characterized by an increased intimal sensitivity to mitogens. Specifically, the intima proliferates with infusion of endothelin, TGF-β, bFGF, and Ang II (32). Proliferation and intimal size can be inhibited by blockade of the angiotensin II receptor (45,46) or endothelin receptors (47,48).

SMC migration is modulated by factors from platelets, specifically PDGF. PDGF is liberated at the time of platelet degranulation as well as synthesized and secreted by vascular wall cells (49). Intimal thickening in rats rendered thrombocytopenic is largely blocked even though the initial wave of SMC mitogenesis persists (50). Furthermore, blockade of PDGFR-β can inhibit intimal development in both the rat and the baboon (36,51). There are five known active forms of PDGF: PDGF AA, AB, BB, CC, and DD (52,53). Dimerization is required for high-affinity binding to the α and β receptor subunits. PDGF-BB is thought to play a critical role in arterial injury response, but the role of the other isoforms is largely unknown (23).

Many novel approaches to inhibiting or reversing neointimal hyperplasia involve the concept of negative growth control. SMCs in normal human arteries have a very low rate of proliferation (0.01% per day), which translates into turnover once every 30 years. Only upon injury do SMCs begin to proliferate. The inhibitory factors that prevent SMC growth can be isolated from the endothelium, SMCs, inflammatory cells, and the matrix.

Certainly the endothelium is critical in modulating SMC quiescence. In the rat, upon regeneration of the endothelium, SMCs cease proliferating (22). Nitric oxide produced by endothelial cell nitric oxide synthase (eNOS) may be an important molecule in regulating SMC growth. With removal of the endothelium and its associated NOS, the SMCs of the intima proliferate. In contrast, in endothelializaed baboon grafts, a change from high to normal shear stress downregulates eNOS and mitogenesis occurs within the intima. Other possible endothelial-derived inhibitors of SMC proliferation include COX-2 (54) and prostaglandins I_2 and E_2. T cells within the intima secrete interferon gamma, which induce MHC II antigens and suppress SMC replication (55).

The matrix secreted in the intima helps maintain the quiescent state of vessel wall SMCs. Within the matrix, heparan sulfates such as perlecan inhibit SMC migration and proliferation in vitro (56–58). Perlecan has been proposed to bind to heparin-binding mitogens, such as fibroblast growth factor-2 (FGF-2), and to prevent them from stimulating smooth muscle cells (59). Matrix-mediated SMC inhibition may also occur via heparin-mediated blockade of mitogen-associated protein kinases as well as cell-cycle genes (e.g., c-myb) and proteases necessary for matrix degradation (60).

Approaches to the treatment of intimal hyperplasia target SMC migration and proliferation. An alternative approach is treatment directed at lesions that already exist. This approach would be applicable to the large number of patients currently suffering from complications related to intimal hyperplasia. The baboon vascular graft model has

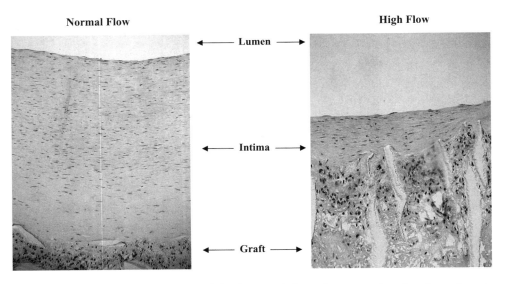

Normal Flow   **High Flow**

Lumen

Intima

Graft

Figure 2 Intimal regression induced by increased flow, demonstrating the dynamic nature of intimal hyperplasia (H&E staining, × 40.) After 12 weeks of normal flow, the graft on the left developed a significant intima. After 8 weeks of normal flow and then 4 weeks of high flow, the intima lining the graft on the right atrophied significantly.

demonstrated the dynamic nature of intimal hyperplastic lesions (13). For example, with the placement of an arteriovenous fistula distal to a vascular graft lined with an intima, shear stress increases through the graft and induces intimal atrophy (61) (Fig. 2). The atrophy is associated with a reduction in matrix content and cell number, with an associated increase in intimal SMC apoptosis. Thus, matrix degradation and SMC apoptosis are also potential targets for pharmacological manipulation.

Apoptosis is an important event in vasculogenesis and vascular injury response. In the rat carotid artery injury model, even though SMCs continue to proliferate at the surface of vessels lacking an endothelium, no net increase in SMC number occurs in these areas (25). In addition, an increase in SMC apoptosis can be detected in these areas. Finally, apoptosis can not only be induced by increases in shear stress but it also may be responsible for the termination of intimal thickening after injury (62–64). In all, control of apoptosis may be a potential strategy for inducing intimal atrophy.

V. THERAPEUTIC APPROACHES TO INTIMAL HYPERPLASIA

A. Mechanical Approaches

The most widely used treatment for intimal hyperplasia is catheter-based direct mechanical manipulation of hyperplastic lesions, generally by balloon dilation. It is estimated that this approach is used for 150,000 coronary lesions annually (65). Balloon angioplasty of a restenotic lesion within a stent is a safe short- and long-term approach for coronary and peripheral lesions with inadequate initial expansion of the stent or focal neointimal growths (66). In these procedures, of the total luminal enlargement, 56% is attributable to further stent expansion, while 44% is from extrusion–axial redistribution of the intima (67). In contrast, balloon treatment of diffuse intimal lesions in well-expanded stents has poor intermediate and long-term outcomes (68). In such lesions, novel approaches have been used such as atherectomy, in which blades excise the in-stent lesion. Unfortunately, all of these mechanical approaches cause additional vascular wall injury in a patient predisposed to intimal hyperplasia. Thus, even though mechanical approaches may initially be effective, they do not address the injury response and stenosing intimal lesions readily recur (69,70).

B. Cell Cycle–Directed Therapies

As discussed earlier, in response to vascular injury, SMCs enter the cell cycle and proliferate. Cell-cycle inhibitors are therefore potential agents to prevent intimal hyperplasia. Generally, these agents must be locally delivered in order to prevent systemic toxicity.

The best-studied antiproliferative approach is vascular brachytherapy. Clinically relevant approaches entail placement of "hot" intravascular catheters or stents. These devices emit either gamma or beta radiation. Ionizing radiation induces nonspecific breaks in chromosomal DNA and is a potent antiproliferative if the cells are actively dividing at the time of exposure. Initial trials have shown effective prevention of angiographic restenosis and reduced need for repeat revascularization (71–73). Unfortunately, vascular brachytherapy has multiple drawbacks. The first is that the procedure can be technically laborious and both the patient and the operators are at a significant risk of exposure to ionizing radiation. In addition, there may be an increased risk of late stent thrombosis, since the radiation prevents endothelial regeneration (74). Finally, the most significant limitation of vascular brachytherapy is the phenomenon of "candy wrapper" restenosis

(75). In areas adjacent to a radioactive stent, intimal hyperplasia may actually be induced, resulting in a patent stent with critical stenoses proximally and distally to the stent edge. This phenomenon is due to lower doses of radiation delivered to the stent ends in the setting of vessel wall balloon injury, leading to intimal hyperplasia and pathological remodeling. Thus, after several years of research, it seems unlikely that radioactive stents will soon become clinically useful tools with broad application.

Initially developed as a macrolide antibiotic and later used as an immunosuppressant, Sirolimus (rapamycin) is a potent inhibitor of both SMC proliferation and migration. This agent binds FK506-binding protein and inhibits TOR (target of Rapamycin), a kinase that regulates cell cycle progression. Recent results from a phase I study using rapamycin-coated stents in 30 patients have been encouraging. No significant toxicity was noted and only 10% of the patients had >15% stenosis from intimal hyperplasia 4 months following stent placement (76). Rapamycin may prove to effectively reduce intimal hyperplasia, though more study of this novel approach is needed.

Another approach to antiproliferative therapy was used in the Project of Ex-vivo Vein graft Engineering via Transfection (PREVENT) study (77). This ongoing trial examines the delivery of E2F transcription factor decoy oligonucleotides as a means to inhibit vein graft stenosis after peripheral bypass surgery. Phase I trials are encouraging with respect to cellular access and were associated with minimal complications and a measurable decrease in vein graft stenosis one year after peripheral vascular bypass.

Paclitaxel(Taxol) and related drugs are used as cancer chemotherapeutic agents. They have diverse mechanisms of action on SMCs, including microtubule stabilization, arrest of cell mitosis, and retardation of cell migration (78,79). Sustained local delivery of paclitaxel by coating of intravascular stents prevented early in-stent restenosis in animal models (80,81), but this inhibition was not maintained over the long term in one study (82). Paclitaxel-coated stents have demonstrated encouraging results in one small human trial (83), but there is a report of acute thrombosis of a paclitaxel-coated stent seven months after implantation (84). A randomized, controlled human trial with taxol coated coronary stents is in progress.

There are many approaches to introduce exogenous genetic material into the vascular system. Current approaches involve primarily adenoviral vectors and cell-based gene transfer. The complexity of vector optimization and techniques of transfection are beyond the scope of this chapter. Nonetheless, gene therapy–based models have provided critical tools in the study of vessel injury response and offer therapeutic promise. Many gene therapy approaches to intimal hyperplasia focus on either inhibiting cell-cycle entry (cytostatic approach) or causing death to cells that have entered the cell cycle (cytotoxic approach) (85).

Several genes have been targeted to induce SMC cytostasis at the site of injury. One approach is to overexpress a constitutively active mutant form of the retinoblastoma protein (RB), which complexes with the E2F family of transcription factors to block entry into the cell cycle (86). SMC proliferation and intimal development in a rat following balloon injury has been inhibited by overexpression of the endogenous cyclin kinase inhibitor protein p21 (87). This protein inhibits cyclin-dependent kinases and thus inhibits S-phase entry. Other genes that have shown cytostatic properties in in vivo models include the homeodomain gene *gax* (88) and dominant-negative mutants of *ras* (89).

The cytotoxic approach generally involves the expression of enzymes capable of converting nucleoside analogues into toxic metabolites that interrupt DNA replication. The result is death of transduced cells entering S phase in the presence of the nucleoside analogue (86). Intimal hyperplasia has been inhibited in animal models using a thymidine kinase isozyme derived from the herpes simplex viral genome, which phosphorylates the inactive drug gancyclovir and interrupts DNA synthesis (90,91). Induction of apoptosis is another cytotoxic approach. As SMC apoptosis in the setting of arterial injury is better understood, novel gene therapy approaches involving modulation of apoptosis will likely develop.

There is growing evidence for a role of stem cells in arterial injury response. Statin drugs may benefit patients with coronary artery disease by increasing the pool of circulating bone marrow–derived endothelial progenitor cells (92). Vascular trauma induces the release of circulating endothelial precursor cells (93). Such precursor cells may be involved in endothelial regeneration at the site of vascular wall injury. Stem cell technology offers many new approaches for preventing restenosis, but the field is too new to foresee clinical applicability in the near future.

C. Growth Factor Inhibition and Matrix Modulation

Many growth factors modulate the vascular injury response (Table 2). These growth factors are responsible for SMC migration and proliferation and act as survival signals preventing initiation of the apoptotic cascade. Blocking antibodies, antisense strategies, or gene therapy approaches can modulate these growth factors.

The most extensively studied growth factor system is PDGF. In multiple arterial injury and vascular graft models, blockade of the PDGFR-β has been shown to inhibit intimal hyperplasia (36,51,94,95). Blockade of the PDGFR-β is thought to function by inhibiting the migration of SMCs into the intima. A human coronary stent trial using a chimeric PDGFR-β–blocking antibody has failed to demonstrate significant angiographic improvements in stent patency (P.W. Serruys, personal communication). Atherosclerotic arteries likely express a larger quantity of PDGFR-α than the healthy vessels used in animal models. In vitro, blockade of both the PDGFR-α and -β simultaneously inhibits migration and mitogenesis more than blockade of the PDGFR-β alone. In vivo studies to block both receptors are ongoing in baboons.

The complexity of the injury response is evidenced in the number of potential therapeutically targeted growth factors. Additional potential targets include IGF-I and -II, thrombin, epidermal growth factor (EGF), heparin binding-EGF (HB-EGF), b-FGF,

Table 2 Summary of Growth Factors Relevant in Intimal Hyperplasia and Associated Inhibitors that Have Demonstrated Efficacy at Inhibiting Intimal Hyperplasia in Vivo

Growth factor	Growth factor inhibitor
PDGF AA, AB, BB, CC, DD	Antibody to PDGFR α or β (36,37,51)
	PDGF chain aptamers (107)
	PDGF-receptor tyrosine kinase inhibitors (108)
EGF, HB-EGF	Antibody to EGFR[a]
Endothelin	Endothelin (A/B) receptor antagonists (47,48)
bFGF	Antagonists to FGFR (109,110)
MMP-3 and MMP-9	Tissue inhibitor of MMP-1 (111,112)
TGF-β1, TGF-β2, TGF-β3	Antibody to TGF-β (113)
	Recombinant TGF-beta RII (114)

[a] Chan A. Clowes A, unpublished observation.

NOS, fibroblast growth factor I (FGF-I), and transforming growth factor β1 (TGF-β). In addition, over-expression of NOS and local release of NO can inhibit SMC proliferation. Modulation of the intimal matrix is another approach to inhibit intimal growth. Smooth muscle cells transduced with replication-defective retrovirus encoding tissue inhibitor of matrix metalloproteinase-1 (TIMP-1), when seeded onto the surface of the artery, suppress intimal thickening (40). MMP-2 and MMP-9 are expressed in smooth muscle cells following injury. Blockade of these MMPs either with an active site inhibitor drug or local overexpression of the natural inhibitor (TIMP-1), suppresses proteolytic activity and migration of smooth muscle cells.

D. Antiplatelet and Anticoagulation Agents

Adhesion of platelets and thrombus formation at the site of vascular wall trauma is involved in the response to injury. Theoretically, prevention of early platelet adhesion and thrombus formation and the resultant exposure of the activated SMCs to the multitude of growth factors within platelet granules and thrombus may have long-term effects on patency. Multicenter randomized trials have shown that an aspirin with or without dipyridamole increased the long-term patency of aortocoronary saphenous vein grafts (96,97). Similarly, ticlopidine improves the long-term patency of saphenous vein bypass grafts in the legs (98). Unfortunately, vessels likely need exposure to these drugs immediately following the injury, which may be associated with increased bleeding complications from surgical sites.

In addition, heparin alone inhibits intimal formation in animals following arterial injury (99,100). The potential mechanisms include regulation of extracellular matrix composition (101), inhibition of SMC migration and proliferation, inhibition of nuclear transcription factors (102), and primary anti-inflammatory effects. Oral delivery of heparin has recently shown promising results in animals in the prevention of in-stent restenosis (103). Human trials have not demonstrated a similar inhibition of intimal growth following balloon angioplasty using systemic delivery of either unfractionated (104) or low-molecular-weight heparin (105). The poor results from these human trials may be due to the inappropriate or inadequate dosing of heparin to the study patients. A recent human trial with local delivery of low-molecular-weight heparin has demonstrated a significant inhibition of intimal hyperplasia in coronary stents (106).

VI. CONCLUSIONS

Animal and clinical studies over the past two decades have documented that intimal hyperplasia is a response to injury and a complication of all forms of arterial reconstruction. Although pathological remodeling (inward remodeling) is a more important mechanism for luminal narrowing in vessels treated with balloon angioplasty, intimal hyperplasia followed by stenosis or restenosis is the principal cause of failure in vein and synthetic grafts as well as stented arteries. Until recently, symptomatic restenosis of a stented artery or stenosis of a bypass graft could not be treated and usually required further surgical reconstruction.

Encouraging results have been obtained with brachytherapy and mechanical interventions. Novel therapies should be compared to these treatments. Preliminary trials using paclitaxel- and rapamycin-coated stents have generated very encouraging results.

The intimal lesion is composed primarily of SMCs. Unfortunately, most of the currently investigated therapeutic approaches are not SMC specific and also inhibit endothelial regeneration and function. It is possible that failure of endothelial regeneration will have significant implications such as late thrombosis. Adjuvant therapy currently under development and targeted specifically at SMCs (e.g., PDGF or EGF) would be expected to circumvent this problem.

REFERENCES

1. Williams DO, Holubkov R, Yeh W, et al. Percutaneous coronary interventions in the current era compared with 1985–1986: The National Heart, Lung, and Blood Institute Registries. Circulation 2000; 102:2945–2951.
2. Grondin CM, Campeau L, Lesperance J, Enjalbert M, Bourassa MG. Comparison of late changes in internal mammary artery and saphenous vein grafts in two consecutive series of patients 10 years after operation. Circulation 1984; 70(supp 1):208–212.
3. Bourassa MG, Enjalbert M, Campeau L. Progression of atherosclerosis in coronary arteries and bypass grafts: Ten years later. Am J Cardiol 1984; 52:102C–107C.
4. Dalman RL, Taylor LM Jr. Basic data related to infrainguinal revascularization procedures. Ann Vasc Surg 1990; 4:309–312.
5. Thatte HS, Khuri SF. The coronary artery bypass conduit: I. Intraoperative endothelial injury and its implication on graft patency. Ann Thorac Surg 2001; 72:S2245–S2252.
6. Gibson KD, Gillen DL, Caps MT, Kohler TR, Sherrard DJ, Stehman-Breen CO. Vascular access survival and incidence of revisions: A comparison of prosthetic grafts, simple autogenous fistulas, and venous transposition fistulas from the United States Renal Data System Dialysis Morbidity and Mortality Study. J Vasc Surg 2001; 34:694–700.
7. Dilley JR, McGeachie JK, Prendergast FJ. A review of histologic changes in vein to artery grafts, with particular reference to intimal hyperplasia. Arch Surg 1988; 123:691–699.
8. DePalma RG, Chidi CC, Sternfeld WC. Pathogenesis and prevention of trauma provoked atheromas. Surgery 1977; 74:931–944.
9. Bonchek LI. Prevention of endothelial damage during preparation of saphenous veins for bypass grafting. J Thorac Cardiovasc Surg 1980; 79:911–915.
10. Cox JL, Chiasson DA, Gotlieb AI. Stranger in a strange land: The pathogenesis of saphenous vein graft stenosis with emphasis on structural and functional differences between veins and arteries. Prog Cardiovasc Dis 1991; 144:45–68.
11. Davies MG, Klyachkin ML, Dalen H, Svendsen E, Hagen PO. Regression of intimal hyperplasia with restoration of endothelium-dependant relaxing factor-mediated relaxation in experimental vein grafts. Surgery 1993; 114:258–271.
12. Zwolak RM, Adams MC, Clowes AW. Kinetics of vein graft hyperplasia: Association of tangential stress. J Vasc Surg 1987; 5:126–136.
13. Kohler T, Kirkman TR, Clowes AW. The effect of external rigid support on vein graft adaptation to arterial circulation. J Vasc Surg 1991; 9:277–285.
14. Veith FJ, Gupta SK, Ascer E. Six year prospective randomized comparison of autologous saphenous vein and expanded polytetrafluoroethylene grafts in infrainguinal arterial reconstructions. J Vasc Surg 1986; 3:104–111.
15. Clowes AW. Intimal hyperplasia and graft failure. Cardiovasc Pathol 1993; 2:179S–1786S.
16. Clowes AW, Kirkman TR, Reidy MA. Mechanism of arterial graft healing: Rapid transmural capillary ingrowth provides a source of intimal endothelium and smooth muscle cell in porous PTFE prostheses. Am J Pathol 1986; 123:220–230.
17. Kimura T, Kaburagi S, Tamura T, et al. Remodeling of human coronary arteries undergoing angioplasty or atherectomy. Circulation 1997; 96:475–483.
18. Post Mj, Borst C, Kuntz RE. The relative importance of arterial remodeling compared with intimal hyperplasia in lumenal renarrowing after balloon angioplasty: A study in the normal rabbit and the hypercholesterolemic Yucatan micropig. Circulation 1994; 89:2816–2821.

19. Mondy JS, Williams JK, Adams MR, Dean RH, Geary RL. Structural determinants of luminal narrowing after angioplasty in atherosclerotic non-human primates. J Vasc Surg 1997; 26:875–883.

20. Zalewski A, Shi Y. Vascular myofibroblasts: Lessons from coronary repair and remodeling. Arterioscler Thromb Vasc Biol 1997; 17:417–422.

21. Ormiston JA, Stewart FM, Roche AH, et al. Late regression of the dilated site after coronary angioplasty: A five year quantitative angiographic study. Circulation 1997; 96:468–474.

22. Fingerle J, Au YP, Clowes AW, Reidy MA. Intimal lesion formation in rat carotid arteries after endothelial denudation in absence of medial injury. Arteriosclerosis 1990; 10:1082–1087.

23. Allaire E, Clowes AW. Endothelial cell injury in cardiovascular surgery: The intimal hyperplasitc response. Ann Thorac Surg 1997; 63:582–591.

24. Nikkari ST, Jarvelainen HT, Wight TN, Ferguson M, Clowes AW. Smooth muscle cell expression of extracellular matrix genes after arterial injury. Am J Pathol 1994; 144:1348–1356.

25. Clowes AW, Clowes MM, Reidy MA. Kinetics of cellular proliferation after arterial injury. Endothelial and smooth muscle cell growth in chronically denuded vessels. Lab Invest 1986; 54:295–303.

26. Kuntz RE, Baim DS. Prevention of coronary restenosis: Evolving evidence base for radiation therapy. Circulation 2000; 101:2130–2133.

27. Mehran R, Dangas G, Mintz GS, et al. Patterns of in stent restenosis: Angiographic classification and implications for long-term clinical outcome. Circulation 1999; 100:1872–1878.

28. Farb A, Sangiorgi G, Carter AJ, Walley VM, Edwards WD, Schwartz RS, Virmani R. Pathology of acute and chronic coronary stenting in humans. Circulation 1999; 99:44–52.

29. Grewe P, Deneke T, Machraoui A. Acute and chronic tissue response to coronary stent implantation: Pathologic findings in human specimen. J Am Coll Cardiol 2000; 35:157–163.

30. Clowes AW, Schwartz SM. Significance of quiescent smooth muscle cell migration in the injured rat carotid artery. Circ Res 1985; 56:139–145.

31. Hanke H, Strohschneider T, Oberhoff M, Betz E, Karsch KR. Time course of smooth muscle cell proliferation in the intima and media of arteries following experimental angioplasty. Circ Res 1990; 67:651–659.

32. Schwartz SM, dsBlois D, O'Brien ERM. The intima: Soil for atherosclerosis and restenosis. Circ Res 1995; 77:445–465.

33. Olson NE, Chao S, Linder V, Reidy MA. Intimal smooth muscle proliferation after balloon catheter injury: The role of basic fibroblast growth factor. Am J Pathol 1992; 140:1017–1023.

34. Ebbecke M, Unterberg C, Buchwald A, Stohr S, Wiegand V. Antiproliferative effects of c-myc antisense oligonucleotide on human arterial smooth muscle cells. Basic Res Cardiol 1992; 87:585–591.

35. Simons M, Edelman ER, Rosenberg RD. Antisense proliferating cell nuclear antigen oligonucleotides inhibit intimal hyperplasia in a rat carotid artery injury model. J Clin Invest 1994; 93:2351–2356.

36. Ferns GAA, Raines EW, Sprugel KH, Motani AS, Reidy MA, Ross R. Inhibition of neointimal smooth muscle accumulation after angioplasty by antibody to PDGF. Science 1991; 253:1129–1132.

37. Jawien A, Bowen-Pope DF, Lindner V, Schwartz SM, Clowes AW. Platelet-derived growth factor promotes smooth muscle migration and intimal thickening in a rat model of balloon angioplasty. J Clin Invest 1992; 89:507–511.

38. Nabel EG, Yang Z, Liptay S, San H, Gordon D, Haudenschild CC, Nabel GJ. Recombinant platelet-derived growth factor B gene expression in porcine arteries induce intimal hyperplasia in vivo. J Clin Invest 1993; 91:1822–1829.

39. Bendeck MP, Zempo N, Clowes AW, Galardy RE, Reidy MA. Smooth muscle cell migration and matrix metalloproteinase expression after arterial injury in the rat. Circ Res 1994; 75:539–545.

40. Forough R, Koyama N, Hasenstab D, Lea H, Clowes M, Nikkari ST, Clowes AW. Over-expression of tissue inhibitor of matrix metalloproteinase-1 inhibits vascular smooth muscle cell functions in vitro and in vivo. Circ Res 1996; 79:812–820.

41. Majesky MW, Linder V, Twardzik DR, Schwartz SM, Reidy MA. Production of transforming growth factor β-1 during repair of arterial injury. J Clin Invest 1993; 92:2952.

42. Viswanathan M, Stromberg C, Seltzer A, Saavedra JM. Balloon angioplasty enhances the expression of angiotensin II AT1 receptors in neointima of rat aorta. J Clin Invest 1992; 90: 1707–1712.

43. Cercek B, Fishbein MC, Forrester JS, Helfant RH, Fagin JA. Induction of insulin like growth factor I messenger RNA in rat aorta after balloon denudation. Circ Res 1990; 66: 1755–1760.

44. Rectenwald JE, Moldawer LL, Huber TS, Seeger JM, Ozaki CK. Direct evidence for cytokine involvement in neointimal hyperplasia. Circulation 2000; 102:1697–1702.

45. Yuda A, Takai S, Jin D, Sawada Y, Nishimoto M, Matsuyama N, Asada K, Kondo K, Sasaki S, Miyazaki M. Angiotensin II receptor antagonist, L-158,809, prevents intimal hyperplasia in dog grafted veins. Life Sci 2000; 68:41–48.

46. Virone-Oddos A, Desangle V, Provost D, Cazes M, Caussade F, Cloarec A. In vitro and in vivo effects of UP 269-6, a new potent orally active nonpeptide angiotensin II receptor antagonist, on vascular smooth muscle cell proliferation. Br J Pharmacol 1997; 120:488–494.

47. Azuma H, Sato J, Masuda H, Goto M, Tamaoki S, Sugimoto A, Hamasaki H, Yamashita H. ATZ1993, an orally active and novel nonpeptide antagonist for endothelin receptors and inhibition of intimal hyperplasia after balloon denudation of the rabbit carotid artery. Jpn J Pharmacol 1999; 81:21–28.

48. Marano G, Palazzesi S, Bernucci P, Grigioni M, Formigari R, Ballerini L. ET(A)/ET(B) receptor antagonist bosentan inhibits neointimal development in collared carotid arteries of rabbits. Life Sci 1998; 63:PL259–PL266.

49. Battegay EJ, Raines EW, Colbert T, Ross R. TNF-alpha stimulation of fibroblast proliferation. Dependence on platelet-derived growth factor (PDGF) secretion and alteration of PDGF receptor expression. J Immunol 1995; 154:6040–6047.

50. Fingerle J, Johnson R, Clowes AW, Majesky MW, Reidy MA. Role of platelets in smooth muscle cell proliferation and migration after vascular injury in rat carotid artery. Proc Natl Acad Sci USA 1989; 86:8412.

51. Davies MG, Owens EL, Mason DP, Lea H, Tran K, Vergel S, Hawkins SA, Hart CE, Clowes AW. Effect of platelet-derived growth factor receptor-alpha and -beta blockade on flow-induced neointimal formation in endothelialized baboon vascular grafts. Circ Res 2000; 86(7): 779–786.

52. Bergsten E, Uutela M, Li X, Pietras K, Ostman A, Heldin CH, Alitalo K, Eriksson U. PDGF-D is a specific, protease-activated ligand for the PDGF beta-receptor. Nat Cell Biol 2001; 3:512–516.

53. Uutela M, Lauren J, Bergsten E, Li X, Horelli-Kuitunen N, Eriksson U, Alitalo K. Chromosomal location, exon structure, and vascular expression patterns of the human PDGFC and PDGFC genes. Circulation 2001; 103:2242–2247.

54. Topper JN, Cai J, Falb D, Gimbrone MA. Identification of vascular endothelial genes differentially responsive to fluid mechanical stimuli: cyclooxygenase-2, manganese superoxide dismutase, and endothelial nitric oxide synthase are selectively up-regulated by steady laminar shear stress. Proc Natl Acad Sci USA 1996; 93:10417–10422.

55. Hansson GK, Holm J. Interferon-gamma inhibits arterial stenosis after injury. Circulation 1991; 84:1266–1272.

56. Bingley JA, Campbell JH, Hayward IP, Campbell GR. Inhibition of neointimal formation by natural heparin sulfate proteoglycans of the arterial wall. Ann NY Acad Sci 1997; 811:238–242.

57. Han RO, Ettenson DS, Koo EW, Edelman ER. Heparin/heparin sulfate chelation inhibits control of vascular repair by tissue engineered endothelial cells. Am J Physiol 1997; 273: H2586–H2595.

58. Nugent MA, Nugent HM, Iozzo RV, Sanchack K, Edelman ER. Perlecan is required to inhibit thrombosis after deep vascular injury and contributes to endothelial cell-mediated inhibition of intimal hyperplasia. Proc Natl Acad Sci USA 2000; 97:6722–6727.

59. Forsten KE, Courant NA, Nugent MA. Endothelial proteoglycans inhibit bFGF binding and mitogenesis. J Cell Physiol 1997; 172:209–220.

60. Au YPT, Kenagy RD, Clowes MM, Clowes AW. Mechanisms of inhibition of heparin of vascular smooth muscle cell proliferation and migration. Haemostasis 1993; 23(suppl 1):177–182.

61. Mattson EJR, Kohler TR, Vergel S, Clowes AW. Increased blood flow induces regression of intimal hyperplasia. Arterioscler Thromb Vasc Biol 1997; 17:2245–2249.

62. Schwartz SM, Bennett MR. Death by no other name. Am J Pathol 1995; 147:229–234.

63. Schwartz SM. Cell Death and the caspase cascade. Circulation 1998; 97:227.

64. Bennett MR, Evan GI, Schwartz SM. Apoptosis of rat vascular smooth muscle cells is regulated by p-53 dependant and independent pathways. Circ Res 1995; 77:266–273.

65. Di Mario C, Marisco F, Adamian M, Karvouni E, Albiero R, Colombo A. New recipes for in-stent restenosis: Cut, grate, roast, or sandwich the intima? Heart 2000; 84:471–475.

66. Wolf A, Schwarz F, Hoffmann M, et al. Repetitive balloon angioplasty for recurrent in-stent restenosis: results of first and second PTCA in focal and diffuse stenosis [abstr]. J Am Coll Cardiol 1999; 33:26A.

67. Mehran R, Mintz G, Popma J. Mechanisms and results of balloon angioplasty for the in-stent restenosis. Am J Cardiol 1996; 78:618–622.

68. Eltchaninoff H, Koning R, Tron C, et al. Balloon angioplasty for the treatment of coronary in-stent restenosis: Immediate results and 6 months angiographic recurrent restenosis rate. J Am Coll Cardiol 1998; 32:980–984.

69. Harrington RA, Califf RM, Holmes DR Jr, Pieper KS, Lincoff AM, Berdan LG, Thompson TD, Topol EJ. Is all unstable angina the same? Insights from the Coronary Angioplasty Versus Excisional Atherectomy Trial (CAVEAT-I). The CAVEAT-Investigators. Am Heart J 1999; 137:199–203.

70. Cohen EA, Sykora K, Kimball BP, Bonan R, Ricci DR, Webb JG, Laramee L, Barbeau G, Traboulsi M, Corbett BN, Schwartz L, Adelman AG. Clinical outcomes of patients more than one year following randomization in the Canadian Coronary Atherectomy Trial (CCAT). Can J Cardiol 1997; 13:825–830.

71. Teirstein PS, Massullo V, Jani S, et al. Catheter-based radiotherapy to inhibit restenosis after coronary stenting. N Engl J Med 1997; 336:1697–1703.

72. Waksman R, White RL, Chan RC, et al. Intra-coronary gamma irradiation therapy after angioplasty inhibits recurrence in patients with in-stent restenosis. Circulation 2000; 101:2165–2171.

73. Leon MB, Teirstein PS, Moses J, et al. Localized intra-coronary gamma-radiation therapy to inhibit the recurrence of restenosis after stenting. N Engl J Med 2001; 344:250–256.

74. Seabra-Gomes R. Radioactive stents to reduce restenosis: Time for an epitaph? Eur Heart J 2001; 22:621–623.

75. Albiero R, Adamian M, Kobayashi N, et al. Short and intermediate term results of ^{32}P radioactive β-emitting stent implantation in patients with coronary artery disease. The Milan dose response study. Circulation 2000; 101:18–26.

76. Sousa JE, Costa MA, Abizaid A, et al. Lack of neointimal proliferation after implantation of sirolimus-coated stents in human coronary arteries. Circulation 2001; 103:192–195.

77. Mann MJ, Whittemore AD, Donaldson MC, et al. Ex-vivo gene therapy of human vascular bypass grafts with EF2 decoy: The PREVENT single center, randomized, controlled trial. Lancet 1999; 354:1493–1498.

78. Rowinsky EK, Donehower RC. Paclitaxel (Taxol). N Engl J Med 1995; 332:1004–1014.

79. Axel DI, Kunert W, Goggelmann C, et al. Paclitaxel inhibits arterial smooth muscle cell proliferation and migration in vitro and in vitro using local drug delivery. Circulation 1997; 96:636–645.

80. Drachman DE, Edelman ER, Seifert P, et al. Neointimal thickening after stent delivery of paclitaxel: Change in composition and arrest of growth over six months. J Am Coll Cardiol 2000; 36:2325–2332.

81. Heldman AW, Cheng L, Jenkins M. Paclitaxel stent coating inhibits neointimal hyperplasia at 4 weeks in a porcine model of coronary restenosis. Circulation 2001; 103:2289–2295.

82. Farb A, Heller PF, Shroff S, et al. Pathological analysis of local delivery of paclitaxel via a polymer-coated stent. Circulation 2001; 104:473–479.

83. de la Fuente LM, Miano J, Mrad J, Penaloza E, Yeung AC, Eury R, Froix M, Fitzgerald PJ, Stertzer SH. Initial results of the Quanam drug eluting stent (QuaDS-QP-2) Registry (BARDDS) in human subjects. Catheter Cardiovasc Intervent 2001; 53:480–488.

84. Liistro F, Colombo A. Late acute thrombosis after paclitaxel eluting stent implantation. Heart 2001; 86:262–264.

85. DeYoung MB, Dichek DA. Gene therapy for restenosis: Are we ready? Circ Res 1998; 82: 306–313.

86. Baek S, March KL. Gene therapy for restenosis: Getting nearer the heart of the matter. Circ Res 1998; 82:295–305.

87. Chang MW, Barr E, Lu MM, Barton K, Leiden JM. Adenovirus mediated overexpression of the cyclin/cyclin dependant kinase inhibitor, p21, inhibits vascular smooth muscle cell proliferation and neointimal formation in the rat carotid artery model of balloon injury. J Clin Invest 1995; 96:2260–2268.

88. Smith RC, Branellec D, Gorski DH, Guo K, Perlman H, Dedieu JF, Pastore C, Mahfoudi A, Denefle P, Isner JM, Walsh K. p21CIP1-mediated inhibition of cell proliferation by over-expression of the gax homeodomain gene. Genes Dev 1997; 11:1674–1689.

89. Ueno H, Yamamoto H, Ito S, Li JJ, Takeshita A. Adenovirus-mediated transfer of a dominant-negative H-ras suppresses neointimal formation in balloon injured arteries in vivo. Arterioscler Thromb Vasc Biol 1997; 17:904–989.

90. Ohno T, Gordon D, San H, Pompili VJ, Imperiale MJ, Nabel GJ, Nabel EG. Gene therapy for vascular smooth muscle cell proliferation after arterial injury. Science 1994; 265:781–784.

91. Simari RD, San H, Rekhter M, Ohno T, Gordon D, Nabel GJ, Nabel EG. Regulation of cellular proliferation and intimal formation following balloon injury in atherosclerotic rabbit arteries. J Clin Invest 1996; 98:225–235.

92. Vasa M, Fichtlscherer D, Adler K, Aicher A, Martin H, Zeiher AM, Dimmeler S. Increase in circulating endothelial progenitor cells by statin therapy in patients with stable coronary artery disease. Circulation 2001; 103:2885–2890.

93. Gill M, Dias S, Hattori K, Rivera ML, Hicklin D, Witte L, Girardi L, Yurt R, Himel H, Rafii S. Vascular trauma induces rapid but transient mobilization of VEGFR2$^+$ AC133$^+$ endothelial precursor cells. Circ Res 2001; 88:167–174.

94. Hart CE, Kraiss LW, Vergel S, Gilbertson D, Kenagy R, Kirkman T, Crandall DL, Tickle S, Finney H, Tarranton G, Clowes AW. PDGFβ receptor blockade inhibits intimal hyperplasia in the baboon. Circulation 1999; 99:564–569.

95. Sirois MG, Simons M, Edelman ER. Antisense oligonucleotide inhibition of PDGF-β receptor subunit expression directs suppression of intimal thickening. Circulation 1997; 95:669–676.

96. Chesebro JH, Clements IP, Fuster V, et al. A platelet-inhibitor drug trial in coronary artery bypass operations: benefit of perioperative dipyridamole and aspirin therapy on early postoperative vein graft patency. N Engl J Med 1982; 307:73–78.

97. Lorenz RL, Schacky CV, Weber M, et al. Improved aorto-coronary bypass patency by low dose aspirin (100mg daily): Effects on platelet aggregation and thromboxane formation. Lancet 1984; 1:1261–1264.

98. Becquemin JP. Effect of ticlopidine on the long-term patency of saphenous-vein bypass grafts in the legs. N Engl J Med 1997; 337:1726–1731.

99. Clowes AW, Karnovsky MJ. Suppression by heparin of smooth muscle cell proliferation in injured arteries. Nature 1977; 265:625–626.
100. Clowes AW, Clowes MM. Kinetics of cellular proliferation after arterial injury: II. Inhibition of smooth muscle cell growth by heparin. Lab Invest 1985; 52:611–616.
101. Snow AD, Bolender RP, Wright TN, et al. Heparin modulates the composition of the extracellular matrix domain surrounding arterial smooth muscle cells. Am J Physiol 1990; 137: 313–330.
102. Pukac LA, Castellot JJ, Wright TJ, et al. Heparin inhibits c-fos and c-myc mRNA expression in vascular smooth muscle cells. Cell Regulation 1990; 1:435–443.
103. Welt FGP, Woods TC, Edelman ER. Oral heparin prevents neointimal hyperplasia after arterial injury. Circulation 2001; 104:3121–3124.
104. Ellis SG, Roubin GS, Wilentz J, et al. Effect of 18 to 24 hour heparin administration for prevention of restenosis after uncomplicated coronary angioplasty. Am Heart J 1989; 117: 777–782.
105. Faxon DP, Spiro TE, Minor S, et al. Low molecular weight heparin in prevention of restenosis after angioplasty. Results of the Enoxaparin Restenosis (ERA) Trial. Circulation 1994; 90:908–914.
106. Kiesz RS, Buszman P, Martin JL, Deutsch E, Rozek MM, Gaszewska E, Rewicki M, Seweryniak P, Kosmider M, Tendera M. Local delivery of enoxaparin to decrease restenosis after stenting: Results of initial multicenter trial: Polish-American Local Lovenox NIR Assessment study (The POLONIA study). Circulation 2001; 103:26–31.
107. Floege J, Ostendorf T, Janssen U, Burg M, Radeke HH, Vargeese C, Gill SC, Green LS, Janjic N. Novel approach to specific growth factor inhibition in vivo: Antagonism of platelet-derived growth factor in glomerulonephritis by aptamers. Am J Pathol 1999; 154: 169–179.
108. Bilder G, Wentz T, Leadley R, Amin D, Byan L, O'Conner B, Needle S, Galczenski H, Bostwick J, Kasiewski C, Myers M, Spada A, Merkel L, Ly C, Persons P, Page K, Perrone M, Dunwiddie C. Restenosis following angioplasty in the swine coronary artery is inhibited by an orally active PDGF-receptor tyrosine kinase inhibitor, RPR101511A. Circulation 1999; 99: 3292–3299.
109. Neschis DG, Safford SD, Hanna AK, Fox JC, Golden MA. Antisense basic fibroblast growth factor gene transfer reduces early intimal thickening in a rabbit femoral artery balloon injury model. J Vasc Surg 1998; 27:126–134.
110. Chen C, Mattar SG, Hughes JD, Pierce GF, Cook JE, Ku DN, Hanson SR, Lumsden AB. Recombinant mitotoxin basic fibroblast growth factor-saporin reduces venous anastomotic intimal hyperplasia in the arteriovenous graft. Circulation 1996; 94:1989–1995.
111. Forough R, Koyama N, Hasenstab D, Lea H, Clowes M, Nikkari ST, Clowes AW. Overexpression of tissue inhibitor of matrix metalloproteinase-1 inhibits vascular smooth muscle cell functions in vitro and in vivo. Circ Res 1996; 79:812–820.
112. Kanamasa K, Otani N, Ishida N, Inoue Y, Ikeda A, Morii H, Naito N, Hayashi T, Ishikawa K, Miyazawa M. Suppression of cell proliferation by tissue plasminogen activator during the early phase after balloon injury minimizes intimal hyperplasia in hypercholesterolemic rabbits. J Cardiovasc Pharmacol 2001; 37:155–162.
113. Wolf YG, Rasmussen LM, Ruoslahti E. Antibodies against transforming growth factor-beta 1 suppress intimal hyperplasia in a rat model. J Clin Invest 1994; 93:1172–1178.
114. Smith JD, Bryant SR, Couper LL, Vary CP, Gotwals PJ, Koteliansky VE, Lindner V. Soluble transforming growth factor-beta type II receptor inhibits negative remodeling, fibroblast transdifferentiation, and intimal lesion formation but not endothelial growth. Circ Res 1999; 84:1212–1222.

5
The Healing Characteristics, Durability, and Long-Term Complications of Vascular Prostheses

Glenn C. Hunter

University of Texas Medical Branch, Galveston, Texas, U.S.A.

David A. Bull

University of Utah Health Sciences Center, Salt Lake City, Utah, U.S.A.

Arterial and venous autografts remain the materials of choice to replace diseased or damaged blood vessels. However, because of their limited supply, there is an increasing need to develop arterial substitutes that are durable, are readily incorporated by host tissues, possess a non- or hypothrombogenic flow surface, have compliance characteristics that closely approximate the native vessel, are resistant to infection, and are easily sutured (1,2). Although none of the currently available prostheses manifests all of the desired characteristics of the ideal arterial replacement, large-diameter Dacron grafts used to replace the abdominal aorta have proved adequate, with 5-year cumulative patency rates of 85–90% (3–5). Late patency rates of 74 and 70% at 10 and 15 years, respectively, have been reported by Nevelsteen et al. (5). Unfortunately, the longevity of small-diameter prosthetic grafts (6 mm in internal diameter or less) is limited by the development of anastomotic intimal hyperplasia and consequent thrombosis of the grafts. When small-diameter prosthetic grafts such as those fabricated from polytetrafluoroethylene or Dacron are placed above the knee, cumulative patency rates range from 37.9 to 71%; below the knee, they range from 30 to 57% (6–9).

The increasing longevity of the population and the more frequent execution of bypass procedures to the more distal vessels of the extremity have resulted in increases in both the number and complexity of the bypass procedures now performed. It is estimated that approximately one-third of patients will require additional surgery related to their bypass graft within 2 years of the initial procedure (10). Furthermore, complications resulting from errors in technique or deterioration of the graft fabric are not uncommon, and the risk of reoperation is increased substantially by the progression of ischemic heart disease and other associated atherosclerotic risk factors in these patients. Reoperative mortality rates of up to 5% and major limb loss rates of 20% have been reported (11). As a consequence, patients in whom complications related to their grafts develop may be unable to withstand the secondary operations needed to replace them. These changes in the demographics of the patients requiring repeated arterial reconstructive procedures and the limited supply of autogenous graft material have increased the need for durable arterial substitutes that will continue to function satisfactorily throughout the patient's remaining life.

In this chapter we discuss the fabrication, healing characteristics, clinical indications, and complications related to grafts fabricated from polyethylene terephthalate (Dacron), polytetrafluoroethylene (PTFE), polyurethane, and the commonly used biological grafts— human umbilical vein grafts, cryopreserved allografts, and bovine xenografts.

I. DACRON GRAFTS

Dacron is the most common prosthetic material used to replace diseased segments of the aorta and its major branches. Although there are numerous variations in construction, all Dacron grafts can be grouped into several major categories: woven versus knitted and smooth versus veloured surfaces. Woven grafts have functioned satisfactorily when used for repair of thoracic and abdominal aortic aneurysms, aortic replacement in patients with known bleeding diatheses, or in the occasional patient who bleeds through the interstices of a preclotted knitted graft immediately after restoration of flow. Knitted grafts are used to bypass occlusive lesions of the aorta, and the iliac, common femoral, and superficial femoral arteries. They have also been used successfully for axillofemoral or femorofemoral bypass grafting.

Long-term patency rates of 85–90% for aortoiliac or aortofemoral bypass grafts and 5-year primary patency rates of 78–88% for axillofemoral, 71% for above-knee, and 57% for below-knee femoropopliteal externally supported Dacron grafts have been reported (3–5, 7, 12–14). The recent study by Robb et al. has demonstrated greater long-term patency of aortofemoral grafts if both the superficial femoral and profunda femoris arteries are patent (15).

A. Fabrication

A knowledge of the fabrication of Dacron grafts is essential for an understanding of the factors that influence healing and/or contribute to the late failure of these grafts.

1. Woven

Woven grafts constructed by interlacing two sets of yarn at right angles to each other are the strongest prosthetic fabric grafts. About 45% of grafts implanted each year fall into this category (1,2). Nonveloured woven grafts are dimensionally stable, relatively impervious to blood, noncompliant, and of high tensile strength. However, they are difficult to suture and tend to fray at their cut edges. The velour component, which can be added to woven grafts by incorporating additional nontextured yarns that are interlaced less frequently than the textured ground yarns, permits a reduction in tightness of the weave without altering permeability. This results in a softer graft that is easier to suture.

2. Knitted

Knitted grafts are of two basic types and are constructed with a set of yarns that are interlooped rather than interlaced. Weft-knitted grafts are formed from one set of yarns interlocked in a circular fashion; warp-knitted grafts are fabricated from several sets of yarns interlooped in a zigzag pattern. Warp-knitted grafts, although more compliant than woven grafts, are less compliant than weft-knitted grafts. Unlike woven grafts they do not run, unravel, or fray at their cut edges.

Even though the walls of knitted grafts are thicker than woven (600 vs. 200 μm), they are more porous because of their construction and as a result readily permit cellular ingrowth through their interstices (2). The interlooping yarns used in the construction of knitted grafts permit greater expansion of the yarn circumferentially than longitudinally; consequently they have reduced dimensional stability and a tendency to dilate (1).

Unlike woven grafts, the greater porosity of knitted grafts requires that they be made impervious to blood before implantation. This can be achieved either (a) by preclotting the graft with blood (2) or by coating the luminal surface with proteinaceous sealants, such as bovine collagen (16,17), gelatin (18,19), or albumin (18–20), or (b) by autoclaving the graft in albumin or blood [as advocated by Bethea and Reemsta (21) and modified by Cooley et al. (22)]. When first introduced, coated grafts were stiffer than uncoated prostheses, making suturing difficult. In addition, the sealants were not uniformly applied, resulting in unpredictable porosity, cracking, peeling, and embolization of the coated material (19). A critical requirement for all coated prostheses is that the rate of absorption of the sealant occur within a precise time frame so that it provides hemostasis without impairing healing. The use of sealant-coated grafts has proved to be particularly advantageous when replacing portions of the thoracic aorta or when repairing ruptured aortic aneurysms, in which intraoperative interstitial and anastomotic bleeding are important causes of morbidity and mortality.

Knitted (Gelseal) and woven Dacron (Gelweave) and, more recently, PTFE (seal PTFE) grafts have all been impregnated with gelatin. The Hemashield graft is a warp-knitted, double-velour graft impregnated with type 1 collagen. Although these grafts can readily be implanted without bleeding in the majority of patients, significant needle-hole bleeding has been observed in some patients having these grafts placed while on cardiopulmonary bypass (23).

B. Healing Characteristics

The body attempts to incorporate the implanted Dacron graft by two distinct cellular processes: (a) *anastomotic pannus ingrowth*, which extends approximately 1–2 cm from the divided artery and is composed of smooth muscle and endothelial cells derived from components of the arterial wall, and (b) *perigraft fibrous tissue*, which encircles the entire external surface of the graft, resulting in encapsulation of the graft. Anastomotic pannus ingrowth, however, does not possess any significant intrinsic tensile strength; hence the anastomotic bond between graft and artery is entirely dependent on the suture material for its integrity. Cells from the outer fibrous capsule readily invade the interstices of the graft but seldom penetrate beyond the midportion of the wall of the prosthesis (24,25). The addition of a veloured component to these grafts to enhance cellular ingrowth may induce excessive proliferation of perivascular fibrous tissue, which decreases the compliance of the graft or contributes to stenosis of an adjacent structure.

The flow surface of a well-healed patent graft is characterized by a layer of compacted, relatively acellular hypothrombogenic pseudointima, which is uniformly present except in areas adjacent to anastomoses or at bifurcations. If initially a prosthesis of too large a diameter has been used or if the diameter of the prosthesis has increased substantially over time, the thickness of this layer tends to increase, so that the lumen of the graft approximates in size that of the outflow vessel. The addition of an internal velour lining may further increase the thickness of this layer and contribute to the ultimate failure of the graft. Poor healing characterized by incomplete covering of the luminal surface has been observed in explants from diabetic patients and those in poor general health (10).

Guidoin et al. (25) noted that the differences in the healing characteristics among the various types of Dacron prostheses could be related solely to the varying thicknesses of the internal fibrous pseudointimal layer and that of the external capsule. The thicknesses of the inner and external linings of the grafts were minimal with woven grafts, moderate in knitted grafts, and greatest for grafts with veloured surfaces (25). We have observed more perigraft tissue ingrowth and greater thrombus adherence in coated grafts than in uncoated prostheses. Reoperation for limb occlusion is technically difficult because of the dense external capsule surrounding the graft. Removal of thrombus with thrombectomy catheters or endarterectomy strippers is difficult and often incomplete. Catheter-directed lytic therapy for graft limb occlusion has also been less successful in these patients than in those with uncoated Dacron grafts. The use of albumin-coated grafts has been associated with inconsistencies in graft porosity, cellular infiltration, and dissection or embolism of the albumin layer and has largely been abandoned (19).

In a histological evaluation of collagen-coated graft explants in humans, Anderson (26) has observed that the collagen component remains intact for up to 8 days after implantation. Grafts removed beyond 1 year were characterized by a cellular pseudointimal layer with numerous capillary loops and periadventitial infiltration of the graft. Experimental and clinical studies indicate that the gelatin sealant on gelatin-coated grafts is resorbed within 1–2 weeks (27). During the first week after implantation, fibrous thrombi and polymorph neutrophils are present on the flow surface. By 2 weeks, most of the gelatin has been reabsorbed, accompanied by a mild inflammatory response and return of the prostacyclin/thromboxane ratio to 1, indicating that the healing process is well advanced (27,28).

Although direct comparisons between collagen-coated and gelatin-impregnated grafts have shown no differences in patency, experimental studies suggest that gelatin-sealed prostheses may be more resistant to infection with *Staphylococcus epidermidis* than uncoated knitted velour polyester (29). In a prospective comparison between collagen-coated, gelatin-impregnated, and stretch PTFE aortofemoral grafts, Prager et al. found no statistical differences in patency (30). When the two Dacron grafts were compared collectively with PTFE, they had a higher infection rate (3 vs. 0%) than the PTFE grafts. The potential for both collagen-coated and gelatin-impregnated grafts to stimulate an immune response after implantation appears low (31).

C. Complications

To date there have been no systematic follow-up studies of all Dacron grafts in otherwise asymptomatic patients; most of the reports in the literature are confined to anecdotal case studies of complications. The noninfectious complications associated with the implantation of these prostheses include (1) dilatation, (2) para-anastomotic aneurysms, and pseudoaneurysms (3) anastomotic stenosis, (4) ureteric obstruction, and (5) neoplasia. Some 90% of such failures occur within the first 3–5 years after implantation.

1. Dilatation

Dilatation, defined as a permanent increase in the diameter of a graft caused by pulsating stresses, has been reported with both arterial homografts and prosthetic grafts used as arterial conduits (1,32–42). Dilatation may involve the entire length of the graft or be confined to isolated portions, resulting in diffuse or focal aneurysmal change.

Significant dilatation of implanted grafts has been documented with all currently available prosthetic materials, including knitted and woven Dacron, nylon, Teflon, Orlon, and PTFE (37–42). However, dilatation is more commonly observed with knitted Dacron because of its inherent structural properties and its more frequent use as an arterial substitute (Fig. 1). Woven grafts have a high initial modulus and therefore are resistant to extension compared with knitted grafts, which have very little resistance to extension because of their loop structure. Consequently, their interlocking loops straighten very easily in the direction of greatest stress, resulting in an increase in diameter. The incidence of graft dilatation reported in the literature, ranging from 1–3%, probably underestimates the true incidence, since only symptomatic patients are likely to undergo imaging (43,44).

In a 30-year review of 390 cases of graft failure, Pourdeyhimi and Wagner (1) found dilatation in 147 (38%), structural defects in 76 (20%), suture line defects in 56 (14%), and graft infection or bleeding in 30 (8.9%). These complications are often interrelated because

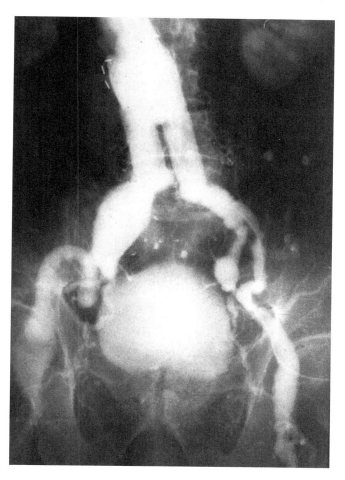

Figure 1 Abdominal aortogram showing dilation of an aortoiliac knitted graft with a right common iliac aneurysm.

graft dilatation may predispose the patient to pseudoaneurysm formation, perforation, or rupture.

Using Doppler ultrasound, Nunn and colleagues (45) studied 95 Dacron aortic grafts implanted for periods ranging from 2 weeks to 138 months in symptomatic patients. They observed dilatation ranging from 0–84% (mean, 17.6%) in 85 of the 95 grafts. Dilatation appeared more pronounced in hypertensive patients (21 vs. 15%). Lundqvist et al. (46), in a study comparing 36 patients with symptomatic graft dilatation and 65 asymptomatic patients, detected graft dilatation of between 25 and 50% in 42 of 101 patients (42%) evaluated. In 12 patients, the diameter of the dilated graft exceeded the preimplantation diameter by more than 50%. Four of these patients had false aneurysms. Furthermore, the incidence of dilatation was greater in symptomatic patients, who also had a higher incidence of false aneurysm formation compared with asymptomatic patients (14 vs. 3%). Berman et al. (47) evaluated 178 aortic grafts implanted for 0.2–233 months (mean 43.3 $\pm$ 3.2 months) with computed tomography (CT). A total of 143 Dacron prostheses (74 woven, 69 knitted) and 35 PTFE prostheses were evaluated. The mean percentage dilatation was 49.2 $\pm$ 4 for knitted prostheses, 28.5 $\pm$ 3.0 for woven prostheses, and 20.6 $\pm$ 1.9 for PTFE. The authors observed a significant correlation between graft dilatation of >50% and knitted grafts.

Etiology.   Permanent deformation of the fabric structure and fatigue of the yarn appear to be important factors in the pathogenesis of graft dilatation. Dilatation of 10–22% occurs when knitted grafts are bench tested at static pressures of 120–200 mmHg for 1 min (1). This corresponds to the initial dilatation seen when these grafts are exposed to arterial pressure. Whether this increase in diameter reflects restoration of the initial diameter (reduced by chemicals and heat used during the crimping process) or simply represents straightening of the interlacing loop structure is unclear. Although bench testing is a fairly reliable predictor of early dilatation, it does not accurately predict late dilatation related to fiber elongation or yarn fatigue.

A number of factors are believed to contribute to deformation of fabric structure and yarn fatigue of Dacron grafts. They include hypertension (45), mechanical or chemical degradation of Dacron fibers (48–51), undetected flaws from the manufacturing process, performance deformation or creep of the fabric due to loss of stitch density (knitted) or fabric count (woven) (44,52), and damage inflicted by the injudicious application of instruments intraoperatively. The contribution of any one of these factors to failure of a given graft often is difficult to ascertain in the individual patient. Microscopic fracture of the fibers with fibrillation (50) is typical of mechanical failure due to cyclical bending or tension or torsion stresses on the graft.

In a comprehensive review of Dacron graft explants removed at autopsy or reoperation, the most consistent finding observed by Guidoin (10) was a time-dependent loss of stitch density found in all prostheses examined. The rate of loss of stitch density depends on the type of fabric construction. Weft-knitted fabrics therefore would be less stable than the warp-knitted ones. As a result of this loss of stitch density, the fabric is susceptible to irreversible dilatation when exposed to arterial blood pressure. Clagett et al. (52) observed a similar loss in stitch density in five patients with dilated grafts. Of considerable interest is the size of the grafts implanted in the patients Clagett et al. (52) studied. The diameters of the grafts used were 19 × 9.5 mm (four patients) and 25 × 12.5 mm (one patient), considerably larger than would be chosen today. One can only speculate as to the contribution of initial graft size to eventual failure.

Chemical biodegradation may further exacerbate the dilatation initially induced by a loss of stitch density. King et al. (50), in a study of 19 prosthetic Dacron explants in residence for intervals ranging from a few hours to 14 years using infrared spectroscopy, observed a decrease in molecular weight and an increase in the content of carboxyl groups proportional to the duration of implantation. It has been postulated that immunologically active macrophages and monocytes that infiltrate the graft as part of the healing process may also contribute to chemical deterioration of these grafts by recruitment of biologically active cells that ingest the individual Dacron fibers (52) (Fig. 2).

Variations in the fabrication of grafts also have been implicated in cases of late fiber deterioration and graft dilatation. In a study of 493 grafts, Berger and Sauvage (44) found that graft dilatation between 17 and 43% was present in 15 cases that had been implanted for 3–15.3 years. The authors postulated that reductions in fiber diameter and/or acute

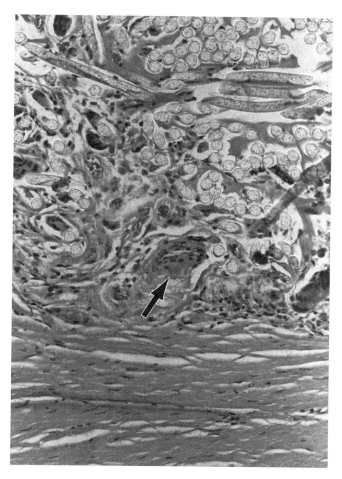

Figure 2 Photomicrograph of the outer surface of a Dacron graft covered with a layer of firmly adherent connective tissue. Foreign-body giant cells and macrophages surrounding and ingesting the Dacron fibers are present. (Original magnification × 200.)

breaks of individual filaments resulting from overheating during the crimping process, frictional wear, or biodegradation were responsible for these changes.

Finally, damage to the graft can occur during implantation from careless handling with instruments. Isolated areas of damaged fibers suggestive of vascular clamp injury have been observed in graft explants (10). Thus careful handling during implantation is essential to avoid damage that may increase later susceptibility to deterioration (44).

Diagnosis. Dilatation of Dacron grafts appears to be a biphasic phenomenon. Early dilatation of approximately 10–22%, commencing immediately after the graft is exposed to arterial blood pressure, plateaus within the first year (Fig. 3) (1). Late dilatation, caused by yarn slippage or breakage, usually is seen within 2–3 years of implantation. Because of the biphasic nature of graft dilatation, evaluation of abnormal dilatation appears unwarranted within the first year after implantation of the graft, since this early dilatation is largely attributed to restoration of the initial diameter of the graft. Late graft dilatation, however, is progressive. Once dilatation is detected, such patients should be carefully monitored for life.

Ultrasound. B-mode ultrasound is widely available, relatively inexpensive, and particularly useful for assessing early and late complications of vascular grafts. Gooding and coworkers (53), in a study of 87 patients with aortofemoral grafts, were able to successfully image the anastomotic sites in 84% of the grafts. The authors discovered 23 unsuspected anastomotic aneurysms (2 aortic and 21 femoral), and perigraft accumulation of fluid or blood was observed in 16 patients. In a study of 127 patients with Dacron grafts, Clifford et al. (54), using Doppler imaging and real-time ultrasound, found graft dilatation of 15–70% in five grafts. More recently we have studied patients with dilated grafts using color-flow Doppler imaging and have observed nonlaminar turbulent flow patterns

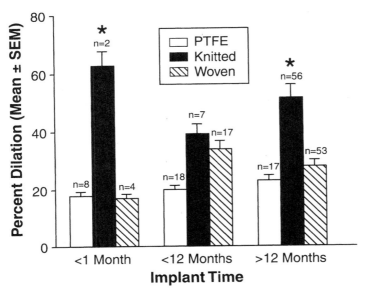

Figure 3 Histogram showing time course of aortic graft dilatation. Knitted Dacron compared with PTFE and woven Dacron. * = p < 0.01 by Anova.

within the grafts reminiscent of those seen in patients with aortic aneurysms. Although this may explain the progressive increase in the pseudointimal lining in these grafts, to date relatively few patients have been studied and no definitive conclusions can be drawn.

Ideally, color-flow Doppler imaging of all asymptomatic aortofemoral grafts should be performed at 1 year and then at 5 years. If no significant alteration in the diameter of the prosthesis is identified at 5 years after implantation, it seems unlikely that significant dilatation will occur and the frequency of follow-up can be reduced. However, once dilatation has been detected, continuing surveillance is indicated to detect anastomotic aneurysms or an increase in luminal pseudointima, either of which may threaten the long-term patency of the graft.

Computed Tomography. Contrast-enhanced computed tomography (CT) is helpful in accurately assessing the size of anastomotic aneurysms and in excluding other complications such as perigraft collections of fluid or air. Unlike ultrasound, CT can be used to evaluate grafts implanted in the abdomen or chest (Fig. 4) (26). Qvarfordt et al. (55), Brown et al. (56), Berman et al. (57), Nunn (45,58), and Kalman (59) have described the usefulness of CT scans for detecting early and late complications of prosthetic grafts. CT scanning of aortic grafts has demonstrated dilatation up to 367% of the aortic portion of knitted prostheses. Dilatation can occur in the body and each of the limbs of an aortic bifurcated graft but may not occur uniformly throughout the graft (Fig. 5). It can also occur in Dacron grafts implanted in other locations such as femoropopliteal bypasses (Fig. 6). Berman et al. (47) reported a complication rate of 13.5%. Kalman et al. found aneurysmal dilatation of the abdominal or thoracic aorta in 13.8% of patients and dilatation of the iliac arteries in patients with tube grafts in 15.4% (59). However, cost and attendant radiation exposure make CT less desirable for routine follow-up and CT should be limited to the evaluation of symptomatic patients or for those instances in which ultrasound examination fails to adequately delineate the graft.

Complications. Progressive increases in diameter of prosthetic grafts have been implicated in anastomotic aneurysm formation, thrombosis, and rupture of the affected grafts (46,51,56). Embolization from a dilated graft containing laminated luminal thrombus also must be considered a potential risk; however, the frequency of this event is a matter of speculation since its occurrence has not been well documented in the literature.

2. Para-Anastomotic Aneurysms and Pseudoaneurysms

Aortic Para-Anastomotic Aneurysms. Para-anastomotic aneurysms occur in 0.5–15% of patients undergoing aortic operations for occlusive or aneurysmal disease and tend to increase in frequency over time (60–65). The incidence of this complication is probably underestimated, as systematic long-term follow-up of aortic prostheses is not currently undertaken.

These aneurysms can occur at either the aortic, iliac, or femoral anastomosis of bifurcated grafts. They can be either true aneurysms or pseudoaneurysms and occur with varying frequency depending on the indication for aortic replacement. True aneurysms of the parental aorta occur almost entirely in patients undergoing aortic replacement for aneurysmal disease; whereas, progressive dilation of the iliac arteries is usually seen in patients undergoing aortic tube graft replacement. Unrecognized or uncorrected preexisting whereas progressive dilatation of aortic dilatation, ongoing matrix degradation as part of the aneurysmal process, and the use of a prosthesis of too large a diameter are among the factors contributing to the development of true para-anastomotic aneurysms (Figs. 7 and 8).

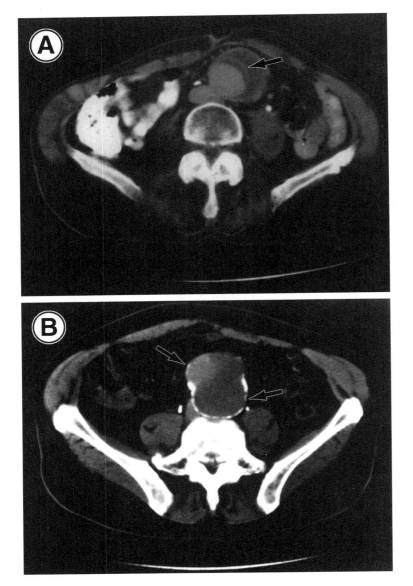

Figure 4 Abdominal CT scans demonstrating (A) a dilated graft (arrow) and the surrounding thrombus from an aortic anastomotic aneurysm and (B) dilatation of the aorta at the site of an end-to-side anastomosis.

In contrast, para-anastomotic pseudoaneurysms are more common following aorto-femoral bypass grafting for occlusive disease and occurs at either the proximal or distal anastomosis with either end-to-end or end-to-side anastomotic configurations. Endar-terectomy of the aortic cuff, suture failure, graft type, defects in the aortic wall, and a mismatch in compliance all contribute to ultimate deterioration of the proximal aortic anastomosis.

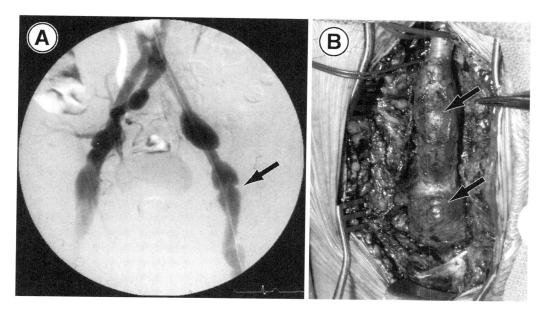

Figure 5   Abdominal arteriogram showing (A) focal dilatations in the limbs of an aortobifemoral graft and (B) operative picture of the focal areas of dilatation seen in A.

The majority of patients with aortic para-anastomotic aneurysms are asymptomatic and are detected incidentally on abdominal ultrasound or CT scanning. A herald bleed or frank rupture in a patient with an aortic prosthesis should alert the surgeon to the possibility of this complication.

The diagnosis is usually confirmed by CT scanning. Careful preoperative evaluation of these patients is essential because of the higher morbidity and mortality rates associated with these reoperative procedures. The size of the aneurysm and the general condition of the patient are among the factors that need to be considered.

The retroperitoneal approach, if not previously used, offers an excellent method of access for repair of these complex lesions. Extension of the graft more proximally, with or without reimplantation of the visceral vessels, is usually required for true aneurysms.

Although endovascular techniques may be applicable for repair of pseudoaneurysms, the small but definite risk of an infectious etiology remains when para-anastomotic aneurysms are repaired surgically. Tissue excised at surgery should be sent for culture and histological examination for the presence of microorganisms.

The operative mortality rates for repair of para-anastomotic aneurysms are high, ranging from 20 to 24% for elective procedures and up to 73% for ruptured aneruysms (62,65).

Whether para-anastomotic aneurysms can be prevented is a matter for debate. However, a few technical precautions at the initial procedure seem prudent. Endarterectomy of the proximal aortic cuff should be avoided and, if necessary, the aorta should be reinforced with Teflon pledgets or placement of a prosthetic cuff overlapping the suture line and the endarterectomized aorta.

Femoral Anastomotic Aneurysms and Pseudoaneurysms.   Anastomotic pseudoaneurysms involving the femoral anastomosis account for more than 80% of cases. A number

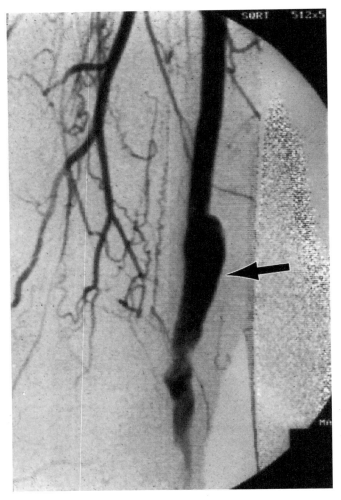

Figure 6 Femoral arteriogram showing diffuse enlargement and focal dilatation (arrow) of a Dacron femoropopliteal graft.

of etiological factors—including weakness of the arterial wall (31%), hypertension (27%), mechanical factors (12%), graft deterioration (12%), impaired wound healing (8%), endarterectomy (7%), and suture failure (3%)—have been implicated in a comprehensive study by Szilagyi et al. (66). Occasionally, there is true dilatation of the common femoral artery at a femoral anastomosis. Here we focus on the contribution of graft dilatation to the development of anastomotic pseudoaneurysms (Fig. 9).

How may dilatation of the prosthesis contribute to the development of anastomotic pseudoaneurysms? Since knitted grafts dilate initially by 10–22%, selection of too large a graft may be an important contributing factor. The diameter of the limbs of the graft should approximate that of the outflow vessel. A graft-to-vessel ratio of 1.2–1.4:1, as suggested by the experimental studies of Kinley et al. (67), may be too generous in view of the inherent propensity of knitted grafts to dilate.

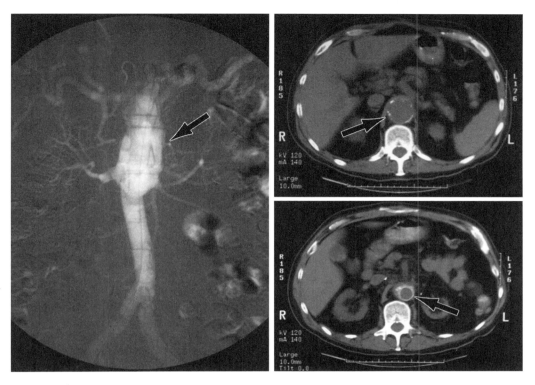

Figure 7 Abdominal aortogram demonstrating a para-anastomotic aneurysm in a patient who had previously undergone repair of an abdominal aortic aneurysm. The abdominal CT scan in the upper panel shows the aneurysm. The PTFE graft used to repair the infrarenal aneurysm is noted in the lower panel (arrow).

The portion of the graft close to the suture line may fail from yarn slippage or breakage. Yarn slippage is common with woven grafts, especially if they are cut on a bias, as is commonly done in performing end-to-side anastomosis. Careful placement of sutures and heat sealing of the cut edges may minimize slippage of the yarn. Yarn breakage was associated more commonly with weft-knitted grafts, which are no longer being manufactured.

Dilatation and anastomotic aneurysms often occur in association (52,68). Kim et al. (68) observed significant graft dilatation ranging from 50 to 150% in the patients they studied. Anastomotic aneurysms were present in all instances. Perhaps suture line stress, minimal when the graft-to-artery ratio is 1.4:1 or less, increases progressively as the graft enlarges. Also, as the graft increases in diameter, it has a tendency to shorten in length, thereby increasing suture line tension even further. Courbier and Aboukhater (69) recently have hypothesized that scarring, caused by the graft exiting beneath the inguinal ligament, may be an additional contributing factor. They recommend prophylactic division of the inguinal ligament. We do not concur with this theory. Although the majority of grafts adhere to the inguinal ligament, most do not exhibit false aneurysm formation. Furthermore, routine division of the inguinal ligament substantially increases the incidence of subsequent inguinal or femoral hernias.

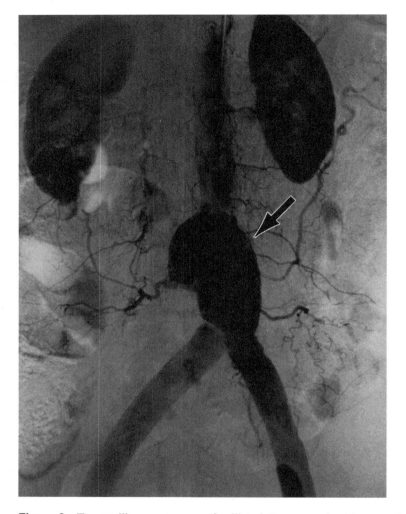

Figure 8   Transaxillary aortogram of a dilated Dacron graft with an aortic anastomotic aneurysm.

In a series of 42 anastomotic aneurysms, Carson et al. (70) found a significant increase in graft-to-artery ratio in 22 of 42 patients (52%), with a mean increase in diameter of 22%. Dilatation and an increase in graft-to-artery ratio (1.3–1.6:1 vs. 1–1.3:1) in patients were significant etiological factors in the recurrence of anastomotic pseudoaneurysms.

Although pseudoaneurysms are subject to the same spectrum of complications as true aneurysms, occlusion of a limb of the graft, especially at the femoral anastomosis, occurs more often than rupture.

Thrombosis.   As the diameter of the graft increases, the fibrous, relatively acellular pseudointimal layer lining the luminal surface of the graft likewise increases progressively, resulting in the simultaneous diminution of the diameter of the lumen to approximate that of the outflow vessel. Dislodgment of this material by trauma or during arteriography or the imposition of distal obstruction by progressive atherosclerosis or anastomotic intimal hyperplasia results in occlusion of the limb (Fig. 10). The management of limb occlusion

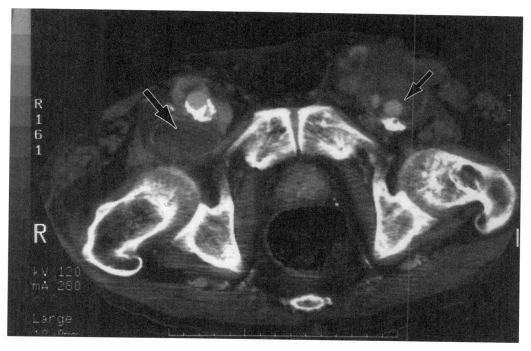

Figure 9 Abdominal CT scan showing large bilateral femoral anastomotic pseudoaneurysms. The outline of the dilated graft limb is indicated by the arrow.

secondary to an anastomotic pseudoaneurysm includes thrombectomy and/or the replacement of a segment of the graft.

Rupture. The final strength of a textile prosthesis is determined by a number of factors including the inherent properties of the basic polymer, the structure and number of filaments as well as the yarn and fabric structure. Grafts manufactured prior to 1981, made with T-62 yarns with trilobar filaments, were significantly weaker than the current fabric grafts made with nontexturized T-56 yarns with cylindrical filaments (71). The guideline, composed of carbon particles, is added to the T-56 yarns during multispinning to both knitted and woven grafts, allowing proper alignment of the graft during implantation (72). The chemical reactions required to insert the guideline results in weakening of the prosthesis and produces a potential site for rupture. Construction of earlier knitted double-velour grafts utilized alternating T-56 yarns twisted in both S and Z configurations. The remeshing line is formed with two simultaneous knitted bands joined together to form the tubular structure of the graft. Both the guidelines and the remeshing lines are potential sites of weakness in Dacron grafts and frequently the sites of rupture. A recent study of 20 human explants by Chakfe et al. (72) demonstrated that ruptures occurred most often in areas of weakness within the prosthesis guideline ($n = 6$), remeshing line ($n = 11$), or both ($n = 3$). Scanning electron microscopy showed major fractures of the tubular filaments, with complete disappearance of the velour in many instances. Ruptures of the prosthesis caused by focal defects within the graft or occasionally disruption of the entire prosthesis are rare but devastating complications. Focal rupture caused by fracture and fragmentation of Dacron fibers or longitudinal tears in grafts manufactured with inadequate tensile strength may result in single or multiple areas of false aneurysm for-

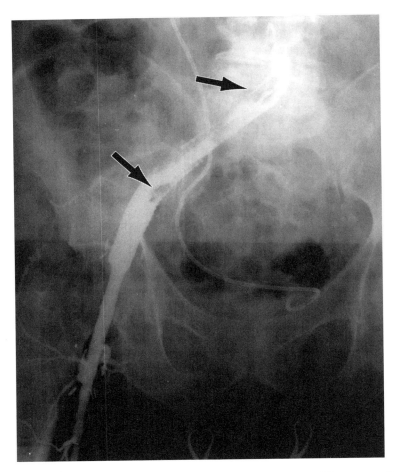

Figure 10   Operative arteriogram demonstrating a dilated Dacron graft limb with irregular pseudointimal tissue lining the graft (arrows). The nondilated PTFE graft used to repair the anastomotic aneurysm is well demonstrated. A stent to decompress the associated ureteral obstruction is present.

mation. These pseudoaneurysms may rupture into a hollow viscus, the retroperitoneum, or freely into the peritoneal cavity (51,73,74). Rupture of an anastomotic pseudoaneurysm, although uncommon in the absence of infection, is a notable cause of morbidity and mortality in patients with prosthetic grafts.

Aortic or iliac anastomotic pseudoaneurysms may rupture into adjacent bowel, most frequently the duodenum. However, other portions of the bowel may be involved also, depending on what portion of the bowel happens to be adjacent to the anastomosis. More rarely, these lesions rupture into the peritoneal cavity or the retroperitoneum.

Rarely do femoral anastomotic aneurysms rupture and usually only in patients with very large, long neglected aneurysms.

Management of Graft Dilatation.   Asymptomatic dilatation of prosthetic grafts without anastomotic pseudoaneurysm formation seldom is detected clinically unless a complication supervenes. Most often the patient presents with a painless groin swelling (the anastomotic aneurysm) and dilatation of the graft is detected during the ensuing workup. Acute or chronic occlusion of one or both of the limbs of an aortobifemoral graft caused by thrombosis of an anastomotic pseudoaneurysm is a less common mode of presentation.

Patients with significant dilatation of their grafts require careful evaluation before operative intervention is undertaken. Significant risk factors increasing operative morbidity and mortality usually are present and reoperation should be tailored to the individual patient. In addition, careful selection of the prosthesis to be used for the repair is essential if additional complications are to be minimized.

The treatment of graft dilatation may entail (a) local repair of anastomotic aneurysms, (b) thrombectomy and profundaplasty in patients with limb occlusion, or (c) graft replacement if the entire graft is dilated more than 50% of its original diameter or if an aortic anastomotic or para-anastomotic aneurysm is present.

A few salient points must be made about the operative techniques for repair of these aneurysms:

1. When an anastomotic aneurysm or pseudoaneurysm associated with graft dilatation is being repaired, a prosthesis that approximates the diameter of the outflow tract, not the dilated proximal graft, must be selected. We prefer to use PTFE in the repair of noninfected anastomotic femoral aneurysms, since this material as currently manufactured does not dilate. Use of another Dacron graft approximating the diameter of the dilated primary graft remains a common practice but may further aggravate the problem, since the new segment of graft likewise is prone to dilatation (Fig. 11).

2. When dilated aortic grafts are being replaced, small segments of the old graft adjacent to the proximal aortic anastomosis may be left in place. This allows replacement of the graft without extensive mobilization of aorta, which is often encased in dense fibrous tissue.

3. The risk of injury to distal vessels may be minimized by using balloon catheter occlusion following isolation of the inflow vessel.

It must be remembered that graft dilatation is a problem inherent with knitted Dacron grafts. Although the tendency to yarn slippage can be minimized by increasing the number of yarns used during manufacture, this is limited by the need to preserve the ability to suture these grafts during implantation.

3. Anastomotic Stenosis

Stenosis caused by neointimal hyperplasia or progression of atherosclerosis occurs with Dacron aortofemoral grafts but with lesser frequency than with PTFE grafts. Progression of atherosclerosis in the profunda femoris or superficial femoral arteries and neointimal hyperplasia are the most frequent causes of graft anastomotic stenosis (75) (Figs. 12 and 13). Stenosis occurring at the proximal aortic anastomosis is usually a result of failure to remove residual atherosclerotic plaque, thrombus, or progression of disease.

These patients usually present with symptoms of acute or chronic limb ischemia caused by occlusion of one or both limbs of the graft. Arteriography delineates the cause of the obstruction and guides direct repair.

Successful management of stenosis or occlusion at the distal anastomosis can be achieved in approximately 90% of patients (75). Surgical repair usually includes thrombectomy of the graft plus endarterectomy of the profunda femoris artery with patch angioplasty (using autogenous vein, endarterectomized segments of the occluded superficial femoral artery, or prosthetic material) (54). Occasionally proximal stenosis may

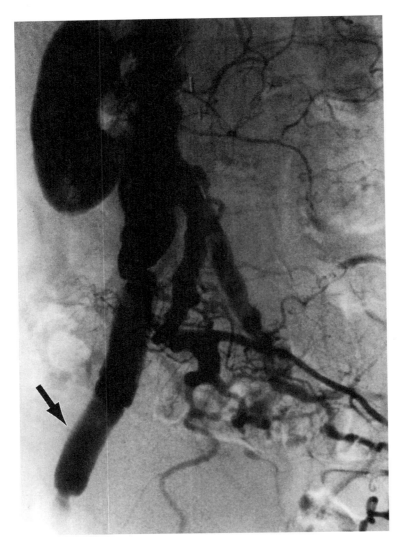

Figure 11 Transaxillary aortogram demonstrating occlusion of the left limb of a dilated aorto-bifemoral graft. The Dacron graft used to repair the right femoral anastomotic aneurysm has subsequently also dilated (arrow).

require replacement of the graft after endarterectomy of the severely narrowed aortic segment. In poor-risk patients with progressively increasing proximal aortic stenosis, placement of a covered stent graft, or axillofemoral bypass grafting may be indicated.

4. Ureteric Obstruction

Ureteric obstruction is a well-recognized complication of aortic reconstructive procedures (Fig. 14). The etiology of hydronephrosis includes ureteric ischemia, kinks, operative trauma, anastomotic aneurysms, graft infection, graft limb thrombosis, and an incidental

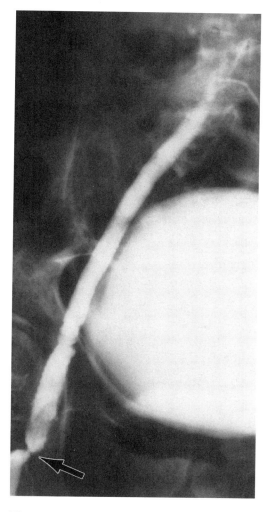

Figure 12 Abdominal aortogram showing a high-grade stenosis at the anastomosis of the Dacron graft at its junction with the profunda femoris artery.

ureteric tumor. In approximately 1% of patients, dense fibrosis, presumably associated with incorporation of the graft, also encases the ureter and results in hydronephrosis (76,77).

Ureteric obstruction may be an incidental finding on workup for some other condition or may present as obstructive uropathy or progressive deterioration in renal function. Evaluation should include measures of renal function and delineation of the site and cause of obstruction by intravenous pyelography, ultrasound, retrograde pyelography, or CT scanning. The position of the ureter relative to the graft is best ascertained by the use of contrast-enhanced CT scanning.

Ureteric obstruction caused by encasement of the ureter by perigraft fibrosis can be avoided by careful positioning of the limbs of the graft posterior to the ureter when performing an aortofemoral bypass. The management of ureteric obstruction depends on

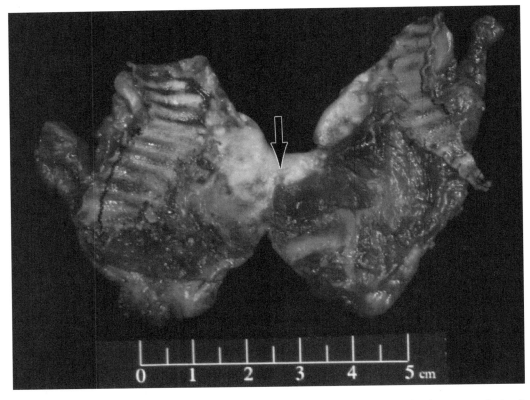

Figure 13 Operative specimen from a patient with anastomotic stenosis due to neointimal thickening.

the physical condition of the patient and the site and cause of the obstruction. Interventional and surgical options include placement of indwelling ureteral stents, division, rerouting and reanastomosis of prosthetic graft limbs if anterior to the ureter, or excision and reanastomosis of the ureter for severe segmental fibrotic stenosis. Infection of the underlying graft remains an ongoing concern with catheter intervention or surgical treatment of ureteric obstruction in these patients.

5. Neoplasia

There are now a few case reports of angiosarcoma developing in patients with Dacron grafts (78–81). The possible contribution of Dacron grafts to the development of angiosarcoma is unclear. Although some experimental evidence links plastic materials with neoplastic change, the evidence in humans is less convincing (81). First, the incidence is extremely low when one compares the number of tumors reported with the number of prosthetic grafts implanted. Second, in the case reported by O'Connell and coworkers (79), the tumor was almost certainly incidental to the Dacron graft in view of the short time interval that elapsed between placement of the graft and diagnosis of the angiosarcoma. However, Fehrenbacher et al. (80) reported an angiosarcoma thought to be related to the use of a Dacron graft implanted 12 years previously. Although the time interval between implantation of the graft and the development of the neoplasm is consistent with a

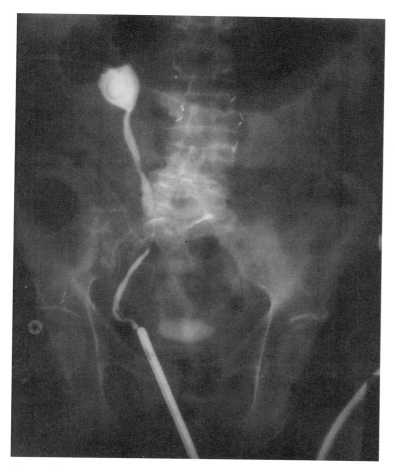

Figure 14   Right retrograde pyelogram shows hydroureteronephrosis with obstruction by the graft limb at the pelvic brim.

possible cause-and-effect relationship, this remains speculative. Nonetheless, although a direct cause-and-effect relationship between the use of Dacron grafts and the development of angiosarcoma cannot be established, continued vigilance seems appropriate.

The diagnosis of angiosarcoma is seldom made antemortem. Progressive stenosis resulting in obstructive or embolic symptoms is the usual clinical presentation. Contrast-enhanced abdominal CT scanning or biplanar arteriography usually will demonstrate an intraluminal filling defect. Excision/grafting and endarterectomy have been advocated for treatment of these lesions. The prognosis is poor; subsequent patient survival usually is only a few months in duration.

II. EXPANDED PTFE GRAFTS

Expanded polytetrafluoroethylene (PTFE) grafts are widely used as arterial substitutes for aortoiliofemoral, axillofemoral, and femorofemoral bypasses. They are also the preferred conduit for carotid subclavian and visceral artery bypasses, dialysis access procedures, and for infrainguinal bypass grafting procedures to the popliteal and tibial vessels when autogenous vein is unavailable. PTFE grafts do not dilate significantly after implantation and thrombus is readily removed with a thrombectomy catheter or lysed by thrombolytic agents. Patency rates at 4–5 years for aortobifemoral grafts range from 91 to 95% (30,82). When used for dialysis access, PTFE grafts have 1-year patency rates of 17–79% (83,84). Primary patency rates for above- and below-knee femoropopliteal bypass grafts range from 39.7 to 61% and 27 to 39%, respectively, between 5 and 8 years (5,7–9). Landry (85) recently has reported a 5-year patency rate of 71% for ringed PTFE grafts placed as axillofemoral bypasses.

A.   Fabrication

Manufactured by mechanical extrusion of the chemically inert carbon fluorine-PTFE, the resulting grafts consist of solid nodes of PTFE interconnected by longitudinally oriented fibrils. The solid-node fibril structure of PTFE comprises only 15 to 20% of the volume of the graft material; the remaining void is filled with air (Fig. 15). Thus PTFE is a porous graft that readily accommodates tissue ingrowth (86).

Continuous deformation, known as "creep," occurs when polymeric materials such as PTFE are subjected to arterial pressure. This was an important factor in aneurysmal dilatation of nonreinforced grafts. Creep occurs in two phases: an initial deformation caused by laxity of the structure is followed by gradual continuous deformation, tending to progress with time (86). Presently, the commercially available PTFE prostheses are made creep-resistant by increasing wall thickness (0.64 vs. 0.5 mm), by increasing the density of the node fibril structure, or by the application of an external reinforcing sheath also of PTFE.

These prostheses demonstrate very little propensity to dilate, hold sutures well, and do not require preclotting; because of their smooth luminal surfaces, thrombus is easily removed.

B.   Healing Characteristics

Although the healing characteristics of PTFE grafts have been studied extensively in experimental animals, few studies of explanted grafts in humans are available, as only occluded grafts are usually analyzed. Experimentally, PTFE grafts are readily incorporated by dense fibrous tissue. The luminal flow surface is covered first by a layer of protein and cellular elements derived from the blood (86,87).

Three distinct processes can be observed at both the proximal and distal anastomoses of small-diameter grafts implanted in experimental animals. In animals with patent grafts, pannus ingrowth originates from the host vessel and extends for approximately 1 cm; neointimal hyperplasia also is often seen. In occluded grafts granulation tissue and thrombus are found at the anastomosis. Clowes and associates (88,89) have demonstrated endothelial cell ingrowth extending approximately 1–1.25 cm from both proximal and distal anastomoses of 4-mm PTFE grafts implanted into baboons at 1 and 3 months postoperatively. Although the tensile strength at an anastomotic suture line between Dacron and the host vessel is entirely dependent on the suture material for its integrity, there is some evidence that healing may occur at anastomoses constructed with PTFE. Quinones-Baldrich et al. (90), using polyglycolic acid suture to construct artery-graft and artery-artery anastomoses in experimental animals, have demonstrated an increase in anastomotic ten-

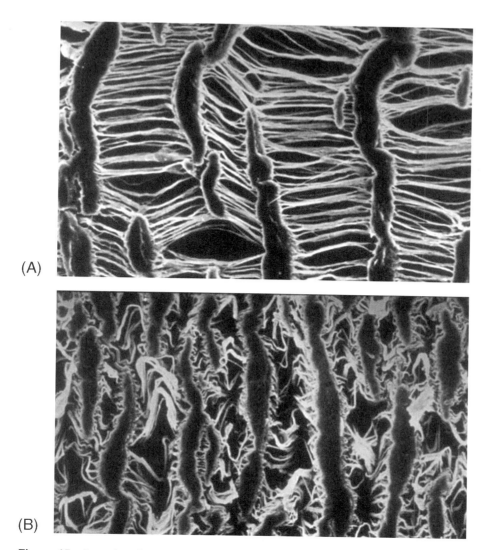

Figure 15 Scanning electron photomicrograph demonstrating (A) node fibril structure of a stretch PTFE graft and (B) the luminal surface of the same graft.

sile strength with PTFE grafts and double-veloured woven Dacron grafts compared with knitted grafts. These data suggest greater anastomotic healing with the former grafts.

Mohring et al. (91) studied explanted PTFE grafts used for dialysis access. They observed distinct differences in the healing between the two commercially available grafts. In nonreinforced grafts, connective tissue ingrowth extending into the interstices of the graft was more pronounced, and these grafts had a noticeably increased cellular internal lining in contrast to the relatively cell-free neointimal lining of reinforced grafts.

PTFE grafts explanted from humans are characterized by an external fibrous capsule of varying thickness, which is present in 39% of explants at 1 month. Thickness of the capsule progressively increases with the length of implantation. Encapsulation, however, is absent in 80% of infected grafts. The interstices of grafts retrieved within the first days after implantation are infiltrated with red cells and fibrin and with proteinaceous material at later time periods. Cellular invasion arising from the external capsule does not occur to any significant degree. Instead, the luminal surface of PTFE grafts is usually covered with an incomplete thin layer of acellular pseudointimal (Figs. 16 and 17). In a scanning electron microscopic study of 298 human graft explants, Guidoin observed bacterial colonization, leukocyte infiltration, and lipid deposition of flow surfaces. Bacterial colonization was present in 56.3% of all grafts examined and leukocytes in 12.7%. Bacteria were only seen in 58.4% of grafts excised for infection. Lipid deposition was usually present in 31.4% of grafts, but cholesterol was detected in only 34.7% of these grafts. In an analysis of 79 explants using Fourier transform infrared spectroscopy, Guidon et al. found no evidence of chemical degradation of PTFE grafts implanted for periods up to 6.5 years. Collagen was detected on the luminal surface of 24 grafts, mainly in the region of the anastomosis. The authors detected anastomotic intimal hyperplasia in only 4 cases (92,93).

The healing response of PTFE grafts used for arteriovenous grafts includes neo-intimal thickening at either the arterial or venous anastomosis, granulation tissue ingrowth along needle puncture tracts, cellular infiltration through the microstructure of the graft, luminal pseudointima formation, and a foreign-body reaction at the graft–host tissue interface (94).

Thrombosis is the major cause of failure of dialysis grafts and is most commonly the result of venous outflow stenosis. Neointimal thickening at the arterial anastomosis, hypercoagulable states, thrombus formation and needle puncture site, pseudoaneurysms, and infection all contribute to the propensity to thrombosis of these grafts.

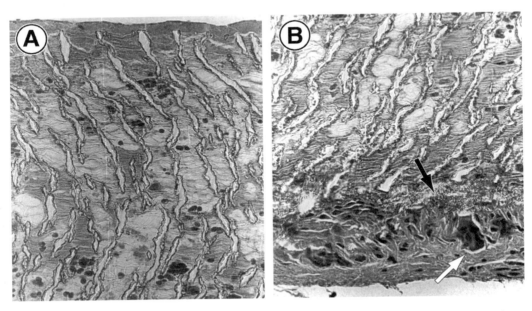

Figure 16 Photomicrograph of the (A) luminal and (B) outer surface of a human PTFE explant. The luminal surface is covered with a pseudointimal layer with occasional cells visible in the graft interstices. Foreign-body giant cells (arrow) are present in the tissue along the external wrap (arrow).

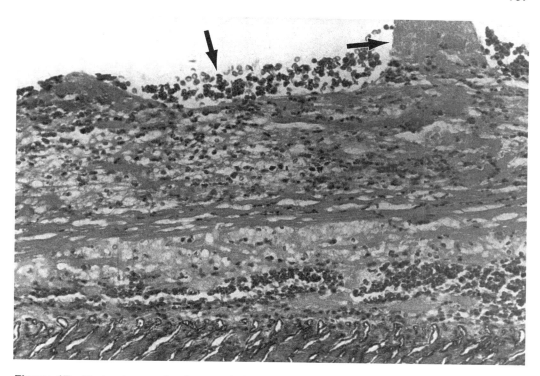

Figure 17 Photomicrograph of an occluded PTFE graft demonstrating thrombus (horizontal arrow) containing neutrophils (oblique arrow) on the luminal surface. No bacteria were observed.

C. Enhancement of Small-Diameter PTFE Graft Patency

The major cause of failure of small-diameter prosthetic grafts is the development of neointimal thickening, most often at the distal anastomosis, resulting in thrombosis of the graft. There are ongoing attempts to improve the long-term patency of small-diameter (<6 mm) prosthetic grafts by modifying either their flow surfaces or configuration of the distal anastomosis. Methods of modifying the luminal flow surface of these grafts include (a) carbon coating, (b) heparin bonding, and (c) endothelial cell seeding. A venous cuff or patch and hooded modification of the graft are among the techniques used to modify the configuration of the distal anastomosis.

1. Reducing Graft Surface Thrombogenicity

Carbon Coating. While carbon impregnation of 25–30% of the wall of PTFE grafts (Carboflow, Impra) has many theoretical advantages in preventing surface thrombus formation, there appears to be no statistically significant benefit over conventional PTFE with regard to their long-term performance (95). Bacourt reported primary and secondary rates of 45 and 53% for carbon-impregnated PTFE compared to 35 and 36% for standard PTFE at 2 years (96).

Heparin Bonding. The development of a thrombus-resistant flow surface to improve the patency of small diameter prosthetic grafts appears desirable. Because of PTFE's electronegative surface properties, it has been difficult to bond heparin to it. Heparin can be bonded onto PTFE using covalent bonding with glutaraldehyde or thermal cross-linking or immobilization onto a Carmeda bioactive surface (97–99). The use of glutaraldehyde has been associated with increased cell toxicity. The heparin content of thermally cross-linked grafts was approximately 0.427 mg/cm^2 in the report by Iwai et al. (98). The walls of thermally bonded heparin grafts are hard, but they become soft when the unbonded gelatin and heparin are removed. Experimentally, heparin-impregnated grafts implanted into the carotid arteries of dogs were associated with increased anastomotic bleeding and a predisposition to perigraft seromas.

Histological examination of heparin-coated grafts at 1 h showed inspissation of interfibril spaces with gelatin and fibrin. By 7 days, cellular infiltration could be observed in coated and uncoated grafts. Only a mild inflammatory response was observed on the outer surface of both heparin-coated and control grafts. One of the theoretical concerns is that the high concentration of heparin may inhibit tissue ingrowth. The heparin immobilized in the fabric of vascular prostheses is released slowly and can still be detected at 5 days (98).

In a recent study comparing patency rates of heparin-bonded Dacron (HBD) with PTFE used to bypass below- and above-knee occlusive disease, Devine et al. reported patency rates of HBD grafts at 1, 2, and 3 years of 70, 63, and 55% compared with 56, 46 and 42% for PTFE. Whether heparin bonding will improve the long-term patency of small diameter prosthetic grafts remains to be determined (99).

Endothelialization of PTFE Grafts.   Following the initial report by Herring et al. (100), there have been numerous attempts to endothelialize the luminal surface of PTFE grafts used for dialysis access or femoropopliteal bypass grafting procedures. The endothelial cells can be obtained from a variety of sources, including human umbilical vein endothelial cells, saphenous, jugular or arm veins, microvascular endothelial cells, omentum, and autologous bone. The cells can be harvested by either mechanical or chemical digestion or liposuction. Cells are either seeded or sodded (ultraheavy seeding) onto the graft surface. Cell retention remains a problem with some of these methods despite the use of enhancing agents such as fibroblast growth factor or fibronectin (101–110).

Endothelialization via transmural ingrowth occurs normally in grafts implanted in canine thoracic aortas by 16 weeks. In humans, endothelialization is limited to the zone of pannus ingrowth within 1–2 cm of the anastomosis. There is usually no transinterstitial full-wall ingrowth. Recently, Wu et al. (111) have elegantly demonstrated endothelial and smooth muscle cells remote from the anastomosis in an explant from a patient with a perigraft seroma, suggesting endothelial cell fallout from the blood.

In humans, mechanically or enzymatically separated endothelial cells (ECs) and microvascular ECs have been used to seed PTFE and Dacron grafts used for dialysis access and infrainguinal bypass grafting in patients with no viable autogenous conduits. Swendenborg (101) evaluated the patency of saphenous vein–derived ECs allowed to grow to confluence on PTFE grafts in sterile culture media and implanted in patients undergoing hemodialysis. In two of the functioning grafts, irregularities developed at needle puncture sites. In a series comparing the patency rates of 10 sodded grafts with 8 control grafts, Berman et al. (112) found no statistical differences in patency between sodded and standard wall PTFE grafts (63 vs. 44%). The characteristic finding in sodded grafts was the marked cellular ingrowth of tissue resulting in a significant reduction of luminal diameter (Fig. 18).

In a phase II study, Zilla et al. reported a 72.9% patency rate for femoropopliteal bypass grafts. This was somewhat lower than the 84.7% 3-year and 73.8% 5-year patency rates reported in phase I of their trial. The inclusion of a larger number of "redo" patients

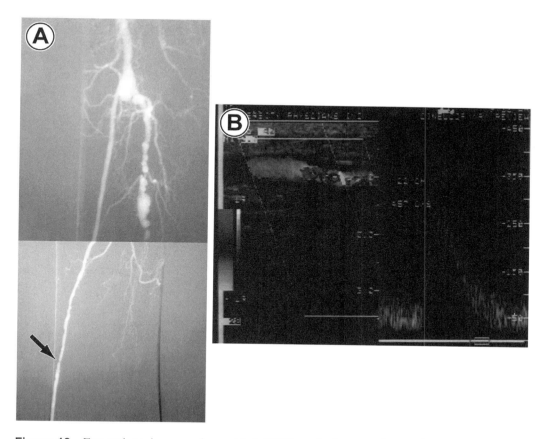

Figure 18 Femoral angiogram of a sodded PTFE graft 4 years after implantation shows irregularity throughout the graft with a focal area of high-grade stenosis. A. The velocities at the site
of stenosis were 457/cm/s. B. The patient refused operative intervention. The graft remained patent
for 3 more years after this angiogram.

and the unavailability of fibronectin for improving cellular adhesions were among the
reasons advanced for the discrepancy in patency rates between the two studies (105).

While technically feasible, endothelialization of prosthetic grafts has not gained
widespread application because of the cumbersome nature of the techniques used.
Furthermore, variable cell adhesion and sterility remain concerns in the cell culture–
dependent procedure.

2. Modification of Anastomotic Configuration

Vein Cuffs and Patches.   Neointimal thickening at either the proximal or, more commonly, the distal anastomosis of PTFE grafts is the major cause of late failure of these
grafts. A number of modifications of the distal anastomosis of such grafts have been used
to alter the flow patterns at this location. There is considerable evidence suggesting that
low wall shear stress, resulting in prolonged particle residence, may be one of the factors
predisposing to anastomotic neointimal thickening. In a study using PTFE aortic grafts in
baboons, Kraiss et al. found that an increase in wall shear stress was associated with a

significant reduction in anastomotic neointimal thickening and smooth muscle cell proliferation (113). Mattsson et al. have shown that high wall shear may actually induce regression of neointimal thickening in the same model (114).

The Linton and Taylor patches, vein interposition cuffs (such as the Miller cuff and Tyrell cuff), and precuffed or hooded grafts are all currently employed to enhance the patency of below-knee PTFE grafts. Taylor reported patency rates of 74 and 58% at 12 and 36 months (Fig. 19) (115–120). Results of the U.K. prospectively randomized trial comparing infrainguinal PTFE bypass grafts with and without vein interposition cuffs showed patency rates for vein cuff and no vein cuff above-knee bypasses of 80 and 84%, respectively, at 1 year and 72 and 70%, respectively, at 2 years (117). In contrast, bypasses to the below-knee popliteal artery showed a significant difference between the cuffed (52%) and noncuffed (29%) grafts at 2 years. Batson et al. showed cumulative patency rates of 65% at 24, 36, and 48 months using the Linton patch (115). In a comparison between distal vein cuff (DVC) and distal arteriovenous fistulas (DAVF), Kreinenberg found 3-year primary patency for DAVF and DVC was 48 and 38%, and secondary patency was 48 and 47%, respectively (121). Neville et al., in an evaluation of 80 PTFE distal bypasses with vein patch, reported 70% primary patency at 3 years and 62.9% at 4 years (120). Current data on the value of patches and cuffs in improving PTFE graft

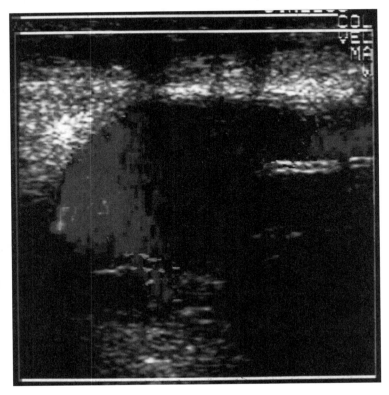

Figure 19   Color duplex scan of a Miller cuff at the distal posterior tibial artery anastomosis of a PTFE bypass graft.

patency are encouraging. Whether the addition of a distal arteriovenous fistula will provide additional improvement in long-term patency awaits further study.

Hooded or Precuffed Grafts.   The results of the hemodynamic studies of Harris et al. have led to the introduction of precuffed (hooded) PTFE grafts (122). Reporting for the North American Prospective Trial Investigations, Panneton found no significant differences in 30- and 10-month patency rates between hooded and PTFE grafts with vein modification (123).

D. PTFE Dialysis Grafts

PTFE is the most commonly used synthetic graft for hemodialysis. Primary patency rates of 17 and 79% at 12 months (stretch grafts) have been reported (83,84,127–134). Secondary patency rates range from 20 to 80%. There are a number of causes of failure of these grafts, including hypercoagulable states, thrombus or stenosis at the arterial anastomosis, and venous outflow stenosis. In addition, needle puncture site trauma (two 15-gauge needles three times a week) results in tearing of the prosthesis, with pseudoaneurysm formation. The needle tracks seal with thrombus and heal by fibrosis and neovascular ingrowth (Figs. 20, 21 and 22). Approximately 220,000 patients undergo dialysis in the United States annually, and this is anticipated to increase by 8–10% per year. Gibson et al., in an analysis of the U.S. Research Data System Dialysis Morbidity and Mortality Wave 2, reported that autogenous fistulas had a higher primary patency rate of 39.8%, versus 24.6% for PTFE at 2 years, and an equivalent secondary patency rate of 64.3 vs. 59.5% (135). In an attempt to improve the longevity of dialysis fistulas, the use of carbon-coated hooded grafts and Taylor and notched vein patches has been employed (128,132,133). Early reports of comparisons between hooded and conventional PTFE grafts show improved primary and secondary patency rates (66.3 and 93.2% for hooded grafts vs. 40.5 and 49.7% for standard wall prostheses). Pipinos et al., in a comparison of the conventional anastomosis Taylor patch and the "notched" vein technique, reported 6-month patency rates of 47, 25, and 41%, which were not statistically different (133).

E. Complications

Early in their use, focal and diffuse dilatation of PTFE grafts was a serious limitation. Although some suggested that hypertension was an important contributing factor, in fact not all patients with dilated grafts were hypertensive. Instead, inherent structural weakness of the prosthesis related to inadequate wall thickness and creep was the most likely causative factor (41,42,86). Modern PTFE prostheses demonstrate very little tendency to dilate (less than 10%).

Late complications of PTFE grafts include anastomotic stenosis or occlusion caused by progression of atherosclerosis or neointimal hyperplasia, thrombosis, and, rarely, pseudoaneurysm formation.

1. Anastomotic Neointimal Hyperplasia

The most frequent cause of failure of PTFE grafts is stenosis or occlusion, most frequently involving the distal anastomosis of femoropopliteal grafts and the venous anastomosis of dialysis access grafts (88). A perplexing problem has been the observation that occlusion may occur suddenly without antecedent symptoms.

Anastomotic neointimal hyperplasia and progression of atherosclerosis are the most frequent pathological findings in occluded grafts (Fig. 23). Careful monitoring at regular

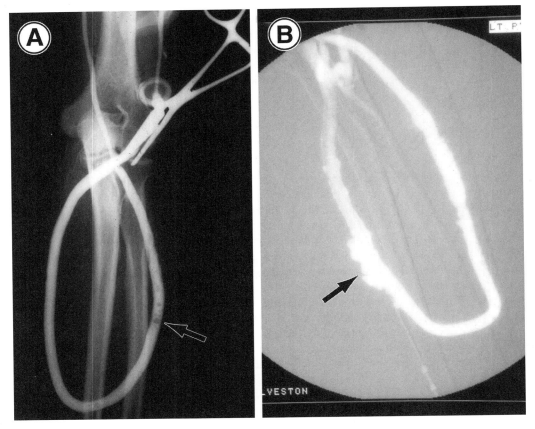

Figure 20   A. Normal intraoperative fistulogram of a recently placed PTFE graft showing some air bubbles. B. Angiogram of a PTFE loop graft demonstrating pseudoaneurysm formation (arrow).

intervals with Doppler-derived pressure indices, flow velocity measurements, and color imaging are essential to detect preocclusive lesions, which are more amenable to correction before thrombosis occurs.

Once thrombosis has occurred, resolution of this occlusive process is essential. This can be achieved either by lysis of the luminal thrombosis with Retavase/Alteplase or by surgical or percutaneous thrombectomy. There have been no prospective randomized trials comparing the efficacy of these newer agents with surgical or percutaneous thrombectomy. Lytic therapy, which successfully delineates the responsible occlusive lesion in approximately 70% of patients with occlusions of less than 14 days' duration, is probably the management of choice in the absence of limb-threatening ischemia (136). There have not been any comparative studies evaluating the efficacy of the newer thrombolytic agents with thrombectomy. The recent practice of combining these agents with a glycoprotein IIb/IIIa inhibitor requires further evaluation (137). Thrombectomy is preferable if the limb is at risk and there has been no significant improvement after 24–48 h of lyric therapy.

A number of interventions are available for managing anastomotic stenoses; here the procedure must, however, be tailored to the prevailing circumstances in each patient.

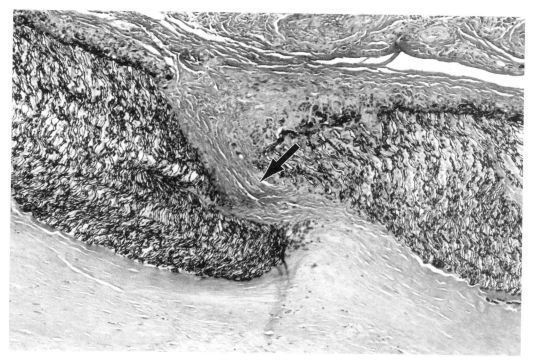

Figure 21 Photomicrograph demonstrating granulation tissue infiltrating a needle puncture site of a PTFE graft (arrow).

Balloon angioplasty and patch angioplasty are the appealing options. However, either procedure is associated with significant reocclusion rates at 3 months. Consequently, our preference is to extend the anastomosis to an uninvolved segment of the vein (for stenosis at the venous end of grafts used for dialysis access) or an uninvolved segment of artery (in patients with occlusion of a femoropopliteal PTFE bypass graft). Construction of an autogenous vein bypass using the saphenous vein or a vein from the arm may be indicated in patients who require a bypass to the tibial vessels.

2. Anastomotic Pseudoaneurysm

Anastomotic aneurysms associated with the use of PTFE grafts are quite uncommon in the absence of infection. Chiesa et al. reported an incidence of femoral anastomotic aneurysms of 1.3% in their series of 2112 patients. An additional patient had an aortic pseudoaneurysm (126). However, we have recently observed several dialysis patients with pseudoaneurysm formation at arteria anastomoses and along the course of PTFE dialysis access grafts resulting from either inadequate compression of needle puncture sites or disruption of node fibril structure.

Retained pieces of PTFE in patients with failed dialysis access grafts or following above- or below-knee amputation are important reservoirs for bacteria. Nonhealing wounds and infected anastomotic aneurysms, which present with local and systemic signs and symptoms of infection, are not infrequent consequences of this practice. If possible, all

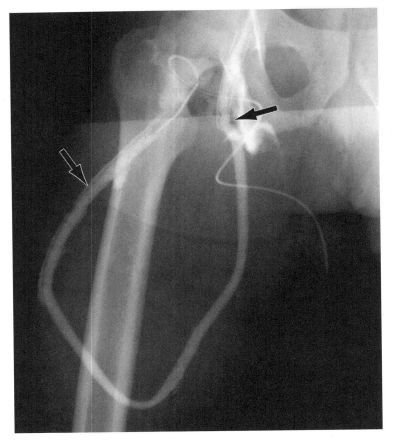

Figure 22 Fistulogram of a PTFE dialysis graft demonstrating the pseudointimal lining the inner surface of the graft (arrow). A stent infiltrated with neointimal ingrowth is present at the venous anastomosis.

residual prosthetic material should be removed from patients with infective lesions in the involved extremity (138).

The principles of evaluation and management of pseudoaneurysm related to the use of PTFE grafts are similar to those for anastomotic aneurysms occurring with the use of fabric or biological grafts.

F. Comparison of Dacron vs. PTFE Bifurcation and Femoropopliteal Grafts

The experience with early PTFE aortic grafts was somewhat limited due to their stiffness, lack of conformability, and bleeding from suture lines. The longitudinally extensible configuration (stretch grafts) has significantly improved handling properties and reduced suture line bleeding.

Prospective randomized trials have not revealed any significant differences in long-term patency between Dacron and PTFE used for aortic reconstruction. Other criteria,

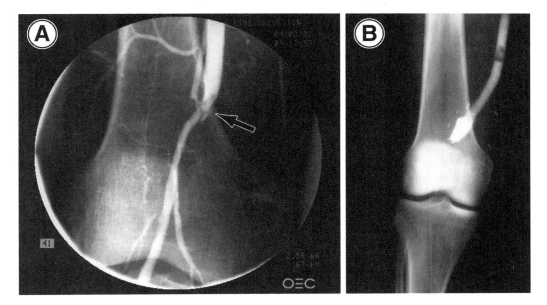

Figure 23 Arteriogram of an above-knee PTFE graft demonstrating (A) neointimal thickening at the distal anastomosis and (B) occlusion of the distal anastomosis. Thrombus is present in the graft.

surgeon preference, graft dilatation, infectability, ease of transection, pseudoaneurysm formation, and propensity to anastomotic intimal hyperplasia are among the factors to be considered in choosing between these two types of prostheses (30,82,124,125).

In a comparison of knitted double-velour Dacron and PTFE grafts, Friedman et al. found that the cumulative patency for PTFE was 95 and 86% for Dacron between 66 and 72 months (125).

In a review of 228 bifurcated PTFE grafts used to reconstruct aortoiliac occlusive disease, Chiesa et al. reported 4 (1.7%) early graft thromboses, 8 (3.3%) late graft limb thromboses, 1 aortic graft infection, 1 femoral graft infection, and 1 aortic and 3 femoral pseudoaneurysms (126).

When using PTFE or aortic reconstruction, the graft edges should be cut with a knife blade so as not to distort the fabric. We prefer to use polypropylene instead of Gore-Tex suture to perform the anastomosis. The graft limbs must be tunneled under slight tension and filled with blood at arterial pressure to minimize elongation and subsequent kinking of the graft. We have encountered very little suture line bleeding except during completion of the second limb anastomosis.

If it has been necessary to do an endarterectomy of the proximal aorta, the proximal anastomosis can be reinforced with a cuff from the body of the graft from which the external wrap has been removed and the graft gently stretched to the desired diameter.

There are few reports of the use of Dacron for femoropopliteal bypass. Massry et al. in a study of 200 grafts reported patency rates of externally supported above-knee Dacron grafts of 76%, 71%, and 50% at 3, 5, and 10 years, respectively. Below-knee grafts had patency rates of 65% and 57% at 3 and 5 years (7).

In a multicenter prospective randomized comparison of Dacron Microvel Hemashield with Gore-Tex, Green et al. (6) reported 5 years primary patency rates of 45% and 43%

and secondary rates of 68% vs. 68%. From the available data, it appears that Dacron and PTFE have similar patency rates when used for femoropopliteal bypass.

G. Perigraft Seroma

The accumulation of fluid around knitted Dacron double-veloured or PTFE grafts, first described by Kaupp et al. (139), is a rare complication of vascular bypass procedures. The incidence of perigraft seroma ranges from 0.2 to 1% of major vascular reconstructions (140). The perigraft reaction is characterized by painless, fluctuant swelling surrounding a portion of the prosthesis or the prosthesis in its entirety, often with erythema of the overlying skin. Grafts placed in extra-anatomic locations (i.e., axillofemoral, femorofemoral, axilloaxillary dialysis access, or subclavian pulmonary bypass grafts) seem particularly prone to this complication and account for 60–75% of cases. Grafts in anatomical positions (aortofemoral, femoropopliteal) account for the remainder (139–149). Persistent perigraft seromas may also occur in association with saphenous vein femoropopliteal grafts, especially in patients with involvement of pelvic lymph nodes due to malignancy or radiation. Ahn et al. (144) documented perigraft seromas in 4.2% of patients with extra-anatomic bypasses, 1.2% with aortofemoral bypasses, and 0.3% with femoropopliteal bypass procedures.

The interval from graft insertion to the clinical presentation of the seroma typically ranges from 1–45 months, with a mean of approximately 25 months (140). Systemic signs of infection are invariably absent and the straw-colored fluid (unless contaminated by repeated attempts at aspiration) is usually bacteriologically sterile. The fluid that resides within a fibrous capsule investing a portion of or the entire graft is biochemically a transudate of serum. In a survey of the members of the North American chapter of the International Society for Cardiovascular Surgery, Blumenberg and coworkers (141) noted that knitted Dacron (54%) and PTFE (34%) grafts were the prosthetic grafts most frequently involved.

Histologically, the tissues surrounding Dacron grafts demonstrate a gradation of changes ranging from an acute inflammatory cell infiltrate at 1 week to mature granulation tissue at 4–6 weeks. Foreign-body giant cells attached to the Dacron fibers are frequently observed. By contrast, the reaction to PTFE grafts is characterized by fibrin deposition with scant giant cell reaction confined almost entirely to the outer surface of the graft (141).

The precise cause of perigraft fluid accumulation is unknown. We have observed two large periaortic fluid collections after use of the stretch PTFE graft, which we believe is related to flushing the graft with heparinized saline to assess the integrity of the proximal anastomosis. CT scan revealed no evidence of para-anastomotic aneurysms (Fig. 24). Needle aspiration of the perigraft collection after an arteriogram to eliminate a para-anastomotic pseudoaneurysm revealed myxomatous tissue and no fluid. Flushing the graft with heparinized saline may be one explanation for the occurrence of perigraft seromas after Blalock Taussig shunts (146). This practice has been discontinued and heparinized blood is currently used to flush the graft to determine if there are major leaks at the proximal anastomosis. However, the fundamental abnormality appears to be failure of incorporation of the graft by the host tissues. Fluid transport through the interstices of the graft, fluid exudation from surrounding tissues, an allergic or immune response, mechanical irritation of the host tissue by repeated motion of the prosthesis, impaired fibrin formation in the graft interstices caused by the use of heparin, and the presence of a fibroblast inhibitory factor in the serum are among the many etiological factors advanced (139–149). Sladen and colleagues (150) have recently demonstrated a human fibroblast inhibitor (molecular

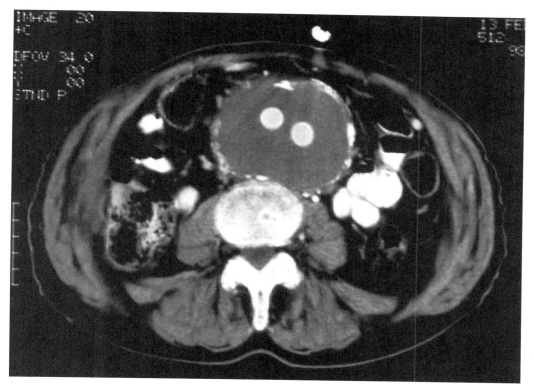

Figure 24 CT scan of a PTFE aortoiliac graft demonstrating perigraft seroma surrounding the limbs of a PTFE bifurcated graft.

weight, 2000 Da) in the serum of patients who develop seromas. Heparin by impairing fibrin formation in the interstices of the graft, may disturb sealing of the graft, resulting in fluid excitation.

Observation or repeated aspiration to control fluid accumulation is successful in approximately two-thirds of patients with perigraft fluid collections; however, secondary infection or graft thrombosis—reported to occur in 5–8% of patients—remains a serious concern (141). Therefore, except in poor-risk patients, removal of the graft and replacement with a prosthesis of different material is recommended. Removal of the prosthesis or plasmapheresis is accompanied by a reduction in the fibroblast inhibitory properties of the serum, suggesting that the graft material may play a role in its induction of the inhibitor. Graft replacement will result in cure of more than 90% of patients. The technique of Lowery et al. (151), in which a communication lined with omentum is fashioned between the graft capsule and the peritoneal cavity, seems a reasonable alternative when the fluid is sterile. Whether modulation of the inhibitor by microfibrillar collagen, ginseng, or high-dose vitamin C will be effective remains to be evaluated (148).

H. Suture Line Failure

The tensile strength of a prosthetic graft-artery anastomosis is dependent entirely on the suture material for its structural integrity. The desirable physical characteristics of the ideal suture material for vascular anastomosis include long-term durability, high tensile strength, a favorable stress-strain relationship, minimal biological reactivity and infection, a low coefficient of friction, and knot security. Healing at the graft-anastomosis interface is limited to pannus ingrowth, which consists of smooth muscle and endothelial cells originating from the arterial wall adjacent to the anastomosis. Although this may extend for approximately 1–2 cm onto the prosthetic graft, it provides little if any, tensile strength. Because silk, nylon, and polyethylene sutures lose tensile strength with time, they should not be used with prosthetic grafts.

Silk sutures were the first used in vascular anastomosis. Moore and Hall (152) reported 25 anastomotic aneurysms associated with the use of silk sutures that were found to be either fractured or absent in their cases. This finding was not surprising, since Cutler and Dunphy (153) had demonstrated deterioration of silk within 2 years of implantation. Anastomotic aneurysms caused by dissolution of silk sutures still may occasionally be encountered in patients who underwent bypass procedures in the early 1960s (Fig. 25).

Braided Dacron and monofilament sutures, such as polypropylene, which do not deteriorate over time, are presently the sutures most often used in constructing vascular anastomosis. However, they will fracture if carelessly handled with instruments (154). Dissolution or fracture of a monofilament suture results in variable disruption of the anastomosis and consequent false aneurysm formation. The latter may rupture or erode

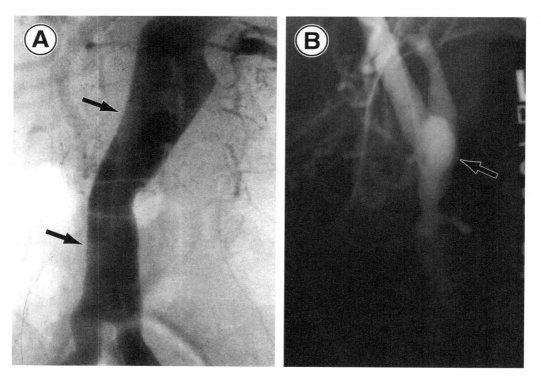

Figure 25 Transfemoral aortogram demonstrating (A) a dilated graft (lower arrow) and an anastomotic aneurysm (upper arrow) in a patient whose anastomosis was constructed with silk sutures in 1966. The femoral anastomotic aneurysm from the same patient is demonstrated in B.

into adjacent bowel, causing graft enteric fistula. Although a polypropylene suture may fracture, this has been extremely rare in our experience (155–158). Careful selection of sutures of appropriate composition and with sufficient tensile strength is an essential first step in ensuring the integrity of an anastomosis.

Polypropylene, the suture material most commonly used to perform vascular prosthetic anastomosis, demonstrates no decrease in tensile strength when subjected to load or exposed to body tissue fluids for prolonged periods of time (154). However, excessive manipulation of the suture with surgical instruments or inadvertent knotting may weaken the suture mechanically and lead to breakage. Indeed, few complications are ascribable to the failure of modern sutures.

PTFE suture is very inert and resistant to degradation by either hydrolysis or tissue enzymes. The inflammatory response, once implanted, is characterized by a mild granulation tissue response composed of a few foreign-body giant cells and a thin capsule, which is usually stabilized at about 30 days (159,160).

I. Carotid Patching

There is increasing evidence that routine carotid patching reduces the incidence of perioperative stroke and late restenosis (161). However, the choice of patch material remains the subject of debate. Saphenous and jugular vein, Dacron, PTFE, and bovine pericardium are among the materials used (162–172).

Proponents of autogenous patches point to their ready availability, ease of suturing and conformability, and a potential reduction in perioperative thrombosis and infection. The major disadvantage of vein patches is the irregularity in their mechanical integrity, which appears to vary with the site of harvest. Another concern is the infrequent but serious complications of aneurysmal dilatation and rupture (163).

Prosthetic and biological patches, while more expensive than autogenous vein, are readily available, resistant to patch dilatation and rupture, and do not have the morbidity associated with vein harvest.

In a prospective randomized study comparing saphenous vein with Dacron in 195 patients undergoing 207 carotid endarterectomies (CEAs), O'Hara et al. found no significant differences in stroke mortality or restenosis rates (162). In a series of 274 patients undergoing CEAs, Hayes et al. found that patients with Dacron patches had a greater number of embolic events than those with a saphenous vein patch. However, there was no difference in the number of patients with >50 emboli between the two groups (163).

In a study of 200 CEAs comparing PTFE with collagen-impregnated Dacron (Hemashield) as the patch material, AbuRahma et al. reported a higher incidence of stroke (0 vs. 7%), carotid thrombosis (0 vs. 5%), and restenosis (2 vs. 5%) in patients treated with the Hemashield patch. The authors concluded that collagen-impregnated Dacron may be more thrombogenic than PTFE. Further prospective studies are necessary to verify the results of this study (164–167).

Comparing primary closure (PC) with PTFE and vein patch closure (VPC), AbuRahma et al. reported an ipsilateral stroke rate of 5% with PC compared to 1% with PTFE and 0% with VPC. The incidence of restenosis and occlusion was 34% for PC versus 2% for PTFE and 9% for VPC. The incidence of restenosis requiring reoperation was 11% for PC, 1% for PTFE, and 2% of VPC (164,165). Archie, in a study comparing vein and Dacron patch angioplasty, reported similar low perioperative thrombosis and stroke rates. Vessels closed with Dacron were more likely to develop a stenoses ≥50% than those closed with vein (168).

There have been few opportunities to evaluate specimens of healed Dacron or PTFE patches in individuals with patent repairs. Shi and colleagues reported complete healing of a carotid Dacron patch in a patient who died of congestive heart failure (169). The specimen was completely incorporated by full-wall tissue ingrowth. The flow surface of the patch, in place for 25 months, was lined by a smooth neointima consisting of smooth muscle and endothelial cells.

Bovine pericardium (BioGuard, Biovascular Inc.) is growing in popularity as a patch material (169,170). In a series of 112 patients treated with a pericardial patch, Grimsley et al. reported no strokes and a 2% incidence of restenosis (>70–99%) (169). The authors conclude that bovine pericardial patches are associated with a low incidence of midterm complications. Reporting on their long-term experience with bovine pericardiual patches, Biasi et al. (170) found no statistically significant differences in stroke rate or restenosis of >60% between vessels closed primarily and those closed with a pericardial patch.

It seems clear that carotid patching is a significant factor in reducing both early thrombotic occlusion and late restenosis in patients undergoing carotid endarterectomy. Each material has some disadvantages: groin wounds (4%), rupture and saphenous nerve injuries with saphenous vein, needle hole bleeding with PTFE, the questionable durability of bovine pericardium over the long term, and the possible increased incidence of thromboembolism and restenosis with coated Dacron (Fig. 26).

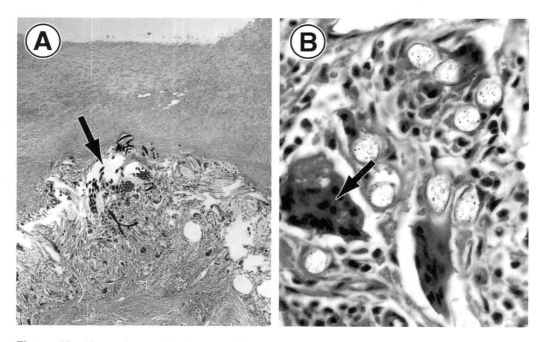

Figure 26 Photomicrograph of a coated Dacron patch removed from a patient with carotid restenosis. Neointimal thickening is present on the luminal surface. The carbon pigment of the guideline is indicated by the arrow. (Original magnification × 100.) Macrophages and multi-nucleated giant cells can be seen ingesting the pigment and Dacron fibrils (arrow). (Original magnification × 200.)

The prosthetic material for "redo" operations is also unclear. In a recent review of 82 carotid reoperations, Rockman et al. reported a higher restenosis rate (2.6 vs. 2.3%) in patients reconstructed with vein than those performed with prosthetic material and recommended prosthetic patch material be used in patients with restenosis (171).

J. Healing of Endovascular PTFE Grafts Used to Treat Occlusive Disease

The use of transluminally placed self-expanding stented grafts has recently been advocated to treat occlusive disease of the aortoiliac and femoropopliteal segments. A study evaluating the safety and efficacy of PTFE-lined nitinol endoprostheses (Hemo Bahn) in 141 limbs in 127 patients reported cumulative patency rates of $98 \pm 3\%$ and $91 \pm 4\%$ for patients treated for iliac lesions and $90 \pm 3\%$ and $79 \pm 5\%$ for femoral artery lesions at 6 and 12 months, respectively (173). These grafts are composed of thin-walled PTFE radially reinforced with nitinol (wall thickness 0.1 mm, pore size 30 μm).

Marin (174), in a series of 26 stented grafts in 21 patients with limb-threatening ischemia, observed that after 3 weeks, organizing thrombus was present on both the intra-luminal surface of the artery and extraluminal surface of the implants. By 6 weeks, the outer surface of the stent graft was firmly adherent to the wall of the native artery. The neointimal lining the lumen of the graft consisted of a thin layer of fibrous tissue with an overlying monolayer of endothelial cells within 2 cm of the graft-to-artery anastomosis. At 3 months, the neointima was present within 1–3 cm of the anastomosis and measured between 40–150 μm in thickness. By 7 months, the graft was well incorporated, with an external capsule. The depth of insertion of the graft–i.e., media or periadventitial plane—determined the extent of healing. Grafts inserted into the media had less mononuclear and foreign-body giant cell reaction than those placed within the periadventitial plane.

Plaque tissue in the iliac or femoral arteries underlying these stents was histologically composed almost entirely of acellular fibrous tissue. In one graft segment, the authors observed extrinsic smooth muscle cell proliferation of sufficient thickness to indent the stent. Van Sambeek et al. noted only minimal luminal changes using intravascular ultrasound to interrogate grafts implanted in the superficial femoral arteries of 12 patients (175).

K. Healing of PTFE Grafts in the Venous System

1. Venal Caval Replacement

Tumors of the liver, kidney, and adrenal gland and soft tissue sarcomas of the retro-peritoneum may all invade the inferior vena cava. Primary or metastatic mediastinal malignancies are the most common cause of obstruction of the superior vena cava (SVC). Mediastinal fibrosis and thrombosis due to central lines and indwelling catheters are the most frequent nonmalignant causes of SVC obstruction. Clinically, upper or lower extremity edema and venous engorgement should suggest the presence of vena caval obstruction. CT used to evaluate these patients has shown that vena caval obstruction may occur in the absence of significant symptoms (176,177). In an attempt to perform a curative resection in patients with tumors invading the inferior vena cava, excision of the vena cava and replacement with ringed PTFE have recently been undertaken. Sarkar et al., in a report of 10 patients, showed that 7 of the 10 grafts were patent or functionally patent at a mean interval of 9 months (176). Although the follow-up period is short and the long-term survival of these patients is presently unknown, vena caval replacement with PTFE does remain patent in the short term. Alimi et al., in a review of SVC reconstruction for nonmalignant disease, reported 30-day primary and secondary patency rates of 79 and

95%, respectively. Significant relief of symptoms was seen in 79% of patients followed long term (177).

2. Portocaval Shunt

Sarfeh et al., in an attempt to reduce portal pressure without abolishing hepatopetal flow, have popularized the use of partial shunts using 8- and 10-mm internal diameter PTFE grafts (178–180). Initially, unsupported grafts were used, but recently almost all grafts used have been ringed, externally supported PTFE grafts. In a series of 46 grafts used in this position, Rypins reported an early thrombosis rate of 15% with PTFE compared to 30–40% reported for Dacron grafts. Thrombosis of these shunts is usually treated nonoperatively with catheter-based interventions (178).

3. Crossover Grafts

PTFE grafts have also been used to bypass obstructed venous segments in the lower extremities in order to relieve symptoms of venous hypertension. The patency or externally supported PTFE grafts can be enhanced by performing an adjunctive arteriovenous fistula. Long-term anticoagulation with warfarin is usually necessary (57,181).

There is not a great deal of information regarding the healing characteristics of prosthetic grafts implanted in the venous system. The desirable qualities of a graft implanted in the venous system include reduced wall thickness, a smooth inner flow surface, and adequate pore size. Patent explants of 60- and 90-μm ePTFE show complete neointimal lining involving the entire extent of the graft. Pannus ingrowth (1–2 cm) is evident at both anastomosis. Endothelial cells originating from perigraft microvessels with widely patent endothelial channels are readily evident (182,183).

In an attempt to improve the patency of venous conduits, investigators have wrapped ePTFE grafts with peritoneum and infused heparin locally. The lined grafts had a similar patency rate at 1 week (86%) as regular PTFE grafts, but patency had decreased to 57% in lined grafts at 8 weeks. Histological examination of the implants removed at 6 weeks showed stenosis of all PTFE grafts due to thrombosis, whereas lined grafts narrowed due to proliferation of granulation and inflammatory tissue between the mesothelial lining and the graft cover (184).

III. POLYURETHANE

The limitations of long-term vascular access using either an autogenous arteriovenous fistula or PTFE interposition graft is that they must mature before they can be accessed. This period of maturation is typically 6 weeks to 6 months for arteriovenous fistula or 10–14 days for a PTFE bridge graft. Because of this delay, a temporary central venous catheter with its incumbent problems is usually required. It is estimated that approximately 2.3 catheters per patient year are needed for the average patient requiring dialysis. In addition to the increased cost of these two-staged procedures, the complications associated with catheter placement, infection, thrombosis, and venous stenosis result in increased morbidity and mortality (185).

Polyurethane grafts, such as Vascugraft/Vectra, offer the potential for early cannulation, thus decreasing cost and morbidity. The Vascugraft comprises randomly oriented microfibers of varying thickness (0.1–5.0 μm), compared to 0.1–1 μm for PTFE, creating pores that communicate throughout the graft wall. Large globules up to 50 μm in diameter are also present. The Vascugraft is thinner than reinforced PTFE (0.46 ± 0.03 vs. 0.86 ± 0.08 μm) and has somewhat less tensile and bursting strength than PTFE. Because of their elasticity, polyurethane grafts show more elongation than PTFE (220 vs. 60%) at their breaking point (186–188).

The Vectra graft has a trilayer design consisting of (a) an inner microporous layer coated with a surface-modifying agent to minimize platelet adhesion; (b) a middle layer of Thoralon to provide strength, flexibility, and sealing properties; and (c) an outer microporous layer to permit tissue ingrowth. In a randomized study of 142 patients comparing the Vectra graft with PTFE, Glickman et al. reported primary patency rates of 55% for Vectra versus 47% for PTFE at 6 months and 44% versus 36% at 12 months, respectively.

Secondary patency rates were 87 and 90% Vectra versus PTFE at 6 months and 78 versus 80% for PTFE at 6 and 12 months, respectively. Some 20–33% of polyurethane grafts were cannulated within 3 days and 53.9% by 8 days. No PTFE grafts were cannulated at 9 days. The authors observed no differences in graft survival between the two grafts (185).

Polyurethane grafts have also been used in the femoropopliteal region, with a primary patency rate of 66% and secondary patency of 80% at 1 year (189). Histological examination of occluded explants revealed that the grafts were surrounded by a capsule of varying thickness. The luminal surface of the grafts were covered with a thin layer of thrombotic material with pannus formation at the anastomosis. There was no evidence of endothelialization of the luminal surface (190) or of any significant chemical changes within the grafts examined.

The major advantage of polyurethane vascular grafts used for dialysis is early cannulation. The disadvantages include the need of a vein of adequate diameter (>3 mm) and the absence of curves or muscle bulk to negotiate. These grafts are technically

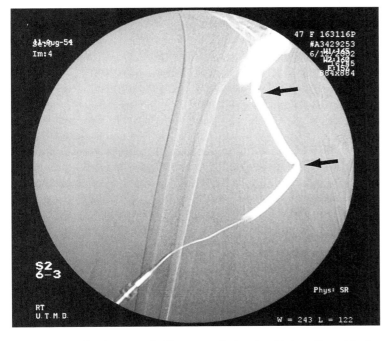

Figure 27   Fistulogram of a Vectra graft showing kinks adjacent to the anastomosis and within the graft.

more difficult to implant; kinking and elongation are commonly encountered. An interposition PTFE segment may be necessary if any turns or bends are encountered in placing these grafts (Fig. 27).

IV. BIOLOGICAL GRAFTS

A. Umbilical Vein Grafts

Glutaraldehyde-stabilized human umbilical vein (HUV) grafts are presently used as alternatives to PTFE grafts for femoropopliteal or tibial bypasses and for dialysis access.

1. Preparation

These grafts are prepared from umbilical cords harvested in the delivery room, which are manually cleaned and stripped. The collagen of cords with acceptable diameter and quality is then cross-linked with glutaraldehyde; soluble proteins and excess Wharton's gel are extracted with ethanol (191). The external surface is covered with a supporting Dacron mesh. Glutaraldehyde starch has been shown to be superior to dialydehyde starch as a cross-linking agent. This results in a more stable graft that is less prone to biodegradation. Five-year primary patency rates range from 53 to 83% for above-knee bypasses. Bypasses to the below-knee popliteal artery and crural vessels have reported secondary patency rates of 71 and 56% (with distal arteriorenous fistulas), respectively (192,193).

2. Healing Characteristics

The healing characteristics of these grafts in humans have been described by Guidoin et al. (194) and more recently by Batt et al. (195) in a study of 39 explants. Macroscopically, they demonstrated irregular thickening of the walls of the grafts, with folds of varying depths involving the luminal surface in virtually all explants. The thrombotic material was present on the luminal surface, especially at anastomosis. The external surfaces of the grafts were covered by fibrous capsules of variable thickness, increasing proportionately with the duration of implantation (194,195).

Scanning electron microscopy demonstrated evidence of lipid deposition in 18 of 39 prostheses; in 13% of the grafts, bacteria were present even though clinical infection was not diagnosed. Cellular infiltrates, most severe when clinical infection was present, were readily demonstrable. Also seen was delamination of the luminal surface (195).

3. Complications

Dilatation. The incidence of aneurysmal dilatation, a not infrequent complication of HUV grafts, increases progressively beyond 5 years. Dilatation of HUV grafts is biphasic: early enlargement of grafts from 4 to 6 mm at the time of implantation to approximately 9 mm in diameter is the norm. Using b-mode ultrasound, Dardik et al. (193) have demonstrated a 21% incidence of dilatation and 36% incidence of focal aneurysms in patients studied beyond 5 years. Cranley et al. (196) found discrete aneurysms (diameter greater than 20 mm) in 11 of 25 patients (44%) surviving with patent grafts for 5 years.

Two morphological variants of aneurysms have been described by Dardik et al. (192) in association with HUV grafts: uniform diffuse dilatation of both the graft and its Dacron mesh or erosion of the graft with rupture of the mesh, resulting in multiple false aneurysms.

The progressive increase in diameter of these grafts beyond 5 years is not entirely unexpected. Reversal of glutaraldehyde-induced cross-linking and immunological mechanisms have been proposed to explain aneurysm formation in these grafts (193). The frequent observation of bacteria within these grafts in the absence of overt infection is intriguing and deserves further study, as it may play a role in aneurysm formation. In their most recent series, Dardik et al. report no aneurysms in 283 bypass grafting procedures performed over a 10-year period.

The guidelines for excision and grafting of aneurysmal HUV grafts are not clear. Dardik et al. (192) state that approximately 6% of these aneurysms in grafts implanted more than 5 years previously are of sufficient size to require surgical excision and repair. However, it appears prudent, from the studies of Cranley et al. (196), to consider resection if the dilated segment exceeds 20–30 mm in size. Excision and grafting of segmental aneurysmal change or replacement of the entire graft if diffusely dilated may be necessary.

Anastomotic Aneurysms. Anastomotic aneurysms have been reported infrequently (1.4%) with the use of HUV grafts and appear to develop more often at anastomotic sites between HUV and dacron grafts (9%) than between HUV host arteries (0.6%) (193). Serial monitoring with duplex imaging, with examinations increasing in frequency beyond the 5-year mark, is essential if significant complications are to be avoided.

Anastomotic Stenosis. Late thrombosis of HUV grafts caused by anastomotic stenosis (in 1.8% of the patients reported by Dardik et al.) is usually associated with neointimal hyperplasia or progression of atherosclerosis at the distal anastomosis (197). Dissection of these grafts can often be extremely difficult because of the dense fibrous reaction that frequently envelops them. If the distal anastomosis can be exposed, a longitudinal arteriotomy is made and extended onto the native vessel beyond the occlusive lesion. Adherent thrombus is removed carefully and the arteriotomy and graftotomy closed with a vein patch. Thrombus within the grafts should be flushed out with heparinized saline solution rather than extracted with a thrombectomy catheter, since these often fracture the luminal surface, thus predisposing the patient to secondary thrombosis. Using these techniques to restore patency to popliteal and crural vessels, Dardik et al. (192) have reported early secondary patency rates of 44–56%. More recently, the authors have used lytic therapy to restore patency to occluded grafts with successful lysis in 85% and limb salvage in 74% of cases (197).

Although bacteria can be demonstrated in significant numbers of HUV graft explants, the incidence of clinical infection nonetheless remains low. In a series of 907 patients, Dardik et al. (192) reported an overall infection rate of 4.3%, which had declined to 3.2% in their most recent update. The incidence was 0.6% in patients undergoing primary revascularization and 3.7% after reoperation. The clinical presentation, evaluation, and management of infection involving HUV grafts are similar to those seen with other prosthetic and biological grafts and are fully discussed elsewhere (192,197).

B. Cryopreserved Allografts

Cryopreserved saphenous and femoral vein allografts are currently used for femoropopliteal bypass grafting, dialysis access, and replacement of thrombosed iliac veins or the inferior or superior vena cava and in patients with peripheral prosthetic graft infections with no other suitable autogenous conduits. Arterial allografts are used to replace the aortic root and thoracic and abdominal aorta in patients with bacterial endocarditis, mycotic aneurysms, or prosthetic graft infection.

1. Preparation and Healing Characteristics

Veins and arteries retrieved from tissue organ donors are carefully rinsed and stored in liquid nitrogen at -120(to -196(C in 15–20% dimethyl sulfoxide (DMSO). Electron microscopy of the vein segments has confirmed their structural integrity after preservation. The endothelial lining of the veins retains its ability to grow in cell culture as well as to produce prostacyclin.

2. Dialysis Grafts

Cryopreserved femoral veins are used for dialysis most often in the presence of infection. In a series of 48 cryopreserved dialysis grafts, Matsuura reported 1-year primary and secondary patency rates of 49 and 75%, respectively, which compared favorably with the 65% primary and 78% secondary patency rates they achieved with brachial artery–to–axillary vein prosthetic grafts (198).

In a study of 22 allograft explants, Johnson et al. (199) demonstrated an intact endothelial lining with evidence of cellular damage and severe rejection as manifested by a lymphocytic infiltrate with CD3, CD8, and CR3 cytotoxic granules in 29% of the explants. The cells lining the lumen and those in the vessel wall were repopulated with cells from the recipient, resulting in either a novel cellular constituency or a mosaic of host and donor cells.

It has been suggested that cryopreserved veins should not be used for dialysis in patients awaiting renal transplantation because a significant number will develop allosensitization. The data, however, appear to be contradictory as to whether use of allografts results in sensitization of the recipient (200).

3. Venous Replacement

There have only been anecdotal reports of the use of cryopreserved femoral veins to bypass occluded segments of the major veins of the upper and lower extremities. Cryopreserved venous valves are presently being evaluated to determine their efficacy in restoring venous competence. In a phase I feasibility study in 10 patients, Dalsing et al. reported 6-month valvular patency rates of 67 and 78% and freedom from valvular incompetence at 56% in patients undergoing femoral and popliteal vein valve transplants (201).

4. Arterial Replacement

Cryopreserved saphenous vein is presently being evaluated by many surgeons as an alternative conduit in patients with inadequate or absent autogenous veins for infrainguinal bypass grafting procedures (202–204).

Patency rates for femoropopliteal or crural bypass procedures range from 36 to 66%. In a recent review of 76 patients undergoing 80 bypass procedures followed for a mean of 17.8 ± 20.9 months, Harris et al. reported primary patency rates of 36.8% at 1 year and 23.6% at 3 years (204).

Patients undergoing femoropopliteal bypass grafting with cryopreserved vein should be anticoagulated with warfarin sodium and antiplatelet agents (203). We have also placed some patients on low-dose prednisone in an attempt to mitigate the immune response. The presently available data suggest that the use of cryopreserved vein in infrainguinal bypass grafting should be limited to those patients with limb salvage or infection with no other autogenous conduit.

5. Cryopreserved Arterial Allografts

Arterial allografts are used to replace the aortic root, thoracic aorta, or abdominal aorta in patients with bacterial endocarditis, mycotic aneurysms, or infected prosthetic grafts (205,206). In a comparison between prosthetic graft replacement and cryopreserved allografts in patients with aortic infection, Vogt et al. reported lower perioperative (6 vs.

18%) mortality and complications rates (24 vs. 63%) in patients with allografts compared to those treated with prosthetic grafts (205). Explanted grafts were acellular, with denudation of the endothelial lining and a low-grade B-cell lymphocyte infiltrate. The elastic tissue was fragmented but the collagen layer was intact.

Lesèche, in a report on 28 patients undergoing treatment for abdominal aortic infection, reported a 17.8% mortality rate and a 67% 3-year survival in patients treated with cryopreserved aortic allografts. Although few complications of the use of cryopreserved arterial conduits are discussed in the literature, anastomotic disruption due to persistent infection and aneurysmal dilatation (3 of 23 Lesèche) remain an ongoing concern (206).

C. Bovine Xenografts

When first introduced, bovine xenografts were used for dialysis access and for femoropopliteal bypass grafting. However, poor long-term patency rates of 50% at 5 years, a 3–6% incidence of aneurysmal dilatation, and a 6–7% incidence of infection when used for infrainguinal bypass grafting have limited their use to dialysis access fistulas (207). There are several advantages to their use for that purpose, including availability, ease of implantation, and immediate use following insertion.

When used for dialysis access procedures, bovine xenografts have a 1-year patency of 26–91% and a 2-year patency between 42 and 83% (208–210) compared with patency rates of 62–93% and 57–85% at 1 and 2 years, respectively, for PTFE grafts (209). Hurt et al. (211), in a study of 140 grafts comparing PTFE grafts and bovine xenografts, were unable to demonstrate any significant difference between the two. Similarly, Reese et al. found no difference in 1-year patency rates (59 vs. 66%) or aneurysmal dilatation (2.2 vs. 2.6%) in a study comparing bovine heterografts and PTFE (212).

The late complications of bovine xenografts used for dialysis access include thrombosis caused by hyperplasia at the venous anastomosis, pseudoaneurysm formation at needle puncture sites, infection that may result in dissolution of segments of the graft, and dilatation of the entire graft. In a comprehensive retrospective analysis of 385 bovine heterografts, Brems and associates (208) reported 160 episodes of thrombosis, 18 cases of dilatation, 18 cases of puncture site pseudoaneurysms, and 8 wound infections.

Thrombosis of bovine heterografts usually necessitates thrombectomy and revision of the venous outflow tract.

Infection occurring within the first month of implantation almost invariably involves the anastomosis, requiring removal of the prosthesis. Since late infection usually occurs at needle puncture sites, replacement of segments of the graft may be undertaken. Dilatation of the entire prosthesis or diffuse pseudoaneurysm may require complete removal of the graft. Focal pseudoaneurysms in the absence of infection can be managed by local excision and placement of an interposition graft to bypass the involved segment.

V. CONCLUSION

The introduction of prosthetic and biological grafts into clinical practice has substantially improved the survival of patients with peripheral vascular disease. However, vascular surgeons generally have not been critical in their evaluation of prostheses used to bypass or replace diseased vessels. The more frequent implantation of grafts into younger patients and the extension of surgical techniques to distal, small-vessel bypasses have heightened the need for durable prostheses and an improved understanding of interactions at the blood–surface interface. It is evident that large-diameter grafts (greater than 8 mm internal diameter), although they generally function well, are nevertheless subject to complications that may lead to loss of life or limb. The long-term patency of small-diameter grafts (less than 6 mm) remains considerably lower than that of their larger-diameter counterparts. Anastomotic intimal hyperplasia and thrombosis of these grafts have not been significantly reduced by the use of antithrombotic and antiplatelet agents. Modification of surface thrombogenicity and modulation of anastomotic wall shear stress by endothelial cell seeding, carbon coating, heparin bonding, or patches and cuffs offers some improvement in patency. However, the long-term efficacy of such measures has not yet been fully established.

A number of changes are presently under way that will influence the long-term results of prosthetic grafts. As greater emphasis is placed on endovascular graft placement, a number of pitfalls loom on the horizon. First, the decision by DuPont to withdraw its polymers from use in implantable devices has removed a stable, reliable source of polyester fabric from the market. The reliability of alternate replacement biomaterials requires careful monitoring. The use of ultrathin prostheses for endovascular grafts ignores the lessons learned from the use of ultrathin implantable Dacron prostheses. In addition, the practice of suturing or welding metals onto Dacron prostheses will result in focal areas of weakness in the material, with a propensity to rupture. Concerted efforts by graft manufacturers to produce durable, nonthrombogenic grafts—along with careful patient selection, operative technique, modification of risk factors, improvement in our understanding of the interaction between the graft and the host tissues, and continued surveillance—are essential if we are to improve the patient's long-term survival and graft function.

REFERENCES

1. Pourdeyhimi B, Wagner D. On the correlation between the failure of vascular grafts and their structural and material properties: A critical analysis. J Biomed Mater Res 1986; 20(3):375–409.
2. Sauvage LR. Biologic behavior of grafts in arterial system. In: Haimovici H, ed. Vascular Surgery 3rd ed. East Norwalk: Appleton and Lange, 1989:136–160.
3. Malone JM, Moore WS, Goldstone J. The natural history of bilateral aortofemoral bypass grafts for ischemia of the lower extremities. Arch Surg 1975; 110(11):1300–1306.
4. Szilagyi DE, Elliott JP Jr, Smith RF, Reddy DJ, McPharlin M. A thirty-year survey of the reconstructive surgical treatment of aortoiliac occlusive disease. J Vasc Surg 1986; 3(3): 421–436.
5. Nevelsteen A, Wouters L, Suy R. Aortofemoral dacron reconstruction for aorto-iliac occlusive disease: a 25-year survey. Eur J Vasc Surg 1991; 5(2):179–186.
6. Green RM, Abbott WM, Matsumoto T, Wheeler JR, Miller N, Veith FJ, et al. Prosthetic above-knee femoropopliteal bypass grafting: Five-year results of a randomized trial. J Vasc Surg 2000; 31(3):417–425.
7. el-Massry S, Saad E, Sauvage LR, Zammit M, Smith JC, Davis CC, et al. Femoropopliteal bypass with externally supported knitted Dacron grafts: A follow-up of 200 grafts for one to twelve years. J Vasc Surg 1994; 19(3):487–494.
8. Johnson WC, Lee KK. A comparative evaluation of polytetrafluoroethylene, umbilical vein, and saphenous vein bypass grafts for femoral-popliteal above-knee revascularization: A prospective randomized Department of Veterans Affairs cooperative study. J Vasc Surg 2000; 32(2):268–277.

9. Quinones-Baldrich WJ, Prego AA, Ucelay-Gomez R, Freischlag JA, Ahn SS, Baker JD, et al. Long-term results of infrainguinal revascularization with polytetrafluoroethylene: a ten-year experience. J Vasc Surg 1992; 16(2):209–217.

10. Guidoin R. A biological and structural evaluation of retrieved Dacron arterial prostheses *US Department of Commerce/National Bureau of Standards Implant Retrieval: Material and Biological Analysis*. 1981.

11. Harris PL. Aorto-iliac-femoral re-operative surgery. Supplementary surgery at secondary operations. Acta Chir Scand Suppl 1987; 538:51–55.

12. el-Massry S, Saad E, Sauvage LR, Zammit M, Davis CC, Smith JC, et al. Axillofemoral bypass with externally supported, knitted Dacron grafts: A follow-up through twelve years. J Vasc Surg 1993; 17(1):107–115.

13. Mii S, Mori A, Sakata H, Kawazoe N. Fifteen-year experience in axillofemoral bypass with externally supported knitted Dacron prosthesis in a Japanese hospital. J Am Coll Surg 1998; 186(5):581–588.

14. Rutherford RB, Patt A, Pearce WH. Extra-anatomic bypass: A closer view. J Vasc Surg 1987; 6(5):437–446.

15. Madiba TE, Mars M, Robbs JV. Aortobifemoral bypass in the presence of superficial femoral artery occlusion: Does the profunda femoris artery provide adequate runoff? J R Coll Surg Edinb 1998; 43(5):310–313.

16. Jonas RA, Schoen FJ, Levy RJ, Castaneda AR. Biological sealants and knitted Dacron: porosity and histological comparisons of vascular graft materials with and without collagen and fibrin glue pretreatments. Ann Thorac Surg 1986; 41(6):657–663.

17. Quinones-Baldrich WJ, Moore WS, Ziomek S, Chvapil M. Development of a "leakproof," knitted Dacron vascular prosthesis. J Vasc Surg 1986; 3(6):895–903.

18. Jonas RA, Ziemer G, Schoen FJ, Britton L, Castaneda AR. A new sealant for knitted Dacron prostheses: Minimally cross-linked gelatin. J Vasc Surg 1988; 7(3):414–419.

19. Kadoba K, Schoen FJ, Jonas RA. Experimental comparison of albumin-sealed and gelatin-sealed knitted Dacron conduits. Porosity control, handling, sealant resorption, and healing. J Thorac Cardiovasc Surg 1992; 103(6):1059–1067.

20. McGee GS, Shuman TA, Atkinson JB, Weaver FA, Edwards WH. Experimental evaluation of a new albumin-impregnated knitted dacron prosthesis. Am Surg 1987; 53(12):695–701.

21. Bethea MC, Reemtsma K. Graft hemostasis: An alternative to preclotting. Ann Thorac Surg 1979; 27(4):374.

22. Cooley DA, Ramagnoli A, Nilam JD, Bossort MI. A method of predisposing woven Dacron grafts to prevent interstitial hemorrhage. Cardiovasc Dis (Bull Texas Heart Inst) 1981; 8:48.

23. Adachi H, Mizuhara A, Yamaguchi A, Murata S, Kamio H, Ino T, et al. Clinical experience of a new gelatin impregnated woven Dacron graft. Japan J Artif Organs 1996; 25(1):214–219.

24. Wesolow A. The healing of arterial prostheses—the state of the art. Thorac Cardiovasc Surg 1982; 30(4):196–208.

25. Guidoin R, Gosselin C, Martin L, Marois M, Laroche F, King M, et al. Polyester prostheses as substitutes in the thoracic aorta of dogs. I Evaluation of commercial prostheses. J Biomed Mater Res 1983; 17(6):1049–1077.

26. Anerson JM. Microvel with hemashield vascular grafts. A preliminary report of the healing response in humans. Angiol Arch Bd 1985; 9:73–77.

27. Drury JK, Ashton TR, Cunningham JD, Maini R, Pollock JG. Experimental and clinical experience with a gelatin impregnated Dacron prosthesis. Ann Vasc Surg 1987; 1(5):542–547.

28. Ukpabi P, Marois Y, King M, Deng X, Martin L, Laroche G, et al. The Gelweave polyester arterial prosthesis. Can J Surg 1995; 38(4):322–331.

29. Farooq M, Freischlag J, Kelly H, Seabrook G, Cambria R, Towne J. Gelatin-sealed polyester resists *Staphylococcus epidermidis* biofilm infection. J Surg Res 1999; 87(1):57–61.

30. Prager M, Polterauer P, Bohmig HJ, Wagner O, Fugl A, Kretschmer G, et al. Collagen versus gelatin-coated Dacron versus stretch polytetrafluoroethylene in abdominal aortic bifurcation

graft surgery: Results of a seven-year prospective, randomized multicenter trial. Surgery 2001; 130(3):408–414.

31. The Canadian Multicenter Hemashield Study GroupImmunologic response to collagen-impregnated vascular grafts: A randomized prospective study. The Canadian Multicenter Hemashield Study Group. J Vasc Surg 1990; 12(6):741–746.

32. Knox WG, Miller RE. Long-term appraisal of aortic and arterial homografts implanted in years 1954–1957. Ann Surg 1970; 172(6):1076–1078.

33. Humphries AW, Hawk WA, DeWolfe VG, Le Fevre FA. Clinicopathologic observations on the fate of arterial freeze-dried homografts. Surgery 1959; 45:59–71.

34. Cooke PA, Nobis PA, Stoney RJ. Dacron aortic graft failure. Arch Surg 1974; 108(1):101–103.

35. Perry MO. Early failure of Dacron prosthetic grafts. J Cardiovasc Surg (Torino) 1975; 16(3):318–321.

36. Blumenberg RM, Gelfand ML. Failure of knitted Dacron as an arterial prosthesis. Surgery 1977; 81(5):493–496.

37. Nucho RC, Gryboski WA. Aneurysms of a double velour aortic graft. Arch Surg 1984; 119(10):1182–1184.

38. Creech OJ, Deterling RA, Edwards S, Julian OC, Linton RR, Schumacker H. Vascular prostheses: Report of the Committee for the Study of Vascular Prostheses of the Society for Vascular Surgery. Surgery 1957; 41:62–80.

39. Eastcott HHG. Rupture of Orlon aortic graft after six years. Lancet 1962; 2:75–76.

40. Hayward RH, White RR. Aneurysm in a woven Teflon graft. Angiology 1971; 22(4):188–190.

41. Campbell CD, Brooks DH, Webster MW, Bondi RP, Lloyd JC, Hynes MF, et al. Aneurysm formation in expanded polytetrafluoroethylene prostheses. Surgery 1976; 79(5):491–493.

42. Roberts AK, Johnson N. Aneurysm formation in an expanded microporous polytetrafluoroethylene graft. Arch Surg 1978; 113(2):211–213.

43. Trippestad A. Dilatation and rupture of Dacron arterial grafts. Acta Chir Scand Suppl 1985; 529:77–79.

44. Berger K, Sauvage LR. Late fiber deterioration in Dacron arterial grafts. Ann Surg 1981; 193(4):477–491.

45. Nunn DB, Freeman MH, Hudgins PC. Postoperative alterations in size of Dacron aortic grafts: An ultrasonic evaluation. Ann Surg 1979; 189(6):741–745.

46. Lundqvist B, Almgren B, Bowald S, Lorelius LE, Eriksson I. Deterioration and dilatation of Dacron prosthetic grafts. Acta Chir Scand Suppl 1985; 529:81–85.

47. Berman SS, Hunter GC, Smyth SH, Erdoes LS, McIntyre KE, Bernhard VM. Application of computed tomography for surveillance of aortic grafts. Surgery 1995; 118(1):8–15.

48. Yashar JJ, Richman MH, Dyckman J, Witoszka M, Burnard RJ, Weyman AK, et al. Failure of Dacron prostheses caused by structural defect. Surgery 1978; 84(5):659–663.

49. Ratto GB, Truini M, Sacco A, Canepa G, Badini A, Motta G. Multiple aneurysmal dilatations in a knitted Dacron velour graft. J Cardiovasc Surg (Torino) 1985; 26(6):589–591.

50. King MW, Guidoin R, Blais P, Gayton A, Cunasekera KR. Degradation of polyester arterial prostheses: A physical or chemical mechanism? In: Fraker AC, Griffen CD, eds. Corrosion and Degradation of Implant Materials. Second Symposium, ASTM STP 859. Philadelphia: American Society for Testing and Materials, 1985:294–307.

51. Rais O, Lundstrom B, Angquist KA, Hallmans G. Bilateral aneurysm of dacron graft following aorto-femoral graft operation. A case report. Acta Chir Scand 1976; 142(6):479–482.

52. Clagett GP, Salander JM, Eddleman WL, Cabellon S Jr, Youkey JR, Olson DW, et al. Dilation of knitted Dacron aortic prostheses and anastomotic false aneurysms: Etiologic considerations. Surgery 1983; 93(1 Pt 1):9–16.

53. Gooding GA, Effeney DJ, Goldstone J. The aortofemoral graft: Detection and identification of healing complications by ultrasonography. Surgery 1981; 89(1):94–101.

54. Clifford PC, Skidmore R, Woodcock JP, Bird DR, Lusby RJ, Baird RN. Arterial grafts imaged using Doppler and real-time ultrasound. Vasc Diagn Ther 1981; 2:43–58.

55. Qvarfordt PG, Reilly LM, Mark AS, Goldstone J, Wall SD, Ehrenfeld WK, et al. Computerized tomographic assessment of graft incorporation after aortic reconstruction. Am J Surg 1985; 150(2):227–231.

56. Brown OW, Stanson AW, Pairolero PC, Hollier LH. Computerized tomography following abdominal aortic surgery. Surgery 1982; 91(6):716–722.

57. Bergan JJ, Yao JS, Flinn WR, McCarthy WJ. Surgical treatment of venous obstruction and insufficiency. J Vasc Surg 1986; 3(1):174–181.

58. Nunn DB, Carter MM, Donohue MT, Pourdeyhimi B. Dilative characteristics of Microvel and Vasculour-II aortic bifurcation grafts. J Biomed Mater Res 1996; 30(1):41–46.

59. Kalman PG, Rappaport DC, Merchant N, Clarke K, Johnston KW. The value of late computed tomographic scanning in identification of vascular abnormalities after abdominal aortic aneurysm repair. J Vasc Surg 1999; 29(3):442–450.

60. Biancari F, Ylonen K, Anttila V, Juvonen J, Romsi P, Satta J, et al. Durability of open repair of infrarenal abdominal aortic aneurysm: A 15-year follow-up study. J Vasc Surg 2002; 35(1):87–93.

61. Edwards JM, Teefey SA, Zierler RE, Kohler TR. Intraabdominal paraanastomotic aneurysms after aortic bypass grafting. J Vasc Surg 1992; 15(2):344–353.

62. Mii S, Mori A, Sakata H, Kawazoe N. Para-anastomotic aneurysms: Incidence, risk factors, treatment and prognosis. J Cardiovasc Surg (Torino) 1998; 39(3):259–266.

63. Locati P, Socrate AM, Costantini E. Paraanastomotic aneurysms of the abdominal aorta: A 15-year experience review. Cardiovasc Surg 2000; 8(4):274–279.

64. Curl GR, Faggioli GL, Stella A, D'Addato M, Ricotta JJ. Aneurysmal change at or above the proximal anastomosis after infrarenal aortic grafting. J Vasc Surg 1992; 16(6):855–860.

65. Allen RC, Schneider J, Longenecker L, Smith RB III, Lumsden AB. Paraanastomotic aneurysms of the abdominal aorta. J Vasc Surg 1993; 18(3):424–432.

66. Szilagyi DE, Smith RF, Elliott JP, Hageman JH, Dall'Olmo CA. Anastomotic aneurysms after vascular reconstruction: Problems of incidence, etiology, and treatment. Surgery 1975; 78(6):800–816.

67. Kinley CE, Paasche PE, MacDonald AS, Marble AE. Stress at vascular anastomosis in relation to host artery: Synthetic graft diameter. Surgery 1974; 75(1):28–30.

68. Kim GE, Imparato AM, Nathan I, Riles TS. Dilation of synthetic grafts and junctional aneurysms. Arch Surg 1979; 114(11):1296–1303.

69. Courbier R, Aboukhater R. Progress in the treatment of anastomotic aneurysms. World J Surg 1988; 12(6):742–749.

70. Carson SN, Hunter GC, Palmaz J, Guernsey JM. Recurrence of femoral anastomotic aneurysms. Am J Surg 1983; 146(6):774–778.

71. Nunn DB. Structural failure of first-generation, polyester, double-velour, knitted prostheses. J Vasc Surg 2001; 33(5):1131–1132.

72. Chakfe N, Riepe G, Dieval F, Le J, Magnen F, Wang L, Urban E, et al. Longitudinal ruptures of polyester knitted vascular prostheses. J Vasc Surg 2001; 33(5):1015–1021.

73. Biedermann H, Flora G. Fatigue problems in dacron vascular grafts. Int J Artif Organs 1982; 5(3):205–206.

74. Watanabe T, Kusaba A, Kuma H, Kina M, Okadome K, Inokuchi K. Failure of Dacron arterial prostheses caused by structural defects. J Cardiovasc Surg (Torino) 1983; 24(2):95–100.

75. Goldstone J. Management of late failures of aorto-femoral reconstructions. Acta Chir Scand Suppl 1990; 555:149–153.

76. Johnston KW. Nonvascular complications of vascular surgery. *Presented at the Seventeenth Annual Symposium on Current Critical Problems and New Horizons in Vascular Surgery*, New York, 1990.

77. Wright DJ, Ernst CB, Evans JR, Smith RF, Reddy DJ, Shepard AD, et al. Ureteral complications and aortoiliac reconstruction. J Vasc Surg 1990; 11(1):29–37.

78. Burns WA, Kanhouwa S, Tillman L, Saini N, Herrmann JB. Fibrosarcoma occurring at the site of a plastic vascular graft. Cancer 1972; 29(1):66–72.

79. O'Connell TX, Fee HJ, Golding A. Sarcoma associated with Dacron prosthetic material: Case report and review of the literature. J Thorac Cardiovasc Surg 1976; 72(1):94–96.

80. Fehrenbacher JW, Bowers W, Strate R, Pittman J. Angiosarcoma of the aorta associated with a Dacron graft. Ann Thorac Surg 1981; 32(3):297–301.

81. Brand KC. Foreign body tumorogenesis, timing and location of preneoplastic events. J Natl Cancer Inst 1971; 47:829.

82. Cintora I, Pearce DE, Cannon JA. A clinical survey of aortobifemoral bypass using two inherently different graft types. Ann Surg 1988; 208(5):625–630.

83. Bacchini G, Del Vecchio L, Andrulli S, Pontoriero G, Locatelli F. Survival of prosthetic grafts of different materials after impairment of a native arteriovenous fistula in hemodialysis patients. Asaio J 2001; 47(1):30–33.

84. Derenoncourt FJ. PTFE for A-V access: six years of experience with 310 reinforced and stretch grafts. In: Henry ML, Ferguson RM, eds. Vascular Access for Hemodialysis—IV. Chicago: Precept Press, 1995:286–291.

85. Landry GJ, Moneta GL, Taylor LM Jr, Porter JM. Axillobifemoral bypass. Ann Vasc Surg 2000; 14(3):296–305.

86. Boyce B. Physical characteristics of expanded polytetrafluoroethylene grafts. In: Stanley JC, ed. Biologic and Synthetic Vascular Prostheses. New York: Grune and Stratton, 1982:553–561.

87. Graham LM, Bergan JJ. Expanded polytetrafluoroethylene vascular grafts: Clinical and experimental observation. In: Stanley JC, ed. Biologic and Synthetic Vascular Prostheses. New York: Grune and Stratton, 1982:536–586.

88. Clowes AW, Gown AM, Hanson SR, Reidy MA. Mechanisms of arterial graft failure. 1. Role of cellular proliferation in early healing of PTFE prostheses. Am J Pathol 1985; 118(1):43–54.

89. Clowes AW, Kirkman TR, Clowes MM. Mechanisms of arterial graft failure. II Chronic endothelial and smooth muscle cell proliferation in healing polytetrafluoroethylene prostheses. J Vasc Surg 1986; 3(6):877–884.

90. Quinones-Baldrich WJ, Ziomek S, Henderson T, Moore WS. Primary anastomotic bonding in polytetrafluoroethylene grafts? J Vasc Surg 1987; 5(2):311–318.

91. Mohring K, Osbach HW, Bersch W, Ikinger U, Schüler PJ. Clinical implications of pathomorphological findings in vascular prostheses. In: Robinson BHB, Hawkins JB, eds. Dialysis, Transplantation Nephrology. London: Pitman, 1978:582–583.

92. Guidoin R, Chakfe N, Maurel S, How T, Batt M, Marois M, et al. Expanded polytetrafluoroethylene arterial prostheses in humans: Histopathological study of 298 surgically excised grafts. Biomaterials 1993; 14(9):678–693.

93. Guidoin R, Maurel S, Chakfe N, How T, Zhang Z, Therrien M, et al. Expanded polytetrafluoroethylene arterial prostheses in humans: Chemical analysis of 79 explanted specimens. Biomaterials 1993; 14(9):–704694.

94. Anderson JM, Bennert KW, Johnson JM. The pathology and healing responses of expanded polytetrafluoroethylene vascular access grafts. In: Wilson SE, ed. Vascular Access Surgery. 2nd ed. Chicago: Year Book, 1988:213–231.

95. Groegler FM, Kapfer X, Meichelbock W. Crural prosthetic revascularization: Randomized, prospective, multicentric comparison of standard and carbon impregnated ePTFE grafts. *27th Global Vascular Endovascular Issues Techniques Horizons Symposium*, New York, 2000:I2.1–I2.3.

96. Bacourt F. Prospective randomized study of carbon-impregnated polytetrafluoroethylene grafts for below-knee popliteal and distal bypass: Results at 2 years. The Association Universitaire de Recherche en Chirurgie. Ann Vasc Surg 1997; 11(6):596–603.

97. Mohamed MS, Mukherjee M, Kakkar VV. Thrombogenicity of heparin and non-heparin-bound arterial prostheses: An in vitro evaluation. J R Coll Surg Edinb 1998; 43(3):155–157.

98. Iwai Y. Development of a thermal cross-linking heparinization method and its application to small caliber vascular prostheses. Asaio J 1996; 42(5):M693–M697.
99. Devine C, Hons B, McCollum C. Heparin-bonded Dacron or polytetrafluoroethylene for femoropopliteal bypass grafting: A multicenter trial. J Vasc Surg 2001; 33(3):533–539.
100. Herring M, Baughman S, Glover J. Endothelium develops on seeded human arterial prosthesis: A brief clinical note. J Vasc Surg 1985; 2(5):727–730.
101. Swedenborg J, Bengtsson L, Clyne N, Dryjski M, Gillis C, Rosfors S, et al. In vitro endothelialisation of arteriovenous loop grafts for haemodialysis. Eur J Vasc Endovasc Surg 1997; 13(3):272–277.
102. Magometschnigg H, Kadletz M, Vodrazka M, Dock W, Grimm M, Grabenwoger M, et al. Prospective clinical study with in vitro endothelial cell lining of expanded polytetrafluoroethylene grafts in crural repeat reconstruction. J Vasc Surg 1992; 15(3):527–535.
103. Deutsch M, Meinhart J, Vesely M, Fischlein T, Groscurth P, von Oppell U, et al. In vitro endothelialization of expanded polytetrafluoroethylene grafts: A clinical case report after 41 months of implantation. J Vasc Surg 1997; 25(4):757–763.
104. Yu H, Wang Y, Eton D, Rowe VL, Terramani TT, Cramer DV, et al. Dual cell seeding and the use of zymogen tissue plasminogen activator to improve cell retention on polytetrafluoroethylene grafts. J Vasc Surg 2001; 34(2):337–343.
105. Zilla P, Deutsch M, Meinhart J, Fischlein T, Hofmann G. Long-term effects of clinical in vitro endothelialization on grafts. J Vasc Surg 1997; 25(6):1110–1112.
106. Sipehia R, Martucci G, Lipscombe J. Transplantation of human endothelial cell monolayer on artificial vascular prosthesis: The effect of growth-support surface chemistry, cell seeding density, ECM protein coating, and growth factors. Artif Cells Blood Substit Immobil Biotechnol 1996; 24(1):51–63.
107. Bellón JM, Garcia-Honduvilla N, Escudero C, Gimeno MJ, Contreras L, de Haro J, et al. Mesothelial versus endothelial cell seeding: Evaluation of cell adherence to a fibroblastic matrix using 111-In oxine. Eur J Vasc Endovasc Surg 1997; 13(2):142–148.
108. Shi Q, Wu MH, Hayashida N, Wechezak AR, Clowes AW, Sauvage LR. Proof of fallout endothelialization of impervious Dacron grafts in the aorta and inferior vena cava of the dog. J Vasc Surg 1994; 20(4):546–557.
109. Scott SM, Barth MG, Gaddy LR, Ahl ET Jr, The role of circulating cells in the healing of vascular prostheses. J Vasc Surg 1994; 19(4):585–593.
110. Birchall IE, Field PL, Ketharanathan V. Adherence of human saphenous vein endothelial cell monolayers to tissue-engineered biomatrix vascular conduits. J Biomed Mater Res 2001; 56(3):437–443.
111. Wu MH, Shi Q, Wechezak AR, Clowes AW, Gordon IL, Sauvage LR. Definitive proof of endothelialization of a Dacron arterial prosthesis in a human being. J Vasc Surg 1995; 21(5):862–867.
112. Berman SS, Jarrell BE, Raymond MA, Kleinert L, Williams SK. Early experience with ePTFE dialysis grafts sodded with liposuction-derived microvascular endothelial cells. Henry ML, Ferguson RM, eds. Vascular Access for Hemodialysis 1995; Vol IV:. Chicago: Precept Press, 1995:292–302.
113. Kraiss LW, Kirkman TR, Kohler TR, Zierler B, Clowes AW. Shear stress regulates smooth muscle proliferation and neointimal thickening in porous polytetrafluoroethylene grafts. Arterioscler Thromb 1991; 11(6):1844–1852.
114. Mattsson EJ, Kohler TR, Vergel SM, Clowes AW. Increased blood flow induces regression of intimal hyperplasia. Arterioscler Thromb Vasc Biol 1997; 17(10):2245–2249.
115. Batson RC, Sottiurai VS, Craighead CC. Linton patch angioplasty. An adjunct to distal bypass with polytetrafluoroethylene grafts. Ann Surg 1984; 199(6):684–693.
116. Taylor RS, Loh A, McFarland RJ, Cox M, Chester JF. Improved technique for polytetrafluoroethylene bypass grafting: Long-term results using anastomotic vein patches. Br J Surg 1992; 79(4):348–354.

117. Stonebridge PA, Prescott RJ, Ruckley CV. Randomized trial comparing infrainguinal poly-tetrafluoroethylene bypass grafting with and without vein interposition cuff at the distal anastomosis. The Joint Vascular Research Group. J Vasc Surg 1997; 26(4):543–550.

118. How TV, Rowe CS, Gilling-Smith GL, Harris PL. Interposition vein cuff anastomosis alters wall shear stress distribution in the recipient artery. J Vasc Surg 2000; 31(5):1008–1017.

119. Kissin M, Kansal N, Pappas PJ, DeFouw DO, Duran WN, HobsonII RW II. Vein inter-position cuffs decrease the intimal hyperplastic response of polytetrafluoroethylene bypass grafts. J Vasc Surg 2000; 31(1 Pt 1):69–83.

120. Neville RF, Tempesta B, Sidway AN. Tibial bypass for limb salvage using polytetrafluoro-ethylene and a distal vein patch. J Vasc Surg 2001; 33(2):266–272.

121. Kreienberg PB, Darling RC III, Chang BB, Paty PS, Lloyd WE, Shah DM. Adjunctive techniques to improve patency of distal prosthetic bypass grafts: Polytetrafluoroethylene with remote arteriovenous fistulae versus vein cuffs. J Vasc Surg 2000; 31(4):696–701.

122. Harris PL, How TV. Haemodynamics of cuffed arterial anastomosis. Crit Ischaemia 9(1)1999;:20–26.

123. Panneton JM. Early results of the Distaflo randomized trial for critical limb ischemia *27th Global Vascular Endovascular Issues Techniques Horizons Symposium*, New York. 2000:I4.1–I4.2.

124. Lord RSA, Nash PA, Raj BT, Stary DL, Graham AR, Hill DA, et al. Prospective randomized trial of polytetrafluoroethylene and Dacron aortic prosthesis. I Perioperative results. Ann Vasc Surg 2(3)1988;:248–254.

125. Friedman SG, Lazzaro RS, Spier LN, Moccio C, Tortolani AJ. A prospective randomized comparison of Dacron and polytetrafluoroethylene aortic bifurcation grafts. Surgery 1995; 117(1):7–10.

126. Chiesa R, Melissano G, Castellano R, Frigerio S. Extensible expanded polytetrafluoro-ethylene vascular grafts for aortoiliac and aortofemoral reconstruction. Cardiovasc Surg 2000; 8(7):538–544.

127. Schuman ES, Standage BA, Ragsdale JW, Gross GF. Reinforced versus nonreinforced polytetrafluoroethylene grafts for hemodialysis access. Am J Surg 1997; 173(5):407–410.

128. Soroma AJ, Hughes CB, McCarthy JT, Jenson BM, Prieto M, Panneton JM, Sterioff S, Stegall MD, Nyberg SL. Prospective, randomized evaluation of a cuffed expanded polytetra-fluoroethylene graft for hemodialysis vascular access. Surgery 2002; 132:135–140.

129. Hakaim AG, Scott TE. Durability of early prosthetic dialysis graft cannulation: Results of a prospective, nonrandomized clinical trial. J Vasc Surg 1997; 25(6):1002–1006.

130. Palder SB, Kirkman RL, Whittemore AD, Hakim RM, Lazarus JM, Tilney NL. Vascular access for hemodialysis. Patency rates and results of revision. Ann Surg 1985; 202(2):235–239.

131. Johnson JM, Anderson JM. Reasonable expectations for PTFE grafts in hemodialysis access. Dialysis Transplant 1983; 12(4):238–240.

132. Escobar FS, Schwartz SA, Aboujoud M, Douzdjian V, Escobar MD, Besarab A, Elliott JP. Comparison of a new "hooded" graft with a conventional ePTFE graft: A preliminary study. In: Henry ML, ed. Vascular Access for Hemodialysis-VI. Chicago: WL Gore & Assoc and Precept Press, 1999:205–212.

133. Pipinos II, Escobar FSI, Anagnostopoulos PV, Elliott JP, Schwartz S. Early experience with Taylor and notched vein patching in the construction of arteriovenous hemodialysis access procedures: Results of a prospective study. Henry ML ed. Vascular Access for Hemodialysis 1998; Vol VI:. Chicago: Precept Press, 1998:213–222.

134. Enzler MA, Rajmon T, Lachat M, Largiader F. Long-term function of vascular access for hemodialysis. Clin Transplant 1996; 10(6 Pt 1):511–515.

135. Gibson KD, Gillen DL, Caps MT, Kohler TR, Sherrard DJ, Stehman-Breen CO. Vascular access survival and incidence of revisions: A comparison of prosthetic grafts, simple autoge-nous fistulas, and venous transposition fistulas from the United States Renal Data System Dialysis Morbidity and Mortality Study. J Vasc Surg 2001; 34(4):694–700.

136. Graor RA, Risius B, Denny KM, Young JR, Beven EG, Hertzer NR, et al. Local thrombolysis in the treatment of thrombosed arteries, bypass grafts, and arteriovenous fistulas. J Vasc Surg 1985; 2(3):406–414.

137. Benenati J, Shlansky-Goldberg R, Meglin A, Seidl E. Thrombolytic and antiplatelet therapy in peripheral vascular disease with use of reteplase and/or abciximab. The SCVIR Consultants' Conference; May 22, 2000; Orlando, FL Society for Cardiovascular and Interventional Radiology. J Vasc Interv Radiol 2001; 12(7):795–805.

138. Rubin JR, Yao JS, Thompson RG, Bergan JJ. Management of infection of major amputation stumps after failed femorodistal grafts. Surgery 1985; 98(4):810–815.

139. Kaupp HA, Matulewicz TJ, Lattimer GL, Kremen JE, Celani VJ. Graft infection or graft reaction? Arch Surg 1979; 114(12):1419–1422.

140. Paes E, Vollmar JF, Mohr W, Hamann H, Brecht-Krauss D. Perigraft reaction: Incompatibility of synthetic vascular grafts? New aspects on clinical manifestation, pathogenesis, and therapy. World J Surg 1988; 12(6):750–755.

141. Blumenberg RM, Gelfand ML, Dale WA. Perigraft seromas complicating arterial grafts. Surgery 1985; 97(2):194–204.

142. Buche M, Schoevaerdts JC, Jaumin P, Ponlot R, Chalant CH. Perigraft seroma following axillofemoral bypass: Report of three cases. Ann Vasc Surg 1986; 1(3):374–377.

143. Bhuta I, Dorrough R. Noninfectious fluid collection around velour Dacron graft: Possible allergic reaction. South Med J 1981; 74(7):870–872.

144. Ahn SS, Machleder HI, Gupta R, Moore WS. Perigraft seroma: Clinical, histologic, and serologic correlates. Am J Surg 1987; 154(2):173–178.

145. Bolton W, Cannon JA. Seroma formation associated with PTFE vascular grafts used as arteriovenous fistulae. Dial Transplant 1981; 10(1):60 (62–63,66).

146. Berger RMF, Bol-Raap G, Hop WJ, Bogers AJ, Hess J. Heparin as a risk factor for perigraft seroma complicating the modified Blalock-Taussig shunt. J Thorac Cardiovasc Surg 1998; 116(2):286–293.

147. LeBlanc JG, Vince DJ, Taylor GP. Perigraft seroma: Long-term complications. J Thorac Cardiovasc Surg 1986; 92(3 Pt 1):451–454.

148. Ahn SS, Williams DE, Thye DA, Cheng KQ, Lee DA. The isolation of a fibroblast growth inhibitor associated with perigraft seroma. J Vasc Surg 1994; 20(2):202–208.

149. Sladen JG, Mandl MA, Grossman L, Denegri JF. Fibroblast inhibition: A new and treatable cause of prosthetic graft failure. Am J Surg 1985; 149(5):587–590.

150. Schneiderman J, Knoller S, Adar R, Savion N. Biochemical analysis of a human humoral fibroblast inhibitory factor associated with impaired vascular prosthetic graft incorporation. J Vasc Surg 1991; 14(1):103–110.

151. Lowery RC Jr, Wicker HS, Sanders K, Peniston RL. Management of a recalcitrant periprosthetic fluid collection. J Vasc Surg 1987; 6(1):77–80.

152. Moore WS, Hall AD. Late suture failure in the pathogenesis of anastomotic false aneurysms. Ann Surg 1970; 172(6):1064–1068.

153. Cutler EC, Dunphy JE. The use of silk in infected wounds. N Engl J Med 1941; 224:101–107.

154. Dobrin PB. Surgical manipulation and the tensile strength of polypropylene sutures. Arch Surg 1989; 124(6):665–668.

155. Calhoun TR, Kitten CM. Polypropylene suture—is it safe? J Vasc Surg 1986; 4(1):98–100.

156. Myhre OA. Breakage of prolene suture. Ann Thorac Surg 1983; 36(1):121.

157. Szarnicki RJ. Polypropylene suture fracture. Ann Thorac Surg 1983; 35(3):333.

158. Aldrete V. Polypropylene suture fracture. Ann Thorac Surg 1984; 37(3):264.

159. Setzen G, Williams EF. Tissue response to suture materials implanted subcutaneously in a rabbit model. Plast Reconstr Surg 1997; 100(7):1788–1795.

160. Gayle RG, Wheeler JR, Gregory RT, Snyder SO Jr. Evaluation of the expanded polytetrafluoroethylene (EPTFE) suture in peripheral vascular surgery using EPTFE prosthetic vascular grafts. J Cardiovasc Surg (Torino) 1988; 29(5):556–559.

161. Moore WS, Kempczinski RF, Nelson JJ, Toole JF. Recurrent carotid stenosis: Results of the asymptomatic carotid atherosclerosis study. Stroke 1998; 29(10):2018–2025.

162. O'Hara PJ, Hertzer NR, Mascha EJ, Krajewski LP, Clair DG, Ouriel K. A prospective, randomized study of saphenous vein patching versus synthetic patching during carotid endarterectomy. J Vasc Surg 2002; 35(2):324–332.

163. Hayes PD, Allroggen H, Steel S, Thompson MM, London NJ, Bell PR, et al. Randomized trial of vein versus Dacron patching during carotid endarterectomy: Influence of patch type on postoperative embolization. J Vasc Surg 2001; 33(5):994–1000.

164. AbuRahma AF, Khan JH, Robinson PA, Saiedy S, Short YS, Boland JP, et al. Prospective randomized trial of carotid endarterectomy with primary closure and patch angioplasty with saphenous vein, jugular vein, and polytetrafluoroethylene: Perioperative (30-day) results. J Vasc Surg 1996; 24(6):998–1007.

165. AbuRahma AF, Robinson PA, Saiedy S, Kahn JH, Boland JP. Prospective randomized trial of carotid endarterectomy with primary closure and patch angioplasty with saphenous vein, jugular vein, and polytetrafluoroethylene: Long-term follow-up. J Vasc Surg 1998; 27(2):222–234.

166. AbuRahma AF, Hannay RS, Khan JH, Robinson PA, Hudson JK, Davis EA. Prospective randomized study of carotid endarterectomy with polytetrafluoroethylene versus collagen-impregnated Dacron (Hemashield) patching: perioperative (30-day) results. J Vasc Surg 2002; 35(1):125–130.

167. AbuRahma AF, Robinson PA, Hannay RS, Hudson J, Cutlip L. Prospective controlled study of carotid endarterectomy with Hemashield patch: Is it thrombogenic?. Vasc Surg 2001; 35(3):167–174.

168. Archie JP. Carotid endarterectomy outcome with vein or Dacron graft patch angioplasty and internal carotid artery shortening. J Vasc Surg 1999; 29(4):654–664.

169. Shi Q, Wu MH, Sauvage LR. Clinical and experimental demonstration of complete healing of porous Dacron patch grafts used for closure of the arteriotomy after carotid endarterectomy. Ann Vasc Surg 1999; 13(3):313–317.

170. Grimsley BR, Wells JK, Pearl GJ, Garrett WV, Shutze WP, Talkington CM, et al. Bovine pericardial patch angioplasty in carotid endarterectomy. Am Surg 2001; 67(9):890–895.

171. Biasi GM, Sternjakob S, Mingazzini PM, Ferrari SA. Nine-year experience of bovine pericardium patch angioplasty during carotid endarterectomy. J Vasc Surg 2002; 36(2):271–277.

172. Rockman CB, Riles TS, Landis R, Lamparello PJ, Giangola G, Adelman MA, et al. Redo carotid surgery: An analysis of materials and configurations used in carotid reoperations and their influence on perioperative stroke and subsequent recurrent stenosis. J Vasc Surg 1999; 29(1):72–81.

173. Lammer J, Dake MD, Bleyn J, Katzen BT, Cejna M, Piquet P, et al. Peripheral arterial obstruction: Prospective study of treatment with a transluminally placed self-expanding stent-graft. International Trial Study Group. Radiology 2000; 217(1):95–104.

174. Marin ML, Veith FJ, Cynamon J, Sanchez LA, Bakal CW, Suggs WD, et al. Human transluminally placed endovascular stented grafts: preliminary histopathologic analysis of healing grafts in aortoiliac and femoral artery occlusive disease. J Vasc Surg 1995; 21(4):595–604.

175. van Sambeek MR, Hagenaars T, Gussenhoven EJ, Leertouwer TC, van der Lugt A, Hoedt MT, et al. Vascular response in the femoropopliteal segment after implantation of an ePTFE balloon-expandable endovascular graft: An intravascular ultrasound study. J Endovasc Ther 2000; 7(3):204–212.

176. Sarkar R, Eilber FR, Gelabert HA, Quinones-Baldrich WJ. Prosthetic replacement of the inferior vena cava for malignancy. J Vasc Surg 1998; 28(1):75–83.

177. Alimi YS, Gloviczki P, Vrtiska TJ, Pairolero PC, Canton LG, Bower TC, et al. Reconstruction of the superior vena cava: Benefits of postoperative surveillance and secondary endovascular interventions. J Vasc Surg 1998; 27(2):287–301.

178. Rypins EB, Conroy RM, Sarfeh IJ. Advantages and disadvantages of polytetrafluoroethylene (PTFE) grafts for portacaval shunting. Vasc Surg 1988; 22(2):88–92.

179. Sarfeh IJ, Rypins EB, Mason GR. A systematic appraisal of portacaval H-graft diameters. Clinical and hemodynamic perspectives. Ann Surg 1986; 204(4):356–363.

180. Sarfeh IJ, Rypins EB. Partial *versus* total portacaval shunt in alcoholic cirrhosis. Results of a prospective, randomized clinical trial. Ann Surg 1994; 219(4):353–361.

181. Sanders RJ, Rosales C, Pearce WH. Creation and closure of temporary arteriovenous fistulas for venous reconstruction or thrombectomy: Description of technique. J Vasc Surg 1987; 6(5): 504–505.

182. Kogel H, Vollmar JF, Cyba-Altunbay S, Mohr W, Frosch D, Amselgruber W. New observations on the healing process in prosthetic substitution of large veins by microporous grafts—animal experiments. Thorac Cardiovasc Surg 1989; 37(2):119–124.

183. Heydorn WH, Geasling JW, Moores WY, Lollini LO, Gomez AC. Changes in the manufacture of expanded microporous polytetrafluoroethylene: Effects on patency and histological behavior when used to replace the superior vena cava. Ann Thorac Surg 1979; 27(2): 173–177.

184. Theuer CJ, Bergamini TM, Theuer HH, Burns CD, Proctor ML, Garrison RN. Vena cava replacement with a peritoneum-lined vascular graft. Asaio J 1996; 42(4):266–270.

185. Glickman MH, Stokes GK, Ross JR, Schuman ED, Sternbergh WC III, Lindberg JS, et al. Multicenter evaluation of a polytetrafluoroethylene vascular access graft as compared with the expanded polytetrafluoroethylene vascular access graft in hemodialysis applications. J Vasc Surg 2001; 34(3):465–473.

186. King MW, Zhang Z, Ukpabi P, Murphy D, Guidoin R. Quantitative analysis of the surface morphology and textile structure of the polyurethane Vascugraft arterial prosthesis using image and statistical analyses. Biomaterials 1994; 15(8):621–627.

187. Huang B, Marois Y, Roy R, Julien M, Guidoin R. Cellular reaction to the Vascugraft polyesterurethane vascular prosthesis: in vivo studies in rats. Biomaterials 1992; 13(4):209–216.

188. Zhang Z, King MW, Guidoin R, Therrien M, Pezolet M, Adnot A, et al. Morphological, physical and chemical evaluation of the Vascugraft arterial prosthesis: Comparison of a novel polyurethane device with other microporous structures. Biomaterials 1994; 15(7):483–501.

189. Bull PG, Denck H, Guidoin R, Gruber H. Preliminary clinical experience with polyurethane vascular prostheses in femoro-popliteal reconstruction. Eur J Vasc Surg 1992; 6(2):217–224.

190. Zhang Z, Marois Y, Guidoin RG, Bull P, Marois M, How T, et al. Vascugraft polyurethane arterial prosthesis as femoro-popliteal and femoro-peroneal bypasses in humans: Pathological, structural and chemical analyses of four excised grafts. Biomaterials 1997; 18(2):113–124.

191. Stanley JC, Lindenauer SM, Graham LM, Zelenock GB, Wakefield TW, Cronenwett JL. Biologic and synthetic vascular grafts. In: Moore WS, ed. Vascular Surgery: A Comprehensive Review. Philadelphia: Saunders, 1990:275–294.

192. Dardik H, Miller N, Dardik A, Ibrahim I, Sussman B, Berry SM, et al. A decade of experience with the glutaraldehyde-tanned human umbilical cord vein graft for revascularization of the lower limb. J Vasc Surg 1988; 7(2):336–346.

193. Dardik H, Ibrahim IM, Sussman B, Kahn M, Sanchez M, Klausner S, et al. Biodegradation and aneurysm formation in umbilical vein grafts. Observations and a realistic strategy. Ann Surg 1984; 199(1):61–68.

194. Guidoin R, Gagnon Y, Roy PE, Marois M, Johnston KW, Batt M. Pathologic features of surgically excised human umbilical vein grafts. J Vasc Surg 1986; 3(1):146–154.

195. Batt M, Gagliardi JM, Avril G, Guzman R, Guidoin R, Hassen-Khodja R, et al. Human umbilical vein grafts as infrainguinal bypasses: Long-term clinical follow-up and pathological investigation of explanted grafts. Clin Invest Med 1990; 13(4):155–164.

196. Cranely JJ, Karkow WS, Hafner CD, Flanagan LD. Aneurysmal dilatation in umbilical vein

grafts. In: Yao JST, Bergan JJ, eds. Reoperative Arterial Surgery. New York: Grune and Straton, 1986:343–358.

197. Dardik H, Wengerter K, Qin F, Pangilinan A, Silvestri F, Wolodiger F, et al. Comparative decades of experience with glutaraldehyde-tanned human umbilical cord vein graft for lower limb revascularization: An analysis of 1275 cases. J Vasc Surg 2002; 35(1):64–71.

198. Matsuura JH, Johansen KH, Rosenthal D, Clark MD, Clarke KA, Kirby LB. Cryopreserved femoral vein grafts for difficult hemodialysis access. Ann Vasc Surg 2000; 14(1):50–55.

199. Johnson TR, Tomaszewski JE, Carpenter JP. Cellular repopulation of human vein allograft bypass grafts. J Vasc Surg 2000; 31(5):994–1002.

200. Benedetto B, Lipkowitz G, Madden R, Kurbanov A, Hull D, Miller M, et al. Use of cryopreserved cadaveric vein allograft for hemodialysis access precludes kidney transplantation because of allosensitization. J Vasc Surg 2001; 34(1):139–142.

201. Dalsing MC, Raju S, Wakefield TW, Taheri S. A multicenter, phase I evaluation of cryopreserved venous valve allografts for the treatment of chronic deep venous insufficiency. J Vasc Surg 1999; 30(5):854–864.

202. Harris RW, Schneider PA, Andros G, Oblath RW, Salles-Cunha S, Dulawa L. Allograft vein bypass: Is it an acceptable alternative for infrapopliteal revascularization? J Vasc Surg 1993; 18(4):553–560.

203. Buckley CJ, Abernathy S, Lee SD, Arko FR, Patterson DE, Manning LG. Suggested treatment protocol for improving patency of femoral-infrapopliteal cryopreserved saphenous vein allografts. J Vasc Surg 2000; 32(4):731–738.

204. Harris L, O'Brien-Irr M, Ricotta JJ. Long-term assessment of cryopreserved vein bypass grafting success. J Vasc Surg 2001; 33(3):528–532.

205. Vogt PR, Brunner-La Rocca HP, Carrel T, von Segesser LK, Ruef C, Debatin J, et al. Cryopreserved arterial allografts in the treatment of major vascular infection: A comparison with conventional surgical techniques. J Thorac Cardiovasc Surg 1998; 116(6):965–972.

206. Lesèche G, Castier Y, Petit MD, Bertrand P, Kitzis M, Mussot S, et al. Long-term results of cryopreserved arterial allograft reconstruction in infected prosthetic grafts and mycotic aneurysms of the abdominal aorta. J Vasc Surg 2001; 34(4):616–622.

207. Rosenberg N. Dialdehyde starch tanned bovine heterografts. In: Sawyer PN, Kaplitt MJ, eds. Vascular Grafts. New York: Appleton-Century-Crofts, 1978:261–270.

208. Brems J, Castaneda M, Garvin PJ. A five-year experience with the bovine heterograft for vascular access. Arch Surg 1986; 121(8):941–944.

209. Andersen RC, Ney AL, Madden MC, LaCombe MJ. Biologic conduits for vascular access: Saphenous veins, umbilical veins, bovine carotid arteries. In: Sommer BG, Henry ML, eds. Vascular Access for Hemodialysis. Chicago: Pluribus Press, 1989:65–83.

210. Sabanayagam P, Schwartz AB, Soricelli RR, Lyons P, Chinitz J. A comparative study of 402 bovine heterografts and 225 reinforced expanded PTFE grafts as AVF in the ESRD patient. Trans Am Soc Artif Intern Organs 1980; 26:88–92.

211. Hurt AV, Batello-Cruz M, Skipper BJ, Teaf SR, Sterling WA Jr, Bovine carotid artery heterografts versus polytetrafluoroethylene grafts. A prospective, randomized study. Am J Surg 1983; 146(6):844–847.

212. Reese JC, Esterl R, Lindsey L, Aridge D, Solomon H, Fairchild RB, et al. A prospective randomized comparison of bovine heterografts versus Impra grafts for chronic hemodialysis. In: Henry ML, Ferguson RM, eds. Vascular Access for Hemodialysis—III. Chicago: Precept Press, 1993:157–163.

6

Anastomotic Aneurysms

Alexander D. Shepard and Gary M. Jacobson*

Henry Ford Hospital, Detroit, Michigan, U.S.A.

An anastomotic aneurysm (AA) is an aneurysm that occurs at an anastomotic interface between a graft and an artery. Although such aneurysms may rarely involve autogenous grafts, they are almost exclusively the result of prosthetic grafting procedures. Historically such aneurysms are believed to be false aneurysms resulting from an anastomotic defect. Extravasation of blood through such a defect leads to a reactive inflammatory response by surrounding tissues and formation of a fibrous capsule. As a result of sustained arterial pressure, the anastomotic defect and associated soft tissue capsule gradually expand resulting in the formation of a false aneurysm. Recently, it has been recognized that an increasing number of AAs may in fact be true aneurysms occurring at the junction of a prosthetic graft and an artery. In this situation the aneurysm results from degeneration of the native arterial wall; this aneurysmal degeneration may be primary (due to inherent structural abnormalities in the arterial wall) or secondary to changes induced by the prosthetic grafting procedure. True aneurysms involving the artery adjacent to an anastomosis have also been termed juxta-anastomotic and lumped together with the more traditional false AAs using the term para-anastomotic. In practice it is frequently difficult to distinguish whether such aneurysms are true or false in nature and the diagnosis and treatment are usually very similar. In the present discussion, the term anastomotic aneurysm (AA) is used to refer to any aneurysm (true or false) occurring at an anastomosis. Regardless of etiology most AAs require repair because of the risk of complications (e.g., rupture, thrombosis) and the resulting potential for loss of life or limb.

I. ETIOLOGY AND PATHOGENESIS

Anastomotic aneurysms may occur as a result of numerous mechanisms or circumstances (Table 1). Typically, there is a failure of technique, graft/suture material, or host arterial wall

---

Current affiliation: Vascular Surgical Associates, P.C., Marietta, Georgia, U.S.A.

Table 1 Proposed Etiological Factors

Patient factors
   Native artery disease
   Infection
   Smoking
   Diabetes
   Hypertension
   Healing complications (e.g., seroma, hematoma)
Material factors
   Graft defects
   Suture degradation or breakage
   Prosthetic graft–arterial wall compliance mismatch
Technical factors
   Inadequate suture bites
   Excessive tension
   Joint motion
   "Redo" procedure
   Endarterectomy

integrity. The most common cause appears to be degeneration of the native artery wall, leading to weakness, fragmentation, and eventual dehiscence of the intact suture line (1). In Szilagyi's 1975 landmark paper on AAs, "deficiency of the arterial wall" was the primary causative factor in more than 30% of patients (1). In essence, the anastomotic sutures simply pull through the degenerated wall—an outcome corroborated by the frequent operative findings of an intact suture line attached to the end of the graft that has completely separated from the native artery. A number of factors can contribute to this degeneration, including aneurysmal disease in the grafted artery, endarterectomy, and hypertension (1–3).

Other patient factors implicated in the formation of AAs include gender, original operative indication, and perioperative complications. In most series, males outnumber females by 9 or 10 to 1, although female gender appears to be a risk factor for recurrent AA (2,4). Patients undergoing aortofemoral bypass for occlusive disease appear to have a higher incidence of AA than patients with aneurysmal disease (2,5,6). Perioperative complications, both local and systemic, are associated with increased rates of AA (1,4,6). Wound complications (e.g., infection, seroma, or lymph leaks) can lead to perigraft fluid collections which prevent full graft incorporation (7). Connective tissue disorders (e.g., Marfan's syndrome) have also been implicated in the genesis of AA following thoracoabdominal aneurysm (TAAA) repair (8).

Infection is an important factor in the development of AAs. By attacking the graft–native artery interface, bacterial proteolytic enzymes weaken and degrade the arterial wall. The possibility of a graft infection should always be considered whenever a suture line aneurysm is encountered. A proximal aortic AA should always alert the clinician to the possibility of an aortoenteric fistula. Seabrook and colleagues have identified occult graft infection as a frequent cause of groin AA (9). They noted a high rate of culture-positive pseudoaneurysms in the absence of clinical signs of infection. Coagulase-negative gram-positive cocci such as Staphylococcus species were the most common isolates. These bacteria have the ability to form biofilms and produce proteolytic enzymes and other destructive substances that degrade host tissues. AAs resulting from infection tend to occur earlier after grafting than do noninfected AAs (3–4 vs. 5–6 years) (1,10).

Material defects, both in graft and suture, are important contributing factors in the formation of AAs. Historically, degradable suture material (silk, braided polyester) is the best-recognized cause of anastomotic disruption (11). In the era of silk suture use (prior to the late 1960s), suture breakdown over time was common, occurring in up to one-quarter of anastomoses. With the advent of modern polypropylene monofilament suture, primary failures are uncommon. However, improper handling of modern monofilament sutures can lead to filament fracture and suture failure. Early textile grafts, which were prone to fragmentation and disruption, are no longer in use, although patients who received them remain at risk for AA development.

Prosthetic graft dilatation predisposes to AA formation. According to LaPlace's law, wall tension increases with increasing vessel diameter. An end-to-side anastomosis effectively doubles the diameter of an artery at the anastomotic site. Dilation of the graft leads to further increases in the effective vessel diameter and may tip the balance of forces in favor of aneurysm formation. Dilatation of Dacron grafts, particularly the knitted designs, is well recognized (12,13). In contrast, expanded polytetraflouroethylene (ePTFE) grafts do not tend to dilate as much (12). Compliance mismatches may subject the anastomosis to forces that predispose to aneurysm formation (14,15). With a relatively stiff, noncompliant prosthesis, there may be preferential dilatation of the artery, resulting in potentially disruptive stresses on the anastomosis. Prosthetic graft materials never completely heal with the adjacent blood vessel. As such, prosthetic graft–to–native artery anastomoses are always more prone to disruption. Autogenous tissues are more resistant to AA complications but are still susceptible if conditions are otherwise unfavorable (e.g., infected field, anastomosis under tension, etc.).

Technical problems are another well-recognized cause of AA. Proper anastomotic technique requires that suture bites pass through a full thickness of healthy arterial wall as well as an adequate margin of graft material. Grafts should be cut to adequate length to avoid excessive tension on the graft–vessel interface. Anastomoses should be tension-free throughout the patient's range of motion. Specific caution must be exercised in high-risk areas (e.g., the proximal anastomosis of an axillofemoral bypass). The mechanical stresses associated with repetitive joint flexion and extension undoubtedly play a role in the genesis of some AAs (e.g., high incidence of femoral AA). Unfortunately these stresses can never be eliminated completely, emphasizing the importance of controlling other risk factors. End-to-side anastomoses are more often associated with AAs than end-to-end anastomoses (2,6,16). As outlined above, an end-to-side anastomosis effectively double the vessel diameter, leading to increased wall tension by LaPlace's law. Sewing to aneurysmal or even mildly dilated arteries should be avoided if practically possible. The risk of juxta-anastomotic aneurysms of the proximal aorta, including visceral patch aneurysms following TAAA repair, may otherwise increase (6,8,10,17,18). The highest incidence of AA in one large study was in patients undergoing bypasses for peripheral aneurysms (14). "Redo" operations also have a higher AA rate (9). Technical errors, along with infection, are associated with early AA formation (1,10).

Regardless of etiology, the presence of an AA at one site is a risk factor for the development of AAs at other sites (2,10,19,20). Schellack and associates noted that 70% of groin AAs after aortofemoral grafting are bilateral, while 17% are associated with an aortic AA (20). Despite the presence of an obvious etiology in many patients, not all patients have identifiable risk factors. The unpredictable occurrence of AAs in such individuals is one reason to maintain lifelong follow-up of all patients undergoing vascular reconstruction, especially when prosthetic materials are utilized.

II. INCIDENCE

The overall incidence of AA ranges from less than 1% to more than 10% of anastomoses at risk (1,2). The type of operation, duration of follow-up, and method of aneurysm diagnosis all contribute to the wide-ranging incidence. In the largest series ever reported, Szilagyi reviewed 4214 arterial reconstructions and found an AA in 3.9% of patients (1.7% of anastomoses at risk). Although AAs can occur anywhere and after any type of bypass grafting, they most commonly occur in the femoral artery as a complication of prosthetic aortic grafting. Iliac and aortic anastomoses are much less frequently involved. In reviewing the Henry Ford Hospital experience with aortic reconstruction for occlusive disease, Szilagyi and associates documented AAs in 5.8% of femoral anastomoses, 2.4% of iliac anastomoses, and only 0.2% of aortic anastomoses (7). Most of these aneurysms were detected by clinical examination. The incidence of aneurysms remained relatively constant over the 30-year span of the study. Others have reported very similar incidences (14). Substantially higher rates of AA, however, have been reported by van den Akker and colleagues in a very similar group of patients undergoing aortic reconstruction—13.6% femoral, 6.3% iliac, and 4.8% aortic (2). By 20 years postoperatively, nearly 50% of patients in this series had developed an AA at one or more anastomoses. The higher incidence of AAs in this report is at least partially due to the incorporation of screening ultrasonography into the follow-up protocol during the last decade of the study.

Others have also reported an increasing incidence of aortic AA (6,16). Utilizing routine ultrasound, Edwards and associates found aortic AAs in 10% of their aortic reconstruction patients at a mean interval of 12 years following initial operation (6). The reasons for this apparent increase are unclear but may well relate to increasing patient longevity in addition to more aggressive screening.

Visceral patch AA following thoracoabdominal aortic aneurysm (TAAA) repair utilizing the Crawford inclusion technique is a type of intra-abdominal AA that has only recently been recognized. A 2001 report from Johns Hopkins documented the presence of such aneurysms in 7.5% of patients (8 of 107) undergoing TAAA repair after a mean follow-up of 6.5 years (8).

Although certain types of AA are being recognized with increasing frequency, the incidence of femoral AA may actually be decreasing. A recent review of our registry revealed a declining number of femoral AA repairs over the last decade despite a steady increase in overall open procedures. Reasons for this decline are unclear but may include improved technique and materials as well as a better understanding of the risk factors associated with AA formation (see Sec. VI, below).

III. CLINICAL PRESENTATION AND DIAGNOSIS

The clinical presentation of AA depends on the location, size, and status of the aneurysm. Symptoms, when they occur, are usually similar to those of degenerative aneurysms at the same location. Femoral AAs most commonly present as an asymptomatic, pulsatile groin mass; patients note an enlarging mass associated with the scar from their previous surgery. Small femoral AAs may be first detected by the clinician during routine follow-up. Rarely do they grow large enough to cause symptoms from nerve compression or venous obstruction. Occasionally femoral AAs present urgently as rapidly enlarging, painful masses or with symptoms of limb ischemia. Ischemic complications result from thromboembolism of associated mural thrombus. Intrabdominal AAs usually remain clinically silent until they grow to a very large size or are detected on cross-sectional imaging studies. Occasionally they present urgently, most frequently with rupture and hemorrhage (2). Because associated scar tissue tends to tether adjacent structures to the prosthetic graft–arterial interface, intrabdominal AAs have a greater tendency to present with fistula formation or compressive symptoms than do degenerative aneurysms. Aortoenteric fistula from erosion of a proximal aortic suture line AA into the overlying, adherent duodenum is the most frequently recognized manifestation of this phenomenon. Hydronephrosis from ureteral entrapment or iliac vein obstruction can result from iliac AAs.

The mean interval from the time of aortic reconstruction to the diagnosis of an AA varies with location. Femoral AAs usually present within 5–6 years, while intrabdominal AAs present 8–10 years after the initial reconstruction (2,6,17,20,21). Earlier presentations are associated with technical error, infection, and recurrent AAs (1,4,10). The presence of risk factors for AA (as discussed above) should heighten one's index of suspicion that an AA may be present. In particular, patients who have developed an AA at one site are at increased risk for developing another AA (2,10,19,20) (Fig. 1). Patients with an AA are overwhelmingly male, with an average age of 62 years (2).

In most patients the diagnosis of a femoral AA is made by physical examination. In questionable cases or obese patients, duplex ultrasound can be helpful in confirming the diagnosis. Even in routine cases, duplex scanning is useful in sizing the aneurysm and documenting the presence of mural thrombus—information that can be helpful in deciding when to intervene. In contrast, intrabdominal AAs are frequently not detectable by physical examination and more commonly present with symptoms (e.g., abdominal or back pain) and/or complications (e.g., rupture, fistula formation) (10,18,21). Ultrasound and cross-sectional imaging studies remain the most commonly employed diagnostic tests. Angiography lacks the sensitivity of other imaging modalities for the diagnosis of AA but is extremely helpful for preoperative planning.

A. Surveillance

The optimal approach to AA is early detection and elective operative repair to avoid the morbidity/mortality associated with urgent presentations. An aggressive screening program is the best way to make an early diagnosis. Our approach combines yearly physical examination with selective ultrasonography or computed tomography (CT) scanning. Since most femoral AAs are detectable on physical examination routine screening with ultrasound is not necessary. In contrast, intra-abdominal AAs are rarely apparent on physical examination unless they are large; routine screening with ultrasonography or CT scanning is necessary (6,10,18). We currently favor CT scanning. Because most intrabdominal AAs occur as a late (8–10 years) complication of aortic grafting, it seems reasonable to obtain a first surveillance study at 5 years. Patients with risk factors for developing an early AA (e.g., previous AA repair, complicated perioperative course) should be screened earlier (2–3 years postoperatively) (10). Subsequent studies can be obtained on an annual or biannual basis depending on circumstances. Observation with surveillance may be reasonable in patients with very small intrabdominal AAs or those who are poor operative candidates.

IV. MANAGEMENT

Treatment is indicated to prevent continuing expansion and rupture or limb-threatening thromboembolic complications. The natural history of AAs differs from that of degenerative aneurysms in that AAs seem to grow more rapidly and unpredictably. The threshold for intervention may therefore be lower than for a degenerative aneurysm of similar size.

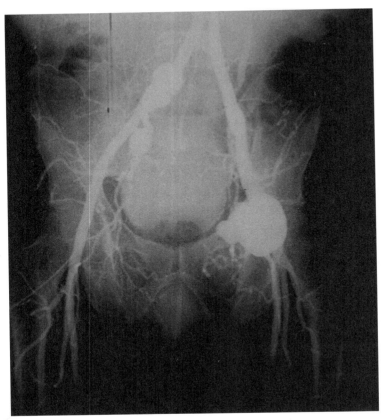

Figure 1 Arteriogram with right aortoiliac and left aortofemoral anastomotic aneurysms and right hypogastric artery true aneurysm.

Many authors feel that the presence of an AA in itself is an indication for repair because of the excess morbidity and mortality associated with conservative follow-up and emergency surgery (5). However, as detailed earlier, not all AAs are false aneurysms and therefore may not be at the same risk for rapid expansion, complications, etc. A selective approach for small AAs may be reasonable assuming that patients are carefully followed at regular intervals (20).

Because complications are uncommon with a femoral AA less than 2 cm in diameter, most authorities do not consider repair of groin AAs until they reach at least 2 cm in diameter (1). Even at this size, if they are stable and without significant intraluminal thrombus, such aneurysms can probably be safely followed with serial duplex scanning. Symptomatic aneurysms or those larger than 2.0–2.5 cm or containing significant mural thrombus should be repaired when diagnosed. Because most intra-abdominal AAs are large when detected, they should also be considered for repair at the time of diagnosis. The management of small intra-abdominal AAs is controversial. Szilagyi has recommended that aortoiliac AAs less than 50% the diameter of the host artery could be safely followed (1). Rapid expansion of small aortic AAs (<4 cm), however, has been reported (21). Patients with an intra-abdominal AA in whom repair is not performed at the time of diagnosis should be followed very closely with imaging studies every 6 months. Occasionally patients with severe comorbidities and limited life expectancy are managed nonoperatively.

Careful preoperative assessment is essential prior to operative intervention. Many patients are a decade older than they were at the time of their original procedure, and associated scarring can greatly increase the technical complexity of operation. High-quality angiography is essential to define the patient's anatomy and allows selection of the optimal surgical approach and method of repair. Cross-sectional imaging studies should be obtained for all intra-abdominal AAs. Besides providing important information on the size and location of the aneurysm, such studies can identify associated pathology, which may alter the conduct of the repair (e.g., perigraft fluid, ureteral entrapment with hydronephrosis). Spiral CT scanning with three-dimensional reconstruction is particularly helpful and has recently eliminated the need for aortography on a high percentage of our abdominal aortic aneurysm patients. Prior to surgery, an attempt should be made to review old operative notes if available. In addition, the operating surgeon should always make a risk assessment as to the chances of graft infection being the cause of the AA. The operative approach for AAs associated with graft infections is much different than that for sterile AAs.

A. Operative Repair

The basic principles of operative management for AAs are the same regardless of their location. The "redo" nature of these procedures makes them technically challenging to perform, even for experienced vascular surgeons. Sharp scalpel dissection is preferred because of the associated, often dense scar tissue. Dissection must be precise to minimize damage to adjacent structures and arterial branches. In severely scarred operative fields, care must be taken to avoid the "easier" dissection plane sometimes found between the adventitia and media; such "exarterectomy" makes subsequent reconstruction extremely difficult. In contrast, dissection of most prosthetic grafts is greatly simplified by entry through an enveloping pseudocapsule that can be stripped from the graft. Proximal control is usually best obtained at a site somewhat removed from the origin of the aneurysm. This approach avoids the most significant scarring, reduces the risk of inadvertent entry into the aneurysm, and provides an adequate cuff of proximal graft or artery for subsequent repair. With severe scarring, distal control is sometimes easier to obtain from within the opened aneurysm using balloon occlusion catheters (or a Foley catheter for the aorta).

During exposure, evidence of graft infection should always be carefully sought (e.g., nonincorporation of the graft, perigraft fluid) and appropriate samples (both fluid and aneursym wall) sent for culture and Gram's stain. We do not routinely sonicate our samples prior to culture unless we are dealing with a recurrent aneurysm (9). Once the aneurysm is open, an attempt should be made to determine the cause of anastomotic disruption if possible. Simple suture repair of a small anastomotic defect can occasionally be considered but is usually not successful in the long term. In the vast majority of cases, the most reliable method of repair is placement of a new interposition graft between the old graft and the host artery.

Segments of healthy, uninvolved artery and graft should be cleared of scar tissue in preparation for anastomosis. In some situations it is simply easier to excise the entire aneurysm and associated scar tissue (e.g., groin AA), while in others such debridement is too risky (e.g., a proximal aortic aneurysm with adherence to bowel). Whenever there is significant concern about the presence of infection, however, more rather than less debridement would seem to be appropriate. The choice of graft material is probably unimportant, although there is some theoretical and clinical support for using ePTFE, which offers improved resistance to infection and less propensity to dilate compared to Dacron (12,22,23). Anastomoses should be tension-free, taking generous, evenly spaced bites into healthy arterial wall. If the arterial lumen is significantly compromised by plaque, endarterectomy should not be avoided because of fears of a recurrent AA; leaving significant plaque behind risks future graft thrombosis. End-to-end anastomoses are preferred over end-to-side for the theoretical reasons discussed above in Sec. I; however, no study has ever shown the superiority of one anastomotic configuration over another in the prevention of recurrent aneurysm formation.

B. Femoral Anastomotic Aneurysms

Most femoral aneurysms can be safely approached through the old groin incision. Occasionally, with larger or acutely expanded aneurysms, it is safer to obtain proximal control through a suprainguinal, extraperitoneal approach. With badly scarred groins, balloon occlusion catheters are helpful not only for distal control but also for controlling bleeding from a patent proximal common femoral artery. Repair is usually easier after excision of the pseudoaneurysm cavity and associated scar, taking care to avoid injury to the femoral vein and nerve. Reconstruction is accomplished with an interposition graft from the transected graft limb proximally to the outflow vessel(s) distally. The profunda femoris is frequently the only outflow vessel and a local endarterectomy or profundoplasty may be needed. Concomitant popliteal/tibial bypass is rarely necessary in our experience (1). Rarely, a patent proximal common femoral artery is supplying critical pelvic perfusion through retrograde flow. In this situation it may be necessary to maintain femoral artery continuity by inserting an interposition graft between the proximal common femoral artery and the distal outflow arteries and suturing a new graft extension to this prosthetic "femoral artery." With large or acutely expanded groin aneurysms, obtaining adequate coverage with healthy skin and soft tissue can be problematic; sartorius myoplasty may be helpful in this situation.

C. Aortoiliac Anastomotic Aneurysms

Proximal aortic suture line aneurysms can be extremely challenging to repair because of their frequent encroachment on the renal arteries and their occasional involvement of the pararenal/visceral aorta. Such aneurysms present problems in terms of optimal exposure, site of proximal aortic clamping, and avoidance of vital organ ischemic complications. A complete discussion of these issues is beyond the scope of this chapter, but a brief description of our approach may be worthwhile. Although some of these aneurysms can be safely accessed through a standard transabdominal inframesocolic approach, more extensive proximal abdominal aortic exposure is frequently needed (Fig. 2). We have found an extended left flank retropertioneal approach invaluable in dealing with these aneurysms (24). This exposure not only provides excellent access to the entire abdominal aorta (from diaphragm to bifurcation) but also allows an approach to the aneurysm through undissected tissue planes, thus minimizing risk to adjacent structures (e.g., duodenum, left renal vein), that may be involved in scar tissue. Aortic cross-clamping at a suprarenal or more proximal level is frequently necessary in the repair of these

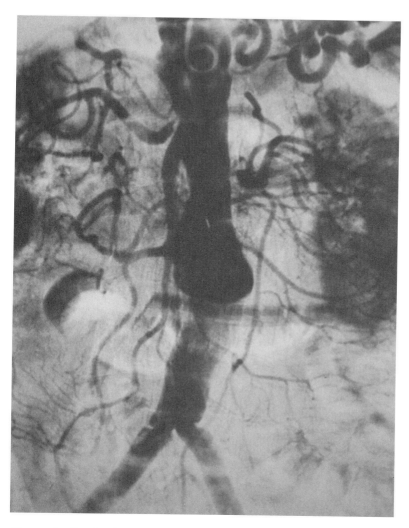

Figure 2 Proximal aortic anastomotic aneurysm.

aneurysms, and appropriate precautions should be taken to minimize the risks of vital organ ischemia and increased cardiac stress (10,17,18). Unless the pararenal aorta is involved in the aneurysmal process, there is usually a short segment of infrarenal aorta available for anastomosis to an interposition graft. If a suprarenal or more proximal aortic clamp has been used, it can be moved on to this graft following completion of this anastomosis to minimize renal (and visceral) ischemia. The distal anastomosis is performed to the old graft after freeing it from its pseudocapsule and resecting any obvious redundancy. No attempt should be made to excise the aneurysm cavity or associated scar because of risk of injury to adjacent structures.

Iliac AAs can be approached either transperitoneally or through an extraperitoneal lower abdominal incision, depending upon size, location, and potential involvement of

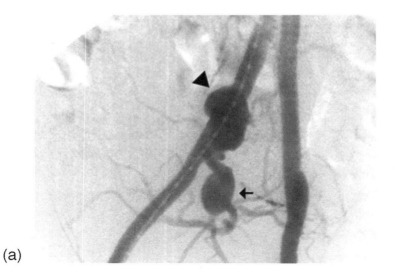

(a)

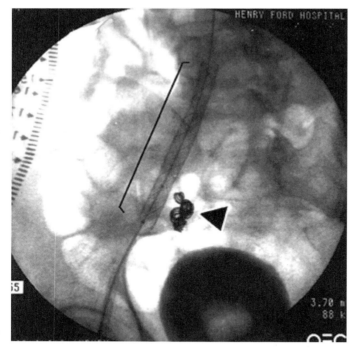

(b)

Figure 3 Endovascular treatment. (a). Iliac anastomotic aneurysm and hypogastric artery true aneurysm. (b). Covered stent (bracket) and embolized coils in hypogastric aneurysm (arrowhead). (c). Completion artiogram with both aneurysms excluded.

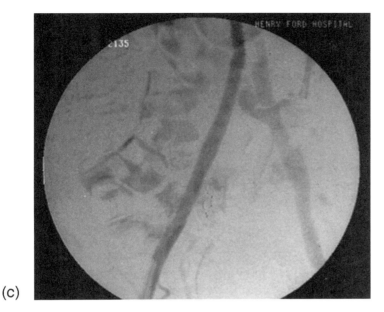

(c)

Figure 3 Continued.

adjacent structures. Because of their proximity to these aneurysms, the ureters are always at risk during operative repair. Routine placement of a ureteral stent on the involved side has proved invaluable in minimizing the risk of injury. Repair follows the guidelines outlined previously. In the rare situation where hypogastric perfusion must be maintained and the aneurysm involves the iliac bifurcation, the interposition graft can be sewn end-to-end to the hypogastric artery distally and the external iliac artery reimplanted into the side of the graft. Again, no attempt should be made to resect or debride the pseudoaneurysmal cavity unless infection is strongly suspected.

D. Endovascular Repair

The repair of some intra-abdominal AAs has been greatly simplified by the recent introduction of endoluminal stent graft techniques. The main anatomical restriction for endovascular repair is the requirement for an adequate proximal "landing zone." While this requirement is not a concern for most iliac AAs, it is necessary for many proximal aortic suture line aneurysms that encroach on the renal arteries. Transrenally based stent grafts may eliminate this constraint for many patients in the future. Currently, in patients with suitable anatomy, this safer and less invasive approach holds great promise to avoid the morbidity and mortality associated with open repairs (25,26). An example of a patient who underwent successful endoluminal repair of an iliac AA is shown in Figure 3.

E. Visceral Patch AA Following TAAA

Perhaps the most technically challenging AAs to repair are those involving the visceral patch following TAAA surgery (Fig. 4). In addition to the scarring associated with any AA, these repairs are also complicated by the extensive exposure and obligatory periods of prolonged vital organ ischemia required. There are several reconstruction options, but all

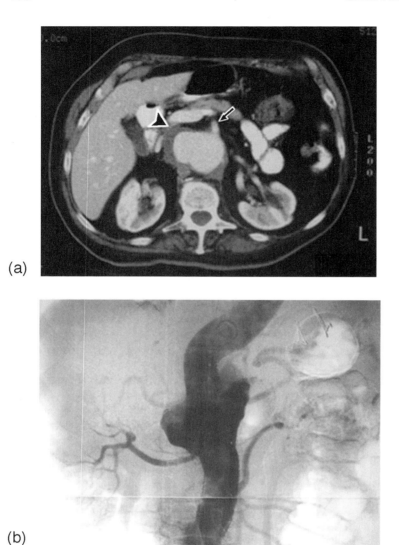

Figure 4 (a) CT scan of a visceral patch aneurysm following type I thoracoabdominal aneurysm repair. Aneurysm wall with mural thrombus (arrowhead) and superior mesenteric artery (arrow). (b) Aortogram of same aneurysm showing right renal artery originating from most distal portion of aneurysm and bypass to left renal artery originating several centimeters lower.

require insertion of a new interposition aortic graft to replace the prosthetic segment involved with the aneurysm. The visceral/renal arteries can be reattached by fashioning a smaller inclusion patch or reimplanting each vessel separately, taking deep bites through their origins to exclude as much aortic wall as possible. The left renal artery can be separately bypassed with a short prosthetic sidearm (8). We have utilized this approach successfully in the one patient with this problem that we have encountered. Alternatively, separate prosthetic bypasses off the new interposition graft can be used to reconstruct all the visceral/renal branches (27). A novel technique employing sequential visceral bypass from the descending thoracic aorta/prosthesis has also been employed with success (28).

V. OUTCOME

The results of femoral AA repair are generally good; the mortality rate is low (3–4%) even when the procedure is performed in acutely symptomatic patients (1,20). Graft limb thrombosis is the most frequent early and late complication, with resulting amputation in less than half the affected patients (1,20). Mulder reported an early limb loss rate of 2.6% (5). Graft infection occurs in up to 5% of patients (20). Recurrent femoral AA is another well-recognized complication, affecting 6–19% of patients (4,5,20). In reviewing our experience, Ernst documented the following risk factors for recurrent groin AAs: female gender, groin wound complications at the time of AA repair, and development of an AA within 4.5 years of the original aortofemoral grafting procedure (4). Repair of recurrent AAs is also associated with good results (4).

   The extensive scarring and frequent need for suprarenal aortic control and renal artery reconstruction combine to increase the risk associated with the repair of proximal aortic AAs. Mortality rates for elective repair average 10–15%, while those for emergent repair exceed 50% (5,10,17,18,21). The morbidity associated with these repairs is also substantial; bleeding, renal dysfunction, and pulmonary insufficiency are the most commonly encountered problems (10,17,18,21). The outcome of iliac artery AA repair is not well documented in the literature, perhaps because this entity is usually lumped with aortic AAs. Risks are certainly less than with aortic AAs, though ureteral scarring can present a problem. Due to the elevated risks associated with emergency open repair, intrabdominal AAs should be repaired on an elective basis at the earliest practical opportunity. Early reports of endovascular treatment of intrabdominal AAs have demonstrated favorable results. The long-term durability and efficacy of this approach, however, has not yet been proven (25,26,29,30).

   Repair of visceral patch AA following TAAA surgery is a morbid undertaking (8). Three of four patients undergoing elective repair in the Johns Hopkins series survived, but only after prolonged intensive care unit and hospital stays (8).

VI. PREVENTION

Reducing the occurrence of AAs requires the application of good surgical technique coupled with a thorough understanding of the associated risk factors. General principles include the construction of a tension-free anastomosis using a monofilament suture and taking generous, evenly spaced bites of healthy arterial wall. Endarterectomy should not be avoided if leaving residual plaque will compromise the outcome of the reconstruction. There is some theoretical evidence that ePTFE grafts are associated with a lower incidence of AA, but the data are not strong enough to recommend one vascular prosthesis over another. There are also theoretical as well as some clinical data to suggest that end-to-end anastomoses are associated with less AAs than end-to-side anastomoses. Unfortunately, in many situations, construction of an end-to-end anastomosis is not possible without risking the interruption of critical arterial perfusion to a specific vascular territory. Placing distal graft limb anastomoses above the inguinal ligament whenever feasible may reduce the mechanical stresses associated with repetitive hip flexion and extension. The importance of avoiding perioperative complications, both local and systemic, is obvious.

Measures to reduce the occurrence of intra-abdominal AAs include placing the proximal aortic anastomosis close to the renals to minimize the risk of aneurysmal degeneration in the retained infrarenal segment. Sewing to aneurysmal or even dilated aorta should be avoided whenever possible. This dictum is particularly important in utilizing Crawford's inclusion technique for reattaching visceral/renal branches to a thoracoabdominal aortic graft. Patches of aorta containing the origins of the renal and visceral vessels should be made as small as possible so as to exclude potentially degenerated aortic wall from the anastomosis. Suture line bites should be taken as close to the ostia of the reimplanted vessels as possible; occasionally it may be necessary to reimplant each vessel separately. To reduce the size of the visceral/renal patch, we routinely reconstruct the left renal artery with a short bypass graft from the aortic prosthesis.

Adoption of these techniques should help reduce the incidence of AAs, though it is unlikely that this common vascular surgical complication will ever be completely eliminated. For the aneurysms that do occur, prompt diagnosis and skilled repair remain the keys for successful management.

REFERENCES

1. Szilagyi DE, Smith FR, Elliot JP, Hageman JH, Dall'Olmo CA. Anastomotic aneurysms after vascular reconstruction: Problems of incidence, etiology and treatment. Surgery 1975; 178:800–816.
2. van den Akker PJ, Brand R, van Schilfgaarde R, van Bockel JH, Terpstra JL. False aneurysms after prosthetic reconstructions for aortoiliac obstructive disease. Ann Surg 1989; 210:658–666.
3. Mii S, Sakata H, Kawazoe N. Para-anastomotic aneurysms: incidence, risk factors, treatment and prognosis. J Cardiovasc Surg 1998; 39:259–266.
4. Ernst CB, Elliott JP Jr, Ryan CJ, Abu-Hamad G, Tilley BC, Murphy RK, Smith RF, Reddy DJ, Szilagyi DE. Recurrent femoral anastomotic aneurysms: A 30-year experience. Ann Surg 1988; 208(4):401–409.
5. Mulder EJ, van Bockel JH, Maas J, van den Akker PJ, Hermans J. Morbidity and mortality of reconstructive surgery of noninfected false aneurysms detected long after aortic prosthetic reconstruction. Arch Surg 1998; 133:45–49.
6. Edwards JM, Teefey SA, Zierler RE, Kohler TR. Intraabdominal paraanastomotic aneurysms after aortic bypass grafting. J Vasc Surg 1992; 15:344–353.
7. Szilagyi DE, Elliott JP, Smith RF, Reddy DJ, McParlin M. A thirty-year survey of the reconstuctive surgical treatment of aortoiliac occlusive disease. J Vasc Surg 1986; 3:421–436.
8. Dardik A, Perler BA, Roseborough GS, Williams GM. Aneurysmal expansion of the visceral patch after thoracoabdominal aortic replacement: An argument for limiting patch size? J Vasc Surg 2001; 34:405–410.
9. Seabrook GR, Schmitt DD, Bandyk DF, Edmiston CE, Krepel CJ, Towne JB. Anastomotic femoral pseudoaneurysm: An investigation of occult infection as an etiologic factor. J Vasc Surg 1990; 11:629–634.

10. Allen RC, Schneider J, Longenecker L, Smith RB, Lumsden AB. Paraanastomotic aneurysms of the abdominal aorta. J Vasc Surg 1993; 18:424–432.
11. Moore WS, Hall AD. Late suture failure in the pathogenesis of anastomotic pseudoaneurysms. Ann Surg 1970; 172:1064–1068.
12. Berman SS, Hunter GC, Smyth SH, et al. Application of computed tomography for surveillance of aortic grafts. Surgery 1995; 118:8–15.
13. Nunn DB, Carter MM, Donohue MT, et al. Postoperative dilation of knitted Dacron aortic bifurcation graft. J Vasc Surg 1990; 12:291–297.
14. Mehigan D, Fitzpatrick B, Browne HI, Bouchier-Hayes DJ. Is compliance mismatch the major cause of anastomotic aneurysms? J Cardiovasc Surg 1985; 26:147–150.
15. Gaylis H. Pathogenesis of anastomotic aneurysms. Surgery 1981; 90:509–515.
16. Mikati A, Marache P, Watel A, Warembourg H Jr, Roux JP, Noblet D, Soots G. End-to-side aortoprosthetic anastomoses: Long-term computed tomography assessment. Ann Vasc Surg 1990; 4:584–591.
17. Hagino RT, Taylor SM, Fujitani RM, Mills JL. Proximal anastomotic failure following infrarenal aortic reconstruction: Late development of true aneurysms, pseudoaneurysms, and occlusive disease. Ann Vasc Surg 1993; 7:8–13.
18. Curl GR, Faggioli GL, Stella A, D'Addato M, Ricotta JJ. Aneurysmal change at or above the proximal anastomosis after infrarenal aortic grafting. J Vasc Surg 1992; 16:855–860.
19. Gautier C, Borie H, Lagneau P. Aortic false aneurysms after prosthetic reconstruction of the infrarenal aorta. Ann Vasc Surg 1992; 6:413–417.
20. Schellack J, Salam A, Abouzeid MA, Smith RB, Steward MT, Perdue GD. Femoral anastomotic aneurysms: A continuing challenge. J Vasc Surg 1987; 6:308–317.
21. Treiman GJ, Weaver FA, Cossman DV, Cossman DV, Foran RF, Cohen JL, Levin PM, Treiman RL. Anastomotic false aneurysms of the abdominal aorta and the iliac arteries. J Vasc Surg 1998; 8:268–273.
22. Schmitt DD, Bandyk DF, Pequet AJ, Towne JB. Bacterial adherence to vascular prostheses. J Vasc Surg 1986; 3:732–740.
23. Carson SN, Hunter GC, Palmaz J, Guernsey JM. Recurrence of femoral anastomotic aneurysms. Am J Surg 1983; 146:774–778.
24. Shepard AD, Tollefson DJF, Reddy DJ, Evans JR, Elliot JP Jr, Smith RF, Ernst CB. Left flank retroperitoneal exposure: A technical aid to complex aortic reconstruction. J Vasc Surg 1991; 14:283–291.
25. Yuan JG, Marin ML, Veith FJ, Ohki T, Sanchez LA, Suggs WD, Cynamon J, Lyon RT. Endovascular grafts for noninfected aortoiliac anastomotic aneurysms. J Vasc Surg 1997; 26:210–221.
26. Morrissey NJ, Yano OJ, Soundararajan K, Eisen L, McArthur C, Teodorescu V, Kerstein M, Hollier L, Marin M. Endovascular repair of para-anastomotic aneurysms of the aorta and iliac arteries: Preferred treatment of a complex problem. J Vasc Surg 2001; 33:503–512.
27. Carrel TP, Signer C. Separate revascularization of the visceral arteries in thoracoabdominal aneurysm repair. Ann Thorac Surg 1999; 68:573–575.
28. Ballard JL. Thoracoabdominal aortic aneurysm repair with sequential visceral perfusion: A technical note. Ann Vasc Surg 1999; 13:216–221.
29. White RA, Donayre CE, Walot I, Wilson E, Jackson G, Kopchock G. Endoluminal graft exclusion of a proximal para-anastomotic pseudoaneurysm following aortobifemoral bypass. J Endovasc Surg 1997; 4(1):88–94.
30. Criado E, Marston WA, Ligush J, Mauro MA, Keagy BA. Endovascular repair of peripheral aneurysms, pseudoaneurysms, and arteriovenous fistulas. Ann Vasc Surg 1997; 11:256–263.

7

Hypercoagulable States and Unexplained Vascular Graft Thrombosis

Jonathan B. Towne

Medical College of Wisconsin, Milwaukee, Wisconsin, U.S.A.

Hypercoagulable states as a cause of unexplained vascular thrombosis present a difficult clinical problem. Most graft failures in the perioperative period are presumed to occur because of technical errors in the construction of the anastomosis, problems with the conduit, or poor patient selection. The diagnosis of an abnormal hypercoagulable state is often made only after all of these other factors have been excluded. Although failure of heparin to prevent clotting in the operative field or immediate thrombosis of a vascular repair suggests abnormal coagulation, the diagnosis can be confirmed only by the blood coagulation laboratory. The clotting disorder must be detected early in the course of the disease to obtain a favorable outcome. Abnormal thrombosis falls into five general categories: (a) heparin-induced platelet aggregation, (b) abnormalities in the antithrombin system, (c) abnormalities of the fibrinolytic system, (d) thrombosis caused by lupus-like anticoagulant, and (e) a miscellaneous category consisting primarily of abnormal platelet aggregation and protein C and protein S deficiency.

I. HEPARIN-INDUCED THROMBOSIS

Paradoxical thrombotic complications of heparin sodium anticoagulant therapy are uncommon but potentially limb-threatening and occasionally fatal. Several investigators have identified a chemically induced, immune thrombocytopenia as the cause of heparin-induced intravascular thrombosis, which usually occurs after 4–10 days of continued exposure to the drug (1–5). The immune factor that triggers the thrombocytopenia has been identified as an IgG antibody, which produced agglutination of normal platelets when either porcine gut or beef lung heparin is added. The IgG protein is stimulated by the heparin/platelet factor 4 complex and activates the platelet via the platelet F_c receptor (6). The thrombi that occur with heparin-induced thrombosis have an unusual grayish white appearance in contradistinction to the red color of most thrombi. The white color is secondary to the creation of fibrin-platelet aggregates, which can be clearly identified on electron microscopy (7).

Rhodes et al. (8) found a heparin-dependent IgG antibody in the serum of several patients by means of the complement lysis inhibition test. They also demonstrated a residual heparin-platelet aggregating effect 12 days to 2 months after patient recovery from the initial exposure to heparin. In these patients, a 24-h infusion of heparin caused a mean reduction of platelet count of $197,000/mm^3$. Since heparin preparations are not pure substances, it is also possible that a high-molecular-weight contaminant not eliminated by the extraction procedure may cause the antiplatelet defect.

Up to 30% of patients may manifest a decrease in their platelet count after starting heparin therapy, but the incidence of significant thrombocytopenia and resulting thrombotic or hemorrhagic complications is approximately 5% (9). Two types of heparin-induced thrombocytopenia are described. Type I, or the acute form, occurs relatively early and results in a benign course with improvement in the platelet count during continued heparin therapy. Type II, or the delayed form, occurs 5–14 days after the institution of heparin therapy in a patient not previously exposed to heparin and after 3–9 days in patients with a history of previous heparin therapy. Type II heparin-induced thrombocytopenia is reported to have a 23–60% thrombotic or hemorrhagic complication rate and a 12–18% mortality rate. Early recognition and treatment results in a significant improvement in the associated morbidity and mortality (10,11). In type I heparin-induced thrombocytopenia, the mechanism of action is thought to be a non-immune-mediated direct effect of heparin on platelets that causes aggregation. Type II heparin-induced thrombocytopenia is due to an immune mediated (IgG and IgM) platelet aggregation.

A. Clinical Presentation

Heparin-induced intravascular thrombosis can occur following a wide variety of indications for heparin administration, including thrombophlebitis with and without pulmonary embolus, perioperative heparin prophylaxis in patients at risk for thrombophlebitis, cardiac surgery, and vascular reconstruction. Platelet aggregation induced by heparin can result from both porcine gut and bovine lung heparin and can affect either the arterial or venous circulation. Both subcutaneous and intravenous heparin administration can produce this phenomenon (12). Even heparin-coated catheters can cause heparin-induced thrombocytopenia. Laster and Silver (12) reported the development of heparin-induced thrombocytopenia in 10 patients whom heparin-coated pulmonary artery catheters were inserted. Despite discontinuation of all other sources of heparin, the thrombocytopenia persisted. Although all of the patient were also given heparin, it is theoretically possible that heparin-coated catheters alone could have caused abnormal platelet aggregation.

The clinical features of this syndrome are often dramatic. In any patient who has had thrombotic complications while receiving heparin therapy, heparin-induced aggregation of platelets should be considered. This is especially important in patients with arterial occlusions who do not have any other evidence of atherosclerotic vascular disease. At operation, the finding of a white clot at thrombectomy should alert the surgeon to the possibility of heparin-induced thrombosis. In contrast to several reports in literature, increased heparin sensitivity rather than increased heparin resistance was noted in several of our patients (7). The cause of this is uncertain, but it is presently believed that it is unrelated to the heparin-induced aggregative immunoglobulin.

It was initially felt that arterial thrombosis was more prevalent than venous thrombosis with this complication. However, some prospective studies by Warkinton et al. demonstrated that there is actually a prevalence of venous to arterial emboli at a 4-to-1 ratio (6). Many of the venous thromboses are not detected unless studies such as duplex scanning doesn't search these out. The most common arterial location of thrombosis is the extremities, primarily the lower extremities, followed by the cerebral circulation, and finally manifesting as myocardial infarctions. The exact cause of this distribution of prevalence of thrombosis is uncertain, but it is certainly the authors' view that the thrombosis occurs more commonly on diseased vessels and that the incidence of diseased vessels in the extremities, particularly the lower extremities, is much higher than in many other vessels. This is followed by carotid bifurcation disease and coronary artery disease.

Skin lesions have been noted in patients with heparin-induced thrombosis. These are often seen at the site of the subcutaneous injection. They can present as a painful erythematous plaques, which can progress to skin necrosis. These can be unaccompanied by thrombocytopenia. With the prevalence of subcutaneous injection, the incidence of these findings has increased (13).

B. Diagnosis

Definitive diagnosis of heparin-induced intravascular thrombosis is obtained by performing platelet aggregation tests. Two patterns of response have been noted. The more common pattern is for the patient's platelet-poor plasma to aggregate donor platelets on the addition of heparin, indicating the presence of a relative nonspecific platelet-aggregating factor in the patient's plasma. The less common pattern is for the patient's plasma to be active against only the patient's platelets and have no effect on donor platelets. Other more sensitive tests include C^{14} serotonin release testing and enzyme-linked immunosorbent essay (ELISA) testing for the antibody to the heparin PF4 complex.

Other clotting factors are usually normal: fibrinogen level is normal, the level of fibrin split products may be mildly elevated but not in the range seen with intravascular coagulation, and prothrombin time is normal or slightly prolonged. All patient have a marked reduction in platelet count of less than $100,000/mm^3$ or a 50% decrease from admission level. In our series (7), the platelet count averaged $37,500/mm^3$ with a range of 6000 to $73,000/mm^3$.

Patients with arterial thrombosis often present with unique angiographic findings. These lesions consist of broad-based, isolated, lobulated excrescences that produce a variable amount of narrowing of the arterial lumen. Usually these findings have an abrupt appearance, with prominent luminal contour deformities in arterial segments that are otherwise normal. This distribution of disease is unusual and distinct from findings commonly seen with atherosclerosis. These changes occur in both the suprarenal and infrarenal portions of the abdominal aorta and represent adherent mural thrombi composed of aggregates of platelets and fibrin incorporating varying amounts of leukocytes and erythrocytes. Platelet aggregation tests should also be performed on any patient in whom recurrent pulmonary embolism developed while he or she was receiving adequate heparin therapy.

The diagnosis of heparin-induced thrombosis is primarily a clinical one. All the current laboratory tests have a relatively high percentage of false-negative rates and the more difficult-to-perform serotonin release and ELISA testing are not available in all hospitals. In a patient in whom the clinical syndrome of low platelet count and abnormal thrombosis is noted and in whom the tests are negative should be treated with a presumptive diagnosis of heparin-induced thrombosis and the tests repeated. Although false-negative tests are reported, false-positive tests are quite unusual.

C.   Treatment

Currently there are three approaches to treating patients with heparin-induced thrombosis (6). The first is the use of danaparoid (a heparinoid), a mixture of glycosaminioglycans (heparin-sulfate) and dermatan sulfate. This is quite effective, but it has a 10–40% cross reactivity with patients having heparin-induced platelet aggregation. Therefore, prior to instituting this therapy, the patient must have a platelet test against danaparoid to make sure that it does not cause platelet aggregation. The second course of therapy is the use of lepirudin, a recombinant form of the medicinal leech salivary protein hirudin, which is a direct thrombin inhibitor that can be quite effective. Patients are monitored by obtaining an activated thromboplastin time (A-PTT), which is kept at the level of 1.5–3 times normal. Following an adequate therapeutic response, the patient can be converted to warfarin for long-term anticoagulation. The third choice is Argatroban, a synthetic direct thrombin inhibitor, derived from L-arginine. Like lepirudin, this is monitored by following activated PTT levels.

When heparin-induced thrombocytopenia is diagnosed, heparin treatment should be reversed immediately with protamine sulfate, and dextran 40 should be administered for its antiaggregating and rheologic effects. Warfarin therapy also should be initiated and continued for several months. In patients with arterial occlusive manifestations of heparin-induced thrombosis, long-term warfarin therapy is recommended because of the possibility of coexisting latent venous occlusive disease.

The response of the platelet count to discontinuation of heparin therapy is usually prompt, often resulting in thrombocytosis, with a platelet count of 500,000 to 6000,000/mm^3 being achieved in several days.

Coagulation tests distinguish heparin-induced platelet aggregation from other clotting disorders. The fibrinogen level and prothrombin time are usually normal. The level of fibrin split products and prothrombin time are normal or slightly elevated. The sole patient in our series with a noticeable elevated level of fibrin split products was the initial patient, in whom the diagnosis was not made antemortem. Heparin therapy was not stopped, and before her death (caused by an intracerebral hemorrhage), she had massive venous thrombosis involving both upper and lower extremities, which resulted in an elevated level of fibrin split products. Early identification of heparin-induced thrombosis is necessary to minimize the catastrophic complications of major limb amputation and death.

This experience suggests that it is imperative, in all patients receiving heparin therapy, to have serial platelet counts done from the fourth day of heparin therapy onward. It is our policy to perform platelet counts every other day starting on the fourth day of heparin therapy. If thrombocytopenia develops, platelet aggregation studies should be performed immediately. With early recognition of complications, the mortality and morbidity of major amputation can be prevented. Morbidity and mortality rates reported in the literature vary from 22 to 61% and 12 to 33%, respectively (14,15).

II.   STRATEGIES FOR PATIENTS WITH HEPARIN-INDUCED PLATELET AGGREGATION

Patients who require subsequent heparin therapy for other vascular or cardiac surgery procedures require special management. In patients in whom heparin-induced platelet aggregation develops, the platelet aggregation tests usually revert to normal from 6 weeks to 3 months. Vascular or cardiac surgery procedures are preferably delayed until these tests revert to normal. We test the patient at 6 weeks and then every 2 weeks thereafter to determine when the platelet aggregation tests are negative. When they are negative, the patient is then admitted to the hospital for surgery. Cardiac catheterization or angiography is done as required without the use of heparin flush solutions, since even small amounts of heparin in the flush solutions can stimulate the development of heparin-induced antiplatelet antibodies. The vascular or cardiac surgery procedure is then performed with the usual administration of heparin. At the conclusion of the procedure, the heparin is reversed with protamine and care is taken during the postoperative period to ensure the patient does not receive heparin inadvertently through the flushing of either central venous catheters or arterial lines. By using this procedure, we have not had any difficulty with reexposure to heparin.

However, a different strategy is necessary for those patients who require an additional vascular or cardiac surgery procedure and who cannot wait until the results from heparin-induced platelet aggregation tests are negative. In patients requiring procedures that can be done without the use of heparin, such as resection of abdominal aortic aneurysm, heparin is not used. However, in patients who require complex lower extremity revascularization or cardiopulmonary bypass, some sort of anticoagulation is necessary. There are basically two approaches. That favored by Laster et al. (16) involves administering aspirin and dipyridamole (Persantine) preoperatively and then using heparin for the operative procedure, as is customary. In addition to aspirin and dipyridamole, we prefer also to use low-molecular-weight dextran, which, in addition to its rheological properties, coats the platelets and interferes with platelet adhesion. In some patients, however, as noted by Kappa et al. (17), the administration of aspirin has no effect on heparin-induced platelet aggregation. Makhoul et al. (18) noted that although aspirin abolished platelet aggregation in 9 of 16 patients with heparin-induced platelet aggregation, it only decreased platelet aggregation in the remaining 7, suggesting that aspirin is not able to reverse abnormal platelet aggregation in all patients. Based on these reports, our procedure is to administer aspirin and dipyridamole for several days before the operative procedure. On the day of operation, the platelet aggregation tests are performed with the addition of heparin. If the heparin causes abnormal platelet aggregation, iloprost can then used to prevent heparin-induced platelet aggregation during the procedure. The use of iloprost can be complicated, particularly since it is a very potent vasodilator and rather large doses of adrenergic agents are often required to support blood pressure. Also, it has been approved for use by the U.S. Food and Drug Administration (FDA) and may be used off label.

Sobel et al. (19) reported an alternate technique in which patients received warfarin anticoagulant combined with dextran as a means of preventing intraoperative thrombosis during reconstruction. This is a reasonable alternative for peripheral vascular reconstructions but is not possible for cardiopulmonary bypass. In the future, different substances may be available to allow for adequate anticoagulation. Makhoul et al. (18) noted in vitro that heparinoids did not cause platelet aggregation. These new anticoagulant agents are being developed in Europe and may, in the future, be available in the United States. Latham et al. have described the use of recombinant hirudin for treatment of a patient who had heparin-induced platelet aggregation and who required cardiopulmonary bypass (20). They were successfully able to anticoagulate the patient and place him on bypass without any untored results.

Cole and Bormanis (21) have reported the use of ancrod, which is made from the venom of the Malaysian pit viper (*Agkistrudon rbodastoma*), as an anticoagulant in patients who have heparin-induced platelet aggregation. Ancrod acts enzymatically on the fibrinogen molecule to form a product that cannot be clotted by physiological thrombin.

III. ANTITHROMBIN DEFICIENCY

Antithrombin III (AT III) is an alpha globulin manufactured in the liver and perhaps by vascular endothelium, with a molecular weight of approximately 60,000 Da and a half-life of 2.8 days (22). It is a serine proteinase inhibitor that binds in equimolar ratios to several enzymes participating in the intrinsic pathway of blood coagulation, including thrombin factors, Ixa, Xa, and Xia (23,24). Heparin significantly accelerates the rate at which AT III neutralizes these enzymes, limiting sequential clotting reactions and preventing fibrin formation. In 1965, Egeberg (19) described a family with an inborn defect of AT III. Subsequent research has confirmed the genetic transmission of this deficiency (25–28). The frequency of this defect is approximately 1 in 2000 to 1 in 5000 in the general population (29,30). There are probably at least two types of AT III deficiency. In the classic form, both the protein level of AT III (as determined by measurement of its protein concentration) and its activity level are reduced in the patient's plasma (31). However, there are other patients in whom the concentration of AT III is normal or even slightly elevated as measured by protein level, but the biological function as measured by activity level tests is abnormal (32). This suggest that these patients are manufacturing a defective antithrombin molecule. Acquired AT III deficiency can occur in patients with severe liver disease, nephrotic syndrome, hypoalbuminemia, malnutrition, and disseminated intravascular coagulation and in some patients taking oral contraceptives. AT III deficiency may be an indicator of significant protein catabolism. Flinn et al. (33) noted low AT III activity. There was low serum albumin (<3 mg/dL) in 48% of these patients, which was associated with an increased incidence of early graft failure.

A. Clinical Presentation

Although AT III deficiency is inherited, it is rare for episodes of thrombosis to be clinically manifest before the second decade of life. Despite continuously depressed levels of AT III in these patients, thrombotic episodes are often related to predisposing factors such as surgery, childbirth, and infection; they rarely occur spontaneously. This deficiency can cause venous thrombosis, pulmonary embolism, dialysis fistula failure, arterial graft occlusion, and spontaneous arterial occlusion. In our initial report, we identified 7 patients (5 men, 2 women; age range, 21–65 years) with antithrombin deficiencies as a cause of thrombosis (34). Three presented with early thrombosis of femorodistal grafts (Fig. 1). In two of these patients the grafts became occluded shortly after surgery in the brief interval between completion of the anastomoses and performance of an operative angiogram. Despite repeated thrombectomies, graft patency could not be obtained for longer than 5 min. Two patients presented with spontaneous arterial thrombosis. One had acute ischemia of the right lower extremity with angiographic demonstration of multiple areas of thrombosis of the distal superficial femoral, popliteal, and tibial systems. The other presented with ischemia of one arm and both legs secondary to extensive thromboses of the brachial artery and its branches of one arm and the femoral, popliteal, and tibial systems of both legs. Extensive arteriography of the entire aorta and cardiac evaluation failed to reveal a proximal origin of embolic material. Another patient had spontaneous thrombosis of the tibial outflow vessels to the foot while undergoing an extended profundoplasty. What distinguishes these patients from those with thrombotic occlusive disease secondary to atherosclerotic disease is the unique history, the distribution of occluded vessels, unusual angiographic findings, and absence of any proximal source of embolic material. Often, clot formation in the operative field despite heparin adminis-

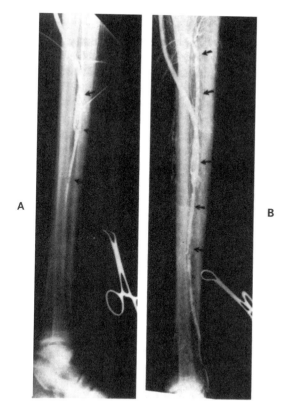

Figure 1 A. Patient with thrombosed femoroperoneal graft the night following surgery. Following graft thrombectomy, patient had evidence of residual thrombi, as noted by arrows. B. Rethrombosis of graft. More widespread residual thrombi are evident. Antithrombin III deficiency was diagnosed and treated, resulting in long-term (>24 months) patency.

tration is the first clue that the patient may have an AT III deficiency. The presence of multiple thrombi on operative angiograms is suggestive of a clotting abnormality.

B. Diagnosis

Results of routing coagulation tests are normal in patients with AT III deficiency. Generally, reductions in AT III are measured by both immunological (tests that measure the total amount of the protein) and functional (tests that measure activity of the AT III molecules) assays. The best screening test is the antithrombin heparin cofactor assay (35,36).

Initially, patients with repeated episodes of venous thrombosis were identified because of the reduction of AT III to levels 50–60% of normal values. Subsequent research has identified patients with arterial thrombosis secondary to low AT II levels. Lynch et al. (37) demonstrated a correlation between low preoperative plasma functional AT III levels and the occurrence of postoperative thrombotic complications following cardiac and vascular surgery. Thrombotic complications included arterial thrombosis, graft thrombosis, deep venous thrombosis (DVT), cerebral vascular thrombosis, spinal infarction, and embolic cortical blindness.

A decrease in AT III levels causes the increase thrombotic tendency in patients taking oral contraceptives. Sagar et al.(38) demonstrated that AT III activity was significantly lower in patients taking oral contraceptives than in control patients. AT III activity fell in both the contraceptive and control groups, but the decline was greater in patients taking oral contraceptives. The only patients in whom DVT developed postoperatively as determined by the (Iodine 125) fibrinogen test were those taking oral contraceptives. Of the 31 patients taking oral contraceptives, 5 had an AT III activity level below 50%; in 3 of these patients, DVT developed.

More recent study has demonstrated that the administration of heparin tends to lower the AT III level. Conrad et al. (39) demonstrated that it is the presence of heparin and not the rate of administration that determines the decrease in AT III; he noted that both subcutaneous and intravenous heparin causes AT III levels to drop the same amount. Since heparin is dependent on AT III for its antithrombotic action, the AT III-lowering effect of heparin in patients with an already low AT III concentration probably indicates that patients are at risk of thrombosis for two reasons. First, heparin is relatively ineffective in patients with low levels of AT III. Second, because heparin binds with AT III, the already low level is decreased even further, possibly to dangerous levels. This is the theoretical basis for the paradoxical thrombotic episodes occasionally seen in patients following cessation of heparin. Since heparin administration decreases the level of AT III, sometimes to significantly dangerous levels, cessation of heparin is followed by a period when the patient is hypercoagulable because the lower AT III level is not counteracted by the heparin. This is why warfarin administration should be overlapped with heparin cessation when treating thrombotic problems. Patients with a congenital AT III deficiency should receive chronic long-term warfarin therapy because of the risk of recurrent thrombolic episodes. In addition to its anticoagulant effect, warfarin increases the level of AT III by an as yet undetermined mechanism. More recently, purified AT III can be obtained by recombinant techniques, which will in the future change the treatment of this deficiency. AT III concentrate was used as factor-specific replacement by Tengborn and Bergquist (40) in patients with AT III deficiency.

IV. DEFECTS IN THE FIBRINOLYTIC SYSTEM

The fibrinolytic system has become better understood in recent years and has been found to be the source of coagulation abnormalities. The components of the fibrinolytic system include plasminogen; plasminogen activators, including human tissue-type plasminogen activator (t-PA) and urokinase, and inhibitors directed against plasminogen activators, plasmin inhibitor (the most important of which is α-antiplasmin) and cellular plasmin inhibitors, which have been identified in platelets and endothelial cells and are very poorly characterized at the present time (41,42). The degradation of fibrin is normally carried out by the proteolytic enzyme plasmin, which is formed from the proenzyme plasminogen by the activation action of plasminogen activators such as t-PA and urokinase. The process is regulated at many levels, resulting in localized plasmin formation at the fibrin surface t-PA is the most important activator and is produced and released from vascular endothelium (43).

Plasminogen is a normal plasma protein consisting of a single polypeptide chain, with a molecular weight of 90,000–94,000 Da (44). Thin-layer gel electro-phoresis coupled with immunofixation can demonstrate up to 10 different forms of plasminogen, with each variant having a glutamic acid as its terminal amino acid. Plasminogen is converted to plasmin by activators, many of which are released from endothelial cells. Plasmin, a serine proteinase, is an important member of the fibrinolytic system that acts by cleaving fibrinogen and fibrin (45–47).

The biosynthesis of plasminogen and fibrinolytic inhibitors is probably under genetic control. In 1978, Aoki et al. (48) reported a patient with recurrent thrombosis who had a hereditary molecular defect of plasminogen. This was followed by similar reports by Kazama et al. (49) in 1981 and Soria et al (50) in 1983. These authors demonstrated that abnormal plasminogen does not have the functional ability of normal plasminogen, resulting in a discrepancy between the biological activity and the amount of plasminogen detected in the serum by radioimmunoassay. These patients had normal concentrations of plasminogen antigen, with approximately one-half of the activity of normal plasminogen. Using electrofocusing techniques coupled with immunofixation and zymograms, they were able to identify ten additional bands, each of which was located on the basic side in close proximity to the corresponding normal band.

Determination of amino acid sequence has demonstrated defects in the arginine 516–valine bond and the substitution of alanine 600 by threonine (51). The major function of the fibrinolytic system in vivo is the limitation of fibrin deposition. A reduction of fibrinolytic activity may provoke a thrombotic tendency by allowing the growth and development of thrombi after the initiating thrombotic event. Most patients with abnormal plasminogen are characterized by a normal antigen concentration and decreased functional activity. Liu et al. (52) reported a plasminogen characterized by both low functional activity and low antigen concentration and called it plasminogen San Antonio.

Ikemoto et al. (53) reported that the genetic characteristics of this disorder follow an autosomal codominant inheritance pattern, with both alleles being completely expressed. The results of the study of two families in our series concur with these findings. The clinical history of recurrent phlebitis in one or our patients and his sister supports the genetic aspect of this disease.

The immunoelectrophoresis technique is quicker, simpler, and less costly than iso-electric focusing and is more applicable to the screening of large groups of patients (54). The significance of abnormal plasminogen is uncertain. It is present in 10% of the normal population and its presence does not ensure that a patient will experience thrombotic complications. More likely, the presence of abnormal plasminogen results in the relative defect of the fibrinolytic system, which places the patient at increased risk should he or she be in a thrombosis-prone situation. Our data suggest, however, that once a thrombotic episode occurs, it is likely to recur, emphasizing the need to identify and treat these patients with long-term warfarin therapy.

A. Clinical Presentation

We have noted thrombosis occurring on both the arterial and venous sides of the circulation in patients with abnormal plasminogen. In our initial report of 8 patients, the age of onset of the first thrombotic episode ranged from 21 to 57 years (54); 3 had venous thrombosis, 2 had spontaneous arterial thrombosis, 2 had occlusion of an arterial reconstruction in the early postoperative period, and 1 had separate episodes of both arterial and venous occlusions.

Thrombosis involving the venous system occurred in 4 patients; 2 had complete obstruction of the iliofemoral venous segment and inferior vena cava, 1 had primarily popliteal vein thrombosis, and the remaining patient had axillary and subclavian vein thrombosis. Of these patients, 2 had concomitant pulmonary emboli, which occurred in 1 patient 4 months after the thrombotic event. Arterial thrombosis occurred in 5 patients; 2 presented with spontaneous thrombosis of the iliofemoral segment. Following thrombectomy with Fogarty catheters, there was no evidence of inflow obstruction, and a complete evaluation for the proximal source of emboli was negative (Fig. 2). Postoperative occlusions of arterial reconstructions occurred in 2 patients. In the first patient, the site of Dacron patch angioplasty of the vertebral artery orifice became occluded the night following surgery. At reexploration, no stricture of the repair was found, and the

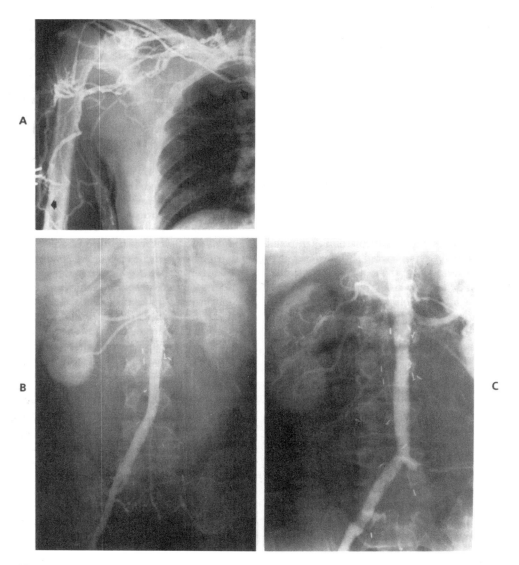

Figure 2 A.Venogram demonstrating subclavian and axillary vein thrombosis in a patient who had separate episodes of arterial and venous thrombosis. B. Angiogram of patient 9 months later, demonstrating occlusion of the left common iliac artery. C. Angiogram obtained 37 months later, showing reocclusion of the common iliac artery. (From Ref. 54.)

thrombosis was limited to the area of the patch angioplasty without distal propagation. In the second patient, thrombosis occurred in a saphenous vein femoral-posterior tibial graft the night following surgery. At reexploration, the thrombus formation was limited to the graft and did not extend to the runoff vessels. Complete angiograms following both initial surgery and reoperation demonstrated technically satisfactory anastomoses. Postoperatively, the graft remained patent with chronic progressive thrombosis of the runoff vessel in both legs. This patient was not diabetic and initially presented with a 6-month history of rest pain in both feet that progressed to digital gangrene. The ankle brachial index (ABI) of the right lower extremity was 0.95, with a toe pressure of 44 mmHg. The ABI of the left leg was 0.65, with a toe pressure of 10 mmHg. Arteriography demonstrated a normal aortoiliac system and a 50% stenosis of the left superficial femoral artery, but occlusion of the pedal and metatarsal arteries was present.

Of the 8 patients in the study of Towne et al. (55), 6 had recurrent thrombosis, 2 had three recurrences, and 4 had two recurrences. The interval between thrombotic episodes ranged from 4 to 36 months. Significantly, 5 patients who had recurrent thrombosis were treated with warfarin following the first episode. Recurrent episodes of thrombosis occurred 2 weeks to several months following cessation of warfarin therapy, and recurrent thrombosis did not develop in any patient while he or she was receiving anticoagulation therapy. We subsequently identified 4 patients who had abnormal plasminogen, as detected by an abnormal arc on immunoelectrophoresis in whom severe thrombosis in the upper extremities developed (Fig. 3) (55). The lack of atherosclerosis in the upper extremities as well as the absence of any proximal embolic source further points out the sometimes catastrophic consequences that patients with abnormal plasminogen may experience. In our experience of over 30 patients in whom we have detected abnormal

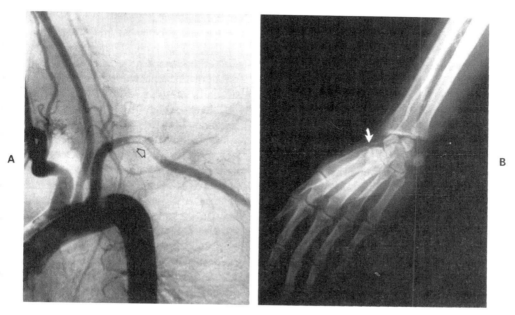

Figure 3 A. Nonoccluding thrombi of subclavian artery occurring several days after carotid angiography from a femoral approach. B. Evidence of distal embolization of the distal radial artery and palmar arch in same patient. (From Ref. 55.)

plasminogen over the last 5 years, recurrent thrombosis has developed in only 1 patient while receiving warfarin therapy.

B. Methods of Testing

A complete coagulation profile on each patient should be performed, including tests of platelet aggregation, prothrombin time, partial thromboplastin time, fibrinogen level, and platelet count. Functional assays of AT III and plasminogen a2 antiplasmin should be performed. Measurements of antigenic activity levels of AT III, plasminogen, a_2 antitrypsin, and a_2 macroglobulins likewise should be obtained. With immunoelectrophoresis, abnormal plasminogen presents as an abnormal band that is separate on the electrophoretic pattern located nearer the anode and distinct from the normal band. We have also noted one patient in whom plasminogen was demonstrated as separate from the main band but was not confined to a distinct band. Indeed this may represent still another species. Several investigators are involved in ongoing studies to further characterize the molecular defect in these plasminogens and to assess the functional impairment. This research requires rather sophisticated techniques to determine amino acid sequencing and to test the functional ability of the various components of the plasminogen molecule.

1. t-Pa and Anti–t-Pa

With the development of a method to measure t-PA, investigators have discovered that levels of t-PA can vary in relation to the occurrence of thrombotic disease (56). Also, the presence of an anti–t-PA that counteracts the effects of t-PA has been detected (57,58). Several studies have identified patients who are thrombosis-prone because of increased levels of anti–t-PA (59–61). Both the mechanisms and the effect of alterations of these mechanisms are poorly understood at the present time. Wiman (56) first developed the test to measure t-PA. In a study of patients with DVT, he found that 40% of his patients had a reduced fibrinolytic potential, which was found to be caused by a reduced capacity to release t-PA or an increased plasma level of an anti–t-PA or a combination of these (60). He also noted a significant correlation between plasma anti–t-PA and the levels of serum triglycerides in patients below the age of 45 with myocardial infarction. Obviously these are primarily data, but they emphasize the need for ongoing investigation to determine more precisely the role of the fibrinolytic system in the pathogenesis of thrombotic disorders.

V. PROTEIN C DEFICIENCY

Protein C is a vitamin K–dependent proenzyme that is involved in the control of clotting and fibrinolysis. Protein C itself is activated by thrombin, but slowly. This activation is increased up to 20,000-fold when thrombin forms a complex with an endothelial cell membrane called thrombomodulin (Fig. 4). Activated protein C combined with phospholipids, calcium, and protein S inactivates the cofactors of the two rate-limiting steps of coagulation, factors Va and VIIa (62–64).

Protein S is likewise a vitamin K–dependent factor. It acts as a cofactor for the anticoagulant activity of activated protein C by promoting its binding to lipid and platelet surfaces, thus localizing protein C activity (65,66). Protein C, in conjunction with protein S, also acts as a profibrinolytic agent by increasing plasmin activity through the inactivation of the major inhibitor of t-PA (62,63).

Heterozygous protein C deficiency is inherited in an autosomal dominant fashion. In hereditary protein C deficiency, the homozygous state is associated with a very high risk of

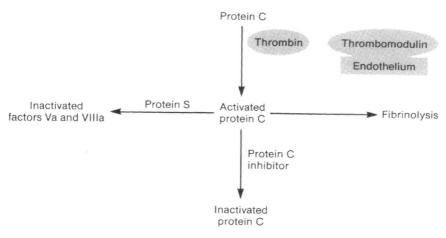

Figure 4 Protein C is produced in the liver and circulates in blood in inactive form. When thrombin becomes bound to endothelial cofactor (thrombomodulin), the complex that is formed rapidly activates protein C. Activated protein C is a potent plasma anticoagulant. It inactivates cofactors of two rate-limiting steps of coagulation (factors Va and VIIIa) and enhances fibrinolysis. These processes require the presence of protein S. Protein C is inactivated by protein C inhibitor in a one-to-one fashion. (From Ref. 71.)

thrombosis (67,68). It usually presents as massive venous thrombosis in the neonatal period and is often fatal. The in utero survival of affected infants may reflect the protection afforded by maternal transfer of protein C or the reduced synthesis of other procoagulants by the fetal liver, which thus compensates for the deficiency of protein C.

In the heterozygous form of the deficiency, a protein C level of 50% is sufficient to predispose individuals to venous thrombosis (69). The incidence of thrombophlebitis in patients who are heterozygous for this deficiency is uncertain. Some kindreds have been identified in which there is a very high incidence of venous thrombosis (up to 80%) by the age of 40, and there are others in which the occurrence of thrombosis is sporadic (69,70). Acquired protein C deficiency can be observed in patients in the acute phase of thrombosis, in patients with disseminating intervascular coagulation, in patients with liver disease, and in postoperative patients.

Protein C deficiency generally manifests itself with venous thrombosis, either as DVT of the lower extremity, often accompanied by pulmonary embolism, or as mesenteric venous thrombosis. We recently reported 5 patients (age range, 28–41 years) with protein C deficiency: 4 had DVT of the lower extremity as the initial thrombotic event and 1 had mesenteric venous thrombosis with small bowel necrosis (71). Two patients had recurrent lower extremity thrombosis, which was bilateral in one. One patient experienced only one clinical episode of DVT, but venous stasis ulceration developed, suggesting multiple episodes of subclinical phlebitis. One patient had a pulmonary embolus. Green et al. (72) evaluated 8 consecutive patients with splanchnic venous thrombosis and demonstrated decreases in the levels of AT III and protein C in all. They were unable to document whether the low levels of protein C and AT III were a result or cause of the thrombosis. Two patients had had a history of venous thrombotic problems, and evaluation of six patients following a period of 1–6 months revealed a persistent low level of protein C, which certainly suggest a congenital etiology. The only case of arterial thrombosis secondary to protein C reduction was reported by Coller et al. (73); they treated a patient who experienced the onset of the first of three episodes of thrombophlebitis at age 23. At age 27, the patient had a pulmonary embolus; at 28, he had a myocardial infarction and superficial femoral artery thrombosis; and at age 31, simultaneous radial and ulnar artery occlusions developed, followed shortly by the development of left ventricular thrombus, which caused embolus to the leg.

A. Methods of Testing

Standard testing includes a radiolabeled Laurell electroimmunoassay to determine human protein C antigen in plasma samples. Normal values should be between 70 and 130% of normal activity. In our patients with venous thrombosis, the level of protein C ranged from 34 to 67% (71). As with the evaluation of all patients with unusual or unexplained thrombosis, measurement of AT III and protein S and routine coagulation studies should be performed simultaneously. We evaluated the family of our patient with mesenteric venous occlusion for protein C deficiency and found the results to indicate an autosomal dominant type of transmission. No thrombotic episodes have been reported by other family members with low protein C levels. Since thrombosis does not develop in all family members with low protein C levels, asymptomatic patients with low levels of protein C should be monitored closely and should not receive prophylactic anticoagulant therapy. However, they should receive prophylactic anticoagulants preoperatively if major surgery or prolonged immobilization is required. In those in whom thrombotic events develop, the onset typically occurs between 15 and 30 years of age. This delay in onset of the first thrombotic episode and the fact that protein C rarely causes arterial thrombosis—as contrasted with our experiences with either abnormal plasminogen or AT III abnormalities—are not well understood. It may be that protein C deficiency requires the slower-moving blood and increased endothelial surface area found in the venous system to manifest itself. However, when protein C deficiency is homozygous, thrombosis is widespread, resulting in death in infancy unless treated.

Because of the risk of recurrent thrombotic events, with the possible sequelae of pulmonary emboli and venous stasis disease, long-term warfarin therapy is recommended. No loading dose should be administered, as this could precipitate warfarin-associated skin necrosis (65,66). Such necrosis occurs 2–5 days following the initiation of warfarin therapy and presents as an erythematous patch on the skin that progresses rapidly to a hemorrhagic area, which can become gangrenous. There is a propensity for involvement of the breasts, abdomen, buttocks, and thighs. The proposed mechanism is one of a transient hypercoagulable state that is created by bolus loading doses of warfarin given to initiate anticoagulation. Because of it short half-life, protein C levels fall faster than levels of factor X and prothrombin; and thus the inhibitory effect of protein C on the coagulation cascade is further diminished. If these levels fall below a critical point, the procoagulant effects of the coagulation cascade proceed unabated and thrombosis ensues. Administration of oral warfarin 5 mg daily should be started to gradually attain a prothrombin time of 1.5–2 times the control value. Heparin therapy and warfarin therapy should overlap by 4–5 days.

VI. PROTEIN S DEFICIENCY

Protein S is a vitamin K–dependent protein that functions as a cofactor of anticoagulant activity of activated protein C. The liver is the major location of synthesis, although more recently the endothelial cells and megakaryocyte were identified as other sites of synthesis. Protein S functions by expediting the binding of activated protein C to the lipid and platelet surfaces. To date, only patients with heterozygous protein S deficiency have been reported (68). Symptomatic patients often have protein S levels 50% of the normal value, and—like protein C deficiency—protein S deficiency primarily causes venous thrombosis (74–76). Protein S deficiency has been estimated by some to be the cause of approximately 10% of cases of spontaneous venous thrombosis. Coller et al. (73) also reported the only known case history of a protein S–deficient patient having arterial occlusive problems. This patient had had recurrent episodes of thrombophlebitis over several years, resulting in venous stasis disease. At age 21, he experienced thrombotic problems in the legs, which resulted in a below-knee amputation. As with patients with protein C problems, patients with protein S deficiency have clotting abnormalities that tend to be recurrent; therefore it is essential that they remain on long-term warfarin therapy. The association of deficiencies in protein C and its cofactor protein S with hypercoagulable states has only recently been appreciated. Data now suggest that the incidence of protein C and protein S deficiencies is more common than either AT III or plasminogen abnormalities. In a recent report evaluating 139 individuals who had at least one major venous thrombotic event, 7% were deficient in protein C, 5% were deficient in protein S, 2% were deficient in plasminogen, and 3% were deficient in AT III (77). A majority (79%), however, had no coagulopathy detectable with current testing methods.

VII. ANTIPHOSPHOLIPID ANTIBODIES

Lupus-like anticoagulants are IgG or IgM antibodies that are directed against phospholipids participating in coagulation disorders. They are present in 16–33% of patients with lupus erythematosus, but they are also associated with a variety of other disorders and are even found in normal individuals (78–80). These antibodies belong to a family of antiphospholipid antibodies that were initially detected because of their effect in vitro on the prolongation of plasma coagulation times. Most commonly, there is a prolongation of activated partial thromboplastin time and, in some patients, also a prolongation of prothrombin time. There have been only rare reports of bleeding tendencies related to the demonstration of a lupus-like anticoagulant; however, in the last decade, there have been an increasing number of reports of the presence of lupus-like anticoagulants associated with abnormal thrombosis in both the arterial and venous systems, spontaneous abortion secondary to placental thrombosis, cerebrovascular accidents, and thrombocytopenia. Lupus-like anticoagulants also cause false-positive tests for syphilis. On occasion, lupus-like anticoagulants can develop after administration of phenothiazines, procainamide, or penicillin; following viral infections in children; and in patients with AIDS suffering from *Pneumocystis carinii* pneumonia.

A. Clinical Presentation

Recurrent thromboses have been reported in about one-third of patients with lupus-like antiocoagulant (81). The most common manifestation is venous thrombosis, usually involving the lower extremities. Pulmonary hypertension caused by recurrent pulmonary emboli or intrapulmonary thrombosis may develop. Repeated strokes have been reported in 15–55% of these patients. Obstetric complications (e.g, spontaneous abortions, intrauterine growth retardation, fetal death) occurring in the second and third trimesters have been reported in 25–35% of women with lupus-like anticoagulant (78–80). Ahn et al. (82) in a study of patients with lupus-like anticoagulant who were undergoing surgery, noted that 9 of 18 vascular surgery procedures were complicated by thrombosis. Seven of these patients suffered multiple postoperative thrombotic complications, resulting in amputation in three. The mechanism of action of lupus-like anticoagulants is not known. Several theories have been suggested, including an inhibitory effect on prostacyclin (PGI_2), which is a potent in vivo inhibitor of platelet aggregation. IgG fractions with lupus-like anticoagulant activity have been shown experimentally to block the production of prostacyclin in rat aortic endothelial cells (83). Other investigators suggest that lupus-like anticoagulant inhibits protein C activation, which is important in preventing thrombosis. Tsakiris et al. (84) believe that the inhibition of the catalytic activity of thrombomodulin might be explained by the direct attachment of lupus-like anticoagulant to thrombomodulin or to adjacent phospholipids of the cell membrane, preventing thrombin and/or protein C from binding to thrombomodulin.

B. Diagnosis

Often the only indication that a patient has lupus-like anticoagulant is an abnormally prolonged activated partial thromboplastin time. On occasion, such a patient can also have a prolonged prothrombin time. An abnormal rabbit brain neutralization procedure and an ELISA for presence of anticardiolipin antibodies can more precisely identify lupus-like anticoagulant (82).

C. Treatment

Because the precise mechanism by which lupus-like anticoagulant causes intravascular thrombosis is not known, treatment has varied, including the administration of antiplatelet medications (aspirin and dipyridamole), anticoagulation with warfarin and heparin, and the administration of steroids. The basis for treatment with antiplatelet medication is that some researchers believe that the lupus-like anticoagulant causes a decrease in the availability of arachidonic acid, which is necessary for the synthesis of prostacyclin inhibitor or platelet aggregation in vessel walls. In obstetric patients, it has been reported that steroid and aspirin administration is effective in preventing spontaneous abortion. Prednisone has been shown to suppress production and/or activity of lupus-like anticoagulant as measured by lessened prolongation of the activated partial thromboplastin time. Until more information is available, we prefer to initiate antiplatelet therapy with aspirin and dipyridamole before surgical procedures. We administer dextran routinely in all vascular reconstructions, and patients are given heparin perioperatively. Postoperatively, heparin therapy was converted to warfarin therapy.

VIII. ACTIVATED PROTEIN C RESISTANCE

A recurring theme throughout this chapter is the fact that the procoagulant and anticoagulant properties of blood are delicately balanced by a complex system of cofactors and inhibitors. The thrombomodulin/protein C anticoagulant pathway is an essential anticoagulant system. As thrombin is generated at sites of vascular injury, it activates and aggregates platelets and clots fibrinogen. It also binds to the endothelial membrane protein thrombomodulin. Upon binding to thrombomodulin, thrombin takes on anticoagulant properties by activating protein C. The activated protein C (APC) cleaves and inactivates factor Va and VIIIa in the presence of protein S. This endothelial-based anticoagulant system allows blood to clot while maintaining intravascular fluidity. Defects in this anti-coagulant pathway can provoke thrombosis; indeed, protein C and protein S deficiencies, discussed previously, are associated with an increased risk of thrombosis in heterozygotes.

A family history of thrombotic events is frequently obtained in young adults with venous thrombosis; however, the inherited deficiencies in anticoagulant proteins, such as protein C and protein S, are found in only about 5% of patients (85). APC resistance is another risk factor for venous thrombosis that is frequently found in these patients. It is, in fact, the most common genetic risk factor for venous thrombosis described to date (86). It is caused by a point mutation in the factor V gene, which causes increased resistance to the anticoagulant effect of activated protein C. This defect was discovered in 1993 by Dahlbäch et al. and has been named factor V Leiden (85).

Dahlbäch originally postulated that defect in the protein C pathway interfered with the anticoagulant action of APC. He devised assays to test this possibility, in which the clotting time of blood was measured in the presence and absence of exogenous APC. In the normal response, the clotting time was prolonged in the presence of APC because of the inactivation of factors Va and VIIIa. A defect was detected as a failure of prolongation of the clotting time resulting from resistance to added APC. Dahlbäch showed that this test detects an autosomal dominant trait associated with thrombosis. Further work done by Bertina and his group demonstrated that the phenotype of APC resistance is associated with a he-terozygous or homozygous single point mutation in the factor V gene, which predicts the synthesis of a factor V molecule that is not properly inactivated by APC (factor V Leiden) (86). Other data confirming these results were published by Zoller and Dahlbäch who studied 50 Swedish families with inherited APC resistance (87). They found that the specific point mutation in the factor V gene was present in 47 of 50 families. In their study, by age 33 years, 20% of the heterozygous and 40% of the homozygous patients had had manifes-tations of venous thrombosis.

Factor V Leiden is present in 3–7% of all Caucasians but is more rare in other ethnic populations (88). It is present in up to 20% of unselected patients with DVT and confers a 5- to 10-fold increased risk of thrombosis in heterozygotes; homozygotes have a 50- to 100-fold increased risk (88).

The laboratory diagnosis is made by measuring the responsiveness of plasma to APC as the ratio of two activated partial thromboplastin times, one in the presence of APC and one in its absence. The APC sensitivity ratio is normalized to the ratio obtained with reference plasma. Resistance to APC is defined by an APC sensitivity ratio of <0.84 (86). A more recent way of identifying this factor V resistance to activated protein C is by a direct assay for the factor V molecule, which is resistant to inactivation by APC (factor V Leiden). The question then arises what can be done about these point mutations, which cause factor V to be resistant to activated protein C. It is clear that this is a major risk factor for thromboembolic disease; however, the majority of patients with these mutant proteins will not suffer thrombosis. The risks of lifelong anticoagulation therapy in an asymptomatic patient must be weighed against the benefit of preventing infrequent but devastating thrombotic attacks. At this point, it would be a logical course of action to treat those patients who have already suffered thrombotic attacks with long-term warfarin therapy.

IX. HYPERHOMOCYSTEINEMIA

Hyperhomocysteinemia is a thiol-containing amino acid derived from the metabolism of methionine. Remethylation of homocysteine with a methyl group from methyltetrahydro-folate (MTHF) reproduces methionine. This reaction is B_{12}-dependent and is catalyzed by methyltetrahydrofolate reductase (MTHFR). Homocysteine can also be metabolized via transulferation to cysteine, a reaction that requires cystathionine synthase and B_6 cofactor. Homozygous deficiency of cystathionine synthase produces classic homocystinurea, in which levels of homocysteine in the blood and urine are quite elevated. This defect is associated with early onset of vascular disease and venous thrombosis; however it is quite rare.

Attention has recently been turned to evaluating other factors that might contribute to elevated levels of homocysteine in the plasma and determining their association with thrombosis. Both a defect in MTHFR or cystathionine synthase can be associated with increased homocysteine levels in the blood. Elevated levels of homocysteine have been found to be present in 10–25% of patients with venous thrombosis, which is approximately 2.5 times the number of control patients with increased homocysteine levels (89,90). In one multicenter trial, homocysteine levels were followed in 264 patients with documented DVT after their 3-month course of oral anticoagulants was stopped. Of these patients, 25% had increased homocysteine levels, and these patients had a 19% recurrence of DVT after 2 years, in comparison to a 6.3% recurrence rate in those patients without increased homocysteine levels (90). It appears that elevated homocysteine levels increase the risk of venous thrombosis up to fourfold (90).

Normalization of homocysteine levels can be accomplished by giving folic acid with or without B_{12}. It remains to be proven, however, that the normalization of homocysteine levels confers any benefit. Treatment, therefore, is unclear. In asymptomatic patients, vitamin supplementation is probably reasonable. In patients who have had DVT, anticoagulation with warfarin or low-molecular-weight heparin should be undertaken, but the time course of this therapy is uncertain. There is evidence that these patients are at high risk for recurrent DVT; for them, lifelong anticoagulation should be considered.

X. UNEXPLAINED THROMBOSIS–GUIDELINE FOR IDENTIFYING HYPERCOAGULABLE PATIENTS

A thorough patient history remains the most important means of identifying patients with potential hypercoagulable disorders. Patients should be asked about previously unexplained thromboses experienced by themselves or by family members. Patients with hypercoagulable syndromes will often report episodes of thrombophlebitis in early adulthood. Of particular importance are those episodes of thrombophlebitis without any contributing factors for their development (e.g., long leg fractures, prolonged immobilization, bed rest because of illness). Hypercoagulable disorders become even more significant in patients with recurrent episodes of thrombophlebitis. Likewise, a history of arterial thrombosis, especially if the episodes occurred at a young age, is an indicator of a coagulation disorder. Eldrup-Jorgensen et al. (91) found a 30% incidence of coagulation abnormalities in patients below 51 years of age undergoing vascular reconstruction. Abnormal clotting syndromes noted were protein S deficiency, protein C deficiency, presence of lupus-like anticoagulants, and plasminogen deficiency. The incidence of arterial graft thrombosis in hypercoagulable patients was 20% at 30 days, which is markedly increased from what one would expect from this type of vascular reconstruction.

A. Clinical Presentation

With experience, one has a sense for what kinds of reconstructions should work and has some expectations concerning the types of problems that can occur. Likewise, one develops a feel for what are typical presentations of atherosclerotic occlusive disease. Unusual or unexplained thromboses (e.g., a thrombosed suprarenal aorta, upper extremity thrombosis, or a total tibial artery occlusion in a patient who is neither diabetic nor has any evidence of atherosclerotic occlusive disease elsewhere) should alert the surgeon to consider a hypercoagulable disorder as the cause. Unusual x-ray findings—in particular, occlusions seen in young patients or in one extremity when the other extremity has no evidence of any disease—should trigger an investigation of the coagulation system.

The role of screening for hypercoagulable states in vascular surgery patients is difficult to ascertain. Donaldson et al. (92) found a 9.5% overall incidence of vascular surgery patients with abnormal test results indicating potential hypercoagulability. The three most common entities demonstrated were heparin-induced platelet aggregation, lupus-like anticoagulants, and protein C deficiency. The incidence of infrainguinal graft occlusion within 30 days was 27% in the hypercoagulable group compared with 1.6% in the noncoagulable group. Currently we do not perform routine screening to detect patients with hypercoagulable states. We depend on patient history and clinical evaluation to identify those patients who may be hypercoagulable, which is probably more cost-effective and efficient than routine screening.

The most difficult experience for a vascular surgeon is dealing with unexplained thrombosis that occurs intraoperatively. Often this occurs during late evening or nighttime hours, when support from the coagulation laboratory is not available. The first step, if indeed heparin has been given, is to determine whether there is clotting in the operative field, which would indicate an AT III deficiency, since AT III is essential for heparin's anticoagulant effect. The anesthesiologist should then test the heparin effect by determining partial thromboplastin time or by performing one of the other variety of tests to measure heparin anticoagulation. The next step is to obtain a platelet count. If it is higher than $100,000/mm^3$ and the activated clotting time (ATC) is not prolonged, the problem is presumed to be the antithrombin system. The patient is then given two units of fresh frozen plasma, with two units given every 12 h for 5 days. AT III deficiency is usually confirmed the next day, with tests done on blood drawn the day before the administration of fresh frozen plasma. Patients with AT III deficiency are maintained on long-term warfarin therapy. If the platelet count is less than $100,000/mm^3$, we presume that heparin-induced platelet aggregation has developed. The patient's history should be carefully examined to try to document the prior administration of heparin. At this time we administer a 50-mL bolus dose of dextran and continue dextran therapy at 25 mL/h. The heparin is reversed with protamine, and platelet aggregation abnormality is confirmed in the morning. Warfarin treatment is continued for 3 weeks to 6 months.

If the platelet count is greater than $100,000/mm^3$ and the ACT is prolonged, we presume that the patient has some other sort of hypercoagulable state, which includes fibrinolytic abnormalities as well as potential problems with protein C, protein S, and lupus-like anticoagulants. In these patients we institute continuous heparin therapy both intraoperatively and postoperatively and give them two units of fresh frozen plasma. Fresh frozen plasma is "shotgun" therapy for a wide variety of coagulation abnormalities.

In the operating room, before the institution of any therapy, blood should be drawn for coagulation tests; it should be kept in mind that many of these tests (e.g., plasminogen electrophoresis and determination of protein C, protein S, and lupus-like anticoagulant) are quite involved, sometimes taking days to a week at some centers. However, if the blood is properly handled, spun down, and frozen, the tests can be done routinely. Our policy is to repeat all abnormal tests in 5 days. One of the problems in diagnosing coagulation abnormalities accurately is that in the process of clotting, clotting factors can be consumed and abnormalities may be the result of clotting and not the cause of it. For all factors that still demonstrate abnormal values at 5–7 days, tests are repeated at 1 month. Patients who have persistently abnormal values are then labeled truly hypercoagulable.

McDaniel et al. (93) have noted the change in coagulation factors with operation. They determined that AT III levels fell on the third postoperative day and subsequently returned to normal by 1 week postoperatively. AT III declined from a mean preoperative level of 110–71% on the third postoperative day. This value returned to normal by the seventh postoperative day, when it was 95% or at the normal.activity level. This variability demonstrates the dynamic aspect of the clotting system and points to the danger of attaching significance to just one isolated laboratory finding. In most patients who sustain complications because of hypercoagulable states, warfarin therapy is instituted in the perioperative and postoperative period. In patients with heparin-induced platelet aggregation, therapy can usually be stopped after 3 months; however, we have recommended prolonged administration in patients with protein C or S deficiency, AT III deficiency, and plasminogen abnormalities because of the risk of recurrent thrombosis.

REFERENCES

1. Babcock RB, Dumper CW, Scharfman WB. Heparin-induced immune thrombocytopenia. N Engl J Med 1976; 295:237–241.
2. Baird RA, Convery RF. Arterial thromboembolism in patients receiving systemic heparin therapy. J Bone Joint Surg 1977; 59:1061–1064.
3. Bell WR, Romasulo PA, Alving BM, et al. Thrombocytopenia occurring during the administration of heparin. Ann Intern Med 1976; 87:155–160.
4. Fratantoni JC, Pollet R, Gralnick HR. Heparin-induced thrombocytopenia: Confirmation of diagnosis with in vitro methods. Blood 1975; 45:395–401.
5. Nelson JC, Lerner RG, Goldstein R, et al. Heparin-induced thrombocytopenia. Arch Intern Med 1978; 138:548–552.
6. Warkentin TE, Levine MN, Hirsh J, et al. Heparin-induced thrombocytopenia in patients treated with low molecular weight heparin or unfractionated heparin. N Engl J Med 1995; 332:1330–1335.
7. Towne JB, Bernhard VM, Hussey C, et al. White clot syndrome. Arch Surg 1979; 114:372–377.
8. Rhodes GR, Dixon RH, Silver D. Heparin-induced thrombocytopenia. Ann Surg 1977; 186:752–758.
9. Silver D. Heparin-induced thrombocytopenia Semin. Vasc Surg 1988; 1:228.
10. Laster J, Ckrit D, Walder N, et al. The heparin-induced thrombocytopenia syndrome update. Surgery 1987; 102:763.
11. Kapsch DN, Adelstein EH, Rhodes GR, et al. Heparin-induced thrombocytopenia, thrombosis, and hemorrhage. Surgery 1979; 86:148–154.
12. Laster J, Silver D. Heparin-coated catheters and heparin-induced thrombocytopenia. J Vasc Surg 1988; 7:667–672.
13. Rosenthanl F. Risk factors for venous thrombosis: Prevalence, risk and interactum. Semin Hematol 1997; 34:171–187.
14. Silver D, Kapsch DN, Tsoi EKM. Heparin-induced thrombocytopenia, thrombosis, and hemorrhage. Ann Surg 1983; 198:301–306.
15. Laster J, Cikrit D, Walker N, et al. The heparin-induced thrombocytopenia syndrome: An update. Surgery 1987; 102:763–770.
16. Laster J, Elfrink R, Silver D. Reexposure to heparin of patients with heparin-associated antibodies. J Vasc Surg 1989; 9:677–682.

17. Kappa JR, Fisher CA, Berkowitz HD, et al. Heparin-induced platelet activation in sixteen surgical patients: Diagnosis and management. J Vasc Surg 1987; 5:101–109.
18. Makhoul RG, Greenberg CS, McCann RL. Heparin-associated thrombocytopenia and thrombosis: A serious clinical problem and potential solution. J Vasc Surg 1986; 4:522–528.
19. Sobel M, Adelman B, Szaboles S, et al. Surgical management of heparin-associated thrombocytopenia. J Vasc Surg 1988; 8:395–401.
20. Latham P, Revelis AF, Joshi GP, Di Maio JM, Jessen ME. Use of recombinant hirudin in patients with heparin-induced thrombocytopenia with thrombosis requiring cardiopulmonary bypass. Anesthesia 2000; 92:263–269.
21. Cole CW, Bormanis J. Ancrod: A practical alternative to heparin. J Vasc Surg 1988; 8:59–63.
22. Abildguard U, Fagerhol MK, Egeberg O. Comparison of progressive antithrombin activity and the concentration of three thrombin inhibitors in human plasma. Scand J Clin Lab Invest 1970; 26:349–354.
23. Seegers WH. Antithrombin III: Theory and clinical applications. Am J Clin Pathol 1978; 69:367–374.
24. Eseberg O. Inherited antithrombin deficiency causing thrombophilia. Thromb Diath Haemorrh 1963; 13:516–530.
25. Brozovic M, Stirling U, Hamlyn AN. Thrombotic tendency and probable antithrombin III deficiency. Thromb Haemost 1978; 39:778–779.
26. Mackie M, Bennett B, Ogstron D, et al. Familial thrombosis: Inherited deficiency of antithrombin III. Br Med J 1978; 1:136–138.
27. Marciniak E, Farley CH, DeSimone PA. Familial thrombosis due to antithrombin III deficiency. Blood 1974; 43:219–231.
28. Sorenson PJ, Dyerburg J, Strotterson E, et al. Familial functional antithrombin III deficiency. Scand J Haematol 1980; 24:105–109.
29. Collen D, Schetz J, DeCock F, et al. Metabolism of antithrombin III (heparin cofactor) in man: Effects of venous thrombosis and of heparin administration. Eur J Clin Invest 1977; 7: 27–35.
30. Odeguard OR, Abildguard U. Antithombin III: Critical review of assay methods. Significance of variations in health and disease. Haemostasis 1978; 7:127–134.
31. Chan V, Chan TK, Wong V, et al. The determination of antithrombin III by radioimmunoassay and its clinical application. Br J Haematol 1979; 41:563–572.
32. Sas G, Blasko G, Banghogyi D, et al. Abnormal antithrombin III (antithrombin Budapest) as a cause of familial thrombophilia. Thromb Diath Haemorrh 1974; 32:105–115.
33. Flinn WR, McDaniel MD, Yao JST, et al. Antithrombin III deficiency as a reflection of dynamic protein metabolism in patients undergoing vascular reconstruction. J Vasc Surg 1984; 1:888–895.
34. Towne JB, Bernhard VM, Hussey C, et al. Antithrombin deficiency—A cause of unexplained thrombosis in vascular surgery. Surgery 1981; 89:735–742.
35. Bick R, Kaplan H. Syndrome of thrombosis and hypercoagulability. Med Clin North Am 1998; 82:409–458.
36. Bick RL, Pergram M. Syndrome of hypercoagualablity and thrombosis. Semin Thromb Haemost 1994; 20(1):109.
37. Lynch DM, Leff, Howe SE. Preoperative AT-III values and clinical postoperative thrombosis: A comparison of three antithrombin III assays. Thromb Haemost 1984; 52:42–44.
38. Sagar S, Stamatakis JD, Thomas DP, et al. Oral contraceptives, antithrombin III activity and postoperative deep vein thrombosis. Lancet 1976; 1:509–511.
39. Conrad J, Lecompte T, Horellou MH, et al. Antithrombin III in patients treated with subcutaneous or intravenous heparin. Thromb Res 1981; 22:507–511.
40. Tengborn L, Bergqvist D. Surgery in patients with congenital antithrombin III deficiency. Acta Chir Scand 1988; 154:179–188.
41. Salem HH, Mitchell CA, Firkin BG. Current views on pathophysiology and investigations of thrombotic disorders. Am J Haematol 1987; 25:463–474.

42. Towne JB. Hypercoaguable states. Semin Vasc Surg 1988; 1(4):201–215.

43. Wiman B, Ljungberg B, Chmielewska J, et al. The role of the fibrinolytic system in deep vein thrombosis. J Lab Clin Med 1985; 105:265–270.

44. Castellino FJ, Powell JR. Human plasminogen. Methods Enzymol 1981; 80:365–378.

45. Wallen P, Wiman B. Characterization of human plasminogen. Biochem Biophys Acta 1972; 257:122–134.

46. Mullertz S. Fibrinolysis: An overview. Semin Thromb Haermost 1988; 10:1–5.

47. Summaria L, Arzadon P, Bernabe P, et al. Studies on the isolation of the multiple molecular forms of human plasminogen and plasmin by isoelectric focusing methods. J Biol Chem 1972; 247:4691–4702.

48. Aoki N, Moroi M, Sakata Y, et al. Abnormal plasminogen—A hereditary molecular abnormality found in patients with recurrent thrombosis. J Clin Invest 1978; 61:1186–1195.

49. Kazama M, Tohura C, Suzuki Z, et al. Abnormal plasminogen—A cause of recurrent thrombosis. Thromb Res 1981; 21:517–522.

50. Soria J, Soria C, Bertarnd O, et al. Plasminogen Paris I: Congenital abnormal plasminogen and its incidence in thrombosis. Thromb Res 1983; 32:229–238.

51. Scharrer IM, Wohl RC, Hach V, et al. Investigation of congential abnormal plasminogen, Frankfurt I and its relationshiop to thrombosis. Thromb Haemostas 1986; 55:396–401.

52. Liu Y, Lyons RM, McDonagh J. Plasminogen San Antonio: An abnormal plasminogen with more cathodic migration, decrease activation and associated thrombosis. Thromb Haemost 1988; 59:49–53.

53. Ikemoto S, Sakata Y, Aoki N. Genetic polymorphism of human plasminogen in a human population. Hum Hered 1987; 32:296–297.

54. Towne JB, Bandyk DF, Hussey CV, et al. Abnormal plasminogen: A genetically determined cause of hypercoagulability. J Vasc Surg 1984; 1:896–902.

55. Towne JB, Hussey CV, Bandyk DF. Abnormalities of the fibrinolytic system as a cause of upper extremity ischemia. J Vasc Surg 1988; 7:661–666.

56. Wiman B. The role of the fibrinolytic system in thrombotic disease. Acta Med Scand 1986; 715 (suppl):169–171.

57. Chmielewska J, Ranby M, Wiman B. Evidence of a rapid inhibitor to tissue plasminogen activator in plasma. Thromb Res 1983; 31:427–437.

58. Kruithof EKO, Tran-Thang C, Ransijn A, et al. Demonstration of a fast-acting inhibitor of plasminogen activators in human plasma. Blood 1984; 64:907–913.

59. Hamsten A, Wiman B, deFaire U, et al. Increased plasma levels of a rapid inhibitor of tissue plasminogen activator in young survivors of myocardial infarction. N Engl J Med 1985; 313: 1557–1563.

60. Wiman B, Lujungberg B, Chmielweska J, et al. The role of the fibrinolytic system in deep venous thrombosis. J Lab Clin Med 1985; 105:265–270.

61. Wiman B, Chimielewska J, Ranby M. Inactivation of tissue plasminogen activator in plasma. J Biol Chem 1984; 259:3644–3647.

62. Marlar RA. Protein C in thromboembolic disease. Semin Thromb Hemost 1985; 11:387–393.

63. Clouse LH, Comp PC. The regulation of hemostasis: The protein C system. N Engl J Med 1986; 314:1298–1303.

64. Stenflo J. Structure and function of protein C. Semin Thromb Hemost 1984; 10:109–121.

65. Kazmier FJ. Thromboembolism, coumarin necrosis, and protein C. Mayo Clin Proc 1985; 60:673–674.

66. Peterson CE, Kwaan HC. Current concepts of warfarin therapy. Arch Intern Med 1986; 146:581–584.

67. Branson HE, Kate J, Marble R, et al. Inherited protein C deficiency and coumarin-responsive chronic relapsing purpura fulminans in a newborn infant. Lancet 1983; 2:1165–1168.

68. Salem HH, Mitchell CH, Firkin BG. Current views on pathophysiology and investigations of thrombotic disorders. Am J Hematol 1987; 25:463–474.

69. Broekmans AW, Veltkamp JJ, Bertina RM. Congenital protein C deficiency and venous thromboembolism: A study of three Dutch families. N Engl J Med 1983; 390:340–344.

70. Griffen JG, Evan B, Zimmerman TS, et al. Deficiency of protein C in thrombotic disease. J Clin Invest 1981; 68:1370–1373.

71. Tollefson DFJ, Friedman KD, Marlar RA, et al. Protein C deficiency: A cause of unusual or unexplained thrombosis. Arch Surg 1988; 123:881–884.

72. Green D, Ganger DR, Blei AT. Protein C deficiency in splanchnic venous thrombosis. Am J Med 1987; 82:1171–1173.

73. Coller BS, Owen J, Jesty J, et al. Deficiency of plasma protein S, protein C, or antithrombin III and arterial thrombosis. Atherosclerosis 1987; 7:456–462.

74. Comp PC, Esmon CT. Recurrent venous thromboembolism in patients with a partial deficiency of protein S. N Engl J Med 1984; 311:1526–1528.

75. Schwarz HP, Fischer M, Hopmeir P, et al. Plasma protein S deficiency in familial thrombotic disease. Blood 1984; 64:1297–1300.

76. Rodgers GM, Shurman MA. Congenital thrombotic disorders. Am J Hematol 1986; 21:419–430.

77. Gladson CL, Griffen JH, Hach V, et al. The incidence of protein C and protein S deficiency in 139 young thrombotic patients. Thrombosis 1985; 66:350a.

78. Espinoza LR, Hartmann RC. Significance of the lupus anticoagulant. Am J Hematol 1986; 22:331–337.

79. Tabechnik-Schor NF, Lipton SA. Association of lupus-like anticoagulant and nonvasculitic cerebral infarction. Arch Neurol 1986; 43:851–852.

80. Shi W, Kriis SA, Chong BH, et al. Prevalence of lupus anticoagulant and anticardiolipin antibodies in a healthy population. Aust NZ J Med 1990; 20:231–236.

81. Dührsen U, Brittinger G. Lupus anticoagulant associated syndrome in benign and malignant systemic disease. Klin Wochenschr 1987; 65:818–822.

82. Ahn SS, Kalunian K, Rosove M, et al. Postoperative thrombotic complications in patients with lupus anticoagulant: Increased risk after vascular procedure. J Vasc Surg 1988; 7:749–756.

83. Greenfield LJ. Lupus-like anticoagulants and thrombosis. J Vasc Surg 1988; 7:818–819.

84. Tsakiris DA, Settas L, Makris PE, et al. Lupus anticoagulant-antiphospholipid antibodies and thrombophilia: Relation to protein-C and protein-S thrombomodulin. J Rheumatol 1990; 17: 785–789.

85. Svensson PJ, Dahlbäch B. Resistance to activated protein C as a basis for venous thrombosis. N Engl J Med 1994; 330:517–521.

86. Bertino RM, Koelemon BP, Kosta, et al. Mutation in blood coagulation factor V associated with resistance to activated protein C. Nature 1994; 369:64.

87. Zeller B, Svensson PJ, Xuhua H, Dahlbäch B. Identification of the same factor V gene mutation in 47 out of 50 thrombosis-prone families with inherited resistance to activated protein C. J Clin Invest 1994; 94:2521.

88. Rosenthaul F. Risk factors for venous thrombosis: Prevalence, risk and interaction. Semin Hematol 1997; 34:171–187.

89. Bos G, Den Heijer M. Hyperhomocysteinemia and venous thrombosis. Semin Thromb Hemost 1998; 24:387–391.

90. Elchinger Stumpflen A, Hirschl M, et al. Hyperhomocysteinemia is a risk factor of recurrent venous thromboembolism. Thromb Haemost 1998; 80:566–569.

91. Eldrup-Jorgensen J, Flanigan DP, Brace l, et al. Hypercoagulable states and lower limb ischemia in young adults. J Vasc Surg 1989; 9:334–341.

92. Donaldson MC, Weinberg DS, Belkin M, et al. Screening for hypercoagulable states in a vascular surgery practice: A preliminary study. J Vasc Surg 1990; 11:825–831.

93. McDaniel MD, Pearce WH, Yao JST, et al. Sequential changes in coagulation and platelet function following femoro-tibial bypass. J Vasc Surg 1984; 1:261–268.

8

Complications and Failures of Anticoagulant and Antithrombotic Therapy

John R. Hoch

University of Wisconsin Medical School, Madison, Wisconsin, U.S.A.

The development of effective anticoagulation strategies was critical to the establishment of vascular surgery as a specialty. Today, we are fortunate to have established anticoagulant agents such as heparin and warfarin, which have proven effective for the prevention and treatment of most thromboembolic disorders. In addition, there are numerous exciting new pharmacological options currently undergoing clinical trials; these may ultimately improve on the effectiveness of current agents and their safety profiles. Vascular surgeons must be knowledgeable about the pharmacology of each agent, its indications for use, and how the effect of the agent is monitored. Most failures in anticoagulant therapy arise from improper choice of agent or administration of insufficient or excessive amounts of the anticoagulant. The major complication of anticoagulation therapy is hemorrhage; however, other, less common adverse effects may affect the survival of life and/or limb.

The surgeon's choice of anticoagulant or antithrombotic agent is dependent upon the nature of the thrombus. Major classes of anticoagulants and antithrombotics include (a) heparins, which induce inhibition of activated coagulation proteins by their interaction with the natural anticoagulant antithrombin (AT, formerly known as antithrombin III); (b) vitamin K antagonists, such as warfarin (Coumadin); (c) direct thrombin inhibitors, such as lepirudin, bivalirudin, and argatroban; (d) factor Xa inhibitors, such as fondaparinux; and (e) platelet function inhibitors, which include aspirin, the thienopyridines (ticlopidine and clopidogrel), and the platelet glycoprotein IIb/IIIa (GPIIb/IIIa) receptor inhibitors. Each class has a different mode of action and indication for use in the treatment or the prophylaxis of thromboembolic disease.

I. UNFRACTIONATED HEPARIN

Unfractionated heparin (UFH) is the anticoagulant of choice for the management of most acute thromboembolic disorders because of its rapid anticoagulant effect when administered intravenously. UFH is an effective prophylaxis for patients at high risk for deep venous thrombosis (DVT) as well as for the treatment of venous thrombosis and pulmonary embolism (PE). Intravenous UFH is indicated for patients undergoing cardiac surgery and vascular surgery as well as coronary and peripheral artery angioplasty. Low-molecular-weight heparins (LMWHs), which were introduced over 25 years ago, have proven to be safe and offer similar or superior efficacy compared to UFH in the management and prophylaxis of thromboembolism. LMWHs offer the advantages of ease of administration, improved bioavailability, and predictable anticoagulation.

A.   Pharmacology

UFH is a mixture of straight-chain glycosaminoglycan sulfate esters with molecular weights ranging from 3000 to 30,000 Da. UFH has a mean molecular weight of 15,000 Da. and contains 10–90 saccharides per molecule (1). Beef lung and porcine intestinal mucosa are the traditional sources for commercial UFH. They have different ratios of high- and low-molecular-weight fractions, with differing anticoagulant activities. Because of this variation in activity, heparin is dispensed in international units (IU) rather than by weight.

Heparins anticoagulant effect is dependent on a plasma cofactor, the proteinase inhibitor antithrombin (AT). Heparin binds to and potentiates the activity of AT via a specific glucosamine unit contained within a pentasaccharide sequence (1,2). Only one-third of UFH molecules contain this specific pentasaccharide sequence. The remaining two-thirds of heparin molecules in UFH preparations contain minimal anticoagulant activity (3). At higher than usual clinical doses of heparin, both fractions of heparin with high and low affinity for antithrombin potentiate the antithrombin effects of a second serine protease inhibitor, heparin cofactor II (4).

The major mechanism responsible for the anticoagulant effect of UFH is the action of the heparin-AT complex, which inactivates activated coagulation proteins thrombin (factor IIa), factor IXa, factor Xa, factor XIa, and factor XIIa. Thrombin and factor Xa are most sensitive to the effects of the heparin-AT complex. Heparin combines with AT in a 1:1 stoichiometric ratio and produces a conformational change in AT that fully activates its serine protease-inhibitory site. Heparin molecules with molecular weights greater than 5000 Da, composed of sequences at least 18 saccharides long, form a ternary complex composed of heparin, AT, and an activated coagulation factor (thrombin, factor IXa or factor XIa) (5). Heparin molecules with molecular weights less than 5,000 Da, composed of sequences less than 18 saccharides long, cannot bind to thrombin (1,2,5). These small fragments, containing a high-affinity pentasaccharide sequence, form a binary complex with AT capable of inactivating factor Xa and factor XIIa (2,5). Heparin may disassociate from the complex and catalyze other thrombin-AT interactions once the AT has neutralized an activated coagulation factor (6). The success of low-dose heparin for venous thromboembolic prophylaxis has been attributed to the inhibition of thrombin production by the heparin-AT complex inhibition of factor Xa. Just 1 μg of the binary heparin-AT complex is able to inhibit 32 U of factor Xa, which is equivalent to the inhibition to 1600 U of thrombin. In contrast, 1000 μg of AT would be required to directly inactive a similar amount of thrombin without the presence of heparin (6).

UFH has also been shown to induce secretion of tissue factor pathway inhibitor by endothelial cells (7). Tissue factor pathway inhibitor (TFPI) inhibits factor VIIa–tissue factor (TF)–induced factor X activation, leading to decreased thrombin generation (7).

Decreased thrombin production by this pathway and by thrombin inactivation by the heparin-AT complex leads to the inhibition of thrombin-induced activation of factor V and factor VIII, potentiating the antithrombotic effect of heparin (8).

Heparin has been shown to bind to platelets and impede their function, causing a prolongation of bleeding time in humans (9). The higher-molecular-weight heparin fractions that have a lower affinity for AT seem to be primarily responsible for heparin's effect on platelet function (10). Heparin's antihemostatic effects may be secondary to its interaction with platelets as well as its anticoagulation effects.

Intravenous infusion of heparin is necessary to achieve an immediate anticoagulant effect, as its availability is decreased by the subcutaneous route (11). After intravenous injection, heparin rapidly binds to the endothelium, macrophages, and UFH-binding plasma proteins (12). Heparin's affinity for plasma proteins is partly responsible for the variability of the anticoagulant response to UFH. The mechanism of heparin clearance is complex. At low and therapeutic doses of heparin, clearance is achieved by binding to receptors on endothelial cells and macrophages where depolymerization occurs. This rapid, saturable mechanism of clearance is responsible for the nonlinear anticoagulant response seen with UFH in the therapeutic range. A second slower, unsaturable mechanism of UFH clearance is kidney-dependent. This mechanism of heparin clearance primarily acts at very high plasma concentrations of heparin. The average half-life of circulating heparin in the therapeutic range is approximately 90 min. Renal failure does not affect the anticoagulant half-life or clearance of UFH when it is administered in a therapeutic range. Hepatic insufficiency has no effect on heparin clearance but may affect anticoagulant activity by reducing the availability of AT and other clotting factors.

Several methods are available to monitor the anticoagulant effect of heparin. The activated partial thromboplastin tine (APTT) is most widely used, with maintenance of the APTT in the range of 1.5–2 times the control values associated with inhibition of intravascular coagulation without excessive risk of hemorrhage (13). The ATT is sensitive to the inhibitory effects of heparin on thrombin, factor Xa, and factor IXa. The APTT should be measured 4–6 h after an initial bolus dose of heparin, the hourly intravenous dose of UFH being adjusted accordingly. The activated clotting time (ACT) may also be used and has the advantage of a linear response to increasing doses of heparin (21). Maintenance of the ACT in the range of 150–200 s provides adequate levels of anticoagulation in the treatment of DVT or acute pulmonary embolism (13); ACT in the range of 200–250 s is recommended for arterial surgery and/or peripheral or coronary endovascular intervention (13).

B. Clinical Application

Multiple studies have documented the effectiveness of low-dose heparin (5000 U subcutaneously 2 h before surgery and every 8–12 h postoperatively until the patient is ambulatory) in reducing the incidence of postoperative DVT and fatal pulmonary embolism. In a review of randomized trials involving more than 15,000 surgical patients, perioperative prophylaxis with UFH was shown to significantly reduce the incidence of DVT by approximately 60%, the incidence of pulmonary embolism (PE) by 47%, and total mortality in the series by 21% compared with control patients (14).

For patients with DVT and PE, the goal of anticoagulation is to prevent clot propagation and new clot formation. Today, LMWH is the anticoagulant of choice for the majority of patients with confirmed DVT and PE (15). Extensive iliofemoral DVT is our primary indication for using intravenous UFH in the management of patients with venous thromboembolism. Although multiple clinical trials comparing UFH with LMWH in the treatment of venous thromboembolism have shown similar efficacy and safety, patients with extensive iliofemoral DVT were usually excluded from these trials because of the large thrombus burden and high levels of activated clotting factors. We recommend a large heparin bolus of 200 U/kg of body weight. The heparin bolus is followed by continuous intravenous infusion of heparin that is adjusted frequently to maintain the APTT at twice the control value. Continuous intravenous heparin infusion is maintained at therapeutic levels for 7–10 days in this subgroup of patients. Oral anticoagulation with warfarin should be started on the first day of unfractionated heparin treatment. Heparin infusion should be continued until the prothrombin time international normalized ratio (INR) has been prolonged into the therapeutic range for at least 4 days (16). UFH can be easily reversed with protamine and has a shorter plasma half-life than LMWH, making it the anticoagulant of choice for patients preparing to undergo surgical or endovascular procedures who require pre- and postoperative anticoagulation.

Intravenous UFH is used by vascular surgeons on a daily basis during arterial reconstructive surgery as well as in performing percutaneous endovascular procedures. Our bias at this time is to give arterial reconstructive patients an intravenous bolus of 100 IU/kg of UFH immediately prior to arterial clamping or balloon angioplasty. Adequacy of anticoagulation is assessed by hourly ACTs. If the ACT falls below 200 s, an additional 1000-U bolus of heparin is administered.

Heparin is used in the management of acute arterial thromboembolic disease to prevent thrombus propagation and to permit collaterals to develop. Whether maintenance of intravenous UFH is necessary following successful thrombolectomy is controversial (17). Our practice is to maintain heparin infusion for 3–4 days following surgery and then to convert to warfarin anticoagulation for those patients identified to have mural thrombus on echocardiogram or atrial fibrillation.

C. Complications

The most common complication of heparin therapy is hemorrhage, which may vary from mild mucosal oozing or hematuria to extensive intracranial, gastrointestinal, retroperitoneal, or urinary bleeding. The risk of hemorrhage from prophylactic low-dose subcutaneous heparin therapy is small. The incidence of wound hematomas in patients placed on prophylactic heparin therapy postoperatively is less than 15% if 15,000 IU or less of heparin is administered daily (18). The incidence of hemorrhage requiring transfusion in these postoperative patients is less than 4% (18). There is a 6–10% risk of bleeding complications when anticoagulation is in the therapeutic range (19). The incidence of hemorrhage, however, may approach 50% in patients with renal failure, underlying hemostatic defects, or thrombocytopenia (19). Patients with severe hypertension, ongoing bleeding, recent neurosurgical operation, or those undergoing percutaneous endovascular procedures are at heightened risk. With close monitoring of the APTT (range of 1.5–2 times control), patients without these risk factors have a small risk of major bleeding complications.

Hemorrhage that is not life-threatening is best managed by discontinuation of heparin therapy. If bleeding continues, heparin may be neutralized with protamine sulfate. The amount of protamine sulfate required can be calculated from results of a protamine titration test or the ACT. If the tests cannot be done, 1–1.5 mg of protamine is usually required to neutralize 100 U of heparin. Portions of the calculated dose, 30–50%, are given slowly intravenously to reduce the risk of hypotension, bradycardia, and peripheral vasodilatation. Excessive administration of protamine should be avoided, as protamine may also act as an anticoagulant via its interaction with platelets and serum proteins (19).

A second potentially life- or limb-threatening complication of heparin is the development of heparin-induced thrombocytopenia (HIT) syndrome. Approximately 1–5% of patients receiving heparin develop heparin-associated antiplatelet antibodies (HAAbs) (21,22). HIT antibodies bind to the antigen composed of a complex of heparin and platelet factor 4 (PF4). The heparin-PF4-IgG immune complexes bind to platelet FcIIa receptors leading to platelet aggregation. Thrombin is generated, possibly as a consequence of antibody damage leading to expression of tissue factor (12,21). The result is the potential for devastating arterial and venous thrombotic complications.

The development of HIT occurs after 4–5 days of UFH therapy in patients exposed to heparin for the first time; thrombocytopenia may develop as early as 24 h in patients who have been reexposed to heparin who have had recent exposure to heparin and have circulating HAAbs (23). Patients characteristically exhibit a drop in platelet count greater than 50% from their baseline, platelets often falling to less than $50,000/mm^3$ (23). Importantly however, 10–15% of patients will have a platelet counts that remain above $150,000/mm^3$. In addition to monitoring the platelet count, patients who demonstrate increasing resistance to anticoagulation with UFH, or new or progressive hemorrhagic or thrombotic complications while on heparin should be screened for HAAbs.

HIT has been associated with a 23% mortality and a 61% morbidity (24). However, with early recognition and treatment, mortality and morbidity can be reduced to 12 and 22.5% respectively (22). Once patients are suspected of HIT, all heparin therapy must be discontinued; this includes even "minor" sources of heparin, including intravenous flushes and heparin-coated catheters. Patients should be administered an appropriate platelet function inhibiting agent (aspirin or clopidogrel) pending diagnosis of HIT. The diagnosis of HIT should be confirmed by either a functional test or an antigen assay. Available functional tests include the serotonin release assay as well as heparin-induced platelet aggregation assays (25,26). The heparin-PF4 enzyme linked immunosorbent assay is an antigen assay in which patient's serum is tested for the presence of antibodies to heparin-PF4. This assay results in a very low number of false-negative results; however, its specificity is lower than that of the functional assays (27,28).

Management of patients with ongoing anticoagulation requirements who have HAAbs is difficult. In centers that have access to heparin-induced platelet aggregation assays, one can test LMWHs against the patient's antibodies to look for cross-reactivity. Cross-reactivity rate with LMWH varies from 20–61% depending on which LMWH is tested (28,29). If all LMWHs cross-react with the patient's antibodies or if a platelet aggregation assay is not available at your hospital, then the recommended management of HIT in patients who require anticoagulation is with intravenous direct thrombin inhibitors (30).

Sensitivity reactions consisting of bronchiole constriction, lack of lacrimation, or urticaria may occur in 2–5% of the patients receiving heparin. Anaphylaxis with circulatory collapse is a rare complication of heparin administration.

Long-term administration of heparin may be associated with alopecia and osteoporosis. The incidence of alopecia is higher in patients who are also receiving warfarin. Hair growth usually resumes once heparin administration is discontinued. Heparin is known to suppress osteoclast formation and to activate osteoblasts that may promote bone loss (12). Osteoporosis and pathological fractures of the vertebral column and long bones have been reported in patients receiving heparin for more than 6 months in dosages exceeding 10,000 U/day (31).

D. Failures

Most failures of heparin therapy are iatrogenic and are related to (a) the use of heparin in patients with contraindications, (b) the administration of insufficient amounts of heparin, (c) not beginning the prophylactic heparin regimen early enough, and (d) and on rare occasions the development of sensitivities to heparin or a congenital or acquired AT deficiency. Prophylactic regimens consisting of low-dose UFH must be initiated either before or concomitantly with the event placing the patient at risk for thromboembolic complications. Low-dose subcutaneous UFH has shown equal efficacy as a prophylactic agent for the prevention of venous thromboembolism even in high-risk general surgery patients compared to LMWHs (32). However, low-dose UFH is not recommended as a venous prophylactic agent in patients undergoing major orthopedic surgery, those with acute spinal cord injury, or in patients with multiple trauma (32). LMWH is the prophylactic agent of choice for these patients unless heparin is contraindicated (32).

Patients who fail to achieve therapeutic levels of anticoagulation with increasing amounts of heparin or require a higher than average doses of heparin to prolong the APTT into the therapeutic range are designated "heparin resistant." Surgeons should become concerned if the daily dose of intravenous UFH exceeds 35,000 U per 24/h (33). Possible causes of heparin resistance include the presence of AT deficiency, the development of HIT, and elevations of factor VIII, fibrinogen, and PF4 (57–62). Factor VIII and fibrinogen levels have been shown to be elevated during many acute illnesses and during pregnancy. Increased levels of factor VIII act to limit the response of the APTT to heparin; however; the in vivo antithrombotic effect is not diminished (33). Thus patients proven to have elevated factor VIII levels should have their heparin anticoagulation monitored by measuring anti-Xa activity (33). It is recommended that for patients who require greater than 35,000 U of UFH per 24 h, the dose should be adjusted to maintain the anti-Xa levels of 0.35–0.70 IU/mL (12,33).

Heparin has limited anticoagulant activity in patients with congenital or acquired AT deficiencies. AT concentrations may decrease during heparin therapy, with up to a 12% decrease 4 h after initiation of therapy and a 33% decrease with continued therapy. Patients with preexisting AT deficiency may experience even greater decreases in circulating in AT concentrations with prolonged heparin administration (34). Fresh frozen plasma or cryoprecipitate can be utilized to replenish deficient levels of AT and allow continued use of UFH. Alternatively, intravenous direct thrombin inhibitors can be utilized if continued anticoagulation is necessary in patients with heparin resistance.

II. LOW-MOLECULAR-WEIGHTS HEPARINS

LMWHs reached the clinical arena in the late 1970s with the promise of several clinical advantages over UFH, including superior bioavailability when administered subcutaneously, equivalent or lower incidence of bleeding complications, lower risk of HIT; predictable dose response, and fixed-dose administration without monitoring (35). LMWH has clearly shifted the paradigm for care of patients with venous thromboembolism. Its rapid adoption by clinicians is primarily because of its pharmacokinetic advantages over UFH.

A. Pharmacology

Commercial LMWHs are prepared by acidic hydrolysis, esterification, enzymatic depolymerization, or fractionation of UFH (36). LMWHs have an average molecular weight of 4500–6000 Da. Over half of the saccharide units in LMW preparations are less than 18 U long. These smaller fragments contain the high affinity pentasaccharide sequence and are able to catalyze the inhibition of factor Xa by AT, but they cannot bind AT and thrombin (1,5). LMWHs have a relatively higher anti–factor Xa and lower anti–factor IIa activity compared to UFH. Commercial LMWH differ in their Xa:IIa affinity ratios. Like UFH, LMWH can induce the secretion of tissue factor pathway inhibitor by vascular endothelial cells, whose action reduces the procoagulant activity of the TF-factor VIIa complex (37).

LMWHs have clear pharmacokinetic advantages over UFH preparations. LMWHs have superior bioavailability when administered subcutaneously and a longer half-life compared to UFH (Table 1). LMWH also has a more predictable dose response allowing clinicians to administer weight adjusted doses of LMWH without laboratory monitoring (39). The greater bioavailability and more predictable dose response of LMWH is attributed to their decreased affinity in binding to plasma proteins, macrophages, and endothelial cells (40). Compared with UFH, LMWHs have reduced binding to platelets and PF4 which explains the lower incidence of HIT associated with LMWHs (41).

LMWH is usually administered as a fixed dose without monitoring. Patients with renal insufficiency, and who are morbidly obese or pregnant, however, require factor Xa monitoring. The most commonly employed laboratory assay for assuring adequacy of anticoagulation with LMWHs is the chromagenic anti-Xa assay (42). When LMWH is administered once daily, an anti-Xa assay should be performed 4 h after the initial dose with a therapeutic range between 1.0 and 2.0 IU/mL (42). When LMWH is administered twice daily, an anti-Xa level ranging from 0.6 to 1.0 IU/mL is recommended (42).

LMWHs are cleared by the kidneys in a dose-independent fashion (12). Because of the renal clearance of LMWHs, it is recommended that anti-Xa assays be utilized in patients

Table 1 A Comparison of the Pharmacokinetic Differences Between Low-Molecular-Weight Heparins (LMWHs) and Unfractionated Heparin (UFH)

Characteristic	UFH	LMWH
Molecular weight	3,000–30,000/Da	4,000–6,000/Da
Plasma half-life	1–2 h	4–6 h
Anti-Xa:anti–IIa activity	1:1	2:1–4:1
Platelet inhibition	Yes	Less than UFH
Reversal of anticoagulation	Protamine	Protamine less effective
Clearance	Endothelial cell and Macrophage binding Renal (at high doses)	Renal (dose-independent)
Administered	Intravenous and subcutaneous	Subcutaneous
Laboratory monitoring	APTT or ACT	- Fixed dose - Serum anti–factor Xa[a]

[a] Serum anti–factor Xa level monitoring recommended for patients with renal insufficiency, pregnancy, and obesity.

with renal insufficiency. This is prudent, as many of the clinical trials that led to approval by the U.S. Food and Drug Administration (FDA) of the LMWHs excluded patients with renal failure.

B. Clinical Application

In the United States, the LMWHs dalteparin and enoxaparin have been approved for use as prophylactic agents for the prevention of venous thromboembolism in patients undergoing abdominal surgery and orthopedic surgery (Table 2). The ability of LMWH and low-dose UFH to prevent DVT in general surgery patients has been studied in numerous large trials and analyzed by metanalysis (43). LMWH proved to be efficacious at preventing DVT in general surgery patients (43,44). Metanalyses revealed that there is a clear dose-response effect of LMWH on bleeding complications (44). There is more bleeding with LMWH if doses of greater than 3400 IU of anti-Xa are given daily, in comparison to low-dose UFH, in a dose of 5000 IU bid or tid. Equivalent bleeding risk is evident if LMWH is administered at less than 3400 U of anti-Xa daily. Cost-effectiveness analyses have been performed for patients undergoing abdominal surgery comparing the cost of LMWHs with low-dose UFH. The authors concluded that in North America prophylaxis with lose-dose UFH was equally efficacious and more economical than LMWH (43).

Subcutaneous LMWH is rapidly replacing intravenous UFH for the initial treatment of patients with uncomplicated venous thromboembolism. Metanalyses have found that unmonitored, weight-adjusted, subcutaneous LMWH is as least as effective as intravenous UFH in preventing recurrent venous thromboembolism (45,46). Early metanalyses, published soon after FDA approval, concluded that the treatment of venous thromboembolism by LMWH was safer and more effective than treatment by UFH (47). Recent

Table 2 FDA-Approved Indications for LMWH Therapy

LMWH	Indication	Dose (Subcutaneous)
Dalteparin	DVT prophylaxis	
	Abdominal surgery	2500 IU anti–factor Xa q 24 h
	Higher-risk abdominal surgery; Hip replacement	5000 IU anti–factor Xa q 24 h
	Treatment of unstable angina/ non-Q-wave MI	120 IU/kg anti–factor Xa q 24 h
Enoxaparin	DVT prophylaxis	
	Abdominal surgery	40 mg[a] q 24 h
	Hip and knee replacement	40 mg q 24 h; initiate $12(\pm 3)$ h preop or 30 mg q 12 h
	Outpatient DVT treatment, without PE	1 mg/kg q 12 h
	Inpatient DVT treatment, with or without PE	1.5 mg/kg q 24 h *or* 1 mg /kg q 12 h
Tinzaparin	Treatment of DVT, with or without PE	175 IU anti–factor Xa q 24 h

Abbreviations: LMWH, low-molecular-weight heparin; MI, myocardial infarction; DVT, deep venous thrombosis; PE, pulmonary embolism.
[a] Enoxaparin I mg = 100 anti–factor Xa IU.

metanalyses however, demonstrate a decrease in overall mortality with LMWH but only a trend toward superiority of LMWH over UFH in preventing recurrent thromboembolism. Gould et al. analyzed 11 randomized, controlled trials designed to compare the safety and efficacy of LMWH compared to UFH for the treatment of acute DVT (45). Thromboembolic events occurred in 5.4% of all patients treated with UFH, compared to 4.6% of patients treated with LMWH. Recurrent thromboembolic events were less common in patients who received LMWH, but the difference was not statistically significant (absolute risk reduction of 0.88%). Importantly, LMWHs reduced mortality rates over 3–6 months of follow-up, compared with the UFH patients (29% relative risk reduction). Dolovich et al. utilized metanalysis to examine 13 studies in which patients were randomized to receive either LMWHs or intravenous UFH for the treatment of acute venous thromboembolism (46). The incidence of recurrent venous thrombosis or pulmonary embolism was similar between UFH and LMWHs groups, but patients treated with LMWH experienced a 24% reduction in the risk of total mortality compared to patients treated with intravenous UFH. Once-daily therapy with LMWH was found to be as safe and effective as twice-daily dosing of LMWH.

While management of DVT with LMWHs has become the standard of care across the United States, clinicians have been slower to adopt LMWH therapy for the management of patients with PE. In the early trials demonstrating efficacy of LMWH for the management of venous thrombosis, patients with PE were either excluded or represented in very small numbers. Recently, LMWH has been evaluated in the treatment of submassive pulmonary embolism in randomized trials (48,49). Simonneau et al. reported the results of a randomized study of 612 patients with symptomatic pulmonary embolism who received either subcutaneous LMWH (once-daily in a fixed dose), or adjusted dose, or intravenous UFH followed by at least 3 months of oral anticoagulation therapy (49). The investigators examined the outcomes of recurrent thromboembolism and death at 8 and 90 days from the initiation of therapy and found no differences between groups. Hull et al. conducted a double-blind, randomized trial comparing LMWH with intravenous heparin treatment in patients with documented proximal DVT who were found on subsequent perfusion lung scan to have a high probability of pulmonary embolism (48). No patient in the LMWH group experienced recurrent venous thromboembolism, compared to 6.8% of patients in the UFH group ($p = 0.009$). The authors concluded that once-daily subcutaneous LMWH treatment was no less effective and probably more effective than use of dose-adjusted intravenous UFH for preventing recurrent venous thromboembolism in patients with nonhemodynamically compromising PE and associated proximal DVT. There are no prospective data demonstrating the efficacy and safety of LMWH treatment for patients who are hemodynamically unstable with massive PE. Therefore it is our practice to manage these patients in the hospital with very closely monitored intravenous UFH.

Although not proven, many obstetricians have a strong sense that pregnant women are at higher risk of developing venous thromboembolism than nonpregnant women. Women with thrombophilic disorders such as deficiencies of antithrombin, protein C, or protein S have an approximately eightfold increased risk of venous thromboembolism during pregnancy (50). Sixty percent of one series of women who developed venous thromboembolism during pregnancy tested positive for factor V Leiden (51). Therefore, with patients with known thrombophilia, consideration should given for the use of prophylactic LMWH, plus postpartum anticoagulation (51). For patients with multiple prior episodes of venous thromboembolism or women already receiving long-term anticoagulation prior to pregnancy, adjusted-dose LMWH is recommended, followed by resumption of long-term oral anticoagulation therapy postpartum. For patients who develop venous thromboembolism during pregnancy, adjusted-dose LMWH is recommended. Anticoagulation with warfarin is contraindicated, as warfarin crosses the placenta. There is strong evidence that LMWHs do not cross the placenta and are safe for the fetus (51). The pharmacokonetics of LMWH change in pregnancy, resulting in a shorter plasma half-life and larger volume distribution. Therefore, monitoring of anti–factor Xa levels is necessary (50,51).

Clinicians are now beginning to investigate the potential role for LMWH in patients undergoing arterial revascularization and/or percutaneous transluminal angioplasty. Historically, on an anecdotal basis, vascular surgeons have used intravenous UFH intraoperatively and have utilized postoperative intravenous UFH in patients who have undergone difficult distal reconstructive procedures. Edmondson et al. compared the effect of postoperative daily injection of LMWH versus a combination of aspirin and dipyridamole every 8 h for 3 months following femoral-to-popliteal bypass grafting (52). The randomization occurred approximately 1 week postoperatively with all patients receiving LMWH during the first week after surgery. At 12 months, graft patency was 78% in the LMWH group, compared to 64% in the aspirin-with-dipyridamole group. Significant improvement in graft patency was seen in the LMWH subgroup of patients undergoing limb salvage surgery, while no benefit was appreciated in patients presenting with claudication. Simama et al. enrolled 201 consecutive patients scheduled for femorodistal reconstructive surgery in an open randomized trial comparing intraoperative and postoperative LMWH with UFH (53). Intraoperatively, the LMWH group received enoxaparin, 75 IU/kg anti-Xa intravenously, while the UFH group received 50 IU/kg, also intravenously. Postoperatively, patients received subcutaneous administration of enoxaparin (75 IU/kg anti-Xa) or UFH (150 IU/kg) beginning 8 h after the initial intravenous dose and then every 12 h for 10 days. Graft thrombosis occurred by 10 days in 8% of patients in the LMWH group, compared with 22% of patients in the UFH group ($p = 0.009$). Major hemorrhages occurred in 12% of patients in each group and there was no difference in mortality rates between groups. Hingorani et al. retrospectively identified 169 patients who postoperatively received intravenous UFH and 161 patients who receive enoxaparin 1 mg/kg every 12 h as a bridge to adjusted dose warfarin therapy (54). Both groups of patients received intravenous UFH for 24 h after surgery. There was no standardization of the length of postoperative LMWH prior to conversion to warfarin. The authors found no difference in the incidence of postoperative complications except for an increased incidence of return to surgery for graft thrombosis, failing grafts, and debridement in patients who received UFH. The authors caution the reader not to draw the conclusion that these retrospective data suggest a decreased incidence of graft thrombosis with LMWH (54).

Plaque rupture leads to tissue factor expression and subsequent activation in a coagulation cascade and generation of factor Xa (55). As LMWHs target factor Xa to a far greater extent than thrombin, their use has been extensively investigated for the management of patients with unstable angina/non-Q-wave myocardial infarction (MI). Metanalyses have shown the superiority of LMWH over placebo in the setting of unstable angina and recently LMWHs have been found to be superior to UFH in this patient population (56). Several clinicians have investigated the role of LMWH as the sole anticoagulant during percutaneous coronary intervention (PCI) (57). Further prospective trials will be necessary to determine the optimal level of anticoagulation; however, similar safety and efficacy outcomes with LMWH compared with UFH have been shown with target anti-Xa levels higher than 0.5 IU/mL (57).

The use of LMWHs for the management of patients undergoing peripheral percutaneous transluminal angioplasty is only now being investigated (58). Schweizer et al. randomized 172 patients who had undergone iliac or superficial femoral artery angioplasty with subsequent extensive dissections to receive either UFH or LMWH for a 7-day period after angioplasty, followed by a 6 month course of aspirin (58). For this group, no significant treatment-related differences in the degree of restenosis were found at 3 weeks, and 3 and 6 months postprocedurally. However, when angioplasty was performed in the superficial femoral artery, the degree of restenosis was significantly lower in the LMWH group compared to the UFH group at all three time points. Further prospective evaluation of the use of LMWH in patients undergoing peripheral angioplasty is warranted.

C. Complications and Failures

Similar to UFH, the most common complication of LMWH is hemorrhage. When LMWH is used for prophylaxis of venous thrombosis, risk of bleeding is small and comparable to low-dose heparin (59). Recent metanalyses also demonstrate comparable risk between LMWHs and UFH for both major and minor bleeding in patients being treated for venous thrombosis and pulmonary embolism (45,46,48). Overdosing patients with LMWH is problematic because protamine is less effective at neutralizing the antithrombin activity of LMWH compared to its effect on UFH (60). Protamine does not neutralize all the Xa-inhibiting activity of LMWH even at protamine/heparin ratios of more than five. Resistance of a specific LMWH to protamine neutralization is a function of not only the LMWHs molecular size but also their degree of sulfonation (60).

In 1997, the FDA issued a public health advisory in order to alert physicians of the increase risk of spinal and epidural hematoma associate with the use of LMWHs (61). At that time, 43 patients in the United States had developed perispinal hematoma, with over half the patients suffering significant neurological impairment. The 6th ACCP Consensus Conference on Antithrombotic Therapy made several recommendations in an attempt to improve the safety of neuroaxial in patients receiving LMWH (32). Some of the recommendations include the following: (a) avoid LMWH if patients have known bleeding disorder, (b) delay spinal needle insertion 8–12 h after LMWH, (c) avoid DVT prophylaxis with LMWH if there is a "bloody tap," (d) remove epidural catheter when anticoagulant effect is at minimum, and (e) delay LMWH prophylaxis for 2 h after needle withdrawal (32).

LMWHs is less likely than UFH to cause HIT antibody formation (41). HIT antibodies bind to the antigen composed of a complex of heparin and PF4. Because 12–14 saccharide units are necessary to form the antigenic complex with PF4, LMW molecules greater than 4000 Da can cause HIT. LMWHs are generally not a treatment option for patients developing HIT secondary to UFH, unless platelet aggregometry is available to test patient serum against specific LMWHs. The management of HIT for patients receiving LMWH is identical to the treatment algorithms developed for patients receiving UFH.

Patients receiving either heparin or LMWH for prolonged periods are at risk for developing heparin-induced osteoporosis. The risk of heparin-induced osteoporosis is related to the length of exposure. The indications for the use of LMWH have been expanding and long-term use of LMWH is indicated for patients with recurrent venous thromboembolism while they are adequately anticoagulated with oral anticoagulant therapy (62,63). There is clinical evidence that LMWHs carry a lower risk of osteoporosis than UFH as well as rat data suggesting that LMWH causes less osteopenia than UFH (64).

As with UFH, failures of LMWH therapy are usually iatrogenic. Clinicians need to be aware that fixed-dose administration of LMWH may at times result in inadequate anticoagulation in selective patients. Patients, who receive LMWH during pregnancy require periodic monitoring of anti-Xa levels because the volume of distribution for LMWH changes as the pregnancy progresses. Options include weight-adjusted dosing or the weekly performance of serum anti–factor Xa levels (51). For morbidly obese patients, the use of weight-adjusted dosing is recommended. Patients with renal failure should have their anti-Xa levels monitored because of the renal clearance of LMWH. In this group of patients, we recommend more frequent monitoring of anti-Xa levels than in the morbidly obese patient.

III. VITAMIN K ANTAGONISTS

A. Pharmacology

Warfarin, first synthesized in 1944 at the University of Wisconsin, is the most popular oral anticoagulant. Gastrointestinal absorption of warfarin is complete, with peak plasma concentrations being 2–12 h after a single oral dose. Warfarin is bound (97%) to albumin and has a circulating half-life of 36–40 h. Oral anticoagulants are principally metabolized by the microsomal fraction of the hepatacyte; metabolites are excreted in the urine.

Warfarin interferes with the action of vitamin K in the synthesis of clotting factors II, VII, IX, and X by the liver. Vitamin K is a cofactor in the reaction that converts glutamyl residues of clotting factor precursors to the carboxyglutamyl residues necessary for the binding of calcium. Patients receiving warfarin produce antigenically similar clotting factors that do not have procoagulant activity because of their abnormal calcium-binding characteristics (65).

Anticoagulation with warfarin is dependent on the reduction of the concentrations of all affected clotting factors and may take 3–5 days to achieve. The time required to reach therapeutic levels of anticoagulation is affected by the rate of "turnover" of the clotting factors, which is directly related to their circulating half-lives. Factor VII and IX zymogens have half-lives of 6–24 h respectively, whereas prothrombin (II) has a half-life of approximately 96 h (66). Early reduction of factor VII and IX zymogens results in an anticoagulant effect reflected by prolongation of the prothrombin time (PT). This early laboratory anticoagulant effect does not translate into an in vivo antithrombotic effect. The antithrombotic effect of warfarin is tied to the reduction of prothrombin, which usually occurs 4 or 5 days after the initiation of warfarin therapy. This is the basis for overlapping heparin or LMWH with warfarin until the INR has been prolonged into the therapeutic range for at least 4 days. Warfarin also inhibits carboxylation of the natural anticoagulant proteins C and S. Protein C's half-life is only 4–6 h; thus those are reduced early and warfarin therapy, creating the potential for transient procoagulant state. Thus these issues—the early drop in protein C activity, and the delayed reduction in prothrombin levels—support the use of a maintainance dose of warfarin rather than a loading dose during the initiation in therapy (67).

The biological effects of warfarin may be potentiated by hepatic insufficiency, malnutrition, or hypermetabolic states such as fever or hyperthyroidism. Many common therapeutic agents may alter the response of the coagulation system to warfarin due to decreased absorption from the gastrointestinal tract, displacement of the drug from its binding site on albumin, increases in the rate at which it is metabolized by the liver, decreased vitamin K availability, or decreases or increases in the plasma half-lives of the affected clotting factors (Table 3).

Warfarin is known to cross the placental barrier and therefore should not be given during pregnancy. During the first trimester, warfarin has a known teratrogenic effect. LMWH is the anticoagulant of choice during pregnancy.

B. Clinical Application

Warfarin has been shown to be an effective prophylactic agent for the prevention of venous thrombosis after hip surgery and major general surgery at a target INR of 2.0–3.0 (68). Although the risk of major hemorrhage in this range of INR is low, the use of warfarin for venous thrombosis prophylaxis is reserved for patients of very high risk because of its complexity of administration.

Randomized trials have demonstrated that warfarin is effective at preventing recurrent venous thromboembolism (VTE) when administered after a course of either UFH or LMWH for acute VTE (68). Warfarin should be started once adequate anticoagulation is obtained with either UFH or LMWH; heparin should be continued for at least 4 days after achieving an INR in the range of 2.0–3.0.

Warfarin therapy is indicated for at least 3 months for patients with proximal DVT or pulmonary embolism if the risk factors leading to the VTE have been corrected. In patients with so-called idiopathic proximal DVT in which no clear risk factors have been identified, warfarin therapy is continued for 6 months. Lifelong warfarin therapy is indicated for patients with recurrent idiopathic venous thromboembolism; antiphospholipid antibody syndrome; deficiencies of protein C, protein S, or antithrombin; and in those with VTE associated with the homozygous factor V Leiden gene type (63,69). Ridker et al. recently reported the early termination of a randomized trial of patients with idiopathic VTE who were assigned to either placebo or low-intensity warfarin (target INR, 1.5–2.0) after first completing full-dose warfarin anticoagulation for a median of 6.5 months (69). The study's endpoints were recurrent venous thromboembolism, major hemorrhage, and death. The study was terminated early after 508 patients had been randomized and followed for a

Table 3 Drug Interactions Affecting Vitamin K Antagonist Activity

Potentiate		Inhibit
Acetaminophen	Micronazole	Barbiturates
Acetylsalicylic acid	Nalidixic acid	Carbamazeprine
Alcohol	Norfloxacin	Cholestyramine
Amiodarone	Ofloxacin	Chlordiazepoxide
Anabolic steroids	Omeprazole	Cyclosporine
Ciprofloxacin	Phenylbutazone	Dicloxacillin
Clofibrate	Phenytoln	Griseofulvin
Cotrimoxazole	Piroxicam	Nafcillin
Disulfiram	Propafenone	Rifampin
Erythromycin	Propranolol	Sucralfate
Fluconazole	Quinidine	Trazodone
Itraconazole	Sulfinpyrazone	
Lovastatin	Tamoxifen	
Metronidazole	Tetracycline	

mean of 2.1 years. Patients treated with low-intensity warfarin had a 64% reduction in the risk of recurrent VTE compared to the placebo group ($p < 0.001$). Low-intensity warfarin was associated with a 48% reduction in the composite endpoint of recurrent VTE, major hemorrhage, or death. Thus there is a role for long-term low-intensity warfarin therapy.

Following heart valve replacement, patients benefit from lifelong anticoagulation to decrease the risk of systemic embolization. The American College of Chest Physicians 1998 guidelines recommend an INR of 2.5–3.5 for most patients with mechanical prosthetic valves and 2.0–3.0 for those with bioprosthetic valves (68). Warfarin therapy has also proven effective for decreasing the risk of stroke in patients with chronic atrial fibrillation. A pooled review of five trials that addressed anticoagulant therapy for the prevention of stroke in atrial fibrillation patients treated with warfarin showed a 69% reduction in the risk of stroke (70). Patients who are able to continue taking their warfarin on a daily basis benefited from an 80% stroke risk reduction.

Retrospective reviews have implied that patients undergoing peripheral arterial bypass procedures may benefit from long-term warfarin therapy (71). The effect of warfarin plus aspirin (WASA) versus aspirin alone (ASA) on peripheral artery bypass patency rates and patient mortality and morbidity was investigated in a multicenter, prospective, randomized trial (72). Patients were randomized to receive aspirin (325 mg/day) versus WASA (target INR 1.4–2.8). The data for patients undergoing vein bypass was analyzed separately from those undergoing prosthetic bypass. Patency rates in patients undergoing vein bypass were unaffected. In the prosthetic bypass group, there was no significant difference in patency rate in patients receiving an 8-mm bypass; however, there was a significant improvement in patency rates in patients in the WASA group who received 6 mm femoral-popliteal bypasses compared to the ASA group (5-year assisted primary patency; 71.4% WASA, 57.9% ASA group, $p = 0.02$). However, the mortality rate for all patients in the WASA group was significantly higher (31.8%) than that for patients in the ASA group (23.0%; $p = 0.0001$). Warfarin did not provide any greater benefit than ASA for the risk of cerebral events, myocardial infarction, or thromboembolic events. Major hemorrhagic complications were more common in the WASA group than the ASA group. The authors conclude that low-dosage warfarin therapy may provide some additional patency benefit for patients who undergo femoropopliteal prosthetic bypass, but at the added cost of an increased risk of mortality and hemorrhagic events.

C. Complications

Hemorrhage is the most common complication of warfarin therapy. Frequency of hemorrhage with warfarin varies widely but is a function of the level of anticoagulation. Patients treated with warfarin to prevent recurrent venous thromboembolism with a target INR of 2.0–3.0 achieve similar efficacy to patients whose target INR is adjusted to 3.0–4.5, but with significantly less bleeding complications (total bleeding 4.3%, INR 2.0–3.0; 22.4%, INR 3.0–4.5; $p = 0.015$) (73). When bleeding complications occur, warfarin should be discontinued. The effects of warfarin may be reversed within 24 h by intravenous administration of 20 mg of vitamin K. Life-threatening hemorrhage is best managed with rapid reversal using infusions of fresh frozen plasma with or without administration of vitamin K. A prothrombin complex concentrate (PCC) has recently been shown to be more effective than vitamin K treatment in rapidly correcting increased INR levels in patients receiving warfarin (74). The use of PCC without vitamin K may, however, result in a repeated increase of INR, leading investigators to recommend concomitant vitamin K use with PCC.

Other than hemorrhage, the adverse effects of warfarin are rare; they include alopecia, dermatitis, fever, nausea, diarrhea, abdominal cramping, and hypersensitivity reactions. A rare complication of warfarin therapy is extensive dermal gangrene, the risk of which is increased if loading-dose regimens are used for initiating therapy. This occurs early after warfarin administration when protein C levels are decreased while the intrinsic coagulation pathway remains intact; patients with congenital or acquired protein C deficiency are therefore at greater risk for this complication. The skin in the thigh, breast, and buttocks is most often involved. Simultaneous heparin administration at the beginning of warfarin treatment prevents this complication (75).

D. Failures

Failure with warfarin therapy—that is, the inability to inhibit coagulation—is most frequently caused by the use of insufficient amounts of warfarin. Individuals have been identified with an inherited resistance to warfarin, which causes them to require 5- to 20-fold higher than average amounts of warfarin to achieve an acceptable INR. Because the plasma warfarin level required to achieve anticoagulation is elevated, it is likely that there is altered affinity of the receptor for warfarin (76). Variation in the dose response to warfarin may also be secondary to a common mutation in the gene coding for one of the common cytochrome P450 enzymes (2C9) responsible for the oxydative metabolism of the warfarin S isomer (77). As previously described, drugs and dietary factors can interfere with the effectiveness of warfarin therapy. Increased consumption of foods high in vitamin K or vitamin K containing supplements has been shown to reduce the anticoagulant response to warfarin.

Antiphospholipid antibody syndrome is an acquired autoimmune disorder associated with both venous and arterial thromboses (50,51,63). While the precise mechanism leading to the hypercoagulable state remains unclear, patients are noted to have elevated levels of lupus anticoagulants and anticardiolipin antibodies (50,51,63). Intravenous UFH is not a good choice for management of these patients, as lupus anticoagulants cause prolongation of the APTT. There is growing evidence that many patients with antiphospholipid thrombosis syndrome will develop recurrent thromboembolic episodes even in the face of therapeutic levels of anticoagulation with warfarin. Current recommendations are to manage patients with LMWH concomitantly with a platelet function inhibiting drug such as aspirin or clopidogrel (63).

IV. DIRECT THROMBIN INHIBITORS

Direct thrombin inhibitors are molecules that interact with thrombin and act to block its interaction with substrates. This is in contrast to the indirect thrombin inhibitors UFH and LMWH, which require the cofactor antithrombin in order to inhibit thrombin's activity. The development of direct thrombin inhibitors parallels the increasing recognition by clinicians of the heparin-induced thrombocytopenia syndrome. The FDA has approved two of the commercially available direct thrombin inhibitors as the anticoagulants of choice for patients with HIT who require continued anticoagulation. A second reason for the development of direct thrombin inhibitors pertains to the inability of the heparin-antithrombin complex to deactivate thrombin-bound to fibrin clots. This may be important clinically in the setting of acute coronary syndromes, where heparin may not be able to inactivate active thrombin bound to fibrin. The third commercially available direct thrombin inhibitor, bivalirudin, is indicated for use as an anticoagulant in patients with unstable angina undergoing percutaneous transluminal coronary angioplasty with the concomitant use of ASA. All three of the commercially available direct thrombin inhibitors are administered intravenously. Ximelagatran is an orally active direct thrombin inhibitor currently under investigation. The pharamacokinetics, clinical use, and complications associated with these direct thrombin inhibitors are reviewed below.

A. Lepirudin

Hirudin is a potent direct inhibitor of thrombin that was originally isolated from the salivary glands of the medicinal leech *Hirudo medicinalis*. Lepirudin and bivalirudin are recombinant proteins derived from the structure of hirudin. Lepirudin is a recombinant hirudin derived from yeast cells; it is a polypeptide composed of 65 amino acids and is identical to natural hirudin except for several amino acid substitutions. Hirudin binds noncovalently to thrombin's active site, yet the strength of this bond is such that hirudin is only very slowly reversible. Lepirudin has a plasma half-life of 40 min after intravenous administration and approximately 120 min after subcutaneous injection (78). After intravenous infusion, peak levels occur rapidly; then lepirudin is cleared by the kidneys, with clearance proportional to the glomerular filtration rate. Thus dose adjustment is recommended based on the patient's creatinine clearance.

Lepirudin has been shown to be an effective treatment for HIT based on prospective trials (79). Patients with normal renal function are given a bolus dose of 0.4 mg/kg followed by an infusion of 0.1–0.15 mg/kg/h to maintain the APTT at 1.5–2.5 times normal control values. APTT values are known to increase in a dose-dependent fashion. Some investigators have noted poor linearity in reproducibility of the APTT for monitoring of direct thrombin inhibitors. The ecarin clotting time (ECT) is currently under clinical investigation for monitoring patients receiving direct thrombin inhibitors. Ecarin, a snake venom enzyme, converts prothrombin to meizothrombin, which is then neutralized by hirudin resulting in a dose-dependent prolongation of clotting time. The ECT has been shown to have a linear correlation with plasma hirudin concentrations whereas both the ACT and APTT have poor correlations (80). Lepirudin has been shown in anecdotal series to be an effective alternative to heparin during cardiopulmonary bypass in patients with HIT (81).

Metanalysis of two prospective trials that investigated the use of intravenous lepirudin to manage patients with HIT demonstrated a clear advantage of lepirudin therapy over historical controls. Lepirudin-treated patients had significantly lower incidences of the combined endpoints of death, limb amputation, and thromboembolic complications compared to historic controls ($p = 0.004$) (82). The primary complication of lepirudin treatment is hemorrhage. The total incidence of bleeding was 42% at 35 days in the lepirudin-treated group compared to 23.6% among historical controls ($p = 0.001$). Common sites of hemorrhage include intracranial, retroperitoneal, and gastrointestinal bleeding. Although lepirudin does not cross-react with HIT antibodies, antihirudin antibodies develop in between 56 and 74% of patients treated for longer than 5 days (81). Hirudin-antihirudin antibody complexes, while not affecting activity, prolongs the renal clearance of lepirudin, which can potentiate its anticoagulation effect. While prospective trials have shown decreased thromboembolic complications in patients with HIT receiving parental lepirudin compared to historic controls, lepirudin unfortunately is not completely protective in this setting. Of 113 patients evaluated, 6.2% of the patients underwent limb amputation, 10.6% experienced a new thromboembolic complication, and the mortality rate was 9.7% (82). The major limitation of lepirudin treatment is that it is contra-indicated in patients with significant renal insufficiency. Whereas lepirudin may have a slight effect on the INR when warfarin is initiated, its effect is not as pronounced as seen with argatroban. Thus transition to warfarin therapy is less complicated with lepirudin than with argatroban.

B. Bivalirudin

Bivalirudin is a recombinant protein based on hirudin which, unlike hirudin, produces only a transient inhibition of the active site of thrombin. Once bivalirudin is bound to thrombin, it is converted into a lower-affinity inhibitor (78). The onset of action is rapid after intravenous administration, with a peak response seen within 15 min. Bivalirudin has a plasma half-life of 25 min, with clearance by renal mechanisms and proteolytic cleavage. Patients with renal insufficiency require adjustment in the rate of administration of bivalirudin; patients with glomerular filtration rates less than 30 mL/min require a reduction in dose of approximately 68% (83). Bivalirudin inhibits both free and clot-bound thrombin. The manufacturer's recommendations are to monitor bivalirudin's anticoagulation affect using APTT, as plasma concentrations of bivalirudin correlated with APTT at all levels of renal function (83).

Clinical trials have demonstrated that bivalirudin is as least as effective as high-dose heparin when combined with ASA at preventing ischemic complications in patients under-going percutaneous transluminal angioplasty for unstable angina (84). In the study that led to FDA approval, patients received what is now the recommended clinical dose of bivalirudin prior to angioplasty. The recommended dose is an intravenous bolus of 1 mg/kg followed by a continuous infusion of 2.5 mg/kg/h for 4 h, with an additional 0.2 mg/kg/h for up to 20 h if needed. Patients in the heparin group in this double-blind, random-ized trial received a high-dose heparin regimen consisting of a bolus dose of 175 IU/kg followed by an 18- to 24-h infusion at a rate of 15 IU/kg/h (84). ACTs were measured at 5 and 45 min after administration of the heparin bolus, with ACTs kept greater than 350 s by periodic rebolusing with heparin. The primary endpoint of the study was in-hospital death, MI, rapid clinical deterioration, or abrupt vessel closure. There was not a significant difference in the incidence of the primary endpoint between groups; however, there was a lower incidence of bleeding (3.8% bivalirudin vs. 9.8% heparin; $p < 0.001$). In the bivalirudin group, patients who presented with postinfarction angia who were randomized to bivalirudin therapy did demonstrate a lower incidence of the primary endpoint (9.1 vs. 14.2%, $p = 0.04$) and a lower incidence of bleeding (3% vs. 11.1%, $p < 0.001$) compared with the group treated with high-dose heparin. There was no difference, however, in the cumulative rate of death between groups at 6 months. These data later contributed to the FDA's decision to approve the use of bivalirudin when combined with ASA in patients with unstable angia or postinfarction angina undergoing coronary angioplasty. Bivalirudin has shown a benefit in preventing DVT in patients undergoing orthopedic surgery and as an adjunct to streptokinase in patients with acute myocardial infarction, although these are not approved indications (78).

C. Argatroban

Argatroban is a small, synthetic molecule derived from arginine that binds reversibly and specifically to the catalytic domain of thrombin (85). Argatroban has the ability, because of its small size, to be an effective inhibitor of thrombin bound to surfaces as well as in solution.

Argatroban is about 50% protein-bound and 50% free in plasma and has an elimination half-life of 39–51 min (86). Argatroban is metabolized in the liver and is not cleared by the kidney, therefore renal function does not affect argatroban's pharmacokinetics (85, 86). Like lepirudin, argatroban does not cross-react with heparin-associated antibodies; however, unlike lepirudin, drug-specific antibodies to argatroban have not been identified. Argatroban is indicated in the United States for the treatment and prophylaxis of HIT.

A prospective, historically controlled study examined the efficacy of argatroban to reduce the endpoints of death, amputation, and new thromboembolic events compared to historic controls (86). Patients received 2 μg/kg/min of argatroban and had the rate of administration adjusted to maintain the APTT at 1.5–3 times baseline levels. The composite endpoint was significantly reduced in the argatroban-treated patients versus control patients with HIT (25.6 vs. 38.8%, $p = 0.014$). The incidence of major bleeding episodes was not different between patient groups. Argatroban has also been approved in the United States for use during percutaneous interventions in patients with HIT. In this setting, argatroban is given as an intravenous bolus of 350 μg/kg followed by continuous infusion at 15–40 μg/kg/min. The infusion rate was adjusted to maintain a target ACT of 300–450 s. Lewis et al. reported a series of 91 HIT patients who underwent 112 percutaneous coronary interventions using intravenous argatroban (87). All patients received aspirin (325 mg) 2–24 h before angioplasty. Sheaths were removed no sooner than 2 h after cessation of argatroban and when the ACT was less than 160 s. Satisfactory outcome of the procedure was attained in 94.5% of the group, and 97.8% achieved adequate anticoagulation. The major bleeding rate was 1.1%, with a minor bleeding rate of 32%. All patients remained free of the major acute complication of death, emergent coronary bypass graft surgery, and Q-wave MI. There are favorable anecdotal reports in the literature reporting successful outcomes in patients undergoing cardiopulmonary bypass with argatroban anticoagulation (88). Although this is not an approved indication for the use of argatroban in the United States, the authors cite the advantage of argatroban over lepirudin for patients with renal insufficiency and a history of HIT requiring cardiopulmonary bypass.

Hemorrhage is the major complication of all direct thrombin inhibitors. There have been no direct comparisons between agents. There is no antidote to the anticoagulation effects of the direct thrombin inhibitors. Other commonly reported complications of argatroban use include diarrhea in 11% of patients, pain in 9%, and rash in 2% (87). Among direct thrombin inhibitors, argatroban alone can cause significant prolongation of the INR. The INR is affected by the argatroban concentration and the degree of warfarin-induced factor activity depletion. Thus it is difficult to transition patients requiring prolonged anticoagulation from argatroban to warfarin.

D. Ximelagatran/Melagatran

Melagatran is a dipeptide direct thrombin inhibitor that binds to the active site of thrombin in a competitive yet reversible manner (89). Melagatran can be administered intravenously or subcutaneously, but it is not well absorbed orally. Ximelagatran is an oral direct thrombin inhibitor currently under investigation for the prevention and treatment of thromboembolism. Ximelagatran can be taken by mouth and is then converted to melagatran the active agent. Peak plasma concentrations of melagatran are attained 2 h after ximelagatran oral administration. Plasma half-life ranges from 2.5 to 3.5 h (90). Melagatran is not metabolized and is cleared primarily by the kidneys; plasma half-life is doubled in patients with renal failure.

Laboratory monitoring does not appear necessary for the clinical use of ximelagatran. The pharmacokinetics, pharmacodynamics, and clinical effects of oral ximelagatran were analyzed in patients with PE and DVT (89). Patients received a fixed-dose of 48 mg oral ximelagatran twice daily for 6–9 days. APTT correlated with plasma melagatran concentrations, peaking at approximately two times the baseline APTT. Clinical symptoms improved in all 12 patients and no deaths or severe bleeding occurred. Thus fixed-dose ximelagatran demonstrated reproducible pharmacokinetics and pharmacodynamics in patients with PE without routine coagulation monitoring.

A randomized, double-blind study examined the dose-response of subcutaneous melagatran followed by oral ximelagatran as thromboprophylaxis in patients undergoing total hip or knee replacement. Efficacy and safety were compared to those of dalteparin (91). A significant dose-dependent decrease in venous thromboembolism was seen with melagatran/ximelagatran. The incidence of venous thromboembolism was significantly lower in the highest-dose melagatran/ximelagatran group compared to dalteparin (15.1 vs. 28.2%, $p < 0.0001$). Although ximelagatran remains in clinical trials and its safety profile and complication risks are still to be defined, it appears to have future promise for the management of patients with thromboembolism as an oral direct thrombin inhibitor that does not require laboratory monitoring.

V. FACTOR Xa INHIBITORS

Fondaparinux sodium is a synthetic pentasaccharide that is an indirect inhibitor of factor Xa. Fondaparinux is an analogue to the pentasaccharide sequence found on small heparin and LMWH molecules (<18 saccharides) that acts to catalyze the inhibition of factor Xa by antithrombin (92). By inhibiting factor Xa selectively, fondaparinux inhibits thrombin generation without a direct effect on thrombin activity. Unlike UFH and LMWH, fondaparinux does not cause the release of TFPI from endothelial cells, and there is minimal binding to plasma proteins. Fondaparinux bioavailability is excellent when administered subcutaneously, with peak concentrations 2 h postdosing. Its plasma half-life is 14–20 h. There is no metabolism of the drug prior to renal excretion. This pharmacokinetic profile allows for once-daily subcutaneous administration with no need for laboratory monitoring or dose adjustment in the majority of patients.

In December 2001, the FDA approved the use of fondaparinux sodium for reducing the risk of VTE after orthopedic surgery for hip fracture, hip replacement, and knee replacement. Four multicenter, randomized, double-blind trials in patients undergoing elective hip replacement, extensive knee surgery, and surgery for hip fracture have compared the efficacy and safety of fondaparinux to that of enoxaparin for the prevention of VTE (93). Patients received either once-daily subcutaneous injections of fondaparinux (2.5 mg) beginning 6 h after surgery or subcutaneous enoxaparin according to approved protocols for the prevention of VTE (93). Metanalysis revealed that fondaparinux significantly reduced the incidence of VTE by day 11 (6.8%) compared to enoxaparin (13.7%, $p < 0.001$). Although fondaparinux achieved an overall 55% reduction in the risk of VTE disturbingly, major bleeding occurred more frequently than with the enoxaperin regimens ($p = 0.008$). Subsequent analyses indicate that administration of fondaparinux earlier than 6 h postoperatively is associated with an increased incidence of major bleeding (94). Fondaparinux is contraindicated in patients with active bleeding, thrombocytopenia, body weight less than 50 kg, and severe renal insufficiency because of an increased risk of major bleeding in these groups. Concern over the perceived increased risk of bleeding complications with fondaparinux led to the evaluation of strategies to reverse its anticoagulation effects. A placebo-controlled randomized trial examined the ability of recombinant factor VIIa (rFVIIa) to reverse the effects of fondaparinux in healthy adults (95). Prolongation of the APTT and PT caused by fondaparinux was reversed with a single intravenous bolus of rFVIIa (90 μg/kg). Thrombin-generation time returned to normal by 6 h after rFVIIa injection. These data suggest the potential for the use of rFVIIa to reverse the anticoagulation effect of fondaparinux in the event of major bleeding complications.

VI. PLATELET FUNCTION INHIBITORS

A. Pharmacology

1. Aspirin

Aspirin (ASA) produces an irreversible inactivation of the cyclooxygenase (COX) activity of COX-1 and COX-2 by acetylating critical serine residues, blocking access of substrate to the enzymes' active site. Inactivation of COX activity interferes with platelet aggregation due to the inhibition of thromboxane A_2 (TXA$_2$). TXA$_2$ induces platelet aggregation and vasoconstriction. Platelets are anucleate, thus inhibition of TXA$_2$ is permanent. ASA is 50- to 100-fold more potent at inhibiting platelet-associated COX-1 than monocyte-associated COX-2 (96). TXA$_2$ is primarily derived from the action of COX-1. The plasma half-life of aspirin is 15–20 min; thus ASA targets COX-1. Considering that only 10% of circulating platelets are replaced daily, once-a-day dosing with aspirin is effective at blocking TXA$_2$.

2. Cilostazol

Cilostazol is a quinolinone derivative that is a potent phosphodiesterase type III inhibitor (97). Phosphodiesterase III inhibition causes elevation of intracellular cAMP levels in platelets and vascular smooth muscle cells, resulting in vasodilatation and inhibition of platelet aggregation. In addition, cilostazol has been reported to inhibit smooth muscle proliferation and to increase levels of HDL cholesterol (97). Cilostazol also inhibits adenosine uptake, leading to increased cAMP in platelets and smooth muscle but decreased cAMP in the heart. Thus the effect of adenosine uptake inhibition on the heart may in part offset the increase in cAMP and the cardiotonic effect attributed to phosphodiesterase III inhibition. Although cilostazol's approved use in the United States is for the management of claudication, it is also an effective platelet inhibitor. Clinicians must be cognizant of this, as many claudicators are already on platelet inhibitors. In healthy volunteers, after a single 100-mg dose of cilostazol, peak plasma levels occurred at 3.6 h; the maximum inhibition of platelet aggregation was 31.1% at 6 h (98).

3. Thienopyridines

The thienopyridines—ticlopidine and clopidogrel—are structurally related potent platelet inhibitors. They are adenosine diphosphate (ADP) receptor antagonists, which inhibit ADP induced platelet aggregation without affecting the arachidonic acid metabolism (99). Both are metabolized in the liver to active metabolites that cause irreversible alterations in ADP receptors. Ticlopidine and clopidogrel cause dose- and time-dependent inhibition in platelet aggregation. After the initiation of therapy, bleeding times reach a peak of 1.5–2 times baseline values over a period of 3–7 days. Recovery of platelet function occurs slowly, over about the same length of time it took to achieve platelet inhibition. When combined, ASA and ticlopidine or clopidogrel act synergistically to inhibit platelet aggregation.

4.   Platelet Glycoprotein IIb/IIIa Inhibitors

Regardless of the stimulus leading to platelet activation, the platelet glycoprotein IIb/IIIa (GPIIb/IIIa) receptors act as the final common step leading to platelet aggregation. Fibrinogen and von Willebrand factor bind to the GPIIb/IIIa receptor, leading to platelet aggregation and thrombus formation. Glycoprotein IIb/IIIa inhibitors compete with fibrinogen and von Willebrand factor to occupy the receptor (100). Currently three GPIIb/IIIa inhibitors are available: abciximab, tirofiban, and eptifbatide. The goal of therapy is to achieve greater than 80% receptor blockade, which will effectively abolish platelet aggregation.

Abciximab is a monoclonal antibody fragment to the GPIIb/IIIa receptor (101). It is a large molecule that binds to the receptor rapidly and tightly, accounting for the short 30-min plasma half-life yet prolonged dissociation from the receptor (40 min). A bolus dose of 0.25 mg/kg blocks greater than 80% of receptors, prolonging the bleeding time; bleeding times return to normal values after 12 h. After the bolus, an infusion of abciximab at 0.125 µg/kg/min can effectively inhibit platelet aggregation for 12 h. Platelet transfusion can reverse the effect of abciximab on platelets. Dosage adjustment for renal insufficiency is not necessary for abciximab.

Tirofiban is a small nonpeptide molecule; it is a reversible antagonist of fibrinogen binding to GPIIb/IIIa receptor (102). Eptifibatide is a synthetic cyclic heptapeptide that is also a competitive inhibitor of GPIIb/IIIa receptor (103). Both of these agents have very rapid rates of dissociation from the GPIIb/IIIa receptor (10–20 s), so that platelet inhibition is dependent on the plasma drug level. Once drug is stopped, bleeding times return to normal within 2–4 h (104). Tirofiban and eptifibatide require dose adjustments for patients with renal insufficiency.

B.   Clinical Applications

Antiplatelet therapy has been proven to decrease adverse cardiovascular events in patients with atherosclerosis. Metanalysis by the Antithrombotic Trialists' Collaboration has shown that antiplatelet therapy in patients at high risk—defined as having previous stroke/TIA, previous MI or acute MI—results in a 25% proportional reduction in serious vascular events (vascular death, MI, and stroke) (105). ASA was the primary antiplatelet therapy in the majority of patients. An earlier metanalysis had not shown a significant benefit for ASA in patients with peripheral arterial disease (PAD) (106). There was a proportional 23% reduction in serious vascular events in the 9214 patients with PAD in the most recent metanalysis, which included trials with other antiplatelet agents such as clopidogrel. The thienopyridines have proven effective agents for patients with peripheral arterial disease. The Swedish Ticlopidine Multicentre Study (STIMS) demonstrated a 29.1% lower mortality in the ticlopidine group compared to placebo (107). The Clopidogrel versus Aspirin in Patients at Risk of Ischaemic Events (CAPRIE) trial compared clopidogrel to aspirin in patients with symptomatic atherosclerosis regardless of symptom location (coronary, cerebral, or peripheral) (108). Based on the first occurrence of ischemic stroke, MI, or vascular death, patients treated with clopidogrel showed a relative risk reduction of 8.7% over and above the 25% reduction currently accepted with ASA. However in patients with PAD, there was a 24% risk reduction in serious vascular events in the clopidogrel group compared to ASA. Cilostazol and the GPIIb/IIIa inhibitors have not been studied in secondary prevention trials.

The management of acute stroke with platelet inhibitors and/or anticoagulants is appealing in concept (i.e., to decrease the risk of ongoing thrombosis), yet the consequences of hemorrhagic complications can be devastating. Metanalysis reveals that ASA therapy results in four fewer nonfatal strokes and five fewer vascular deaths per 1000 patients presenting with acute stroke (105). Accepting that there is an increased risk of hemorrhage with ASA, patients benefit from ASA in the setting of acute stroke if computed tomography reveals the absence of intracranial hemorrhage. Metanalysis of clinical trials evaluating the addition of anticoagulation strategies to ASA during acute stroke reveals a significant increase in mortality and rate of intracranial hemorrhage in the anticoagulation group (109). GPIIb/IIIa inhibitors are under investigation for use in the management of acute ischemic stroke. Preliminary data from a dosing study imply a trend toward improved outcomes versus placebo (110).

Platelet inhibitors decrease the risk of bypass graft occlusion in patients undergoing peripheral artery reconstructive surgery. The Antithrombotic Trialists' Collaboration metanalysis of trials designed to assess the effect of platelet inhibitors on the fate of arterial or graft patency found that the platelet inhibitor groups had a significantly lower rate of graft occlusion (16%) than controls (25%, $p < 0.0001$) (111). The majority of trials used ASA as their platelet inhibitor. While clopidogrel's affect on graft patency has not been evaluated, ticlopidine has been prospectively evaluated in patients undergoing femoropopliteal or femorotibial saphenous-vein bypass grafts. A total of 243 patients were randomly assigned to receive either ticlopidine (250 mg twice a day) or matching placebo for 2 years. The 2-year cumulative patency rate was 82 % in the ticlopidine group and 63 % in the placebo group ($p = 0.002$) (112).

Platelet inhibitors clearly benefit patients experiencing acute coronary syndromes and improve outcomes following percutaneous transluminal coronary angioplasty (PTCA) and stenting. The Clopidogrel in Unstable Angina to Prevent Recurrent Ischaemic Events Trial (CURE) randomized over 12,500 patients to receive in a double-blind manner, either placebo or clopidogrel (113). All patients received ASA (75–325 mg daily), while the clopidogrel arm received an initial 300-mg loading dose of clopidogrel followed by a 75-mg daily dose. Compared to ASA alone, the combination of ASA and clopidogrel reduced the composite risk of cardiovascular death, stroke, and MI, with a relative risk reduction of 20% ($p < 0.001$). The protective effect of clopidogrel was apparent within 2 h of initiation of therapy, and this benefit was consistent at 30 days and after long-term treatment. The Clopidogrel for the Reduction of Events During Observation (CREDO) trial evaluated the effect of ASA and clopidogrel dual therapy following PTCA and stent placement in a randomized, double-blind trial enrolling 2116 patients (114). Patients received either a preprocedure bolus of 300 mg clopidogrel followed by 75 mg daily for 12 months or a placebo bolus and clopidogrel for 28 days. At 1 year, long-term clopidogrel therapy was associated with a 26.9% relative reduction in the combined risk of death, MI, or stroke ($p = 0.02$) The risk of major bleeding at 1 year increased in the long-term group, but not significantly (8.8 vs. 6.7%, $p = 0.07$).

Cilostazol combined with ASA has been studied as a platelet inhibitor for the prevention of coronary stent occlusion and restenosis (115). When cilostazol was compared to ticlopidine, there were no differences in the rate of early stent occlusion, but the incidence of long-term restenosis was reduced with cilostazol (13%) compared to ticlopidine (31%, $p < 0.05$). A recent metanalysis of 19 randomized, placebo-controlled trials was done to evaluate the impact of intravenous antagonists of the GPIIb/IIIa receptor on the survival of patients undergoing PTCA and stenting (116). Mortality and MIs were significantly reduced in the GPIIb/IIIa group at 30 days and 6 months. Major bleeding was increased only in the trials that continued intravenous heparin after the procedure.

The role of platelet inhibitors during peripheral arterial angioplasty/stent placement has been studied in only a limited fashion. Applying the data from the coronary system to the peripheral arteries, clinicians have adopted an antithrombotic strategy of periprocedural use of ASA/clopidogrel and heparin. We recommend 325 mg of ASA at least 24 h prior to the procedure and clopidogrel 75 mg daily for 3–5 days prior to the procedure or 300 mg of clopidogrel at least 6 h preoperatively. During the intervention, heparin is given to maintain an activated clotting time greater than 200 s. Use of GPIIb/IIIa inhibitors in high-risk patients undergoing carotid stent placement has been compared, in a nonrandomized fashion, to intravenous UFH in lower-risk patients and found to decrease the incidence of ischemic stroke (3 vs. 12%, n.s.) (117). However, 5% of the GPIIb/IIIa-treated patients suffered intracranial hemorrhage. GPIIb/IIIa inhibitors all appear to have the ability to disaggregate acute platelet-rich thrombi (118). We have used GPIIb/IIIA inhibitors selectively to treat peripheral artery dissection during angioplasty procedures and have witnessed disaggregation of acute thrombi. Controlled clinical trials are warranted.

C. Complications and Failures

All platelet inhibitors place patients at risk for developing bleeding complications. A decision must be weighed for each patient, balancing the patient's risk of thromboembolic event with the risk of the platelet inhibitor. The antithrombotic effect of ASA appears to be independent of the dose (75 to 1300 mg) (104). The recent Antiplatelet Trialists' Collaboration metanalysis of patients with vascular disease demonstrated that a low dose of ASA (75–160 mg) offers the same protection against thrombotic events as higher doses, yet with a lower risk of gastrointestinal hemorrhage (105). The higher a patient's risk of cardiovascular complications, the more favorable is ASA's safety profile. Ticlopidine and clopidogrel have a potential similar to that of ASA to cause bleeding complications in patients with cardiovascular disease, but they are less likely to cause gastrointestinal hemorrhage (119). In the CURE trial, the overall risk of major bleeding was increased in the clopidogrel-plus-ASA group compared to the placebo (ASA) group (3.7 vs. 2.7%, $p = 0.001$), but the incidence of life-threatening bleeding (2.2 vs. 1.8 %, $p = 0.13$) or hemorrhagic strokes (0.1 vs. 0.1%) was similar (113). As clopidogrel has gained wider acceptance, many surgeons have anecdotally reported their experience with prolonged needle-hole bleeding. Hongo et al. prospectively compared patients undergoing coronary artery bypass graft surgery whom had clopidogrel exposure within 7 days prior to surgery to those patients never exposed to clopidogrel (120). The clopidogrel patients had a 10-fold higher rate of reoperation for bleeding and significantly increased chest tube output and as well as greater transfusion requirements.

Along with the hope that GPIIb/IIIa receptor inhibitors would improve patient outcomes in interventions with a high likelihood of thromboembolism has come concern regarding their potential for significant bleeding complications. The EPIC trial first demonstrated that GPIIb/IIIa therapy combined with traditional antithrombotic therapy (ASA and UFH) decreased ischemic events in patients undergoing PTCA (121). However, the incidence of major bleeding was increased in the abciximab treated patients (14%) compared to those receiving placebo (7%, $p = 0.001$). All the GPIIb/IIIa inhibitors share this heightened bleeding risk; bleeding risk can be decreased with early cessation of intravenous UFH, careful sheath management, and the use of reduced, weight-adjusted doses of heparin (116).

Gastrointestinal side effects are frequent with ASA. The gastrointestinal toxicity of ASA is dose-related (122). The overall relative risk of upper gastrointestinal complications associated with ASA is between 2.2 and 3.1% (122). Diarrhea, nausea, and vomiting can occur in up to 30–50% of patients using ticlopidine (99). Patients using clopidogrel experience far fewer gastrointestinal side effects than those using ticlopidine. Patient complications in the CAPRIE trial included rash (0.26%), diarrhea (0.23%), upper gastrointestinal discomfort (0.97%), and gastrointestinal hemorrhage (0.52%) (108).

Ticlopidine and clopidogrel have both been reported to cause thrombocytopenia and thrombotic thrombocytopenic purpura (99,123). Drug withdrawal usually reverses TTP; periodic monitoring of platelet counts is recommended at the initiation of therapy. Ticlopidine has also been associated with neutropenia and aplastic anemia, while neutropenia is rare with clopidogrel (104). Neutropenia is the most serious side effect of ticlopidine treatment, occurring in 2.1% of patients (99). Cases usually develop during the first 3 months of therapy; thus complete blood counts and platelet counts are recommended every 2 weeks during this period.

Thrombocytopenia is a significant complication of GPIIb/IIIa receptor inhibitor therapy. Abciximab can cause drops in platelet counts to <50,000/µL in 1–2% of patients, with counts dropping 0.5–1.0% in the first 2 h after the start of treatment (104). Thrombocytopenia is reversible with withdrawal of therapy, but this may take several days. Both tirofiban and eptifibatide can cause equally dramatic reversible thrombocytopenia; in their case, the mechanism appears immune-mediated (104,124).

Headache is a common side effect of cilostazol, occurring in 34% of cilostazol-treated patients compared to 14% of placebo-treated patients. Discontinuation of drug because of headache occurred in 3.7% of cilostazol-treated patients compared to 1.3% of placebo-treated patients (125). Other common side effects included palpitations in 10% and diarrhea in 19%. When the FDA approved cilostazol for clinical use, a prior history of heart failure was a contraindication. This recommendation was based on the increased mortality rate seen in patients with heart failure using older phosphodiesterase inhibitors. Pratt pooled the safety data from eight phase III clinical trials evaluating cilostazol (125). He reported that the cardiovascular morbidity and all-cause mortality was 6.5% for cilostazol (100 mg bid) compared to 7.7% for placebo groups.

Most failures of platelet function inhibitors are related to inappropriate clinical application, incorrect dosage, or delayed initiation of therapy. Future improvements to facilitate the monitoring of platelet function, hopefully at the bedside, will likely improve our clinical outcomes.

REFERENCES

1. Rosenberg RD, Bauer KA. The heparin-antithrombin system: A natural anticoagulant mechanism. In: Colman RW, Hirsh J, Marder VJ, et al, eds. Hemostasis and Thrombosis: Basic Principles and Clinical Practice. 3rd ed. Philadelphia: Lippincott, 1994:837–860.
2. Casu B, Oreste P, Torri G, Zoppetti G, Choay J, Lorneau JC, Petitou M, Sinay P. The structure of heparin oligosaccharide fragments with high anti-(factor Xa) activity containing the minimal antithrombin III-binding sequence. Biochem J 1981; 97:599–609.
3. Lam LH, Silbert JE, Rosenberg RD. The separation of active and inactive forms of heparin. Biochem Biophys Res Commun 1976; 69:570–577.
4. Tollefsen DM, Majerus DW, Blank MK. Heparin cofactor II: Purification and properties of a heparin-dependent inhibitor of thrombin in human plasma. J Biol Chem 1982; 257:2162–2169.
5. Choay J. Structure and activity of heparin and its fragments: an overview. Semin Thromb Hemost 1989; 15:359–364.

6. Haas S, Bluemel G. An objective evaluation of the clinical potential of low molecular weight heparins in the prevention of thromboembolism. Semin Thromb Hemost 1989; 15:424–434.

7. Lupu C, Poulsen E, Roquefeuil S, Westmuckett AD, Kakkar VV, Lupu F. Cellular effects of heparin on the production and release of tissue factor pathway inhibitor in human endothelial cells. Arterioscler Thromb Vasc Biol 1999; 19:2251–2262.

8. Ofosu FA, Sie P, Modi GJ, Fernandez F, Buchanan MR, Blajchman MA, Boneu B. The inhibition of thrombin-dependent feedback reactions is critical to the expression of anti-coagulant effects of heparin. Biochem J 1987; 243:579–588.

9. Ockelford PA, Carter CJ, Cerskus A, Smith CA, Hirsh J. Comparison of the in vivo hemor-rhagic and antithrombotic effects of a low antithrombin III affinity heparin fraction. Thromb Res 1982; 27:679–690.

10. Salzman EW, Rosenberg RD, Smith MH, Lindon JN, Favreau L. Effect of heparin and heparin fractions on platelet aggregation. J Clin Invest 1980; 65:64–73.

11. Hull RD, Raskob GE, Hirsh J, Jay RM, Leclerc JR, Geerts WH, Rosenbloom D, Sackett DL, Anderson C, Harrison L. Continuous intravenous heparin compared with intermittent sub-cutaneous heparin in the initial treatment of proximal-vein thrombosis. N Engl J Med 1986; 315:1109–1114.

12. Hirsh J, Warkentin TE, Shaughnessy, Anand SS, Halperin JL, Raschke R, Granger C, Ohman EM, Dalen JE. Heparin and low-molecular-weight heparin. Mechanisms of action, pharmaco-kinetics, dosing, monitoring, efficacy, and safety. Chest 2001; 119:64S–94S.

13. Tolleson TR, O'Shea JC, Bittl JA, Hillegass WB, Williams KA, Levine G, Harrington RA, Tcheng JE. Relationship between Heparin anticoagulation and clinical outcomes in coronary stent intervention: observations from the ESPRIT trial. J Am Coll Cardiol 2003; 41:386–393.

14. Collins R, Scrimgeour A, Yusuf S, Peto R. Reduction in fatal pulmonary embolism and venous thrombosis by perioperative administration of subcutaneous heparin. Overview of results of randomized trials in general, orthopedic, and urologic surgery. N Engl J Med 1988; 318:1162–1173.

15. Hirsh J, Lee AY. How we diagnose and treat deep vein thrombosis. Blood 2002; 99:3102–3110.

16. Hirsh J, Dalen JE, Anderson DR, Poller L, Bussey H, Ansell J, Deylon D. Oral antico-agulants: Mechanism of action, clinical effectiveness, and optimal therapeutic range. Chest 2001; 119:8S–21S.

17. Forbes TL, DeRose G, Harris KA. Is long-term anticoagulation after acute thromboem-bolic limb ischemia always necessary? Can J Surg 2002; 45:337–340.

18. Kakkar VV. Prevention of venous thromboembolism. Clin Hematol 1981; 10:543–583.

19. Kapsch DN, Silver D. Complications in failures of anticoagulation therapy. In: Bernhard VM, Towne JB, eds. Complications in Vascular Surgery. New York: Grune and Stratton, 1985:405–419.

20. Calaitges JG, Silver D. Antithrombotic therapy. In: Rutherford RB, et al., eds. Vascular Surgery 5th ed. Philadelphia: Saunders, 2000.

21. Aster RH. Heparin-induced thrombocytopenia and thrombosis. N Engl J Med 1995; 332: 1374–1376.

22. Laster J, Cikrit D, Walter N, Silver D. The heparin-induced thrombocytopenia syndrome: an update. Surgery 1987; 102:763–770.

23. Mureebe L, Silver D. Heparin-induced thrombocytopenia: pathophysiology and manage-ment. Vasc Endovasc Surg 2002; 36:163–170.

24. Silver D, Kapsch DN, Tsoi EDM. Heparin-induced thrombocytopenia, thrombosis and hemorrhage. Ann Surg 1983; 198:301–306.

25. Greinacher A, Amiral J, Dummel V, Vissac A, Kiefel V, Mueller-Eckhardt C. Laboratory diagnosis of heparin-associated thrombocytopenia and comparison of platelet aggregation tests, heparin-induced platelet activation tests and platelet factor 4/heparin enzyme-linked immunosorbent. Transfusion 1994; 34:381–385.

26. Pouplard C, Amirral J, Boug J, Laporte-Simitsiclis S, Delahouse B, Gruel Y. Decision analysis

for use of platelet aggregation test common carbon 14-0 tonin release assay, and heparin-platelet factor 4 enzyme-linked immunosorbent assay for diagnosis of heparin-induced thrombocytopenia. Am J Clin Pathol 1999; 111:700–706.

27. Lindhoff-Last E, Gerdsen F, Ackermann H, Bauersach SR. Determination of heparin-plate factor 4-IgG antibodies improves diagnosis of heparin-induced thrombocytopenia. Br J Haematol 2001; 113:886–897.

28. Kikta MJ, Keller MP, Humphrey PW, Silver D. Can low molecular weight heparins and heparinoids be safely given to patients with heparin-induced thrombocytopenia syndrome? Surgery 1993; 114:705–710.

29. Slocum MM, Adams JG Jr, Teel R, Spadone DP, Silver D. Use of enoxaparin in patients with the heparin-induced thrombocytopenia syndrome. J Vasc Surg 1996; 23:839–843.

30. Kaplan KL, Francis CW. Direct thrombin inhibitors. Semin Hematol 2002; 39:187–196.

31. Jaffe MD, Willis PW. Multiple fractures associated with long-term sodium heparin therapy. JAMA 1965; 193:152–154.

32. Gerrts WH, Heit JA, Clagett GP, Pineo GF, Colwell CW, Anderson FA, Wheeler HB. Prevention of venous thromboembolism. Chest 2001; 119:132S–175S.

33. Levine MN, Hirsh J, Gent M, Turpie AG, Cruickshank M, Weitz J, Anderson D, Johnson M. A randomized trial comparing activated thromboplastin time with heparin assay in patients with acute venous thromboembolism requiring large daily doses of heparin. Arch Intern Med 1994; 154:49–56.

34. Thomas DP. Heparin. Clin Hematol 1981; 1:443–458.

35. Hirsh J. Low-molecular-weight heparin: A review of the results of recent studies of the treatment of venous thromboembolism and unstable angina. J Circ 1998; 98:1575–1582.

36. Nielsen JI, Ostergaard P. Chemistry of heparin and low molecular weight heparin. Acta Chir Scand Suppl 1988; 534:52–56.

37. Altman R, Scazziota A, Rouvier J. Efficacy of unfractionated heparin, low molecular weight heparin, and both combined for releasing total and free tissue factor pathway inhibitor. Haemostasis 1998; 28:229–235.

38. Wheitz JI. Low-molecular-weight heparins. N Engl J Med 1997; 337:688–698.

39. Levine M, Gent N, Hirsh J, Leclerc J, Anderson D, Weitz J, Ginsberg J, Turpie AG, Demers C, Kovacs M. A comparison of low-molecular-weight administered primarily at home with unfractionated heparin administered in the hospital for proximal-deep vein thrombosis. N Engl J Med 1996; 334:677–681.

40. Young E, Wells P, Holloway S, Weitz J, Hirsh S. Ex-vivo and in-vitro evidence that low molecular weight heparins exibit less binding to plasma proteins than unfractionated heparin. Thromb Haemost 1994; 71:300–304.

41. Warkentin TE, Levine MN, Hirsh J, Horsewood P, Roberts RS, Gent M, Kelton JG. Heparin-induced thrombocytopenia in patients treated with low molecular weight heparin or unfractionated heparin. N Engl J Med 1995; 332:1330–1335.

42. Laposata M, Green D, Van Cott EM, Barrowcliffe TW, Goodnight SH, Sosolik RC. The clinical use in laboratory monitoring of low molecular weight heparin, danaparoid, hirudin and related compounds, and argatroban: College of American Pathologists Conference X XXI on laboratory monitoring of anticoagulant therapy. Arch Pathol Lab Med 1998; 122:799–807.

43. Etchells E, McLeod RS, Geerts W, Barton P, Desky AS. Economic analysis of low-dose heparin versus the low-molecular-weight heparin enoxaparin for prevention of venous thromboembolism after colorectal surgery. Arch Intern Med 1999; 159:1221–1228.

44. Koch A, Boughes S, Ziegler S, Dinkel H, Daures JP, Victor N. Low-molecular-weight heparin and unfractionated heparin in thrombosis prophylaxis after major surgical intervention: update of previous meta-analyses. Br J Surg 1997; 84:750–759.

45. Gould MK, Dembitzer AD, Doyle RL, Hastie TJ, Garber AM. Low-molecular-weight heparins compared with unfractionated heparin for treatment of acute deep vein thrombosis. A meta-analysis of randomized, control trials. Ann Intern Med 1999; 130:800–809.

46. Dolovich LR, Ginsberg JS, Douketis JD, Holbrook AM, Cheah G. A meta-analysis com-

paring low-molecular-weight heparins with unfractionated heparin in the treatment of venous thromboembolism. Examining some unanswered questions regarding location of treatment, product type, and dosing frequency. Arch Intern Med 2000; 160:181–188.

47. Siragusa S, Cosmi B, Piovella F, Hirsh J, Ginsbert JS. Low-molecular-weight heparins and unfractionated heparin in the treatment of patients with acute venous thromboembolism: Results of a meta-analysis. Am J Med 1996; 100:269–277.

48. Hull RD, Raskobe GE, Brant RF, Pineo GF, Elliot G, Stein PD, Gottschalk A, Valentine KA, Mah AF. Low-molecular-weight heparin versus heparin in the treatment of patients with pulmonary embolism. American-Canadian Thrombosis Study Group. Arch Intern Med 2000; 160:229–236.

49. Simonneau G, Sors H, Charbonnier B, Page Y, Laaban JP, Azarian R, Laurent M, Hirsch JL, Ferrari E, Bossom JL, Mottier D, Beau B. A comparison of low-molecular-weight heparin with unfractionated heparin for acute pulmonary embolism. THESEE Study Group. Tinzaparine ou heparine standard: evaluations dans l'envolie pulmonaire. N Engl J Med 1997; 337:663–669.

50. Friederich PW, Sanson BJ, Simioni P, et al. Frequency of pregnancy related venous thromboembolism in anticoagulant factor deficient women: implications before prophylaxis. Arch Intern Med 1996; 125:955–960.

51. Ginsberg JS, Grer I, Hirsh J. Use of antithrombotic agents during pregnancy. Chest 2001; 119:122S–131S.

52. Edmondson RA, Cohen AT, Das SK, Wagner MB, Kakkar VV. Low molecular weight heparin versus aspirin and Dipyridamole after femoropopliteal bypass grafting. [Published erratum appears in Lancet 1994; 344: 1307]. Lancet 1994; 344:914–918.

53. Simama CM, Gigou F, Ill P. Low molecular weight heparin versus unfractionated heparin in femorodistal reconstruction surgery: a multi-center open randomized trial. Enoxart Study Group. Ann Vasc Surg 1995; 9(suppl):S45–S53.

54. Hingorani A, Gramse C, Ascher E. Anticoagulation with enoxaparin versus intravenous unfractionated heparin in postoperative vascular surgery patients. J Vasc Surg 2002; 36:341–345. Comment in: J Vasc Surg 2003; 37:700–701. Author replies 701.

55. Ardissino D, Merlini PA, Aarlens R, Coppola R, Bramucci E, Lucreziotti S, Repetto A, Fetiveau R, Mannucci PM. Tissue factor in human coronary atherosclerotic plaques. Clin Chim Acta 2000; 291:235–240.

56. Antman EM, Cohen M, Radley D, McCabe C, Rush J, Premmereur J, Braunwald E. Assessment of the treatment effect of Enoxaparin for unstable angina/non-Q-wave myocardial infarction: TIMI 11 B-ESSENCE meta-analysis. Circulation 1999; 100:1602–1608.

57. Wong GC, Giugliano RP, Antman EM. Use of low molecular weight heparins in the management of acute coronary artery syndromes and percutaneous coronary intervention. JAMA 2003; 289:331–342.

58. Schweizer J, Muller A, Forkmann L, Hellner G, Kirch W. Potential use of low-molecular-weight heparin to prevent restenosis in patients with extensive wall damage following peripheral angioplasty. Angioplasty 2001; 52:659–669.

59. Nurmohamed MT, Rosendaal FR, Buller HR, Dekker E, Hommes DW, Vandenbroucke JP, Briet E. Low-molecular-weight heparin versus standard heparin in general and orthopedic surgery: a meta-analysis. Lancet 1992; 340:152–156.

60. Crowther MA, Berry LR, Monagle PT, Chan AK. Mechanisms responsible for the failure of protamine to inactivate low-molecular-weight heparin. Br J Haematol 2002; 116:178–186.

61. Lumpkin MN. FDA Public Health Advisory. Anesthesiology 1998; 88:27A–28A.

62. Luk C, Wells PS, Anderson D, Covacs MJ. Extended outpatient therapy of low molecular weight heparin for the treatment of recurrent venous thromboembolism despite warfarin therapy. Am J Med 2001; 111:270–273.

63. Bick RL. Antiphospholipid thrombosis syndromes. Hematol Oncol Clin North Am 2003; 17:115–147.

64. Muir JM, Hirsch J, Weitz JI, Andrew M, Young E, Shaughnessy SG. A histomorphometric

comparison of the effects of heparin in low molecular weight heparin on low cancellous in bone in rats. Blood 1997; 89:3236–3242.

65. Suttie JW. Oral anticoagulant therapy: The biosynthetic basis. Semin Hematol 1977; 14:365–374.

66. Zivelin A, Rao VM, Rapaport SI. Mechanisms of the anticoagulant effect of warfarin as evaluated in rabbits by selective depression of individual procoagulant vitamin-K dependent clotting factors. J Clin Invest 1993; 92:2131–2140.

67. Harrison L, Johnston N, Massicotte MP, Crowther M, Moffat K, Hirsh J. Comparison of 5-mg and 10-mg loading doses in initiation of warfarin therapy. Ann Intern Med 1997; 126:133–136.

68. Hirsch J, Fuster V. Guide to anticoagulant therapy. Part 2: Oral anticoagulants. American Heart Association. Circulation 1994; 89:1469–1480.

69. Ridker PM, Goldhaber SZ, Danielson A, Rosenberg Y, Evy CS, Deitcher SR, Cushman M, Moll S, Kessler CM, Elliott CG, Paulson R, Wong T, Bauer KA, Schwartz BA, Miletich JP, Bounameaux H, Glinn RJ. Long-term, low-intensity warfarin therapy for the prevention of recurrent venous thromboembolism. N Engl J Med 2003; 348:1425–1434. E pub 2003 Feb 24. www.nengm.org.

70. Albers GW, Sherman DG, Gress DR, Paulseth JE, Petersen P. Stroke prevention in non-valvular atrial fibrillation: a review of prospective randomized trials. Ann Neurol 1991; 30:511–518.

71. Flinn WR, Arohrer MJ, Yao JS, McCarthy WJ III, Fahey VA, Bergan JJ. Improved long-term patency of infragenicular polytetraflouroethylene grafts. J Vasc Surg 1998; 7:685–690.

72. Johnson WC, Williford WO, and members of the Department of Veteran's Affairs Cooperative Study #362. Benefits, morbidity, and mortality associated with long-term administration of oral anticoagulant therapy to patients with peripheral arterial bypass procedures: a prospective randomized study. J Vasc Surg 2002; 35:413–421.

73. Hull R, Hirsch J, Jay R, Carter C, England C, Gent M, Turpie AG, McLoughlin D, Dodd P, Thomas M, Raskob G, Ockelford P. Different intensities of oral anticoagulant therapy in the treatment of proximal-vein thrombosis. N Engl J Med 1982; 307:1676–1681.

74. Yasaka M, Sakata T, Minematsu K, Naritomi H. Correction of INR by prothrombin complex concentrate and vitamin K in patients with warfarin related hemorrhagic complication. Thromb Res 2002; 108:25–30.

75. Chan YC, Valenti D, Mansfield AO, Stansby G. Warfarin induced skin necrosis. Br J Surg 2000; 87:266–272.

76. Alving BM, Strickler MP, Knight RD, Barr CF, Berenberg JL, Peck CC. Hereditary warfarin resistance. Arch Intern Med 1985; 145:499–501.

77. Mannucci PM. Genetic control of anticoagulation. Lancet 1999; 353:688–689.

78. Kaplan KL, Francis CW. Direct thrombin inhibitors. Semin Hematol 2002; 39:187–196.

79. Greinacher A, Volpel H, Janssens U, Hach-Wunderle V, Kemkes-Matthes B, Eichler P, Mueller-Velten HG, Potzsch B, for the HIT Investigators Group. Recombinant hirudin (lepa-rudin) provide safe and effective anticoagulation in patients with heparin-induced thrombocytopenia—a prospective study. Circulation 1999; 99:73–80.

80. Potzsch B, Madlener K, Seelig C, Reiss CF, Greinacher A, Muller-Berghaus G. Monitoring of small r-hirudin anticoagulation during cardiopulmonary bypass, assessment of the whole blood ecarin clotting time. Thromb Haemost 1997; 77:920–925.

81. Liu H, Fleming NW, Moore PG. Anticoagulation for patients with heparin-induced thrombocytopenia using recombinant hirudin during cardiopulmonary bypass. J Clin Anesth 2002; 14:452–455.

82. Greinacher A, Eichler P, Lubenow N, Kwasny H, Luz M. Heparin-induced thrombocytopenia with thromboembolic complications: meta-analysis of 2 prospective trials to assess the value of parental treatment with leparudin and its therapeutic aPTT range. Blood 2000; 96:846–851.

83. Robson R. The use of bivalirudin in patients with renal impairment. J Invas Cardiol 2000; 12(suppl F):33–36.

84. Bittl JA, Storny J, Brinker JA, Ahmed WH, Meckel CR, Chaitman BR, Maraganore J, Deutsch E, Adelman B, for the Hirulog Angioplasty Study Investigators. Treatment with bivalirudin (hirulog) as compared with heparin during coronary angioplasty for unstable or postinfarction angina. N Engl J Med 1995; 333:764–769.

85. Bush L. Argatroban, a selective potent thrombin inhibitor. Cardiovasc Drug Rev 1991; 9:247–263.

86. Lewis BE, Wallis DE, Berkowitz SD, Matthai WH, Fareed J, Walenga JM, Bartholomew J, Sham R, Learner RG, Ziegler ZR, Rustagi PK, Jang IK, Rifkin SD, Moran J, Hursting MJ, Kelton JG; for the ARG-911 Study Investigators. Argatroban anticoagulant therapy in patients with heparin-induced thrombocytopenia. Circulation 2001; 103:1838–1843.

87. Lewis BE, Matthai WH, Cohen M, Moses JW, Hursting MJ, Leya F, for the ARG-216/310/311 Study Investigators. Argatroban anticoagulation during percutaneous coronary intervention in patients with heparin-induced thrombocytopenia. Cathet Cardiovasc Intervent 2002; 57:177–184.

88. Lubenow N, Selleng S, Wollert HG, Eichler P, Mullejans B, Greinacher A. Heparin-induced thrombocytopenia and pulmonary bypass: perioperative argatroban use. Ann Thorac Surg 2003; 75:577–579.

89. Wahlander K, Lapidus L, Olsson CG, Thuresson A, Eriksson UG, Larson G, Eriksson H. Pharmacokinetics, pharmacodynamics and clinical effects of the oral direct thrombin inhibitor ximelagatran in acute treatment of patients with pulmonary embolism and deep vein thrombosis. Thromb Res 2002; 107:93–99.

90. Eriksson H, Eriksson UG, Frison L, Hansson PO, Held P, Holmstrom M, Hagg A, Jonsson T, Lapidus L, Leijd B, Stockelberg D, Safwenberg U, Taghavi A, Thorsen M. Pharmacokinetics and pharmacodynamics of melagatran, a novel synthetic LMW thrombin inhibitor, in patients with acute DVT. Thromb Haemost Mar 1999; 81:358–363.

91. Eriksson BI, Bergqvist D, Kalebo P, Dahl OE, Lindbratt S, Bylock A, Frison L, Eriksson UG, Welin L, Gustafsson D. Melagatran for Thrombin inhibition in orthopaedic surgery. Ximelagatran and melagatran compared with dalteparin for prevention of venous thromboembolism after total hip or knee replacement: the METHRO II randomised trial. Lancet 2002; 360:1441–1447.

92. Walenga JM, Jeske WP, Samama MM, Frapaise FX, Bick RL, Fareed J. Fondaparinux: a synthetic heparin pentasaccharide as a new antithrombotic agent. Expert Opin Invest Drugs 2002; 11:397–407.

93. Turpie AG, Bauer KA, Eriksson BI, Lassen MR. Fondaparinux vs enoxaparin for the prevention of venous thromboembolism in major orthopedic surgery: a meta-analysis of 4 randomized double-blind studies. Arch Intern Med 2002; 162:1833–1840.

94. Kwong LM, Muntz JE. Thromboprophylaxis dosing: the relationship between timing of first administration, efficacy, and safety. Am J Orthop 2002; 31(suppl):16–20.

95. Bijsterveld NR, Moons AH, Boekholdt SM, van Aken BE, Fennema H, Peters RJ, Meijers JC, Buller HR, Levi M. Ability of recombinant factor VIIa to reverse the anticoagulant effect of the pentasaccharide fondaparinux in healthy volunteers. Circulation 2002; 106:2550–2554.

96. Cipollone F, Patrignani P, Greco A, Panara MR, Padovano R, Cuccurullo F, Patrono C, Rebuzzi AG, Liuzzo G, Quaranta G, Maseri A. Differential suppression of thromboxane biosynthesis by indopufen and aspirin in patients with unstable angina. Circulation 1997; 96:1109–1116.

97. Liu Y, Shakur Y, Yoshitake M, Kambayashi Ji J. Cilostazol (pletal): a dual inhibitor of cyclic nucleotide phosphodiesterase type 3 and adenosine uptake. Cardiovasc Drug Rev 2001; 19:369–386.

98. Woo SK, Kang WK, Kwon KI. Pharmacokinetic and pharmacodynamic modeling of the

antiplatelet and cardiovascular effects of cilostazol in healthy humans. Clin Pharmacol Ther 2002; 71:246–252.

99. Quinn MJ, Fitzgerald DJ. Ticlopidine and clopidogrel. Circulation 1999; 100:1667–1672.

100. Topol EJ, Byzova TV, Plow EF. Platelet GPIIb-IIIa blockers. Lancet 1999; 353:227–231.

101. Tcheng JE, Ellis SG, George BS, Kereiakes DJ, Kleiman NS, Talley JD, Wang AL, Weisman HF, Califf RM, Topol EJ. Pharmacodynamics of chimeric glycoprotein IIb/IIIa integrin antiplatelet antibody Fab 7E3 in high-risk coronary angioplasty. Circulation 1994; 90:1757–1764.

102. Kereiakes DJ, Kleiman NS, Ambrose J, Cohen M, Rodriguez S, Palabrica T, Herrmann HC, Sutton JM, Weaver WD, McKee DB, Fitzpatrick V, Sax FL. Randomized, double-blind, placebo-controlled dose-ranging study of tirofiban (MK-383) platelet IIb/IIIa blockade in high risk patients undergoing coronary angioplasty. J Am Coll Cardiol 1996; 27:536–542.

103. O'Shea JC, Buller CE, Cantor WJ, Chandler AB, Cohen EA, Cohen DJ, Gilchrist IC, Kleiman NS, Labinaz M, Madan M, Hafley GE, Califf RM, Kitt MM, Strony J, Tcheng JE. ESPRIT Investigators. Long-term efficacy of platelet glycoprotein IIb/IIIa integrin blockade with eptifibatide in coronary stent intervention. JAMA 2002; 287:618–621.

104. Patrono C, Coller B, Dalen JE, FitzGerald GA, Fuster V, Gent M, Hirsh J, Roth G. Platelet-active drugs: The relationships among dose, effectiveness, and side effects. Chest 2001; 119 (suppl 1):39–63.

105. Antithrombotic Trialists' Collaboration. Collaborative meta-analysis of randomised trials of antiplatelet therapy for prevention of death, myocardial infarction, and stroke in high risk patients. Br Med J 2002; 324:71–86.

106. Collaborative overview of randomised trials of antiplatelet therapy: I. Prevention of death, myocardial infarction, and stroke by prolonged antiplatelet therapy in various categories of patients. Antiplatelet Trialists' Collaboration. Br Med J 1994; 308:81–106.

107. Janzon L. The STIMS trial: the ticlopidine experience and its clinical applications. Swedish Ticlopidine Multicenter Study. Vasc Med 1996; 1:141–143.

108. CAPRIE Steering Committee. A randomised, blinded, trial of clopidogrel versus aspirin in patients at risk of ischaemic events (CAPRIE). Lancet 1996; 348:1329–1339.

109. Berge E, Sandercock P. Anticoagulants versus antiplatelet agents for acute ischaemic stroke. Cochrane Database Syst Rev 2002; 4:CD003242.

110. The Abciximab in Ischemic Stroke Investigators. Abciximab in acute ischemic stroke: a randomized, double-blind, placebo-controlled, dose-escalation study. Stroke 2000; 31:601–609.

111. Antiplatelet Trialists' Collaboration. Collaborative overview of randomised trials of antiplatelet therapy: II. Maintenance of vascular graft or arterial patency by antiplatelet therapy. Br Med J 1994; 308:159–168.

112. Becquemin JP. Effect of ticlopidine on the long-term patency of saphenous-vein bypass grafts in the legs. Etude de la ticlopidine apres pontage femoro-poplite and the association Universitaire de Recherche en Chirurgie. N Engl J Med 1997; 337:1726–1731.

113. Yusuf S, Zhao F, Mehta SR, Chrolavicius S, Tognoni G, Fox KK. The Clopidogrel in Unstable Angina to Prevent Recurrent Events Trial Investigators. Effects of clopidogrel in addition to aspirin in patients with acute coronary syndromes without ST-segment elevation. N Engl J Med 2001; 345:494–502. Erratum in: N Engl J Med 2001; 345:1506, 1716.

114. Steinhubl SR, Berger PB, Mann JT, Fry ET, DeLago A, Wilmer C, Topol EJ, CREDO Investigators. Clopidogrel for the reduction of events during observation. Early and sustained dual oral antiplatelet therapy following percutaneous coronary intervention: a randomized controlled trial. JAMA 2002; 288:2411–2420. Erratum in JAMA 2003; 289:987.

115. Kamishirado H, Inoue T, Mizoguchi K, Uchida T, Nakata T, Sakuma M, Takayanagi K, Morooka S. Randomized comparison of cilostazol versus ticlopidine hydrochloride for antiplatelet therapy after coronary stent implantation for prevention of late restenosis. Am Heart J 2002; 144:303–308.

116. Karvouni E, Katritsis DG, Ioannidis JP. Intravenous glycoprotein IIb/IIIa receptor antag-

onists reduce mortality after percutaneous coronary interventions. J Am Coll Cardiol 2003; 41:26–32.

117. Qureshi AI, Suri MF, Ali Z, Kim SH, Lanzino G, Fessler RD, Ringer AJ, Guterman LR, Hopkins LN. Carotid angioplasty and stent placement: a prospective analysis of perioperative complications and impact of intravenously administered abciximab. Neurosurgery 2002; 50:466–473. Discussion 473–475.

118. Moser M, Bertram U, Peter K, Bode C, Ruef J. Abciximab, eptifibatide, and tirofiban exhibit: dose-dependent potencies to dissolve platelet aggregates. J Cardiovasc Pharmacol 2003; 41:586–592.

119. Hankey GJ, Sudlow CL, Dunbabin DW. Thienopyridine derivatives (ticlopidine, clopidogrel) versus aspirin for preventing stroke and other serious vascular events in high vascular risk patients. Cochrane Database Syst Rev 2000; 2:CD001246.

120. Hongo RH, Ley J, Dick SE, Yee RR. The effect of clopidogrel in combination with aspirin when given before coronary artery bypass grafting. J Am Coll Cardiol 2002; 40:231–237.

121. Use of a monoclonal antibody directed against the platelet glycoprotein IIb/IIIa receptor in high-risk coronary angioplasty. The EPIC Investigation. N Engl J Med 1994; 330:956–961.

122. Garcia Rodriguez LA, Hernandez-Diaz S, de Abajo FJ. Association between aspirin and upper gastrointestinal complications: systematic review of epidemiologic studies. Br J Clin Pharmacol 2001; 52:563–571.

123. Nara W, Ashley I, Rosner F. Thrombotic thrombocytopenic purpura associated with clopidogrel administration: case report and brief review. Am J Med Sci 2001; 322:170–172.

124. Rezkalla SH, Hayes JJ, Curtis BR, Aster RH. Eptifibatide-induced acute profound thrombocytopenia presenting as refractory hypotension. Catheter Cardiovasc Intervent 2003; 58:76–79.

125. Pratt CM. Analysis of the cilostazol safety database. Am J Cardiol 2001; 87:28D–33D.

9

Gastrointestinal and Visceral Ischemic Complications of Aortic Reconstruction

Daniel J. Reddy and Hector M. Dourron*

Henry Ford Hospital, Detroit, Michigan, U.S.A.

Gastrointestinal complications following aortic reconstructive surgery are well recognized and are associated with a potentially high mortality rate. Contemporary practice, with advances in pre- and postoperative care as well as improvements in operative technique, have contributed to a progressive decline in morbidity and mortality after aortic reconstruction when compared to the past three decades. Nonetheless, maintenance of a low rate of morbidity challenges the vascular surgeon's ability to identify and adopt new strategies to limit perioperative complications. Although an array of gastrointestinal complications (Table 1) have been reported following aortic reconstruction, severe morbidity leading to prolonged hospitalization and death can often be avoided by prompt recognition and expert management. An understanding of the setting in which these complications occur and the influence of patient comorbidities are key. As many as 50% of patients who have gastrointestinal complications require operative intervention, with reported mortality rates ranging from 16–67% (1–3).

Although a number of risk factors for gastrointestinal complications have been identified, splanchnic bed arterial hypoperfusion appears to be the most common final pathological mechanism implicated in most cases. The inferior mesenteric artery (IMA) is commonly divided during aortic reconstruction. The loss of the IMA, reduced hypogastric arterial flow, or hindgut atheroembolization have been implicated in the pathogenesis of ischemic colitis following aortic reconstruction (3). Moreover, atheroemboli may affect the small bowel, kidney, and spinal cord as well as the hindgut. Additional factors that increase the risk of ischemic colitis are listed in Table 2.

Mounting evidence suggests that intestinal ischemia is important in the development of irreversible shock and multiple organ system failure (4). To prevent these complications,

---

* *Current affiliation*: Vascular Surgical Associates, P.C., Austell, Georgia, U.S.A.

Table 1　Gastrointestinal Complications Following Aortic Reconstruction

Paralytic ileus
Upper gastrointestinal bleed
Gastritis
Duodenal ulcer
Gastric ulcer
Clostridium difficile enterocolitis
Acute cholecystitis
Mechanical obstruction
Chylous ascites
Pancreatitis
Colon ischemia
Small bowel ischemia
Visceral ischemia

the vascular surgeon must provide for adequate colonic and pelvic arterial blood supply following aortic reconstruction, along with the many additional requirements of these complex procedures.

I. CLASSIFICATION

Gastrointestinal complications of a functional and ordinarily self-limiting nature occur frequently following aortic reconstruction. Paralytic ileus of the stomach and colon lasting 36–48 h following transperitoneal repair of the aorta is common and seldomly leads to major morbidity or prolonged hospitalization. Bowel manipulation, extensive lysis of adhesions, and hematoma formation may contribute to this problem; particularly in patients with the autonomic neuropathic comorbidity of diabetes mellitus. Postoperative pancreatitis is a less common but potentially more severe gastrointestinal complication following aortic reconstruction. Elevated amylase and lipase levels support the diagnosis, although clinical manifestations of pancreatitis are unusual. Vigorous retraction and more proximal dissection, particularly at the paraceliac level, are considered to play a role in the pathogenesis. The most serious gastrointestinal complication following aortic reconstruction remains ischemic colitis.

The foregut, midgut, hindgut, and pelvis are endowed with a rich collateral arterial bed that, under normal circumstances, protects both solid and hollow viscera from

Table 2　Predisposing Factor for the Development of Ischemic Colitis Following Aortic Reconstruction

Improper IMA ligation
Loss of IMA–hypogastric blood flow
Ruptured aneurysm
Perioperative hypotension
Retractor trauma
Inadequate development of collaterals
IMA to SMA flow in the meandering mesenteric artery

ischemia when axial perfusion is interrupted by disease or operative manipulation. However, patients with aneurysmal or occlusive processes often have diseased collaterals or lack a complete collateral pattern, putting them at greater risk of visceral ischemia. Although the colon or small bowel may be affected, the colon is far more commonly involved. Colonic ischemia following aortic reconstruction is typically secondary to arterial occlusion or atheroembolism. Venous compromise of the colon following aortic reconstruction has been reported but seldom encountered without low flow or hematological disease, particularly in the setting of intra-abdominal sepsis. Colonic ischemia is more commonly associated with aneurysmal rather than arterial occlusive disease owing to the richer collateral beds that develop over time with chronic occlusive disease (5).

Greenwald et al. have provided a practical classification of colonic ischemia (CI) that stratifies specific conditions resulting from ischemic injury to the colon as reversible or irreversible (6). These classes can then be subcategorized further as (a) reversible ischemic colonopathy (submucosal or intramural hemorrhage), (b) reversible or transient ischemic colitis, (c) chronic ulcerative ischemic colitis, (d) ischemic colonic stricture, (e) colonic gangrene, and (f) fulminant universal ischemic colitis. Subcategories a and b are limited to the mucosa. Subcategory c extends to the muscularis and is not reversible. Subcategories e and f are transmural and result in perforation. More than 60% of reported cases involve transmural ischemia. The most common anatomical site for all types of colonic ischemia following aortic reconstruction is the sigmoid colon after inferior mesenteric artery ligation (7). No doubt other factors can play a contributing role in the pathogenesis (Table 2).

II. ANATOMY AND PATHOPHYSIOLOGY

The inferior mesenteric artery (IMA) and its branches serve to bridge the midgut, hindgut, and pelvis via collateral communications with the superior mesenteric artery (SMA) and the hypogastric arterial circulation. Among these three circuits, the IMA is the main axial blood supply to the left colon. The SMA and IMA circuits communicate via the meandering artery and the marginal artery of Drummond, both of which originate from the left branch of the middle colic artery and terminate in the left colic artery or IMA. The meandering artery can typically be found within the mesenteric pedicle and is at risk of injury during retraction for exposure. The marginal artery of Drummond is rather constant along the transverse and descending colons. However, in 5% of individuals, it is lacking in the region of the ascending colon; in 20%, it is absent in the sigmoid colon; and it exists with even greater inconsistency at the rectosigmoid junction (8). Finally, the hypogastric arteries, via the lower rectal branches, provide a bridge between the systemic and visceral circulations. This can further collateralize the left colon by way of the superior rectal branch of the IMA.

The incision and operative approach selected for aortic reconstruction is individualized for each patient. Most authors describe the approach to the infrarenal aorta via a transperitoneal midline incision, although reports are accumulating detailing certain patient factors that favor a retroperitoneal approach to reduce gastrointestinal complications (9). In a 1987 nonrandomized comparison of the retroperitoneal and transabdominal approaches from Sicard et al., 6% of patients with transperitoneal repair were found to have a prolonged ileus (more than 96 h), while none were noted in the retroperitoneal group (10). In a later prospective randomized trial reported by these same authors, 10% of patients with aortic repair by the transabdominal approach experienced prolonged ileus and 6% had small bowel obstructions, of which more than 50% required operative intervention (11). Furthermore, no patients in the retroperitoneal approach group required reoperation for gastrointestinal complications.

Colonic ischemia becomes clinically evident in a variety of stages of severity. In the mildest cases, mucosal ischemia may lead to an inflammatory reaction of the submucosa, with mucosal sloughing and eventual complete healing. A moderate ischemic injury can extend to the muscularis mucosa, and these cases generally heal with some degree of stricture. The most severe cases of ischemia involve transmural necrosis with perforation of the bowel wall. The mortality rate of colonic infarction after aortic reconstruction has been reported as high as 80–100% (12). Therefore knowledge of and provision for the anatomical collateralization pathways supplying the viscera is of vital importance during aortic reconstruction. Avoidance of injury to collateral pathways or reimplantation or bypass of vital arterial branches is key to the prevention of intestinal ischemia and lowering of morbidity following aortic reconstructive surgery.

III. CLINICAL MANIFESTATIONS AND DIAGNOSIS

A high index of suspicion will facilitate early diagnosis of postoperative colonic ischemia and avoid potentially fatal complications. Clinical evidence of ischemic colitis is seen in approximately 2% of elective infrarenal aortic reconstructions (13–15) and in up to 32% of patients who survive repair of a ruptured aortic aneurysm (16). Prospective studies with colonoscopy suggest ischemic mucosal changes in 7–35% of patients undergoing elective aortic procedures (17) and up to 60% of patients with ruptured aortic aneurysms (18). Clearly, not all of these patients manifest clinical signs of colonic ischemia; therefore it is the vascular surgeon's challenge to identify the subgroup of patients with insufficient collateral circulation to maintain colon viability. The classic clinical presentation for colonic ischemia is bloody diarrhea in the early postoperative period. Nonetheless, only 29–36% of patients with documented ischemic colitis will exhibit this feature, making it an insensitive clinical predictor (19,20). Despite its relatively low incidence, bloody diarrhea, when present, is a compelling clinical sign that often predicts transmural colonic ischemia (16). Other clinical signs suggestive of colonic ischemia are listed in Table 3. Clinical suspicion is confirmed by colonoscopy, which should be performed at the bedside of any patient suspected of ischemic colitis. Repeated studies over a 1- to 2-day interval can help clarify resolution or progression of this disease process. Passage of the colonoscope to 40 cm from the anal verge is usually sufficient to detect ischemic colitis in up to 95% of patients (16), as isolated ischemia of the right or transverse colon with no left colonic

Table 3   Clinical Signs of Ischemic Colitis

Fever
Anuria
Hypotension ≤90 mmHg
Abdominal pain
Abdominal distention
Elevated WBC count thrombocytopenia
Postoperative fluid requirements ≥5L
Packed red blood cells ≥6U
Lactic acidemia

involvement is rare (18,20). Early mucosal changes seen on colonoscopy include circumferential petechial hemorrhage and edema. More advanced cases may demonstrate pseudomembranes, erosions, and ulcers. But even in these cases, in the absence of peritoneal signs, conservative management such as bowel rest, fluid administration, and parenteral nutrition may suffice, with the most common sequela being colonic stricture. Beyond these changes, however, the colon will appear yellowish-green, necrotic, and noncontractile. At this point colonic perforation should be considered imminent and operative intervention is advised.

Another method for predicting colonic ischemia is transluminal pH (pH_t) mucosal monitoring (21). The theory behind pH_t is that anaerobic metabolism caused by insufficient oxygen delivery to the gut can be detected by a low pH of the gastric or colonic mucosa. Studies have shown that sigmoid acidosis (pHt below 7.1) signals an early warning and, if not corrected within 2 h, is predictive of major morbidity (22). Barium contrast studies have been used to document late sequelae of ischemic colitis but are of no use for diagnosis in the immediate postoperative period. In summary, frequent reexamination of the abdomen, repeated colonoscopy, and monitoring of hemodynamic parameters are required when ischemic colitis is suspected. We have evaluated other modalities, such as fluorescein injection with Wood's lamp examination, pulse oximetry, and Doppler ultrasound in controlled experimental studies of small bowel ischemia (23). However; none of these modalities have been confirmed by clinical trials of hindgut ischemia.

IV. ISCHEMIC COLITIS FOLLOWING STENT-GRAFT REPAIR OF ABDOMINAL AORTIC ANEURYSMS

Several large series have reported no cases of ischemic colitis following endovascular repair of abdominal aortic aneurysms (AAAs) (24–26). Sandison et al. reported one case of sigmoid necrosis following endovascular repair of an infrarenal aortic aneurysm and attributed the complication to embolization of a patent internal iliac artery (27). Jaeger et al. reported a second case of ischemic colitis following endorepair, which, on postmortem, was attributed to cholesterol emboli (28). Kalliafas et al. reported a partial-thickness colonic ischemia after stent-graft placement with inadvertent exclusion of an internal iliac artery during the procedure (29). Kalliafas identified 12 additional patients in his series who had internal iliac exclusion but did not develop colonic ischemia. Miahe et al. reported two episodes colonic ischemia after endovascular aortic repair (30). The first patient was found to have mild mucosal changes after exclusion of a patent inferior mesenteric artery with preservation of both internal iliac arteries. The second patient, who had previously undergone a Whipple procedure and pelvic radiation therapy for prostate cancer, required colectomy. Finally, Marin et al. reported a case of mild ischemic colitis following stent graft repair of an iliac aneurysm in which the contralateral iliac artery was occluded during the procedure (31). In a recent study, Rhee et al. prospectively followed 49 patients who underwent iliac artery coverage with or without coil embolization of one or both internal iliac arteries during aortic endovascular reconstruction (32). They reported that internal iliac arteries can be covered by extending the graft across the internal iliac orifice into the external iliac artery with minimal adverse consequences in patients who have common iliac arteries unsuited for deployment of endografts. They further recommend that if bilateral internal iliac arteries orificial openings are to be covered or occluded, one of these should be revascularized if possible. From these reports the calculated incidence of ischemic colitis following aortic stent graft repair is 1.4%. This low reported incidence of colonic ischemia following stent graft placement awaits confirmation, as the inferior mesenteric artery is found to be patent in a large number of elective open aortic repair, procedures, and stent graft repair occludes direct flow into the inferior mesenteric artery. Risk factors for the development of colonic ischemia after aortic stent graft placement include significant superior mesenteric artery occlusive disease and inadequate pelvic collateral perfusion. Additionally, as endovascular repair of the aorta becomes more common, further risk factors for colonic ischemia will likely be identified. As experience is gained, the magnitude of the potential problem will come into sharper focus and future clinical trials should prompt the development of practice guidelines.

V. PREVENTION

Preoperative evaluation of the blood supply to the colon as well as intraoperative assessment of colonic perfusion by Doppler ultrasound or pH_t may help to identify those patients who would benefit from mesenteric reconstruction. In order to minimize the morbidity and mortality associated with ischemic colitis, a high index of suspicion will assist in making an earlier diagnosis. Proper ligation of the IMA, avoidance of perioperative hypotension, careful placement of retractors, and finally reimplatation of an IMA

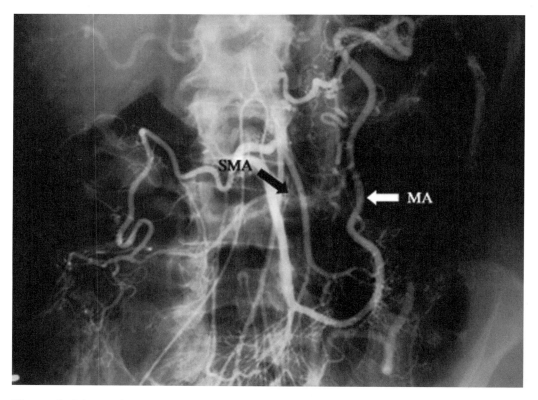

Figure 1 Mesenteric angiogram. Retrograde filling of superior mesenteric artery through a meandering mesenteric artery from the inferior mesenteric artery. (SMA, superior mesenteric artery; MA, meandering mesenteric artery.)

with inadequate collateral development should greatly reduce the incidence of this devastating complication.

VI. ARTERIOGRAPHY

Aortography has been used for many years in the preoperative evaluation of patients undergoing aortic reconstruction. It is particularly indicated in patients with a history or physical signs of intestinal angina. Visualization of a meandering mesenteric artery may alert the clinician to significant superior or inferior mesenteric arterial disease (Fig. 1). Reversal of flow in the meandering mesenteric artery from the inferior to the superior mesenteric artery warrants further study by way of a lateral aortic view to document superior mesenteric artery stenosis as, these patients are at considerable without associated superior mesenteric artery reconstruction or reimplatation of the inferior mesenteric artery, these patients are at considerable risk of small bowel ischemia.

VII. OPERATIVE TECHNIQUES AND TREATMENT

One common factor in most cases of ischemic colitis is ligation of the inferior mesenteric artery. Inappropriate or improper ligation may be the most important pitfall for surgeons to avoid. The inferior mesenteric artery begins to branch shortly after its origin from the aorta. A proper ligation involves dissection of the artery to within 2 cm of its origin and suture ligation at this point, thus avoiding interruption of important collaterals. An alternative and perhaps better technique is IMA ligation at its orifice from within the aneurysmal sac. Many diseased aortas contain either intramural thrombus or unstable mural plague, which can easily be dislodged and embolize. Broadcast of this debris can lead to ischemic events in multiple organs and is avoided through judicious handling during dissection. In dealing with a ruptured aortic aneurysm, the surgeon faces additional challenges. Often the patient is found to have a large hematoma within the mesentery. This should not be evacuated, as doing so can cause disruption of vital collateral pathways. Interruption of collateral pathways may also occur with overvigorous retraction. Antegrade restoration of flow to the hypogastric arteries or through other pathways preserves the pelvic collateral circulation and minimizes the development of ischemic colitis. Clinical prediction of the viability of bowel is unreliable; the surgeon is advised to rely on more objective data to determine whether the bowel has adequate collateral perfusion without restoration of the inferior mesenteric artery. Several tests of bowel perfusion have been described, including inferior mesenteric artery stump pressure, radioisotope scanning, fluorescein dye, colonic serosal photoplethysmography, Doppler interrogation in the colonic mesentery, and tonometric measurement of colonic mucosal pH. However, these methods are often time-consuming, they require experience, and are some are currently experimental and therefore impractical in the clinical setting. Additionally, most techniques determine adequacy of colonic collateral blood flow in the operating room when overall perfusion is optimized and do not predict maintenance of flow in the postoperative period, when inadequate resuscitation can often a cause hypotension and induce ischemia. The advantages of Doppler interrogation in the colonic mesentery and tonometric measurement of colonic mucosal pH are that the Doppler is available and easy to use and that the tonometric measurement can be continued well into the postoperative period.

Hypotension and hypoperfusion in the operative as well as postoperative period are major causes of morbidity following aortic reconstruction. The colonic collateral circulation is susceptible to periods of hypotension once the inferior mesenteric artery has been ligated. Monitoring of the patient's overall fluid status using central venous and pulmonary wedge pressures is necessary in critically ill and high-risk patients.

An alternative approach to the prevention of colonic ischemia after aortic reconstruction is to reimplant all patent inferior mesenteric arteries. This methodology has been practiced by the University of Florida, where 151 patients undergoing aortic reconstruction from 1986–1989 had patent mesenteric arteries reimplanted. No patients suffered colonic ischemia requiring operative intervention, and there were no deaths attributable to colonic ischemia (33).

VIII. SUMMARY

Gastrointestinal complications following standard or endovascular techniques of aortic reconstruction continue to be an important problem. In view of the potential severity of these complications following aortic reconstruction, early identification of patients at risk is important. The early diagnosis of ischemic colitis hinges on a high index of suspicion and prompt action to optimize the patient's hemodynamic status. Once the diagnosis of ischemic colitis is entertained, it is the surgeon's responsibility to confirm this either through prompt fiberoptic colonoscopy or tonometric measurement of colonic mucosal pH. For patients with mild to moderate ischemic changes, conservative management with fluid resuscitation and close monitoring is appropriate. However, in more severe cases, aggressive management, including early colonic resection, is the best method by which to lower the mortality due to these devastating complications.

REFERENCES

1. Christenson JT, Schmuziger M, Maurice J, Simonet F, Velebit V. Gastrointestinal complications after coronary artery bypass grafting. J Thorac Cardiovasc Surg 1994; 108:899–906.
2. Mercado PD, Farid H, O'Connell TX, Sintek C, Pfeffer T, Khonsari S. Gastrointestinal complications associated with cardiopulmonary bypass proceduces. Am Surg 1994; 60:789–792.
3. Ernst CB. Prevention of intestinal ischemia following abdominal aortic reconstruction. Surgery 1983; 96:102–106.
4. Antonsson J, Fiddian-Green RG. The role of the gut in shock and multiple system organ failure. Eur J Surg 1991; 157:3–12.
5. Ernst CB. Intestinal ischemia following abdominal aortic reconstruction. In: Bernard VM, Town JB, eds. Complications in Vascular Surgery. New York: Grune & Stratton, 1985:325–350.
6. Greenwald DA, Brandt LJ, Reinus JF. Ischemic bowel disease in the elderly. Gastroenterol Clin North Am 2001; 30(2):445–473.
7. Farkas JC, Calvo-Verjat N, Laurain C, et al. Acute colorectal ischemia after aortic surgery: Pathophysiology and prognostic criteria. Ann Vasc Surg 1992; 6:11.
8. Steward JA, Rankin FW. Blood supply of the large intestine:Its surgical considerations. Arch Surg 1933; 26:843.
9. Shepard AD, Tollefson DF, Reddy DJ, Evans JR, Elliott JP, Smith RF, Ernst CB. Left flank retroperitoneal exposure: A technical aid to complex aortic reconstruction. J Vasc Surg 1991; 14:283–291.
10. Sicard GA, Freeman MB, VanderWoude JC, Anderson CB. Comparison between the transabdominal and retroperitoneal approach for reconstruction of the infrarenal abdominal aorta. J Vasc Surg 1987; 5:19–27.

11. Sicard GA, Reilly JM, Rubin BG, Thompson RW, Allen BT, Flye MW, Schechtman KB, Young-Beyer P, Weiss C, Anderson CB. Transabdominal versus retroperitoneal incision for abdominal aortic surgery: Report of a prospective randomized trial. J Vasc Surg 1995; 21:174–183.

12. Kim MW, Hurdahl SA, Dang CR, McNamara JJ, Staehly CJ, Whelan TJ. Ischemic colitis after aortic aneurysmectomy. Am J Surg 1983; 145:392–394.

13. Johnson WC, Nasbeth DC. Visceral infaction following aortic surgery. Ann Surg 1963; 86:65–73.

14. Young JR, Humphries AW, deWolf VG, LeFevre FA. Complications of abdominal aortic surgery: II. Intestinal ischemia. Arch Surg 1963; 86:51–59.

15. Papadopoulos CD, Mancini HW, Marino WM Jr. Ischemic necrosis of the colon following aortic aneurysmectomy. J Cardiovasc Surg 1974; 15:494–500.

16. Bandyk DF, Florence MG, Johansen KH. Colon ischemia accompanying ruptured abdominal aortic aneurysm. J Surg Res 1981; 30:297–303.

17. Fry PD. Colonic ischemia after aortic reconstruction. Can J Surg 1988; 31:162–164.

18. Hagihara PF, Ernst C, Griffen WO. Incidence of ischemic colitis following abdominal aortic reconstruction. Surg Gynecol Obstet 1979; 149:571–573.

19. Longo WE, Lee TC, Barnett MG, et al. Ischemic colitis complicating abdominal aortic aneurysm surgery in the U.S. veteran. J Surg Res 1996; 60:351–354.

20. Bjorck M, Bergqvist D, Troeng T. Incidence and clinical presentation of bowel ischemia after aortoiliac surgery—2930 operations from a population-based registry in Sweden. Eur J Vasc Endovasc Surg 1996; 12:139–144.

21. Schiedler MG, Cutler BS, Fiddian-Green RG. Sigmoid intramural pH for prediction of ischemic colitis during aortic surgery. A comparison with risk factors and inferior mesenteric artery pressures. Arch Surg 1987; 122:881–886.

22. Björck M, Hedberg B. Early detection of major complications after abdominal aortic surgery: Predictive value of sigmoid colon and gastric intramucosal pH monitoring. Br J Surg 1994; 81:25–30.

23. Tollefson FJ, Wright DJ, Reddy DJ, Kintanar EB. Intraoperative determination of intestinal viability by pulse oximetry. Ann Vasc Surg 1995; 9:357–360.

24. Makaroun MS. The AnCure endografting system: An update. J Vasc Surg 2000; 33(S):129–134.

25. Matsumara J, Katzen BT, Hollier LH, et al. Update on the bifurcated Excluder endoprosthesis: Phase I results. J Vasc Surg 2001; 33:150–153.

26. Zarins CK, White RA, Hodgson KJ, et al. for the AneuRx Clinical Investigators. Endoleak as a predictor of outcome following endovascular aneurysm repair: AneuRx multicenter clinical trial. J Vasc Surg 2000; 32:90–107.

27. Sandison AJ, Edmondson RA, Panayiotopoulos YP, et al. Fatal colonic ischemia after stent graft for aortic aneurysm. Eur J Vasc Endovasc Surg 1997; 13:219–220.

28. Jaeger HJ, Mathias KD, Gissler HM, et al. Rectum and sigmoid colon necrosis due to cholesterol embolization after implantation of an aortic stent graft. J Vasc Intervent Radiol 1999; 10:751–755.

29. Kalliafas S, Albertini JN, Macierewicz J, et al. Incidence and treatment of intraoperative technical problems during endovascular repair of complex abdominal aortic aneurysms. J Vasc Surg 2000; 31:1185–1192.

30. Mialhe C, Amicabile C, Becquemin JP. Endovascular treatment of infrarenal abdominal aneurysm by the stentor system: Preliminary results of 79 cases. Stentor Retrospective Study Group. J Vasc Surg 1997; 26:199–209.

31. Marin ML, Veith FJ, Lyon RT, et al. Transfemoral endovascular repair of iliac aneurysms. Am J Surg 1995; 170:179–182.

32. Rhee RY, Muluk SC, Tzeng E, Carroll N, Makaroun MS. Can the internal iliac artery be safely covered during endovascular repair of abdominal aortic and iliac artery aneurysms? Ann Vasc Surg 2002; 16:29–36.

33. Burress Welborn M III, Seeger JM. Prevention and management of sigmoid and pelvic ischemia associated with aortic surgery. Sem Vasc Surg 2001; 14:255–265.

10

Spinal Cord Ischemia

Alfio Carroccio and Nicholas J. Morrissey

Mount Sinai School of Medicine, New York, New York, U.S.A.

Larry H. Hollier

Louisiana State University Health Sciences Center School of Medicine, New Orleans, Louisiana, U.S.A.

Spinal cord ischemia with a resulting neurological deficit remains a devastating complication following thoracoabdominal aortic surgery. It has been reported to occur in 0–40% of patients undergoing aortic surgery, depending upon the type of pathology present as well as circumstances present at the time of operation (1–8). Clinical presentation can range from somatosensory loss to complete flaccid paralysis immediately following surgery or delayed presentation up to several weeks postoperatively.

An appreciation of the anatomy as well as the mechanism of ischemic injury has led to various strategies attempting to reduce the impact of the ischemia. Such measures include intercostal artery reimplantation, cerebrospinal fluid drainage, hypothermia techniques, distal perfusion techniques, pharmacotherapy, and mechanisms of ischemic preconditioning. Although these adjuncts have been evaluated in multiple human as well as animal research protocols and appear promising, the problem has yet to be resolved. This chapter focuses on determinants of spinal cord ischemia as well as the various measures utilized in avoiding the resulting neurological deficit.

I. ANATOMY

The predominant blood supply to the spinal cord derives from the longitudinally oriented spinal arteries. The single anterior spinal artery supplies the gray matter as well as the anterior white matter. The paired posterior spinal arteries supply the dorsal columns as well as the posterior white matter (9–11). Ischemia from interruption of the anterior spinal artery may result in paralysis, sphincter dysfunction, and decreased pain and temperature sensation, while vibratory sensation and proprioception may be affected by interruption of the posterior circulation.

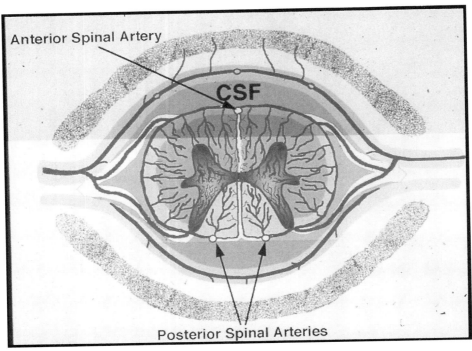

Figure 1 Spinal cord cross-sectional diagram demonstrating single anterior and double posterior spinal arteries with contribution from segmental arteries.

The posterior spinal arteries are more continuous; they are supplied by 12 dorsal medullary arteries (Fig. 1). The anterior spinal artery may have a more segmental or discontinuous path, with contribution from radicular arteries from the thoracic and lumbar regions (11,12). The most prominent of the radicular arteries, the artery of Adamkiewicz, can originate anywhere from T8 to L3; however, it is most often in the region of T9-T12 (13). Additional collateral blood supply is provided by the internal thoracic, long thoracic, intercostal, scapular, and proximal radicular arteries (14). In the lower aortic region, collateral blood flow from lumbar, iliolumbar, and lateral sacral arteries may prove critical and therefore require preservation of the hypogastric circulation. The lower incidence of neurological consequences following aortic coarctation surgery (0.41%) as compared to traumatic aortic rupture (19%) is a good demonstration of the protective benefit of collaterals in the more chronic disease states (15).

II. PHYSIOLOGY OF ISCHEMIA

Neuronal tissue damage may result from two phases of ischemic insult. The first or initial phase of acute ischemia results from interruption of neural tissue perfusion. The second insult occurs following reperfusion of the neural tissue with the inherent byproducts of reperfusion injury.

A. Acute Ischemia

The acute ischemic phase can result in neural infarct if the duration and severity of ischemia is prolonged (16). Like other cells, neurons depend on high-energy substrate to function. In particular, the gray matter, which relies on a microvascular blood supply, has increased cellular and mitochondrial density, requiring greater oxygen concentration. Therefore this is the first area of neuronal death under ischemic conditions (17). Diminished energy substrate delivery results in decreased cellular activity as well as an acidic environment following anaerobic energy utilization (18,19). In this anoxic environment, depolarization of neurons releases excitatory amino acids such as glutamate and aspartate (20), which have been retrieved at elevated levels in the cerebrospinal fluid of patient with ischemic spinal cord injury following aneurysm repair (21). These excitatory messengers bind and activate N-methyl D-aspartate (NMDA) and non-NMDA receptors, with a resulting influx of calcium and activation of second messengers and production of prostaglandins and thromboxanes. In concert, these mediators induce constriction of smooth muscle cells and increased resistance, with further ischemia. This cycle is initiated by the release of excitatory amino acids, with a resulting positive feedback that can result in cell death beyond the area of critical ischemia.

B. Reperfusion Injury

In the second phase of reperfusion injury, with the reintroduction of oxygen where there is already preexisting vasoconstriction, tissue swelling, and metabolites, oxygen radicals are formed. These by-products destroy cells via lipid peroxidation, with membrane breakdown and further release of excitatory amino acids (17). Reperfusion also introduces inflammatory cells, such as activated leukocytes, which adhere to the microvasculature and release cytotoxic mediators (22). The cellular damage induced by this reperfusion process functions as debris in further occluding the microvasculature and propogating the ischemic insult.

III. DETERMINANTS OF SPINAL CORD ISCHEMIA

A. Aortic Pathology

As the spinal cord blood supply is often segmental and dependent on a contribution from collateral arteries, the need for extensive aortic replacement requires interruption of an increasing number of branch vessels providing spinal cord perfusion and thus a higher risk of ischemia (Fig. 2). The more extensive type II thoracoabdominal aneurysms have been reported to have a 31% paraplegia rate, whereas in the less extensive type IV aneurysms, paraplegia occurred in only 4% (6,7). In patients with aortic dissection, the rate rose to 40% among type II aneurysms. The study also identified a poorer neurological outcome for thoracic aneurysms as compared to abdominal aneurysms. Aortic dissection has been associated with an increased risk of neurological injury. While dissection is often reported as a risk factor for spinal cord injury, a more recent study of patients undergoing thoracoabdominal aortic aneurysm repair using contemporary methods identified the acute dissections as more predictive of neurological injury (23).

B. Aortic Cross-Clamp Time

The length of aortic cross-clamp time of is often cited as a critical factor in determining risk of paraplegia (2,24–27), where the risk rises linearly as the time progresses beyond

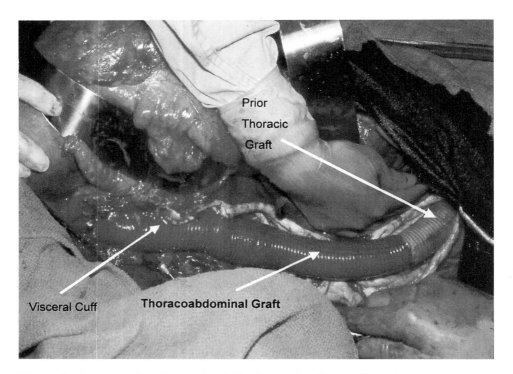

Figure 2 Intraoperative photographs following repair of a type II aortic aneurysms.

20–30 min of aortic occlusion (Fig. 3). The impact of clamp time has been disputed by some (28,29); the suggestion is that it should be viewed with consideration of other co-existing variables such as distal perfusion, operative experience, and adjunctive techniques. Spinal cord protective measures, such as cerebrospinal fluid drainage and distal aortic perfusion, may decrease the risk of spinal cord ischemia at a given cross-clamp time as compared to the same clamp time without the utilization of these adjunctive measures.

C. Proximal Hypertension

Cerebral perfusion pressure equals the mean arterial pressure minus the cerebrospinal fluid (CSF) pressure. Maintaining adequate cerebral perfusion, therefore, may be influenced by fluctuation in these variables. Placement of a proximal aortic clamp can interfere with the autoregulatory response, with resulting fluctuations in cerebral and spinal blood flow. In an animal study, lowering of proximal aortic pressure caused a significant decrease in CSF oxygenation; restoration of mean proximal aortic pressure caused a recovery of CSF oxygen tension (30).

Control of proximal hypertension following aortic cross-clamping maintains autoregulation in the coronary or cerebral circulation. Proximal hypertension, however, can cause an increase in CSF pressure, and use of nitroprusside can result in increased CSF production. A diminished mean arterial pressure with an unchanged or possibly increased CSF pressure may result in decreased cerebral perfusion pressure of the distal cord.

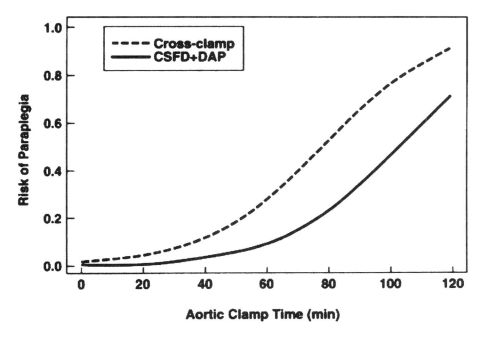

Figure 3 Graph demonstrating association between paraplegia risk and aortic cross-clamp time in patients undergoing repair of type I and II thoracoabdominal aneurysms. The influence of cerebral spinal fluid drainage and distal aortic perfusion is also represented. (From Ref. 2.)

IV. DETECTION OF SPINAL CORD ISCHEMIA

An impetus for intraoperative monitoring of spinal cord ischemia is that measures may be taken to help counteract the ischemic insult and avoid deleterious consequences. One method of detection involves evaluating somatosensory or motor evoked potentials (SEPs or MEPs). By stimulating a peripheral nerve in the lower extremity such as the posterior tibial nerve and measuring the cortical response over time as a tracing, one can follow the parameters of latency and amplitude. Increasing latency and decreasing amplitude can then serve as a marker for neuronal ischemia (31,32). With increasing levels of ischemia, the tracing can disappear. This can be beneficial only if the determined ischemia can be reversed. If, during aortic exclusion, one identifies SEPs with increasing latency and decreasing amplitude, one should consider using a distal perfusion mechanism. While utilizing distal perfusion, changing SEPs may signify that excluded collaterals are critical; therefore the patient may benefit from intercostal reimplantation. Also, fading SEPs with low distal perfusion pressures should encourage measures to increase distal perfusion pressure or a more expeditious completion of an anastomosis (32).

Criticism of the use of SEPs points to the fact that they represent the cord at the posterior column level, influenced by peripheral nerve involvement, and reports have noted paraplegia despite a lack of change in the SEPs (33). Despite the enthusiasm of some, comparison of outcomes resulting from the use of SEP detection versus a clamp-and-sew technique and no SEPs had no bearing on neurological outcome (6). Given the criticism, a more sensitive detection of the anterior horn cells by MEPs has been investigated (34). Use of epidural anesthesia or stimulation of the motor cortex can be followed by measuring peripheral motor nerve action potential response (35), with a decrease in amplitude greater than 25% below baseline serving as an indicator of ischemia. Problems with seizure activity (36) and the need for low-level neuromuscular blockade are difficulties occurring at this level of detection.

In a study comparing the utilization of motor evoked potentials (MEPs) with somatosensory evoked potentials (SEPs) during aortic surgery, MEPs proved more beneficial (37). In comparison to monitoring with MEPs, SEPs showed delayed detection of ischemia and a high rate of false-positive results.

V. PREVENTION

A. Intercostal Artery Reimplantation

Prevention of spinal cord ischemia by the reimplantation of intercostal arteries using a Carrel patch or interposition graft during aortic aneurysm repair is a measure that has supporters as well as detractors (Fig. 4). Evidence for the benefit of this technique may rely first on the basic concept of providing an adequate blood supply to the spinal column,

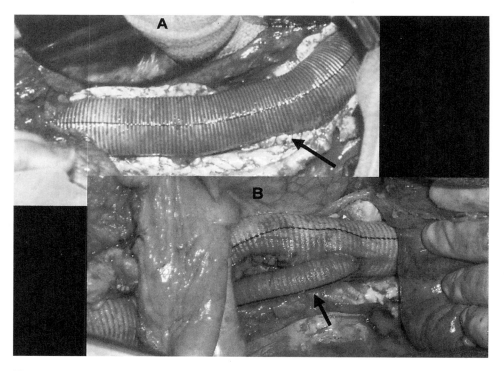

Figure 4 Intraoperative photos following thoracoabdominal aortic aneurysm repair. A. Arrow indicates intercostal artery reimplantation via a carrel patch. B. Arrow indicates intercostal artery reimplantation via an interposition graft.

which may be dependent on collateral blood flow from the intercostal arteries. Animal studies utilizing a baboon model have identified a spinal cord blood flow of 15–20 mL/100g of tissue per minute at baseline. Following a cross-clamp time of 60 min, the flow had dropped to 1.5 mL/100g of tissue per minute. No evidence of ischemic injury was noted when the blood supply was maintained ≥10 mL/100 g/min, while paraplegia resulted from flow <4mL/100 g/min (38).

The ability of intercostal reimplantation to supply adequate spinal cord blood flow, thus avoiding ischemic consequences, is based on observed changes in SEPs following selective reimplantation of various excluded intercostal branches (39,40).

The decision for intercostal reimplantation has also been described based upon evaluation of preoperative angiography (41–43). Arteries deemed critical because of their size and location may require reattachment.

Although studies evaluating paraplegia following aortic replacement have been reported to reveal the benefit of reimplantation (44,45), others have found the end result to show no difference based upon whether or not intercostals are reimplanted (6,46). A more accurate explanation probably relies on the status of the intercostals during intra-operative assessment. Cases with unidentified or occluded intercostals have been described as less likely to result in paraplegia. Also, a true assessment of the benefits of such a measure is often difficult to describe given the individual circumstances during surgery as well as the effect that other adjunctive measures may have.

More recently, a greater appreciation for the contribution of collateral and intercostal blood supply has emerged from the endovascular treatment of aortic aneurysms (47). In our experience, paraplegia following endovascular thoracic aortic aneurysm repair occurred in 3 of 72 patients (4.2%). After excluding patients who had previous or concommitant open AAA repair, we observed a paraplegia rate of 0%. The neurodeficits may result from interruption of critical intercostal arteries, which become more evident with abdominal aortic replacement and or loss of collateral flow from lumbar arteries.

B. CSF Drainage

As mentioned earlier, cerebral or spinal cord perfusion pressure depends on the difference between mean arterial pressure (MAP) and CSF pressure (CSFP). Regulating a balance requires control not only of arterial pressure but also of of the CSF pressure. Regulation of proximal blood pressure following placement of an aortic cross clamp is necessary to avoid deleterious myocardial and cerebral effects. This may diminish distal aortic perfusion with a relative increase in CSF pressure, which can be regulated by drainage of the CSF fluid. In a study evaluating the benefit of both distal aortic perfusion as well as CSF drainage, the combined adjuncts demonstrated an improved neurological outcome with repair of thoracic and thoracoabdominal aortic aneurysm (48). With numerous animal studies describing the benefit of CSF drainage, a prospective randomized study in humans identified no difference in neurological outcome among patients undergoing CSF drainage compared to those who did not (26). Supporters of this technique criticize the study for having limited the volume of CSF drainage as well as the drainage itself to only the intraoperative time period. More recent randomized studies have shown a significant decrease in paraplegia among patients undergoing CSF drainage (2,49). Interestingly, cases of delayed spinal cord ischemia presenting weeks after aortic aneurysm surgery have shown some benefit from CSF drainage. While the mechanism remains unclear, the benefit of CSF drainage is recognized (50).

C. Hypothermia

The principle that hypothermia diminishes the consequences of spinal cord ischemia is based upon a reduction in the decline of glucose and ATP stores as well as a reduction in the release of excitatory amino acids (18). Methods of achieving hypothermia have included surface cooling, perfusion of cooled blood or saline into the distal occluded aorta, cold perfusion of the subarachnoid space, and profound hypothermia with bypass (8). Generalized or surface cooling risks systemic complications, including coagulopathy; therefore it may be preferable to utilize hypothermia of the paraspinal space. In studies using rabbits, satisfactory spinal cord protection during aortic occlusion can be achieved at moderate regional hypothermia (51). A human study comparing epidural cooling to a previous cohort suggests a benefit of epidural cooling (52). Alternative approaches have included localized hypothermia by perfusion of exposed collaterals (53). Unfortunately, use of epidural cooling in humans has resulted in a small incidence of brainstem infarction, which is obviously quite worrisome.

D. Distal Aortic Perfusion

Various methods of improving distal aortic flow have been utilized. The benefit of sustaining lumbar cord flow and the support it provides to excluded segments of thoracic aorta is unclear (54). Methods of distal perfusion have included both full and partial bypass.

Full cardiopulmonary bypass can provide a more controlled distal perfusion as well as hypothermia; however, the degree of anticoagulation does impose the increased risk of bleeding complications in extensive aortic replacements (15,25,55). The introduction of heparin-bonded shunts (56) were meant to circumvent this problem; however, the small cross-sectional area of the shunt conduits (35) can result in a significant gradient to the distal aorta, with a diminished cardiac output (14). In addition, use of shunts also poses inherent problems with dislodgment and embolization (57).

Partial bypass can provide distal perfusion and control of proximal hypertension without cardiopulmonary arrest. Proximal access can be achieved at the levels of the pulmonary veins, left atrium, or proximal aorta. Distal perfusion can be introduced to the distal aorta and femoral arteries. Additional selective perfusion cannulas can be introduced to the visceral and renal branches when the aortic lumen is exposed, thereby possibly mitigating coexistent visceral and renal ischemia (Fig. 5). The clear benefit of such distal perfusion techniques has yet to be determined (14,25,29). Distal perfusion can also be addressed by extra-anatomic bypass. Preoperative construction of axillofemoral bypass can provide distal flow during aortic exclusion without the need for an external pump or anticoagulation beyond that which is necessary for the aortic replacement (15,29,58).

Cardiopulmonary bypass increases circulating levels of cytokines (59–61). We believe that less cytokine production will result from the use of an accessory graft for perfusion of the visceral segment as opposed to the pump. A technique we have lately utilized in the treatment of type I, II, and III thoracoabdominal aneurysms consists of the incorporation of an accessory bifurcated graft originating from the side of the proximal main graft, with one limb being sutured initially to the left iliac artery. Following the creation of the proximal aortic anastamosis, a cross-clamp is applied to the main graft, distal to the origin of the accessory graft. This allows blood to flow through the new proximal anastamosis into the accessory graft and out the two limbs of this accessory graft. One limb of the accessory graft anastamosed to the common iliac artery will provide pelvic and lower extremity blood flow. The second limb provides flow through selective perfusion catheters

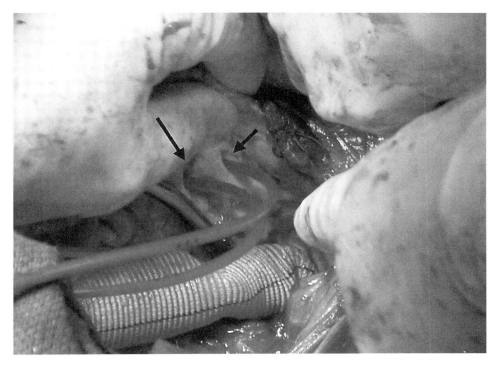

Figure 5 Intraoperative photo during thoracoabdominal aortic aneurysm repair. Arrows indicate orifice of visceral and renal arteries with catheters providing selective perfusion during repair.

to the renal and visceral vessels. Visceral and pelvic ischemia is limited to the time required for creation of the proximal anastamosis. This accesory graft provides distal perfusion while the intercostal, visceral, renal, and distal aortic reconstructions are performed.

E. Selective Visceral Perfusion

Changes in plasma cytokine concentrations were related to the duration of visceral ischemia and the frequency rate of postoperative, single, or multiple-system organ dysfunction in a study examining plasma proinflammatory cytokines after abdominal and thoracoabdominal aortic aneurysm (TAAA) repair (62). In a rabbit model, we identified an association of viscerally derived cytokines and spinal cord ischemia (63). With interruption of aortic and visceral flow, the deleterious effects on the spinal cord were more pronounced than with aortic interruption alone. Currently we are investigating this relationship in a population of patients undergoing thoracoabdominal aneurysm repair. The benefit of selective visceral perfusion during thoracoabdominal aneurysm repair may improve outcome (64). The exact role it may have on spinal cord ischemia has yet to be determined.

F. Pharmacotherapy

The benefit of delineating the physiological mechanism behind spinal cord ischemia is that medicinal intervention at multiple levels may mitigate the consequences of spinal ischemia.

While being investigated predominantly in animal models, areas of interest have included blockage of calcium influx (16), control of vasoconstriction (65), control of platelet aggregation and prostenoid release (66), blocking the release or downstream effects of excitatory amino acids (24,67–69), the decrease of reperfusion injury (17,70,71), inhibiting neutrophil activation after the transient ischemia with activated protein C (72), membrane stabilization and control of apoptosis with steroids (73), and the benefit of growth factors (74,75) as well as ischemic preconditioning (76).

Future means of spinal cord protection may include gene delivery of neurotrophic growth factors. Investigation into the possible protective effect of the glial cell line–derived neurotrophic factor via adenovirus-mediated gene delivery on transient spinal cord ischemia in rabbits has revealed improvement in the survival of motor neurons (77).

VI. SUMMARY

Investigation into the basic elements responsible for spinal cord ischemia has provided a better understanding of this complex process. Despite the many human as well as animal trials to prevent this dreaded complication, no one distinguishing measure seems most beneficial. In addition to extensive surgical experience in aortic surgery, the best current approach appears to be the utilization of multiple adjunctive procedures as determined appropriate on individual bases, with the hope of interrupting the deleterious ischemic cascade at several levels.

REFERENCES

1. Coselli JS, LeMaire SA. Left heart bypass reduces paraplegia rates after thoracoabdominal aortic aneurysm repair. Ann Thorac Surg 1999; 67:1931–1934.
2. Safi HJ, Hess KR, Randel M, Iliopoulos DC, Baldwin JC, Mootha RK, et al. Cerebrospinal fluid drainage and distal aortic perfusion: Reducing neurologic complications in repair of thoracoabdominal aortic aneurysms types II and I. J Vasc Surg 1996; 23:223–229.
3. Cambria RP, Davison K, Carter C, Brewster DC, Chang Y, Clark KA, et al. Epidural cooling for spinal cord protection during thoracoabdominal aneurysm repair: a five-year experience. J Vasc Surg 2000; 31:1093–1102.
4. Katz NM, Blackstone EH, Kirklin JW, Karg RB. Incremental risk factors for spinal cord injury following operation for acute traumatic transection. J Thorac Cardiovasc Surg 1981; 81:669–674.
5. Jacobs MJ, de Mol BA, Elenbaas T, Mess WH, Kalkman CJ, Schurink GW, Mochtar B. Spinal cord blood supply in patients with thoracoabdominal aortic aneurysms. J Vasc Surg 2002; 35(1):30–37.
6. Crawford E, Crawford J, Safi H, et al. Thoracoabdominal aortic aneurysm: Preoperative and intraoperative factors determining immediate and long term results of operation in 605 patients. J Vasc Surg 1986; 3:389–404.
7. Svensson LG, Crawford ES, Hess KR, Coselli JS, Safi HJ. Experience with 1509 patients undergoing thoracoabdominal aortic operations. J Vasc Surg 1993; 17(2):357–370.
8. Kouchoukos N, Rokkas C. Descending thoracic and thoracoabdominal aortic surgery for aneurysm or dissection: how do we minimize the risk of spinal cord injury. Semin Thoracic Cardiovasc Surg 1993; 5:47–54.
9. Svensson L, Klepp P, Hinder R. Spinal cord anatomy of the baboon: comparison with man and implications for spinal cord blood flow during thoracic aortic cross clamping. S Afr J Surg 1986; 24:32–34.

10. Piccone A, Green R, Ricotta J, et al. Spinal cord ischemia following operations on the abdominal aorta. J Vasc Surg 1986; 3:94–103.

11. Szilagyi D, Hageman J, Smith R, Elliot J. Spinal cord damage in surgery of the abdominal aorta. Surgery 1978; 83:38–56.

12. Gharagozloo F, Larson J, Dausmann M, et al. Spinal cord protection during surgical procedures and the descending thoracic and thoracoabdominal aorta. Chest 1996; 109:799–809.

13. Adamkiewicz A. Die Blutgefasse des menschlichen Ruckernmarkes: I. Theil die Gefasse der Ruckenmarksubstanz. Sitzungsb Akad Wissensch Wien Math Naturw Klass 1882; 84:469.

14. Svensson L, Loop F. Prevention of spinal cord ischemia in aortic surgery. In: Yao JST, ed. Arterial Surgery. New York: Grune & Stratton, 1988:273–285.

15. von Oppell U, Dunne T, De Groot M, Zilla P. Spinal cord protection in the absence of collateral circulation: meta analysis of mortality and paraplegia. J Card Surg 1994; 9:685–691.

16. Kwun BD, Vacanti F. Mild hypothermia protects against irreversible damage during prolonged spinal cord ischemia. J Surg Res 1995; 59:780–782.

17. Hall E, Wolf D. A pharmacologic analysis of the pathophysiologic mechanisms of post traumatic spinal cord ischemia. J Neurosurg 1986; 64:951–961.

18. Allen B, Davis C, Osborne D, Karl I. Spinal cord ischemia and reperfusion metabolism: the effect of hypothermia. J Vasc Surg 1994; 19:332–340.

19. Drenger B, Parker S, Frank S, Beattie C. Changes in cerebral spinal fluid pressure and lactate concentrations during thoracoabdominal aortic aneurysm surgery. Anesthesiology 1997; 86: 41–47.

20. Taira Y, Marsala M. Effect of proximal arterial perfusion pressure on function, spinal cord blood flow, and histopathologic changes after increasing intervals of aortic occlusion in the rat. Stroke 1996; 27:1850–1858.

21. Brock MV, Redmond JM, Ishiwa S, Johnston MV, Baumgartner WA, Laschinger JC, Williams GM. Clinical markers in CSF for determining neurologic deficits after thoracoabdominal aortic aneurysm repairs. Ann Thorac Surg 1997; 64(4):999–1003.

22. Clark W, Walsh C, Briley D, Brace C. Neutrophil adhesion in central nervous system ischemia in rabbits. Brain Behav Immun 1993; 7:63–69.

23. Coselli JS, LeMaire SA, de Figueiredo LP, Kirby RP. Paraplegia after thoracoabdominal aortic aneurysm repair: Is dissection a risk factor? Ann Thorac Surg 1997; 63(1):28–36.

24. Rothman S, Olney J. Glutamate and the pathophysiology of hypoxic-ischemic brain damage. Ann Neurol 1986; 19:105–111.

25. Livesay L, Cooley D, Ventemiglia R, et al. Surgical experience in descending thoracic aneurysmectomy with and without adjuncts to avoid ischemia. Ann Thorac Surg 1985; 39:37–46.

26. Crawford E, Svensson L, Hess K, et al. A prospective randomized study of cerebral spinal fluid drainage to prevent paraplegia after high risk surgery on the thoracoabdominal aorta. J Vasc Surg 1990; 13:36–46.

27. Katz N, Blackstone E, Kirklin J, et al. Incrimental risk factors for spinal cord injury following operation for acute traumatic aortic transection. J Thorac Cardiovasc Surg 1981; 81:669–674.

28. Hollier L, Symmonds J, Pairolero P, et al. Thoracoabdominal aortic aneurysm repair: analysis of postoperative morbidity. Arch Surg 1988; 123:871–875.

29. Crawford E, Rubio P. Reappraisal of adjuncts to avoid ischemia in the treatment of aneurysms of the descending aorta. J Thorac Cardiovasc Surg 1973; 66:693–704.

30. Hellberg A, Tulga Ulus A, Christiansson L, Bergqvist D, Thelin S, Karacagil S. Influence of low proximal aortic pressure on spinal cord oxygenation in experimental thoracic aortic occlusion. J Cardiovasc Surg (Torino) 2001; 42(2):227–231.

31. Cunningham JJ, Laschinger J, Merlin H, et al. Measurement of spinal cord ischemia during operations upon the thoracic aorta. Ann Surg 1982; 196:285–296.

32. Marini C, Cunningham J. Issues surrounding spinal cord protection. In: Karp R, Laks H, Wechsler A, eds. Advances in cardiac surgery. St. Louis: Mosby-Year Book, 1993:89–107.

33. Lesser R, Raudzens P, Luder H, et al. Postoperative neurologic deficits may occur despite unchanged intraoperative somatosensory evoked potentials. Ann Neurol 1986; 19:22–25.

34. Agnew W, McCreery D. Considerations of safety in the use of extracranial stimulation for motor-evoked potentials. Neurosurgery 1987; 20:143–147.

35. de Haan P, Kalkman C, de Mol B, et al. Efficacy of transcranial motor evoked myogenic potentials to detect spinal cord ischemia during operations for thoracoabdominal aneurysms. J Thorac Cardiovasc Surg 1997; 113:87–101.

36. Shenaq S, Svensson L. Paraplegia following aortic surgery. J Cardiothorc Vasc Anesth 1993; 7:81–94.

37. Meylaerts SA, Jacobs MJ, van Iterson V, De Haan P, Kalkman CJ. Comparison of transcranial motor evoked potentials and somatosensory evoked potentials during thoracoabdominal aortic aneurysm repair. Ann Surg 1999; 230(6):742–749.

38. Svensson L, Rickards E, Coull A, et al. Relationship of spinal cord blood flow to vascular anatomy during thoracic aortic cross-clamping and shunting. J Thorac Cardiovasc Surg 1986; 91:71–78.

39. Ueda T, Shimizu H, Mori A, Kashima I, Moro K, Kawada S. Selective perfusion of segmental arteries in patients undergoing thoracoabdominal aortic surgery. Ann Thorac Surg 2000; 70(1):38–43.

40. Meylaerts SA, De Haan P, Kalkman CJ, Jaspers J, Vanicky I, Jacobs MJ. Prevention of paraplegia in pigs by selective segmental artery perfusion during aortic cross-clamping. J Vasc Surg 2000; 32(1):160–170.

41. Savader S, Williams G, Trerotola S, et al. Preoperative spinal artery localization and its relationship to postoperative neurologic complications. Radiology 1993; 189:165–171.

42. Bachet J, Guilmet D, Rosier J, et al. Protection of the spinal cord during surgery of thoracoabdominal aortic aneurysms. Eur J Cardiothorac Surg 1996; 10:817–825.

43. Kieffer E, Richard T, Chiras J, et al. Preoperative spinal cord arteriography in aneurysmal disease of the descending thoracic and thoracoabdominal aorta: preliminary results in 45 patients. Ann Vasc Surg 1989; 3:34–46.

44. Shiiya N, Yasuda K, Matsui Y, et al. Spinal cord protection during thoracoabdominal aneurysm repair: Result of selective reconstruction of the critical segmental arteries guided by evoked spinal cord potential monitoring. J Vasc Surg 1995; 21:970–975.

45. Svensson L, Hess K, Coselli J, Safi H. influence of segmental arteries, extent, and aortofemoral bypass on postoperative paraplegia after thoracoabdominal aortic operation. J Vasc Surg 1994; 20:255–262.

46. Schepens M, Boezeman E, Hamerlijnk R, et al. Somatosensory evoked potentials during exclusion and reperfusion of critical aortic segments in thoracoabdominal aortic aneurysm surgery. J Card Surg 1994; 9:692–702.

47. Gravereaux EC, Faries PL, Burks JA, Latessa V, Spielvogel D, Hollier LH, Marin ML. Risk of spinal cord ischemia after endograft repair of thoracic aortic aneurysms. J Vasc Surg 2001; 34(6):997–1003.

48. Estrera AL, Miller CC III, Huynh TT, Porat E, Safi HJ. Neurologic outcome after thoracic and thoracoabdominal aortic aneurysm repair. Ann Thorac Surg 2001; 72(4):1225–1231.

49. Coselli JS, Lemaire SA, Koksoy C, Schmittling ZC, Curling PE. Cerebrospinal fluid drainage reduces paraplegia after thoracoabdominal aortic aneurysm repair: results of a randomized clinical trial. J Vasc Surg 2002; 35(4):631–639.

50. Azizzadeh A, Huynh TT, Miller CC III, Safi HJ. Reversal of twice-delayed neurologic deficits with cerebrospinal fluid drainage after thoracoabdominal aneurysm repair: a case report and plea for a national database collection. J Vasc Surg 2000; 31(3):592–598.

51. Martelli E, Cho JS, Mozes G, Gloviczki P. Epidural cooling for the prevention of ischemic injury to the spinal cord during aortic occlusion in a rabbit model: determination of the optimal temperature. J Vasc Surg 2002; 35(3):547–553.

52. Cambria RP, Davison JK, Carter C, Brewster DC, Chang Y, Clark KA, Atamian S. Epidural

cooling for spinal cord protection during thoracoabdominal aneurysm repair: a five-year experience. J Vasc Surg 2000; 31(6):1093–1802.

53. Coles J, Wilson G, Sima A, et al. Intraoperative management of thoracic aortic aneurysms: Experimental evaluation of perfusion cooling of the spinal cord. J Thorac Cardiovasc Surg 1983; 85:292–299.

54. Svensson L, Patel V, Robinson M, et al. Influence of preservation or perfusion of intraoperatively identified spinal cord blood supply on spinal motor evoked potentials and paraplegia after aortic surgery. J Vasc Surg 1991; 13:355–365.

55. Jex R, Schaff H, Piehler J, et al. Early and late results following repair of dissection of the descending aorta. J Vasc Surg 1986; 3:226–237.

56. Gott V. Heparinazed shunts for thoracic vascular operations (editorial). Ann Thorac Surg 1972; 14:219.

57. Crawford E, Fenstermacher J, Richardson W, Sandiford F. Reappraisal of adjuncts to avoid ischemia in treatment of thoracic aortic aneurysms. Surg 1970; 67:182.

58. Molina J, Cogordan J, Einzigs, et al. Adequacy of ascending aorta-descending aorta shunt during cross clamping of the thoracic aorta for the prevention of spinal cord ischemia. J Thorac Cardiovasc Surg 1985; 90:126–136.

59. Chenoweth DE, Cooper SW, Hugli TE, Stewart RW, Blackstone EH, Kirklin JW. Complement activation during cardiopulmonary bypass: Evidence for generation of C3a and C5a anaphylotoxins. N Engl J Med 1981; 304:497–503.

60. Bruins P, te Velthuis H, Yazdanbakhsh AP, et al. Activation of the complement system during and after cardiopulmonary bypass surgery: postsurgery activation involves C-reactive protein and is associated with postoperative arrhythmia. Circulation 1997; 96:3542–3548.

61. Paparella D, Yau TM, Young E. Cardiopulmonary bypass induced inflammation: pathophysiology and treatment. An update. Eur J Cardiothorac Surg 2002; 21(2):232–244.

62. Welborn MB, Oldenburg HS, Hess PJ, et al. The relationship between visceral ischemia, proinflammatory cytokines, and organ injury in patients undergoing thoracoabdominal aortic aneurysm repair. Crit Care Med 2000; 28(9):3191–3197.

63. Morrissey NJ, Kantonen I, Liu H, et al. The effect of mesenteric ischemia/reperfusion on spinal cord injury following transient aortic occlusion in rabbits. J Endovasc Ther 2002; 9(suppl 2): 1144–1150.

64. Cambria RP, Davison JK, Giglia JS, Gertler JP. Mesenteric shunting decreases visceral ischemia during thoracoabdominal aneurysm repair. J Vasc Surg 1998; 27(4):745–749.

65. Svensson L, Von Ritter C, Groeneveld H, et al. Cross-clamping of the thoracic aorta: influence of aortic shunts, laminectomy, papaverine, calcium channel blockers, allopurinol, and superoxide dismutase on spinal cord blood flow and paraplegia in baboons. Ann Surg 1986; 204:38–47.

66. Lapchak PA, Araujo DM, Song D, Zivin JA. Neuroprotection by the selective cyclooxygenase-2 inhibitor SC-236 results in improvements in behavioral deficits induced by reversible spinal cord ischemia. Stroke 2001; 32(5):1220–1225.

67. Kanellopoulos GK, Xu XM, Hsu CY, Lu X, Sundt TM, Kouchoukos NT. White matter injury in spinal cord ischemia: protection by AMPA/kainate glutamate receptor antagonism. Stroke 2000; 31(8):1945–1952.

68. Lang-Lazdunski L, Heurteaux C, Mignon A, Mantz J, Widmann C, Desmonts J, Lazdunski M. Ischemic spinal cord injury induced by aortic cross-clamping: prevention by riluzole. Eur J Cardiothorac Surg 2000; 18(2):174–181.

69. Lang-Lazdunski L, Heurteaux C, Dupont H, Widmann C, Lazdunski M. Prevention of ischemic spinal cord injury: comparative effects of magnesium sulfate and riluzole. J Vasc Surg 2000; 32(1):179–189.

70. Rahman A, Ustundag B, Burma O, Ozercan IH, Erol FS. Neuroprotective effect of regional carnitine on spinal cord ischemia-reperfusion injury. Eur J Cardiothorac Surg 2001; 20(1):65–70.

71. de Haan P, Vanicky I, Jacobs MJ, Bakker O, Lips J, Meylaerts SA, Kalkman CJ. Effect of

ischemic pretreatment on heat shock protein 72, neurologic outcome, and histopathologic outcome in a rabbit model of spinal cord ischemia. J Thorac Cardiovasc Surg 2000; 120(3): 513–519.

72. Hirose K, Okajima K, Taoka Y, Uchiba M, Tagami H, Nakano K, Utoh J, Okabe H, Kitamura N. Activated protein C reduces the ischemia/reperfusion-induced spinal cord injury in rats by inhibiting neutrophil activation. Ann Surg 2000; 232(2):272–280.

73. Kanellopoulos GK, Kato H, Wu Y, Dougenis D, Mackey M, Hsu CY, Kouchoukos NT. Neuronal cell death in the ischemic spinal cord: the effect of methylprednisolone. Ann Thorac Surg 1997; 64(5):1279–1286.

74. Nakao Y, Otani H, Yamamura T, Hattori R, Osako M, Imamura H. Insulin-like growth factor 1 prevents neuronal cell death and paraplegia in the rabbit model of spinal cord ischemia. J Thorac Cardiovasc Surg 2001; 122(1):136–143.

75. Bowes M, Tuszynski MH, Conner J, Zivin JA, Continuous intrathecal fluid infusions elevate nerve growth factor levels and prevent functional deficits after spinal cord ischemia. Brain Res 2000;17;883(2):178–183.

76. Zvara DA, Colonna DM, Deal DD, Vernon JC, Gowda M, Lundell JC. Ischemic preconditioning reduces neurologic injury in a rat model of spinal cord ischemia. Ann Thorac Surg 1999; 68(3):874–880.

77. Sakurai M, Abe K, Hayashi T, Setoguchi Y, Yaginuma G, Meguro T, Tabayashi K. Adenovirus-mediated glial cell line-derived neurotrophic factor gene delivery reduces motor neuron injury after transient spinal cord ischemia in rabbits. J Thorac Cardiovasc Surg 2000; 120(6):1148–1157.

11

Impotence Following Aortic Surgery

Richard Kempczinski

University of Cincinnati, Cincinnati, Ohio, U.S.A.

Although Leriche and Morel (1) first described the association between impotence and distal aortic occlusion, Harris and Jepson (2) were the first to report erectile dysfunction as a complication of aortic surgery. These studies first called our attention to vasculogenic impotence, but a true appreciation of the magnitude of this problem awaited more refined diagnostic techniques and a better understanding of the mechanism of erection.

Impotence, the inability to achieve or maintain an erection adequate for satisfactory coitus, must be distinguished from *retrograde ejaculation*, which is primarily a neurogenic disorder in which bladder neck closure does not occur and semen is deposited into the bladder. In such cases the patient is still able to complete coitus and achieve orgasm. Although impotence, by the above definition, appears to be a disorder limited to men, women with aortoiliac arterial obstructive disease may complain of insufficient vaginal lubrication and loss of orgasm (3). However, this is a much less common problem, because female genital sensation depends in great part on the integrity of the somatic pudendal nerves and their efferent sensory fibers. These are situated deep within the pelvis and are protected by the thick layer of endopelvic fascia. Furthermore, collateral arterial blood supply to the female sexual organs is quite extensive. As a result, female organic "impotence" is extremely uncommon (4).

This chapter describes the physiology of erection as we currently understand it and explores how the normal interplay of neural and vascular elements can be disturbed by the development of arterial occlusive disease or by surgical attempts to correct it. Because patients with erectile dysfunction often consult vascular surgeons, the various diagnostic techniques that may be necessary in these patients are emphasized. Finally, those technical modifications that should be employed during aortic surgery to prevent iatrogenic impotence, as well as the most effective current treatment for established impotence, are discussed.

I. PHYSIOLOGY OF ERECTION

In the 40 years since Leriche and Morel (1) first described the association between aortoiliac arterial occlusive disease and impotence, medical research has broadened our understanding of the complex interplay between psychological, hormonal, neurological, and vascular elements that is required to achieve an adequate erection.

Satisfactory male sexual function presupposes anatomically normal male genitalia, an appropriate hormonal milieu, intact nerve and blood supply to the genitalia, and appropriate physical and/or psychic stimulation. Absence of any one of these elements or moderate dysfunction in several of them may result in impotence.

A. Neurophysiology

The precise neurophysiological basis for erection remains unknown. The afferent and efferent neural pathways that appear to be involved in erection are depicted in Figure 1. Thoracolumbar sympathetic nerves (TI2-L4) are believed to be important in mediating psychogenic erections, which can occur even in patients with complete sacral cord destructions (5). However, younger individuals undergoing bilateral radical retroperitoneal node dissection, in which both sympathetic nerve chains are usually removed, rarely become impotent (6). Therefore sacral efferent (parasympathetic) outflow appears capable of mediating both psychogenic and reflex erections. Clearly, bilateral resection of the TI 2 -LI sympathetic ganglia can result in retrograde ejaculation. However, this should not be confused with erectile dysfunction.

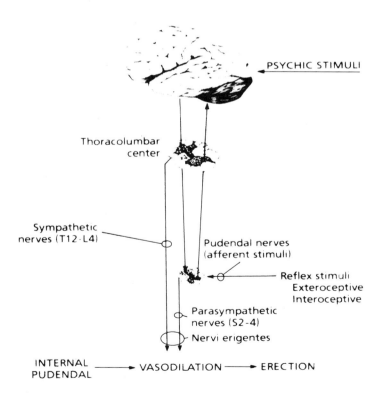

Figure 1 Diagrammatic representation of the neural pathways involved in penile erection. (From Ref. 40.)

Based on current neurophysiological research, erection appears to develop as a result of neural transmissions that reach the genitalia via the pelvic parasympathetic nerves. Destruction of the parasympathetic outflow from the sacral cord will cause impotence. Pelvic operations—such as radical prostatectomy or abdominal perineal resection of the rectum, in which parasympathetic nerve damage often occurs—have been associated with postoperative impotence in 70–100% of cases (7). The final common pathway for this hemodynamic control appears to be the short adrenergic nerves within the penis.

The central nervous system (CNS) loci that initiate erection have not been precisely identified. However, since these signals must reach the genitalia via the spinal cord, injury or transection of the cord may result in impotence. Reflex erections are possible in a high percentage of patients with lesions of the upper spinal cord, but the level of injury largely determines the preservation of erectile potency. These reflex erections appear to require the integrity of the afferent pudendal nerves, since pudendal neurectomies in such patients result in impotence.

Most drugs that produce impotence do so by their actions on these neurophysiological pathways. However, it is difficult to determine whether their actions are peripheral or central. Ganglion-blocking agents, such as hexamethonium, are a well-known cause of impotence and ejaculation disturbances. Propranolol frequently causes impotence when administered in doses greater than 200 mg/day. Drugs such as reserpine, α-methyldopa, and tricyclic antidepressants probably produce impotence by their action on the CNS.

In summary, normal erectile function appears to involve both pelvic parasympathetic nerves and penile corporal short adrenergic receptors. Although both α-adrenergic and β-adrenergic receptors are present within the penis, α-adrenergic receptors are believed to predominate in a 10:1 ratio. In addition, recent studies have suggested that vasoactive intestinal polypeptide, either alone (8) or in synergy with α- adrenergic blockade (9) or acetylcholine (10), may be responsible for erection. Thus erection can no longer be considered to be a purely cholinergic event and acetylcholine is not the final neurotransmitter. Nevertheless, many questions remain regarding the neurophysiology of erection.

B. Penile Blood Supply

When neural pathways are intact, the ability to achieve an erection is largely determined by the adequacy of arterial inflow. The blood supply of the penis arises from the internal pudendal artery, which is one of the terminal branches of the internal iliac artery. The paired internal pudendal arteries enter the male perineum through the lesser sciatic foramina. Each of the internal pudendal arteries, in turn, gives rise to a dorsal penile artery, a more laterally placed deep artery of the penis, which supplies the corpus cavernosum, and a bulbourethral artery, which supplies the corpus spongiosum (Fig. 2). Terminal branches of the penile arteries and the penile vessels themselves appear to communicate with the cavernous spaces via structures previously called polsters, Ebner pads, or coussinets (11).

Recent investigations in animal models and human volunteers have settled some of the long-standing controversies regarding the precise sequence of events in erection (12). In the flaccid state, the arterioles are constricted and the venous sinusoids contracted. Together, they exert maximal resistance against arterial flow, thus allowing only a small amount of nutrient blood to enter the corpora. The venules in the periphery of the corpora run between the adjacent sinusoidal walls, whereas the larger intermediary venules traverse the sinusoidal wall and tunica albuginea for some distance before exiting as the emissary veins. While the sinusoids are contracted, these venules drain freely to extrapenile veins.

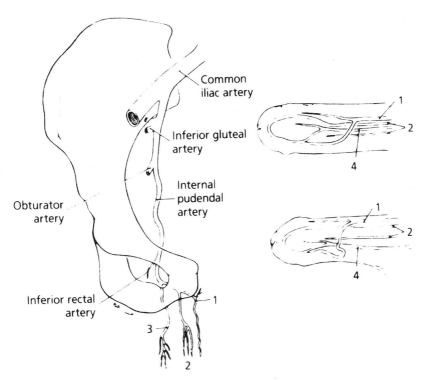

Figure 2 The major blood supply to the penis is from the deep and dorsal penile arteries and the urethral artery. These are branches of the internal pudendal artery, which in turn is branch of the internal iliac artery. 1. Dorsal artery of the penis; 2. deep artery of the penis; 3. perineal artery; 4. urethral artery. (From Ref. 4.)

During erection, the smooth muscles of the sinusoids and arterioles relax, which in turn increases sinusoidal compliance and causes a maximal decrease in peripheral resistance. This results in an immediate increase in arterial flow and filling of the sinusoids. The resulting dilation of the arterial tree not only allows blood to enter rapidly but also permits transmission of approximately 80% of the arterial systolic pressure to the sinusoidal spaces (*vascular or full erection phase*). Subsequent contraction of the bulbocavernous and ischiocavernous muscles either spontaneously or reflexly compresses the proximal corpora and culminates in cavernosal rigidity, with further engorgement of the glans penis as seen during intercourse (*skeletal muscle or rigid erection phase*). In the full erection phase, mean pressure in the corpora cavernosa is approximately 90 to 100 mmHg. In the rigid erection phase, compression of the blood-distended corpora can increase the intracavernous pressure well above arterial systolic pressure.

This proposed sequence of events is further supported by the work of Newman et al. (13), who infused the pudendal arteries of human cadavers at a pressure of 200 mmHg but were unable to produce a normal erection. Subsequently, direct infusion of the corpora cavernosa at rates ranging from 20 to 50 mL/min resulted in a normal erection. Once an erection was obtained, it was possible to maintain turgidity with decreased infusion rates. These results are similar to those of studies by Michal and Pospichal (14), who demonstrated that a mean infusion rate of 90 mL/min directly into the corpora was initially necessary to produce erections in normal human subjects. But once an erection was achieved, a maintenance flow rate of 62 mL/min was satisfactory to maintain erection.

By injecting microspheres into the internal pudendal arteries in cadavers, investigators have confirmed the presence of arteriovenous shunts measuring 1 μm in diameter (13). They also noted that occlusion of the dorsal vein of the penis failed to result in an erection. Thus erection appears to occur as the result of preferential redirection of increased arterial flow into the corporal spaces and active venoconstriction is apparently unnecessary.

C. Psychic Influences

Although recent work has emphasized the frequent organic nature of postoperative impotence, the contribution of psychogenic factors should not be lightly dismissed. Following major surgical procedures, the patient and his sexual partner may be concerned that resumption of normal sexual activity could be potentially harmful, thus resulting in decreased libido and functional impotence. Even if such subconscious fears alone may be inadequate to cause erectile dysfunction, they may be contributory in the presence of marginal penile perfusion. When initial attempts at resumption of normal sexual activity in the postoperative period meet with failure, a reactive depression may result, which can prolong the problem. If appropriate neurological and vascular causes of impotence have been excluded postoperatively, complete evaluation of the patient and, if possible, his sexual partner by a concerned and knowledgeable psychiatrist may be helpful.

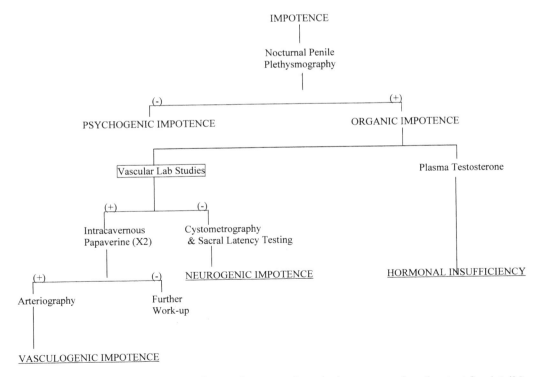

Figure 3 Algorithm suggesting a diagnostic approach to the impotent patient (see text for details). (From Ref. 40.)

II. DIAGNOSIS

Since so many factors can result in erectile dysfunction, a multimodal diagnostic approach to the problem is essential (Fig. 3). Even in those cases where the underlying defect cannot be directly corrected, confirmation of the organic nature of the patient's impotence is vital in preventing the emotional havoc that this problem can wreak on his personal life. Furthermore, once the diagnosis of organic impotence is established, the patient can be referred for a penile implant if appropriate correction of the specific problem is impossible.

III. HISTORY

Although many of the barriers that previously precluded frank discussion of erectile dysfunction have fallen, some patients are still reluctant to broach this problem with their physician. Since 70–80% of patients with aortoiliac arterial occlusive disease in some series have been impotent (15,16) and as many as 50% of diabetic patients under the age of 40 may be similarly disabled (17), vascular surgeons must be prepared to initiate such discussions with their patients. This is especially important preoperatively, not only to permit modification of the operation to relieve impotence when possible but also to document that the condition antedated the surgical procedure.

A careful and detailed history of the patient's sexual dysfunction may suggest its etiology. *Organic impotence* is typically of gradual onset and results in complete inability to achieve erection. It is not partner-specific, and masturbatory and morning erections are absent. The onset of the patient's symptoms cannot be related to any identifiable emotional stress and libido is typically retained. By contrast, *psychogenic impotence* may be rapid in onset, frequently within less than 1 month, and may be intermittent in pattern. Partner specificity may be present, and erection can be achieved during masturbation. Morning erections occur and the onset of the patient's symptoms can frequently be related to an identifiable emotional stress. The presence of normal sexual drive may be quite variable.

In those patients with known organic impotence, certain historical features help to differentiate those with neurogenic versus vasculogenic impotence. Patients suffering from *neurogenic* impotence are usually unable to achieve erections at all and may have decreased testicular sensation on palpation. Ejaculation with masturbation in such patients is generally absent. On the other hand, patients with *vasculogenic* impotence may be able to achieve an erection temporarily, but it is short-lived. Testicular pain on palpation is normal and masturbatory ejaculations are present. In patients with external iliac artery occlusion, the ipsilateral internal iliac artery may be the major collateral blood supply to the lower extremity. Some of these patients may report that they are able to achieve a satisfactory erection during foreplay; however, when thrusting is initiated, the penis becomes flaccid and coitus impossible. Presumably the increased demand for blood by the buttock and thigh muscles during active coitus shunts blood away from the genitalia, causing loss of erection (16).

A. Nocturnal Penile Tumescence

This study is based on the observation that sexually potent men can regularly have erections during the rapid-eye-movement (REM) phase of sleep (18). The complete absence of tumescence during an adequate sleep study is strong evidence of organic impotence. Unfortunately, the failure of erection is often qualitative rather than complete, and it has been difficult to standardize the quality of erections. Such studies are difficult to perform properly and are best carried out on an inpatient basis in specially equipped sleep laboratories (19). Changes in penile circumference are monitored by means of mercury-filled strain gauges and/or video camera characterizations of the quality of the erection. The documentation of normal erections during REM sleep clearly establishes the psychogenic basis of the patient's erectile dysfunction and allows appropriate therapy.

B. Noninvasive Vascular Testing

Canning et al. (20) first emphasized that vascular insufficiency of the pelvic vessels, even in the presence of normal femoral pulses, could result in impotence. They attempted to identify such patients by palpating penile pulses and performing impedance plethysmography. Subsequently, other investigators assessed penile blood flow using mercury strain-gauge plethysmography, spectrographic or ultrasonic measurement of penile systolic pressure, and pulse volume recordings (21–24). When such studies are abnormal and the possibility of vasculogenic impotence is likely, more traditional noninvasive tests to exclude aortoiliac arterial occlusive disease should be performed. Kempczinski (24) studied 134 patients using the Doppler velocity meter to measure penile systolic pressure. This, in turn, was divided by brachial systolic pressure to obtain a penile brachial index (PBI). Pulse volume waveforms (PVW), or penile volume change with each cardiac cycle, were also recorded. The influence of both sexual function and patient age on each of these parameters was then determined.

Age exerted a deleterious influence on all variables of penile blood flow independent of the status of sexual potency. Patients under the age of 40 had a mean PBI of 0.99, compared with a PBI of 0.74 for equally potent men over the age of 40. By contrast, impotent men over the age of 40 had a mean PBI of 0.58 (Fig. 4).

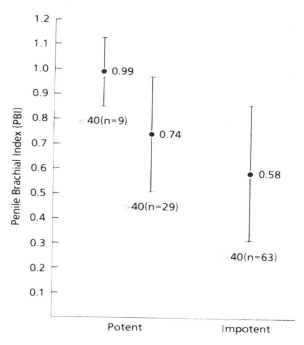

Figure 4   Distribution of penile brachial index (mean ± SD) in patients by age and sexual potency. (Data from Ref. 24.)

The PVW of patients under the age of 40 was of good to fair quality, and no poor-quality waveforms were observed. With increasing age and sexual dysfunction, a greater percentage of patients had poor-quality waveforms, but this difference was not statistically significant. The validity of the findings has been confirmed by numerous investigators, who have emphasized the importance of this type of testing in the evaluation of patients with erectile dysfunction (25,26). However, the diagnosis of vasculogenic impotence cannot be established solely on the basis of such noninvasive measurements. Although mean PBIs differed significantly between the three groups, there was a great deal of overlap, and several patients were fully potent despite PBIs less than 0.6. Other researchers have similarly confirmed a lack of correlation between PBI and the degree of erectile dysfunction (16). Although a low PBI is not sufficient to establish the diagnosis of vasculogenic impotence, the finding of a PBI greater than 0.8 confirms the adequacy of penile blood flow and suggests that vasculogenic impotence is extremely unlikely.

DePalma et al. (27) have placed greater emphasis on the diagnostic importance of the penile PVW. Using a pneumoplethysmographic cuff containing a pressure transducer, they inflated the cuff to mean arterial pressure and recorded waveforms on a polygraph. Waveform amplitude greater than 6 mm and a systolic upstroke rate of 4–6 mm at a speed chart of 25 mm/s were considered normal. Marked flattening of the waveforms with delayed upstroke greater than 6 mm and rounded waveforms were considered abnormal. Although the investigators noted certain borderline categories in which diagnosis is equivocal, the technique was particularly helpful in cases where the PBI was between 0.6 and 0.7.

Recently, Lue et al. (28) reported the use of duplex scanning in the evaluation of vasculogenic impotence. Using a high-resolution 10 MHz ultrasound probe, they were able to clearly visualize the cavernosa arteries, dorsal veins, tunica albuginea, corpora cavernosa, and corpus spongiosum. The diameter of the arterial lumina, the thickness of the arterial walls, and the quality of their pulsations were assessed before and after papaverine injection. Pulsed Doppler was then used to study the blood flow through each of the penile arteries. Since this test can be performed only on the vessels distal to the pubis, further visualization of the pelvic vasculature with internal pudendal arteriography was required when ultrasonography suggested arterial disease.

C. Neurological Testing

Since there are no direct measures of the neural pathways involved in erection, indirect measures must be employed. Fortunately, the autonomic pathways involved in micturition and erection are similar and *cystometrography* with measurement of bladder capacity and residual urine can be used as an indirect measure of penile innervation, assuming that involvement of the appropriate pelvic nerves is reflected by abnormalities in both areas. Using this technique, Ellenberg (17) confirmed neuropathy in 82% of impotent diabetic subjects.

The bulbocavernous reflex may be quantified by indirect measurement of pudendal nerve velocity (*sacral latency testing*). Since this examination requires electrical stimulation of the penile skin with simultaneous electromyographic recording of the response in the bulbocavernous muscle, it must generally be performed with the patient under general anesthesia. The technique has been modified by using surface-mounted perineal electrodes, thus making measurement of somatosensory evoked potentials (SEPs) from the dorsal penile and posterior tibial nerves more comfortable. Values that are three standard deviations above the mean are considered abnormal (27).

D. Intracavernous Papaverine Injection

This technique is useful in differentiating vasculogenic from psychogenic impotence (12). However, it cannot distinguish psychogenic erectile dysfunction from neurogenic or hormonal impotence. It should be used only to supplement a careful history and physical examination, not to supplant it.

In patients with a penis of average size, 60 mg of papaverine diluted with 2–5 mL of normal saline solution is injected into the corpus cavernosum. A rubber band is wrapped tightly around the base of the penis before the injection to ensure that most of the drug remains in the corpus, and it is left in place for 2 min after injection. The dose of papaverine may need to be adjusted in patients with an unusually large or small penis. In patients suspected of neurogenic impotence, an initial test dose of 15 mg of papaverine should be used, since they are prone to suffer priapism.

After the rubber band is removed, the patient is asked to stand so as to increase venous pressure in the pelvis and further reduce the entry of papaverine into the systemic circulation. If a full erection develops within 10 min and it lasts more than 30 min, the arterial, venous, and sinusoidal mechanisms can be assumed to be normal and vasculogenic impotence can be excluded. However, since a full erection may not develop in a nervous or anxious patient under the conditions of testing, a poor response does not infallibly confirm vasculogenic impotence (12). When two or more injections fail to produce an erection, an angiogram should be considered.

E. Angiography

The pelvic vasculature can be visualized using standard angiographic techniques with appropriate oblique projections. This should be the first procedure performed when large-vessel arterial occlusive disease or aortic aneurysm is suspected. Patency of the internal iliac artery on each side should be determined and the presence of significant lesions should be noted. Unfortunately, arteriographic findings correlate poorly with the patient's erectile function. In one study where these were compared, 23% of potent men undergoing aortic operation were noted to have bilateral iliac artery occlusions and an additional 36% had unilateral occlusion (29). This is not surprising, since routine angiograms rarely provide complete definition of the distal penile vasculature and cannot assess the adequacy of collateral blood flow around arterial occlusive lesions.

When no flow-reducing lesions are identified in the hypogastric arteries or their major branches, selective cannulation of the internal pudendal artery with the patient positioned in the appropriate degree of obliquity may be necessary. Since selective cannulation of this vessel may be difficult and the subsequent injection of dye painful, such studies are usually performed with the patient under epidural anesthesia (30). Intra-arterial vasodilators administered before the injection of contrast material are important for improving visualization of the penile arteries (Fig. 5).

Corpus cavernosography, which can usually be performed under local anesthesia, may be used in the assessment of patients with erectile dysfunction, which is thought to be secondary to venous outflow problems. However, pulsed Doppler sonography should routinely be performed in such patients, since only those with a normal sinusoidal system and arterial tree will have a good arterial response to papaverine. If a patient does not achieve a full erection, the problem can be attributed to abnormal venous channels rather than to sinusoidal fibrosis. In addition, patients with congenital or acquired chordee may require cavernosography (31).

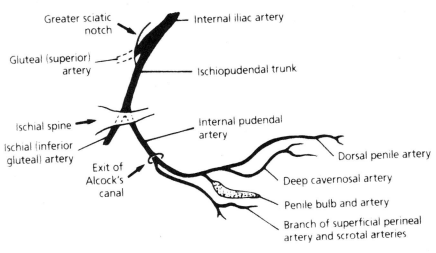

Figure 5 Idealized normal subselective angiogram. Note filling of dorsal and deep penile arteries. The arteries of the corpus spongiosum are not visualized. (From Ref. 27.)

F.   Prevention

In order to ensure preservation of erectile function, surgical correction of aortoiliac occlusive disease must accomplish the following objectives: minimal disturbance of genital autonomic function, maintenance of adequate pelvic blood flow, and successful revascularization of the ischemic extremity. DePalma (32) has popularized a nerve-sparing approach to the infrarenal aorta that emphasizes approaching the abdominal aorta along its right lateral aspect, minimal division of longitudinal periaortic tissues to the left of the infrarenal aorta, avoidance of dissection at the base of the inferior mesenteric artery, and sparing of the nerve plexus that crosses the left common iliac artery (Fig. 6). Using such a nerve-sparing approach, several surgeons have achieved a notable reduction in postoperative impotence (29,33–35).

Although the findings on preoperative angiograms correlate poorly with erectile function, preservation of adequate perfusion into at least one hypogastric artery appears to be a vital component of all operations that are successful in minimizing iatrogenic erectile dysfunction. When possible, direct antegrade perfusion of the internal iliac artery should be ensured. This may require thromboendarterectomy of the hypogastric artery orifice when appropriate. If both external iliac arteries are occluded or stenotic and a bypass into the common femoral arteries is anticipated, proximal aortic anastomosis should be performed in an end-to-side fashion, since retrograde perfusion of the internal iliac artery would be impossible in such circumstances and significant reduction of pelvic blood flow would be likely. When proximal disease is so extensive that thromboendarterectomy is impractical and preoperative noninvasive testing has confirmed decreased penile perfusion, simple aortofemoral grafting may not always restore a pelvic collateral blood flow adequate to relieve vasculogenic impotence. Preoperative recognition of such cases is not easy. However, when the probability seems likely, the surgeon should consider reimplanting the hypogastric artery into one limb of the aortofemoral graft or adding a jump graft into the distal hypogastric artery (36).

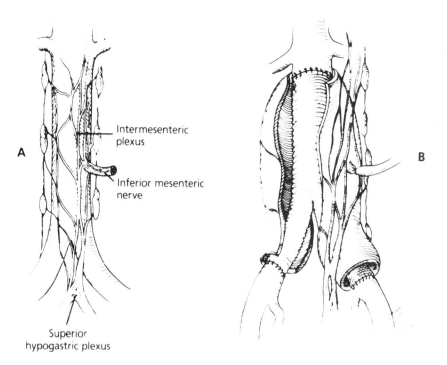

Figure 6 Diagrammatic representation of the autonomic nerve supply to the penis (A) and suggested modification of the surgical approach to the aorta during resection of abdominal aortic aneurysm (B) to minimize damage to these structures. (From Ref. 35.)

In patients with unilateral iliac artery occlusive disease, the objectives of nerve–sparing extremity revascularization and increased hypogastric artery perfusion may all be accomplished using femorofemoral bypass. Several investigators have confirmed the success of this procedure in improving penile blood flow and restoring erection (25,37). Femorofemoral bypass is especially appropriate for young, sexually active men with unilateral disease, since it avoids the necessity for any periaortic dissection.

When direct aortic reconstruction is necessary, it is important to avoid flushing atheromatous debris down the hypogastric artery (29). Operative techniques should be modified to adequately back-bleed the hypogastric arteries before completion of anastomoses. Unfortunately, emergent aortic surgery, such as the resection of a ruptured abdominal aortic aneurysm, rarely allows time for the careful anatomic dissection necessary to avoid nerve damage, and the incidence of iatragenic impotence is accordingly higher (38). Although rarely under the control of the vascular surgeon, emergent operations should be avoided whenever possible.

The impact of *endovascular revascularization* or *endovascular graft implantation* in aortoiliac revascularization on the incidence of iatrogenic impotence has not yet been evaluated. However, the absense of direct dissection near the parasympathetic nerve plexus surrounding the iliac arteries should have a favorable impact on reducing iatrogenic neurogenic impotence. Furthermore, the ability to approach and dilate vessels more distally located within the pelvis may make it possible to revascularize vessels previously unapproachable by traditional, direct vascular surgical techniques.

G. Treatment

Once organic impotence is confirmed, a reasonably precise etiological diagnosis is essential before initiating appropriate therapy. If arteriograms confirm occlusion of the proximal pelvic arteries and the measured PBI is less than 0.6, bypass into a distal patent branch of the hypogastric artery on at least one side should be considered. If the PBI is less than 0.6 but no large-vessel occlusive lesions are identified, selective angiograms of the internal pudendal artery may document more distal occlusive lesions. If deep patent penile or dorsal penile arteries can be confirmed, consideration should be given to direct revascularization of the penis using the inferior epigastric artery and microvascular anastomosis into one of these vessels. Although the long-term durability of such procedures has not been documented, initial success has been reported in approximately 70% of such procedures. The recent popularity of an endovascular approach to previously inaccessible vessels and balloon dilation, with or without the implantation of an endovascular stent, offers the potential for yet another alternative approach to these problems.

When neurogenic impotence appears likely, patients may be managed by teaching them to perform self-injection of intracorporal papaverine or by implantation of a suitable penile prosthesis. The recently proven effectiveness of sildenafil citrate (Viagra®) in treating patients with psychogenic or neurogenic impotence suggests that this form of therapy should be seriously considered in patients with postoperative impotence, especially if vascular laboratory testing documents adequate penile blood flow. Furthermore, since the side effects of Viagra® are minimal, it may be more appropriate to try an empiric course of therapy with this medication when neurogenic impotence is suspected rather than resorting to the complex diagnostic testing, i.e., cystometrography and/or sacral latency testing, which would be required to confirm the diagnosis of neurogenic impotence. Similarly, even if noninvasive vascular laboratory studies suggest borderline penile blood flow, an empiric trial of Viagra® is so much simpler than complex arteriographic studies requiring selective cannulation of the hypogastric arteries that it seems reasonable to consider such a course of action prior to embarking on expensive, potentially harmful diagnostic testing.

In hypertensive patients who require ganglion-blocking drugs to control their disease and in whom impotence develops secondary to such medications, alternate forms of treatment should be found. If the hypertension is secondary to renal artery stenosis, renal revascularization should be considered.

H. Results

In a collected series of 138 patients undergoing aortic reconstruction using standard vascular surgical techniques, Flanigan et al. (29) documented a 25% incidence of iatrogenic impotence. By minimizing periaortic dissection and emphasizing a nerve-sparing technique—along with efforts to ensure perfusion of at least one hypogastric artery during the arterial reconstruction—they completely eliminated iatrogenic impotence. Furthermore, retrograde ejaculation was reduced from 43% in the collected series to only 3% in the control group.

Since 80% of patients who present with aortoiliac arterial occlusive disease already have significant erectile dysfunction, careful planning of the operative reconstruction to ensure hypogastric artery perfusion is essential if this symptom is to be relieved. Excluding patients with diabetes mellitus, in whom neurogenic impotence is most likely, relief of preoperative erectile dysfunction can be anticipated in 30% of patients so afflicted (15,29). Half of the patients who regained potency following revascularization were noted to have bilateral iliac artery occlusion on the preoperative arteriogram (29).

IV. CONCLUSION

A mulitmodal diagnostic approach to the impotent patient is essential to ensure precise etiological diagnosis and appropriate therapy. Furthermore, an understanding of the multiple factors involved in achieving a normal erection is essential if potency is to be preserved during the course of direct aortic surgery. Since nearly 25% of patients undergoing direct aortic reconstruction will suffer iatrogenic erectile dysfunction if appropriate technical modifications are not employed, the problem of iatrogenic impotence is not inconsequential.

When direct aortoiliac revascularization is necessary, appropriate nerve-sparing dissection of the infrarenal aorta and preservation of hypogastric perfusion can virtually eliminate the postoperative development of erectile dysfunction and maximize the chance for improvement in preoperative impotence. If the patient is an appropriate candidate for an endovascular treatment of their arterial lesions, the danger of postoperative neurogenic impotence can be virtually eliminated and the likelihood of improvement in preoperative impotence maximized if preoperative noninvasive testing shows a low PBI and the proposed endovascular procedure can restore flow into at least one of the hypogastric arteries.

When postoperative impotence occurs despite every precaution, an attentive and objective approach can offer much comfort to the patient and his sexual partner. In most cases, an empirical trial of Viagra® seems appropriate. In only a small percentage of such cases will additional revascularization be necessary.

REFERENCES

1. Leriche R, Morel A. The syndrome of thrombotic obliteration of the aortic bifurcation. Ann Surg 1948; 127:193.
2. Harris JD, Jepson RP. Aorto-iliac stenosis: A comparison of two procedures. Aust NZ J Surg 1965; 3:211.
3. DePalma RG, Kedia K, Persky L. Vascular operations for preservation of sexual function. In: Bergan JJ, Yao JST, eds. Surgery of the Aorta and Its Body Branches. Orlando, FL: Grune & Stratton, 1979.
4. Queral LA, Flinn WR, Bergan JJ, Yao JST. Sexual function and aortic surgery. In: Bergan JJ, Yao JST, eds. Surgery of the Aorta and Its Body Branches. Orlando, FL: Grune & Stratton, 1979.
5. Weiss HD. The physiology of human penile erection. Ann Intern Med 1972; 76:793.
6. Kedia KR, Markland C, Fraley EE. Sexual function following high retroperitoneal lymphadenectomy. J Urol 1975; 114:237.
7. Drane RJ, Siroky MB. Neurophysiology of erection. Urol Clin North Am 1981; 8:91.
8. Willis EM, Ottesen B, Wagner G, Sundler F, Fahrenkrug J. Vasoactive intestinal polypeptide (VIP) as a possible neurotransmitter involved in penile erection. Acta Physiol Scand 1981; 113:545.
9. Adaikan PG, Kottegoda SR, Ratnam SS. Is vasoactive intestinal polypeptide the principal transmitter involved in human penile erection? J Urol 1986; 135:638.
10. Benson GS. Penile erection: In search of a neurotransmitter. World J Urol 1983; 1:209.
11. Conti G. L'erection due penis humain et ses bases morphologic vascularies. Acta Anat (Basel) 1952; 14–17.
12. Lue TF, Tanagho EA. Physiology of erection and pharmacological management of impotence. J Urol 1987; 137:829.
13. Newman HF, Northrup JD, Devlin J. Mechanism of human penile erection. Invest Urol 1964; 1:350.
14. Michal V, Pospichal J. Phalloarteriography in the diagnosis of erectile impotence. World J Surg 1978; 2:329.

15. May AG, DeWesse JA, Rob CG. Changes in sexual function following operation on the abdominal aorta. Surgery 1969; 65:41.
16. Nath RL, Menzoian JO, Kaplan KH, McMillian TN, Siroky MB, Krane RJ. The multi-disciplinary approach to vasculogenic impotence. Surgery 1981; 89:124.
17. Ellenberg M. Impotence in diabetes: The neurologic factor. Ann Intern Med 1971; 75:213.
18. Bohlen JG. Sleep erection monitoring in the evaluation of male erectile failure. Urol Clin North Am 1981; 8:119.
19. Karacan I, Salis PJ, Ware JC, Dervent B, Williams RL, Scott FB, Attia SL, Beutler LE. Nocturnal penile tumescence and diagnosis in diabetic impotence. Am J Psychiatry 1978; 135:191.
20. Canning JR, Bowers LM, Lloyd FA, Cottrell TLC. Genital vascular insufficiency and impotence. Surg Forum 1963; 14:298.
21. Abelson D. Diagnostic value of the penile pulse and blood pressure: A Doppler study of impotence in diabetics. J Urol 1975; 111:636.
22. Britt DB, Kemmerer WT, Robison JR. Penile blood flow determination by mercury strain gauge plethysmography. Invest Urol 1971; 8:673.
23. Gaskell P. The importance of penile blood pressure in cases of impotence. Can Med Assoc J 1971; 105:1047.
24. Kempczinski RF. Role of the vascular diagnostic laboratory in the evaluation of male impotence. Am J Surg 1979; 138:278.
25. Merchant RF Jr, DePalma RG. Effects of femorofemoral grafts on postoperative sexual function: Correlation with penile pulse volume recordings. Surgery 1981; 90:962.
26. Queral LA, Whitehouse WM, Flinn WR, Zarins CK, Bergan JJ, Yao JST. Pelvic hemodynamics after aortoiliac reconstruction. Surgery 1979; 86:799.
27. DePalma RG, Emsellem HA, Edwards CM, Druy EM, Shultz SW, Miller HC, Bergsrud D. A screening sequence for vasculogenic impotence. J Vasc Surg 1987; 5:228.
28. Lue TF, Hricak H, Marick KW, Tangaho EA. Vasclogenic impotence evaluated by high-resolution ultrasonography and pulsed Doppler spectrum analysis. Radiology 1985; 155:777.
29. Flanigan DP, Schuler JJ, Keifer T, Schwartz JA, Lim LT. Elimination of iatrogenic impotence and improvement of sexual function after aorto-iliac revascularization. Arch Surg 1982; 117:544.
30. Ginestie JF, Romieu A. Radiologic Exploration of Impotence. The Hague: Martinus Nijhoff, 1978.
31. Fitzpatrick T. The corpus carvenosum intercommunicating venous drainage system. J Urol 1975; 113:494.
32. DePalma RG. Impotence in vascular disease: Relationship of vascular surgery. Br J Surg 1982; 69:514.
33. DePalma RG, Levine SB, Feldman S. Preservation of erectile function after aortoiliac reconstruction. Arch Surg 1978; 113:958.
34. Miles JR, Miles DG, Johnson G. Aortoiliac operations and sexual dysfunction. Arch Surg 1982; 117:1177.
35. Weinstein MH, Machleder HI. Sexual function after aorto-iliac surgery. Ann Surg 1975; 181:787.
36. Biller A, Dagher FJ, Queral LA. Surgical correction of vasculogenic impotence in a patient after bilateral renal transplantation. Surgery 1982; 91:108.
37. Schuler JJ, Gray B, Flanigan DP, Williams LR. Increased penile perfusion and reversal of vasculogenic impotence following femorofemoral bypass. Br J Surg 1982; 67–69.
38. Flanigan DP, Pratt DG, Goodreau JJ, Burnham SJ, Yao JST, Bergan JJ. Hemodynamic and angiographic guidelines in selection of patients for femorofemoral bypass. Arch Surg 1978; 113:1257.
39. Michal V, Kramar R, Hejhal L. Revascularization procedure of the cavernous bodies. In: Zorgomotti AW, Rossi G, eds. Vasculogenic Impotence Proceedings of the First International Conference on Corpus Cavernosum Revascularization. Springfield, IL: Charles C. Thomas, 1980.
40. Kempczinski FR, Birinyi LK. Impotence following aortic surgery. In: Bernhard VM, Towne JB, eds. Complications in Vascular Surgery. 2d ed. Philadelphia: Saunders, 1985:311–324.

12

Complications Following Reconstructions of the Pararenal Aorta and Its Branches

Kenneth J. Cherry, Jr.
Mayo Clinic, Rochester, Minnesota, U.S.A.

I. INTRODUCTION

Operations upon the juxta- and suprarenal aorta and the visceral branches of the upper abdominal aorta are performed much less frequently than reconstructions confined to the infrarenal aorta and its pelvic and extremity branches. There is evidence that more juxtarenal aneurysms are being diagnosed and repaired in absolute numbers (1). The sophistication of modern imaging modalities allows more detailed and easier assessment of the paravisceral aorta than in years past, and there is more of a trend to longitudinal follow-up by vascular surgeons now than previously. In addition, endovascular treatment of infrarenal abdominal aortic aneurysms is currently performed for anywhere from 40–80% of patients undergoing aneurysm repair at referral centers. A larger percentage of the aortic aneurysms now repaired conventionally are juxta- or suprarenal. In the recent series from the Cleveland Clinic, the repair of juxtarenal aneurysms accounted for 10.8% of their total repairs in 1995 and 31.7% in 2000 (2). This relative increase in juxtarenal reconstructions reflects the active endovascular practice of those surgeons for the treatment of infrarenal aortic aneurysms.

Furthermore, failed or failing stent-graft repairs of the infrarenal aorta are frequently necessarily managed with open repair: suprarenal, supramesenteric, or supraceliac clamping is often required.

Endovascular angioplasty and stenting of renal artery lesions has supplanted conventional surgery as the major interventional modality to treat renovascular hypertension for both atherosclerotic and fibromuscular dysplastic lesions around the country. Nonetheless, there exist renal artery lesions that are not well treated by endovascular techniques: atherosclerosis or fibromuscular dysplasia involving major branch vessels, atherosclerotic lesions of extended length, extremely distal lesions or branch vessel lesions, eccentric calcific renal artery plaque, dense aortic calcific disease extending into the renal artery, multiple small stenotic renal arteries not suitable for stenting, aneurysms involving large branch vessels or in distal locations, and complications of endovascular therapy, such as thrombosis, dissection, or perforation. Not all of these require open repair, but many do.

Angioplasty and stenting of the mesenteric arteries has its proponents and enthusiasts, some of whom claim that open surgery is passé. Short segment stenoses of the superior mesenteric artery are well treated by this modality. Stenoses of the celiac artery are more difficult to treat because of the early branching of that vessel, its often short main trunk, and the overlying median arcuate ligament. A "bald aorta" with no demonstrable celiac or superior mesenteric artery ostia, as well as long occlusions of the superior mesenteric artery with reconstitution of the vessel at the infrapancreatic position, are poorly treated by endovascular technique. Furthermore, there are no good data concerning medium- or long-range follow-up for angioplasty and stenting, and that lack of data must temper the enthusiasm for this new modality. Kasirajan et al. at the Cleveland Clinic had a higher recurrence at 3 years in their patients undergoing endovascular repair than in those having open reconstruction; they felt good-risk patients should be offered open repair as a first option (3). In our series of 98 patients, we identified a subset of poor-risk patients greater than 70 years of age who might have been better served by endovascular repair than by open surgery; we felt that the majority were better treated with conventional reconstruction (4). As endovascular technology improves, undoubtedly the percentage of patients with chronic mesenteric ischemia needing conventional operations will decrease. At present, however, the ability to perform conventional operation for chronic mesenteric ischemia remains a necessary part of our education and skill.

Endovascular repair of aortic aneurysmal disease involving the juxta- and suprarenal aorta, or the necessity of providing safe attachment sites proximal to the renal arteries, is in its nascent period. Surgical investigators such as John Anderson in Adelaide, Timothy Chuter in San Francisco, and Larry Hollier and Michael Marin in New York are leading the way, making ingenious advances in applying endovascular techniques to the upper abdominal aorta and its branches (5–8). For most patients, however, juxta- and suprarenal aortic aneurysmal and occlusive disease remain open surgical problems.

Reconstructions of the paravisceral aorta and its visceral branches may be daunting not only because of the relative rarity with which they are performed but also because of the anatomical milieu. There is close proximity, indeed intimacy, of the upper abdominal aorta and its branches with the diaphragm, esophagus, stomach, vagus nerves, spleen, liver, biliary tree, pancreas, proximal small bowel, adrenal glands, and kidneys. Dissection, exposure, and repair are all the more challenging. The choice of incision, choice of approach, site of clamp placement, and proper sequence of clamping and unclamping all contribute heavily to the success or failure of these operations. The need to clamp above the renal arteries or above the mesenteric vessel(s) adds an element of ischemic insult to the solid organs, especially the kidneys, not present with infrarenal aortic repairs. Juxtarenal clamping is also a potential source of renal atheroemboli. Upper abdominal aortic clamping adds further cardiac stress. Pulmonary function may likewise be compromised.

II. OPERATIONS ON THE JUXTA- AND SUPRARENAL AORTA

Operations on the juxta- and suprarenal aorta may be performed utilizing various incisions, approaches, and clamp sites. Classically, type IV thoracoabdominal aortic aneurysm repairs, as well as endarterectomy of the paravisceral aorta and/or mesenteric vessels, were approached through low-lying thoracoabdominal or thoracoretroperitoneal incisions. Those approaches, involving not only abdominal incisions but also incisions of the diaphragm and thoracic cavity were and are occasioned by increased pulmonary and wound problems (9). There are patients, however, who still require the more extensive thoracoretroperitoneal method. Extremely thin or asthenic persons with very narrow costal margins are poorly served by laparotomy and medial visceral rotation, as the ipsilateral lower rib cage prevents the surgeon from obtaining a proper orientation to deal with the upper extent of the aorta or with the mesenteric vessels. At the other extreme, morbidly obese patients or extremely large patients may require thoracoretroperitoneal exposure simply for adequate and comfortable handling of the arteries.

Those anatomical considerations aside, most surgeons dealing with these problems prefer, if possible, to use incisions confined to the abdomen, combined with transperitoneal approaches, retroperitoneal approaches, or medial visceral rotation. Those incisions may be midline, transverse, oblique, or combinations thereof.

The operative results for pararenal aneurysm repair at large referral centers are good to excellent, with mortality ranging from 0 to 15.4% and averaging approximately 5% (Table 1) (2,10–19). In a small series, not included in Table 1, Tordoir et al. had no mortality in their 15 patients with pararenal aortic aneurysms (20). Similarly, Schneider et al., in their series of 23 patients, reported no mortality (17). Qvarfordt et al. had a 1.3% mortality for 77 patients, an even more salutary figure when one considers that 70% of those patients had concomitant renal artery reconstructions (11). Allen and colleagues in a large series from the Washington University–Barnes Hospital had a mortality of 1.5% in their patients and likewise reconstructed the renal arteries (15). Jean-Claude et al., continuing the work from the University of California-San Francisco, reported a mortality of 5.8% in 257 patients (19). The most recent report is from Sarac and colleagues at the Cleveland Clinic, concerning 138 patients with juxtrarenal aneurysms, has a very similar mortality of 5.1%. This was statistically different from the results of their open infrarenal aortic reconstructions (2.8%) (2).

In two other series, not included in Table 1 because of the range of patients analyzed, Shepard et al., at the New England Medical Center, used an extended left flank incision and retroperitoneal exposure in 23 high-risk patients with abdominal aortic aneurysms, 14 of whom required suprarenal and supraceliac clamping for pararenal occlusive and aneurysmal problems. There was only one death (4%) (21). Shepard and coworkers, continuing their work at Henry Ford Hospital, reported the same approach for 85 patients with complex occlusive and aneurysmal aortic problems. The elective mortality in their series was 2.4% (22).

The two large series with the best mortality, those of Qvarfordt et al. and Allen et al., are remarkable not only for the low mortality reported but also for the surgeons' willingness and ability to clamp at the supramesenteric level in addition to the suprarenal and supraceliac levels. Neither study found any increase in morbidity or mortality with that approach (11,15).

The abdominal incisions used are, in the main, surgeons' choices. Body habitus, previous operation, comorbidities, (e.g., pulmonary disease), and the segment of aorta needing repair all impact upon those decisions. Exposure may be infracolic transperitoneal for juxta- and even suprarenal aortic reconstructions and for renal artery repairs. It may be transperitoneal through the lesser omentum for mesenteric reconstructions. It may be retroperitoneal. Darling et al. report few if any problems dealing with even the right renal artery utilizing a retroperitoneal approach (23). That view is shared by the group from Henry Ford (22). For more proximal repairs, medial visceral rotation allows exposure of the entire abdominal aorta; this is our preferred approach for upper abdominal operations. The left kidney may be mobilized anteriorly or left in situ, depending on the work to be done and the anatomy. If superior mesenteric artery reconstruction is to be performed, the kidney is

Table 1 Literature Summary[a]

Study	No. of cases	AAA Type[a] (no.)	Cross-Clamp Level	Mortality Rate	Baseline Elevated Cr	Transient Cr Rise	New-Onset Dialysis	Elevated Cr at Discharge
Crawford et al. (10), 1986	101	JR 88 SR 0 RAOD 13	SC 93 SSMA 0 SR 8	7.9%	18.8%	15.8%	7.9%	ND
Qvarfordt. (11), 1986	77	JR22 SR 24 RAOD 31	SC 13 SSMA 17 SR 45	1.3%	54.5%	23.0%	2.5%	13.0%
Green et al. (12), 1989[b]	52	JR29 SR ? RAOD ?	SC 30 SSMA 0 SR 22	15.4%	ND	ND	11.5%	ND
Poulias et al. (13), 1992	38	JR 32 SR 0 RAOD 6	SC 0 SSMA 0 SR 38	5.3%	15.8%	23.7%	13.2%	13.2%
Breckwoldt et al. (14), 1992[c]	39	Unclear	SC8 SSMA 2 SR 25	2.6%	ND	28.2%	2.6%	12.8%
Allen et al. (15), 1993[d]	65	JR 24 SR 15 RAOD 7	SC 27 SSMA 12 SR 26	1.5%	20.0%	12.3%	3.1%	3.1%
Nypaver et al. (16), 1993	53	JR 41 SR 6 RAOD 6	SC 21 SSMA 4 SR 28	3.8%	17.0%	22.6%	5.7%	7.5%
Schneider et al. (17), 1997	23	SR 23 SR 0 RAOD 0	SC 23 SSMA 0 SR 0	0.0%	ND	26.1%	0.0%	0.0%
Faggioli et al. (18), 1998[e]	50	JR 39 SR 6 RAOD 5	SC 8 SSMA 0 SR 42	7.0% (elective only)	10.0%	ND	ND	0.0%
Jean-Claude et al. (19), 1999	257	JR 122 SR 58 RAOD 77	SR 42 SC 33 SSMA 48	5.8%	31.1%	30.4%	7.0%	10.5%
Sarac et al. (2), 2002	138	JRA 138	SC 43 SR 95	5.1%	15.4%	19.6%	28.3%	5.8%

Abbreviations: AAA, abdominal aortic aneurysm; Cr, creatinine level; JR, juxtarenal; SR, suprarenal; RAOD, renal artery occlusive disease; SC, superceliac; SSMA, supra-superior mesenteric artery; ND, no clear data.

[a] Best estimate of categorization University of California–San Francisco pararenal abdominal aortic aneurysm groups.

[b] Very difficult to put the data in this study into this format; also suprarenal clamp group contained 11 patients who initially had an infrarenal clamp.

[c] Only 33 abdominal aortic aneurysms matched University of California–San Francisco categories.

[d] Only 46 abdominal aortic aneurysms matched University of California–San Francisco categories.

[e] Includes seven ruptured pararenal abdominal aortic aneurysms.

Source: Ref. 19.

better left in situ. Injury to the spleen and kidneys is more likely with upper retroperitoneal exposure and medial visceral rotation than with a transperitoneal approach (9,23).

All three methods of exposure—transperitoneal, retroperitoneal, and medical visceral rotation—offer excellent choices for the correct patient populations. All are subject to complication. Thoracoabdominal incisions and oblique flank incisions, in distinction to classic laparotomy incisions, are subject to flank herniation or laxity of the flank muscles because of division of the nerves. There is also the potential problem of costochondral pain or instability (9,22).

Of considerable import and debate is the choice of the proximal aortic clamp site. It is on this issue that success or failure hinges. Crawford preferred supraceliac clamping and used it almost exclusively (10). As stated previously, the surgeons at UCSF and at Washington University–Barnes applied clamps at suprarenal, supramesenteric and supraceliac sites (11,15). Green et al. from the University of Rochester have recommended against suprarenal clamps (12). That group reported a higher mortality with suprarenal clamps, 32%, in comparison to a 3% mortality for supraceliac clamping and a sevenfold increase in frank renal failure with suprarenal clamping. Of note, 11 patients included in that suprarenal group were initially clamped at an infrarenal level and the clamp level changed during the course of their operations. That fact underscores the absolute necessity for clear and precise judgment in choosing the clamp site and technical excellence in exposing the proper aortic segment in a thorough, gentle manner. Renal artery atheroembolization is the most feared sequela of dissection and exposure and of improper clamp placement; it was felt by Green et al. to account for their poor results with suprarenal clamping. They felt that nonaneurysmal atherosclerosis in the pararenal area was the culprit. Of note again, the authors stated: "The placement of the proximal clamp was dependent on the *operative* findings [italics added]." I would maintain that the route of exposure and the choice of proximal clamp site is dependent on appropriate and accurate *preoperative* imaging and assessment rather than on operative findings. Nonetheless, the concern of Green et al. for atheroembolization is valid and is reinforced in an unexpected way by the most recent finding from Jean-Claude et al. from the University of California–San Francisco, in which 6 of their 15 deaths (40%) were attributed to visceral ischemia or infarction. Those authors felt that atheroembolization was the mechanism of injury in 5 of those 6 patients (19). Parenthetically, they have not experienced this particular complication in the last 10 years (Louis Messina, personal communication). Further, and in contradistinction to Green's findings, they found that atheroembolization was more likely with *supraceliac* clamping or supramesenteric clamping than with suprarenal clamping (9.1, 6.3, and 0.6% respectively). Similarly, Sarac and colleagues from the Cleveland Clinic found supraceliac clamping less safe than suprarenal clamping (2).

Cardiac disease, of course, remains a primary cause of perioperative morbidity and mortality for all vascular patients. Preoperative screening with physiological and anatomical tests; appropriate medical or interventional management; and maximization of intra-operative cardiac status with appropriate pharmacological, anesthetic, and monitoring methods are all paramount to achieving excellent results (24). This chapter does not address that issue further with the exception of cardiac function and site of clamp placement.

III. COMPLICATIONS

In most series, renal insufficiency is the leading complication of juxtarenal aortic operations; it is certainly the most analyzed and the most feared, as evidenced by Table 1. It was the leading complication in the majority of the series cited with transient rises of serum creatinine in 12.3–30.4% of patients and led to the need for new dialysis in 0–28.3% of patients (2,10–19). Preoperative renal dysfunction is felt by most authors to be the most accurate indicator of postoperative decline in renal function (2,15,19), but other authors have not been able to demonstrate that association (14,16). Nypaver et al. felt that postoperative renal insufficiency was more likely when concomitant renal artery operations were necessary or when there was a major intraoperative complication (16). Allen and colleagues at Washington University–Barnes Hospital, on the other hand, felt that attention to renal artery disease improved their results (15). Authors such as Green et al. have implicated suprarenal clamp placement and embolization. Whereas others, such as Allen et al., have found no correlation between clamp placement and complications (12,15). Jean-Claude et al. and Sarac and colleagues at the Cleveland Clinic have implicated supraceliac clamping as the more hazardous maneuver (2,19). Jean-Claude and colleagues also found statistical correlation with cross-clamp time. As 75% of their patients improved, they felt that acute tubular necrosis secondary to cross-clamp-induced ischemia—and not atheroembolization—was the disease mechanism (19). The group from Barnes found no correlation between cross-clamp time and renal insufficiency. They felt that accurate aortic cross-clamping, attention to renovascular disease, and cold perfusion of the renal arteries obviated the deleterious ischemic effects of cross-clamping (15).

Shepard et al. and Poulios and colleagues also use hypothermic renal perfusion, as does the group at Barnes (13,15,22). We also prefer its use. Some surgeons at our institution use a continuous drip, while others perfuse the kidneys with boluses of ice-cold heparinized saline on a periodic basis, such as every 15 min.

Kashyap et al. at Massachusettes General Hospital described renal failure in 183 patients following thoracoabdominal aortic surgery; of these, 29 had type IV thoracoabdominal aortic aneurysms, 17 had suprarenal aortic aneurysms and 12 underwent renal or mesenteric reconstructions (25). Acute renal failure was associated with a preoperative creatinine of 1.5 or higher and a cross-clamp time exceeding 100 min; the complication of acute renal failure was associated with a 10-fold increase in mortality. One-quarter of their patients with preoperative renal insufficiency developed renal failure, but one must remember that this group of 185 patients included 125 patients with type I, II, or III thoracoabdominal aortic aneurysms—groups that are at higher risk for this complication and for death. However, Sarac and colleagues, on the same note, found that supraceliac clamping was the sole predictor of postoperative mortality and that supraceliac clamping, diabetes, and preoperative renal insufficiency were the predictors of postoperative renal insufficiency (2).

Renal dysfunction may result from prolonged ischemia, atheroembolization, renal artery occlusive disease, artery or graft thrombosis, hypovolemia, hypoperfusion, hyperperfusion, shock, or multisystem organ failure, with its cytokine response (26). Acute renal failure is exacerbated by proximal aortic repair, preoperative renal insufficiency, intraoperative complications, and comorbidities. Renal dysfunction is also related to age, cardiac dysfunction, and diabetes. Cherr and Hansen feel that the recovery of renal function is dependent on preoperative renal function, age, and cross-clamp time (27).

When all these studies with their diverse findings are considered, it would seem that renal ischemic issues relate primarily to the patient's preexistent renal and cardiac status, the presence of renovascular disease, placement of the cross-clamp, clamping sequence, cross-clamp time, and the patient's hemodynamic status intraoperatively. Hydration, before angiography and in the preoperative period as well as intraoperatively, with determination and maintenance of the patient's best hemodynamic and cardiac function, and appropriate fluid and blood replacement during the operation are paramount in lessening the chances of renal insufficiency. Pulmonary artery catheters should be used in all patients undergoing upper abdominal and visceral reconstructions. Transesophageal echocardiography may be added to those patients with known cardiac disease. Lasix and mannitol are used. Mannitol is given not only for its osmotic diuresis but also to decrease renovascular resistance and provide free radical scavenging. It also increases the glomerular filtration rate during periods of hypoperfusion (27). Vasodilators are given prior to clamping. Most surgeons, ourselves included, favor the use of intraoperative dopamine in low doses for its dopaminergic type 1 effects. Fenoldopam, if available, may be a better drug, as it has no dopaminergic type 2 effects and is known to be protective of the kidney. Heparin is, of course, used for these repairs. With careful dissection and exposure, judicious clamp placement, and an expeditious, well-planned reconstruction, the ischemic insults may be minimized. Further, if prolonged renal ischemic times are anticipated, ice slush may be placed about the kidney. Cold perfusate is used by many authors when possible, as stated above. The visceral vessels may be clamped prior to applying the aortic clamp so as to minimize the chances of atheroembolization, either temporarily if the clamp is juxtarenal or for the formal reconstruction.

In regard to intraoperative cardiac function, there may be real benefit in applying a supramesenteric rather than a supraceliac clamp if the chosen approach and the aortic and branch vessel anatomy will allow. Jean-Claude et al. have pointed out that they had only one death from myocardial infarction (MI) in their series of 257 patients (19). However, 5.8% of their patients sustained an MI. In analyzing the previous papers on pararenal aneurysm repair, they found that MI accounted for 32% of the deaths in those series. In addition to the usual preoperative cardiac assessment and intraoperative management, those authors felt that vasodilation before placement of the aortic cross clamp was important and helped reduced cardiac-related deaths and that the limited use of supraceliac cross-clamping, confined to 13% of their patients, was beneficial to the group. The increased stress on the heart from supraceliac clamping is mitigated in part by the application of a supramesenteric clamp instead, allowing afterload reduction through the mesenteric circulation (28).

Pulmonary dysfunction is another frequent and serious complication of surgery involving the upper abdominal aorta or aortic branch. Messina of the University of California–San Francisco feels it is the greatest risk facing these patients with pararenal aneurysms (Louis Messina, personal communication). In Reilly et al.'s review from that institution of their 108 operations (87 elective) utilizing medial visceral rotation, 31% of the patients had postoperative pulmonary problems and respiratory failure (9). In the follow-up study by Jean-Claude et al., pulmonary complications—respiratory insufficiency and pneumonia—were the most frequent complications, occurring in 14.4% of patients. Pneumonia was the leading complication in the series of Breckwoldt et al. (14), and ventilator dependence for greater than 48 h was the number one complication in the series from Washington University (15). Nypaver et al. reported that it was the primary complication in their patients (16). In our review of 98 patients undergoing open revascularization for chronic mesenteric ischemia, the number one complication was ventilator dependence or tracheostomy; it occurred in 6 patients (4).

Pulmonary insufficiency is much more likely with a thoracoabdominal incision than it is with a purely abdominal approach (9). Patients known preoperatively to have chronic obstructive pulmonary disease (COPD) may be pretreated with mechanical pulmonary toilet and/or steroids if the latter have been shown to be helpful on preoperative pulmonary function testing. Transverse abdominal incisions, postoperative epidural analgesia, and retroperitoneal exposures are all thought to be of benefit to patients with COPD and are used preferentially for patients with known pulmonary compromise at our institution.

Gastrointestinal complications after upper abdominal aortic surgery occur less frequently than either renal or pulmonary complications. One notable exception is documented in the report from Jean-Claude et al. in their review of 257 patients undergoing repair of juxtarenal aneurysms, suprarenal aneurysms, or aneurysms associated with renal artery occlusive disease (19). Visceral ischemia or infarction was the cause of death in 6 (40%) of the 15 patients dying in the postoperative period. Atheroembolization was felt to be the mechanism of injury in 5 and chronic, unoperated mesenteric occlusive disease caused the other death. Valentine et al., at Parkland, studied the problem of gastrointestinal complications in 120 patients following aortic surgery (29). All of their patients were approached transperitoneally. Gastrointestinal complications occurred in 25 (21%), the most frequent problem being ileus requiring replacement of a nasogastric tube. The occurrence of gastrointestinal complications was associated with intraoperative complications, greater than normal blood loss, and the necessity for more fluid resuscitation. There was an increased prevalence of pulmonary and renal complications in these same patients.

That same group looked at pancreatitis following aortic reconstructions (30). They found that 1.8% of their patients undergoing aortic reconstructions of all types experienced pancreatitis. None died from pancreatitis or its complications per se, and those authors felt this to be a rare, self-limited, and seldom serious complication in their patients following aortic surgery. The great majority of their patients were clamped infrarenally. Four patients did develop complications of pancreatitis, with multiple system organ failure in three and pseudocyst in one. All four of those patients had undergone *suprarenal or higher clamping*. In keeping with this fact, Reilly at al. reported pancreatitis in 6 (6.8%) of their 88 patients undergoing medial visceral rotation and suprarenal clamping, and 2 of those 6 died of pancreatitis or its complications (9). It is probable that the combination of ischemia and local trauma attendant on medial visceral rotation (from dissection, mobilization, and retraction) is responsible for that difference. Great care must be taken with the pancreas no matter what approach is used.

Splenic injury with its usual sequela, splenectomy, is reported for both retroperitoneal exposure and medial visceral rotation (9,23). Anecdotally, it occurs occasionally with a transperitoneal approach but not nearly so frequently.

End-organ failure, including liver failure, has been reported with supraceliac clamping (31,32). It relates directly to ischemia time. Patients with hepatic dysfunction or a history of cirrhosis or hepatitis are particularly susceptible to ischemic liver failure. Selective mesenteric shunting is appropriate for patients with types I to III thoracoabdominal aortic aneurysms but is not entirely applicable for patients with pararenal aneurysms (33). Ballard has developed a trifurcated graft technique, with separate grafts to branch vessels in addition to the aortic replacement graft, to reduce ischemic time (34). His principle may be useful for patients with known liver or renal dysfunction if prolonged supraceliac clamping is anticipated.

Pseudoaneurysm, or anastomotic aneurysm, is the most common long-term problem with aortic grafts, occurring in approximately 4–10% of patients (35). Its exact prevalence is not known. When an aggressive follow-up protocol utilizing new imaging modalities is utilized, recurrence may be higher than has been suspected.

Patients having had thoracic aneurysms repaired are much more likely to develop a subsequent true or false aneurysm than patients whose first operation was for infrarenal aortic aneurysm (35). Whether patients with juxta- or suprarenal aneurysms are more prone to develop pseudoaneurysms than patients with infrarenal aneurysms is not known. Obviously, follow-up for grafts with proximal anastomoses above the level of the renal arteries requires serial computed tomography rather than ultrasound.

Hallett et al., in a population-based study of 307 patients from Olmsted County, Minnesota, having abdominal aortic aneurysm repairs, found graft-related complications in 29 (9.4%) (36). Their study extended out to 36 years with an average follow-up of 5.8 years. Anastomotic pseudoaneurysms occurred in 3%, graft thrombosis in 2%, graft enteric fistulas in 1.6%, infection in 1.3% and other complications in lesser numbers. Biancari et al. from Finland performed a retrospective study of 208 abdominal aortic aneurysm patients operated upon at one hospital and found that there were late graft complications in a very similar 15.4% of their patients (37). Para-aortic anastomic aneurysms developed 2.9%, more distal aneurysms in 8.7%, and bilateral or recurring aneurysms in 3.4%. Their follow-up ranged from 0.1–21.7 years with a median of 8.0 years.

The repair of recurrent juxtarenal aneurysms is attended by higher morbidity and mortality than is primary reconstruction (35).

IV. CONCLUSIONS

Successful operative management of the pararenal aorta and the visceral branches requires thoughtful preoperative planning and meticulous operative technique to reduce the inherent morbidity and mortality to the minimum. Accurate preoperative assessment of the quality of the aorta, especially of the extent and pattern of atherosclerosis in the paravisceral area on the back wall, is probably the single most important step in providing a safe and effective operation upon the pararenal aorta. Lateral views of the aorta, by either conventional angiography or high-resolution reconstructed computed tomography, are mandatory. In closing, I can do no better than to quote as follows:

1. Careful consideration of the route of exposure, location of the proximal aortic clamp, and the preservation of renal function with renal hypothermia and with the repair of significant renal artery lesions will result in minimal morbidity and mortality in patients requiring surgery for juxtarenal with suprarenal abdominal aortic aneurysms (15).

2. Accurate preoperative assessment of the amount of disease in the aorta at the planned level of cross-clamping, correct selection of the optimal cross-clamp level, selection of the optimal approach for the needed exposure, and following the proper clamping and declamping sequence for the aorta and visceral branches are all important factors in reducing the incidence rate of atheroembolization (19).

3. It is the patient whose cross-clamp level is incorrectly chosen who has the highest likelihood of significant complications, usually atheroembolic and often fatal (19).

REFERENCES

1. Taylor SM, Mills JL, Fujitani RM. The juxtarenal abdominal aortic aneurysm. Arch Surg 1994; 129:734–737.
2. Sarac TP, Clair DG, Hertzer NR, et al. Contemporary results of juxtarenal aneurysm repair. J Vasc Surg 2002; 36:1104–1111.
3. Kasirajan K, O'Hara PG, Gray BH, et al. Chronic mesenteric ischemia: Open surgery versus percutaneous angioplasty and stenting. J Vasc Surg 2001; 33:63–67.

4. Park WM, Cherry KJ Jr, Chua HK, et al. Current results of open revascularization for chronic mesenteric ischemia: A standard for comparison. J Vasc Surg 2002; 35:853–859.
5. Anderson JL, Berce M, Hartley DE. Endoluminal aortic grafting with renal and superior mesenteric artery incorporation by graft fenestration. J Endovasc Ther 2001; 8(1):3–15.
6. Faruqi RM, Chuter TA, Reilly LM, et al. Endovascular repair of abdominal aortic aneurysm using a pararenal fenestrated stent-graft. J Endovasc Surg 1999; 6(4):354–358.
7. Chuter TA, Gordon RL, Reilly LM, et al. An endovascular system for thoracoabdominal aortic aneurysm repair. J Endovasc Ther 2001; 8(1):25–33.
8. Burks JA, Faries PL, Gravereaux EC, et al. Endovascular repair of abdominal aortic aneurysms: Stent-graft fixation across the visceral arteries. J Vasc Surg 2002; 35:109–113.
9. Reilly LM, Ramos TK, Murray SP, et al. Optimal exposure of the proximal abdominal aorta: A critical appraisal of transabdominal medial visceral rotation. J Vasc Surg 1994; 19:375–390.
10. Crawford ES, Beckett WC, Greer MS. Juxtarenal infrarenal abdominal aortic aneurysm. Special diagnostic and therapeutic considerations. Ann Surg 1986; 203:661–670.
11. Qvarfordt PG, Stoney RJ, Reilly LM, et al. Management of pararenal aneurysm of the abdominal aorta. J Vasc Surg 1986; 3:84–93.
12. Green RM, Ricotta JJ, Ouriel K, DeWeese JA. Results of supraceliac aortic clamping in the difficult elective resection of infrarenal abdominal aortic aneurysm. J Vasc Surg 1989; 9:124–134.
13. Poulias GE, Doundoulakis N, Skoutas B, et al. Juxtarenal aortic aneurysmectomy. J Cardiovasc Surg 1992; 3:324–330.
14. Breckwoldt WL, Mackey WC, Belkin M, O'Donnell TJ Jr. The effect of suprarenal cross-clamping on abdominal aortic aneurysm repair. Arch Surg 1992; 127:520–524.
15. Allen BT, Anderson CB, Rubin BG, et al. Preservation of renal function in juxtarenal and suprarenal abdominal aortic aneurysm repair. J Vasc Surg 1993; 17:984–959.
16. Nypaver TJ, Shepard AD, Reddy DJ, et al. Repair of pararenal abdominal aortic aneurysms. An analysis of operative management. Arch Surg 1993; 128:803–813.
17. Schneider JR, Gottner RJ, Golan JF. Supraceliac versus infrarenal aortic cross-clamp for repair of nonruptured infrarenal and juxtarenal abdominal aortic aneurysm. Cardiovasc Surg 1997; 5:279–285.
18. Faggioli G, Stella A, Freyrie A, et al. Early and long-term results in the surgical treatment of juxtarenal and pararenal aortic aneurysms. Eur J Vasc Endovasc Surg 1998; 15:205–211.
19. Jean-Claude JM, Reilly LM, Stoney RJ, Messina LM. Pararenal aortic aneurysms: The future of open aortic aneurysm repair. J Vasc Surg 1999; 29:902–912.
20. Tordoir JHM, van de Pavoordt HDWM, Eikelboom BC, et al. Thoraco-abdominal aortic approach for the treatment of pararenal aneurysm. Neth J Med 1988; 40:1–5.
21. Shepard AD, Scott GR, Mackey WC, et al. Retroperitoneal approach to high-risk abdominal aortic aneurysms. Arch Surg 1986; 121:444–448.
22. Shepard AD, Tollefson DF, Reddey DJ, et al. Left flank retroperitoneal exposure: A technical aid to complex aortic reconstruction. J Vasc Surg 1991; 14:283–291.
23. Darling RC III, Shah DM, Chang BB, et al. Retroperitoneal approach for bilateral renal and visceral artery revascularization. Am J of Surg 1994; 168(2):148–151.
24. Elmore JR, Hallett JW Jr, Gibbons RJ, et al. Myocardial revascularization before abdominal aortic aneurysmorrhaphy: Effect of coronary angioplasty. Mayo Clin Proc 1993; 68:637–641.
25. Kashyap VS, Cambria RP, Davison JK, L'Italien GJ. Renal failure after thoracoabdominal aortic Surgery. J Vasc Surg 1997; 26:949–957.
26. Welborn BM, Oldenburg HS, Hess PJ, et al. The relationship between visceral ischemia, proinflammatory cytokines, and organ injury in patients undergoing thoracoabdominal aortic aneurysm repair. Crit Care Med 2000; 28:3191–3197.
27. Cherr SG, Hansen KJ. Renal complications with aortic surgery. Semin Vasc Surg 2001; 14(4):245–254.
28. Roizen MF, Beaupre PN, Alpert RA, et al. Monitoring with two-dimensional transesophageal echocardiography: Comparison of myocardial function in patients undergoing supraceliac, suprarenal-infraceliac, or infrarenal aortic occlusion. J Vasc Surg 1984; 1:300–305.

29. Valentine RJ, Hagina RT, Jackson RM, et al. Gastrointestinal complications after aortic surgery. J Vasc Surg 1998; 28:404–412.
30. Burkey SH, Valentine RJ, Jackson MR, et al. Acute pancreatitis after abdominal vascular surgery. J Am Coll Surg 2000; 191:373–380.
31. Harward TRS, Brooks DL, Flynn TC, Seeger JM. J Vasc Surg 1993; 18:459–469.
32. Harward TRS, Welborne MB III, Martin TD, et al. Visceral ischemia and organ dysfunction after thoracoabdominal aortic aneurysm repair. A clinical and cost analysis. Ann of Surg 1996; 223(6):729–736.
33. Cambria RP, Davison JK, Giglia JS, Gertler JP. Mesenteric shunting decreases visceral ischemia during thoracoabdominal aneurysm repair. J Vasc Surg 1998; 27:745–749.
34. Ballard JL. Thoracoabdominal aortic aneurysm repair with sequential visceral perfusion: A technical note. Ann Vasc Surg 1999; 13:216–221.
35. Cherry KJ. Techniques in the management of recurrent aortic aneurysm. In: Yao JST, Pearce WH, eds. Aneurysms: New Findings and Treatments. Norwalk, CT: Appleton & Langee, 1994:249–258.
36. Hallett JW Jr, Marshall DM, Petterson TM, et al. Graft-related complications after abdominal aortic aneurysm repair: Reassurance from a 36-year- population-based experience. J Vasc Surg 1997; 25:277–286.
37. Biancari F, Ylönen K, Anttila V, et al. Durability of open repair of infrarenal abdominal aortic aneurysm: A 15-year follow-up study. J Vasc Surg 2002; 35:87–93.

13

Complications of Modern Renal Revascularization

Jeffry D. Cardneau and Louis M. Messina

University of California, San Francisco, San Francisco, California, U.S.A.

Renovascular hypertension due to renal artery occlusive disease is the most common cause of secondary hypertension (1,2). Its prevalence in both the general population and the hypertensive population is not known precisely, with estimates ranging from 0.18 (3) to 5% (4,5) of the hypertensive population to 3% of the general population (6). Renal artery occlusive disease may be responsible for up to 16% of patients with end-stage renal disease, and its prevalence appears to be increasing (7). The vast majority of renal artery occlusive disease causing hypertension is due to atherosclerosis, ranging from 67 to 97.8% (8–12).

The benefits of renal revascularization for renovascular hypertension have been known for several decades. A study from the Mayo Clinic published 30 years ago showed that patients who underwent surgical management of hypertension had better long-term survival than did those treated by drug therapy alone. A total of 84% of the surgical group but only 66% of the drug therapy group were alive at a follow-up of 7–14 years (13). Modern-day renal revascularization includes percutaneous renal angioplasty alone, percutaneous angioplasty with stenting, and traditional open surgical techniques. All techniques have associated complications. These complications can, for simplicity, be placed into three categories. These are errors in patient selection, periprocedural complications, and late complications. Late complications should include not only technical problems but also failure to maintain clinical benefit for which the procedure was performed. However, documentation of the durability of improved control of hypertension and preservation of renal function is beyond the scope of this chapter. Therefore this topic is not dealt with here.

I. PATIENT SELECTION

Renal artery stenosis does not inevitably lead to renovascular hypertension. Renal artery stenosis is present in up to 4% of unselected patients and up to 16% of hypertensive patients undergoing aortography (14). Indeed, renal artery stenosis may be present in up to 40% of new cases of end-stage renal disease in the elderly (15). Its mere presence does not establish cause and effect. One study discovered that 45–60% of autopsies of both normotensive and hypertensive patients showed the presence of renal artery stenosis (15). Thus, it is imperative that an appropriate algorithm be employed to identify patients for revascularization. A recent prospective trial failed to show the superiority of angioplasty over best-drug therapy in the management of what was believed to be renovascular hypertension (16). This failure of renal angioplasty in the management may have been due to poor patient selection. Improper patient selection for renal revascularization can expose patients to serious, life-threatening complications. Clinical clues that renal artery stenosis may be the cause of hypertension include abrupt onset of hypertension, particularly at the extremes of age; recently accelerated or malignant hypertension; hypertension refractory to medication (usually at least three medications); unexplained azotemia in the setting of hypertension; azotemia induced by angiotensin-converting enzyme (ACE) inhibitors; or hypertension in a patient with diffuse atherosclerotic disease (coronary, carotid, or peripheral) (1,17). Renovascular hypertension is usually severe, such that there is a low likelihood that a patient with a diastolic blood pressure below 95 mmHg has this process (6). Additionally, an episode of pulmonary edema in a patient with poorly controlled hypertension and renal insufficiency should prompt investigation for the diagnosis of bilateral renal artery stenosis (18).

Some studies have found demographic differences in the prevalence of renovascular hypertension, with a low occurrence in African Americans. In one study of 45 patients with new end-stage renal disease, all 10 patients with renal artery stenosis (RAS) were white while none were African-American (19). Data from the Health Care Finance Administration (HCFA) show that renovascular disease progressing to renal failure is present more commonly in whites than in African Americans at a ratio of 14:1 (20). While these differences may be present in the select population of patients with RAS progressing to end-stage renal disease, the most recent literature suggests that RAS itself shows no ethnic predilection (21).

Arteriography has traditionally been the "gold standard" for the diagnosis of RAS. Certain arteriographic findings are present in renovascular hypertension. These include the presence of collateral vessels and a systolic pressure gradient across the stenosis of at least 10 mmHg (2). It is generally agreed that an angiographic stenosis of about 70% is hemodynamically significant (22). This degree of stenosis corresponds to an approximate 40% drop of renal perfusion pressure, which is necessary to cause a decrease in the glomerular filtration rate (GFR) (15). However, several noninvasive studies have been used successfully to select patients who might benefit from revascularization. Duplex ultrasonography has proven sensitive, with numerous groups reporting sensitivity of greater that 93% (23,24). Duplex criteria for stenosis are listed elsewhere (23). A ratio of peak systolic velocities in the renal artery and aorta of at least 3.5:1 and a peak systolic renal artery velocity of at least 180 cm/s strongly suggests a stenosis of 60% or more. Ultrasonography may be even more useful in determining patients who will benefit from revascularization when using the resistive index (RI) of at least 0.8 as an exclusionary criterion (25). The latter suggests intrinsic renal disease as the cause of renal insufficiency.

Measurement of plasma renin activity after ACE inhibition is another method to diagnose clinically significant RAS. Baseline renin activity is measured, followed by the administration of 25 mg of captopril. Plasma renin activity (PRA) is measured again at 60 min. Accordingly, a post-captopril PRA of greater than 12 ng/mL/h, an increase in PRA of more than 10 ng/mL/h, or an increase of 150% from baseline was highly suggestive of renovascular hypertension (26). The sensitivity and specificity was 100 and 95%, respectively (4). Others have not shown such reliable results. Captopril renal scintigraphy may be a more sensitive study (27). Renal scintigraphy takes advantage of the decreased glomerular filtration rate of radiotracer after the administration of ACE inhibitor. Diagnostic criteria for significant RAS include a delayed time of maximal activity of radiotracer greater than 11 min after captopril, asymmetry of peak activity of each kidney, marked cortical retention of radionuclide after captopril, and marked reduction in the calculated GFR of the kidney (4). Sensitivity ranges from 90 to 93%, while specificity ranges from about 93 to 100%. Since this test takes advantage of differential radionuclide activity due to the stenotic renal artery, its positive predictive value decreases in the setting of bilateral RAS and in patients with moderate renal insufficiency.

Magnetic resonance angiography (MRA), although considerably more expensive than ultrasound, may become the noninvasive procedure of choice for the diagnosis of renovascular occlusive disease and preprocedure planning. Recent series cite sensitivities of 93–100% and specificities of 88–100% when both 3D gadolinium-enhanced and 3D phase-contrast sequences are used (28). Another advantage of MRA for this purpose is the ability to image the aorta and its branches in order to define options for open surgical treatment.

II. PERIPROCEDURAL COMPLICATIONS

A. Percutaneous Procedures

When Gruntzig introduced percutaneous transluminal angioplasty (PTA) of the renal arteries in 1978, a new treatment modality for renovascular hypertension was established. While angioplasty alone has been highly successful for fibromuscular disease (1), it has led to more disappointing results for atherosclerotic lesions, which are far more common. For this reason, angioplasty followed by stent deployment is now more common. Although renal angioplasty and/or stenting is successful technically in the large majority of patients, its overall effectiveness in the management of renovascular hypertension has been questioned. As mentioned previously, the only such prospective randomized trial failed to show renal angioplasty to be more effective than best drug therapy in the management of hypertension (16). Complications for both angioplasty alone and angioplasty with stenting are addressed together below (Table 1), with a few exceptions. Fundamental to the process of transluminal angioplasty is cracking the intimal and medial layers of the artery. Thus, by definition, there will be a dissection at the end of a technically successful procedure. It is only when the arterial wall does not remain compressed that this dissection become flow-limiting and becomes a complication. Usually, when an arterial (flow-limiting) dissection or occlusion occurs, a guidewire is still in place. This complication can almost always be remedied with placement of a stent. Some would therefore argue that these are not complications. The need for unplanned stent placement for dissection or occlusion occurs in 1–3% of renal PTA procedures (5, 29–31). Additionally, PTA can fail technically due to elastic recoil of the vessels, requiring stenting to reduce the stenosis. This is especially common in atherosclerotic ostial lesions occurring in 12–38% of lesions (17,30,32). Rarely, rigid, calcified stenoses are encountered that cannot be dilated by the angioplasty balloon. Other complications in percutaneous procedures are common to both PTA alone and stenting; they are therefore described here collectively. Several studies have shown that the rate of total complications is not significantly different from PTA alone and PTA with

Table 1 Approximate Cited Ranges of Complications After Percutaneous Transluminal Renal Revascularization

Overall	4–50 %
"Minor"	4.5–48
"Major"	5–17
Local	
Hematoma	4–21
Retroperitoneal hematoma	0–6.8
Pseudoaneurysm	0–9.5
Occlusion of access vessel	<1
Femoral arteriorvenous fistula	0–1.6
Renal	
Initial technical failure	<2
Artery dissection	0–2.4
Artery/stent occlusion	0–4.8
Artery pseudo/aneurysm	0–1.5
Transient renal failure	3.4–21
Prolonged azotemia	2
Stent maldeployment	0.2–2.4
Artery perforation/extravasation	0–6.9
Perinephric hematoma	<1.1
Cholesterol atheroemboli	1–8
Need for emergency nephrectomy	<1
Systemic	
Hemorrhage requiring transfusion	0–9.5
Sepsis	<1
Aortic dissection	Rare
Stroke	0–3.3
Myocardial infarction	0–9
Distal emboli (eg: limbs or other organs)	0.1–1.1
Mortality	1

stenting, with incidences ranging from 4.4–50% (5,11,14,29–31,33–40). A recent met-analysis comparing 644 PTA patients with 678 stented patients showed an overall complication rate of 13% for PTA and 11% for stenting (41). Many have subdivided these rates into "major" and "minor" complications, minor complications being exemplified by groin hematomas and major complications including stroke and renal infarction. Reported minor complication rates range from about 4.5–48%, while major complication rates occur in about 5–17% of reported series. Complications have also been previously grouped into three categories: local, renal-related, and systemic (42). This classification is maintained here.

1. Local Complications

These complications are related to the percutaneous access that is required for these procedures. Some of these complications may be minimized using ultrasound guidance for puncture as well as the use of micropuncture techniques with small-gauge needles and coaxial dilating systems.

    Hematoma is often the most common complication listed in series related to transluminal techniques. This usually occurs after the removal of the sheath or catheter. The frequency of this complication can be reduced by using diligent pinpoint digital pressure on the artery entry site. The use of sandbags and diffuse pressure, as with a large pack of gauze, are to be discouraged. The reported incidence is about 4–21%.

In addition to local hematoma formation, retroperitoneal hematomas can occur when the femoral artery is accessed. This often is due to a puncture that is inadvertently high, in the external iliac artery rather than the common femoral artery. This inadvertent puncture thus lies above the inguinal ligament and poses difficulty in compression at the end of the procedure. The incidence of retroperitoneal hematoma may be as high as 6.8%. Pseudoaneurysms can occur at the puncture site, which may require surgical repair. However, smaller, stable pseudoaneurysms can be managed conservatively or with ultrasound-guided compression and thrombin injection. The reported incidence of pseudoaneurysm ranges from 0 to 10%.

Occlusion of the access artery is possible, especially in this setting of patients who have atherosclerosis of the punctured vessel. This can occur in the femoral artery, the iliac artery in which the access sheath is positioned, or the brachial artery when an upper extremity approach is used. Occlusion rates are reduced in modern series with the use of periprocedural heparinization and smaller delivery catheters. Stents of the size appropriate for renal vessels can almost always be delivered on a 5F catheter or smaller and delivered through 5F or 6F sheaths. The incidence of occlusion is less than 1%.

Acute ischemia of a lower limb—or arm in the case of a brachial artery access—can be due to thrombosis of the access vessel, as discussed above, but it also may due to vessel dissection or emboli to the limb. Although rare, acute limb ischemia occurred in 4.1% of patients in one study (43).

2. Renal-Related Complications

These complications are those distant to the percutaneous access site and are related to wire, catheter, or stent manipulation. Dissection of the renal artery is due either to the balloon angioplasty performed (see above) or to a subintimal placement of the guidewire tip during cannulation of the vessel. This dissection may be of no hemodynamic significance but can propagate to cause segmental renal infarction or even complete artery occlusion. Propagation of the dissection can also proceed proximally (Fig. 1). With the more routine use of stents, dissection is less common now than in series of PTA alone. Series report an incidence of dissection with stenting ranging from zero to 2.4% (11,30,31,33,37,43).

Renal artery occlusion can be the result of artery dissection or acute thrombosis due to manipulation, cracking of the atherosclerotic plaque, or the stent placement itself. Systemic heparin is usually given during the procedure; thus acute occlusion is rare. Occlusion occurs in zero–4.8% of cases (30,34,35,37,43). Where it has occurred, it has sometimes been successfully treated with thrombolytics, whereas in other instances an urgent surgical repair was required (37).

Another renal-related complication is impairment of renal function. This can be due to multiple mechanisms. Impaired renal function can manifest itself as a postprocedure rise in serum creatinine, sometimes progressing to dialysis-dependent renal failure. Fortunately, dialysis dependent renal failure is usually transient. Impaired renal function occurs in 3.4–21% of patients (14,30,33,35). In Leertouwer's metanalysis, procedure-related renal failure occurred in 34 of 799 treated arteries (4.2%) (41). Postulated mechanisms for postprocedural renal failure include contrast-induced injury, sudden onset of high pressure within the glomeruli, development of reactive oxygen species after revascularization, and renal atheroemboli from traversing the lesion. Eosinophilia greater

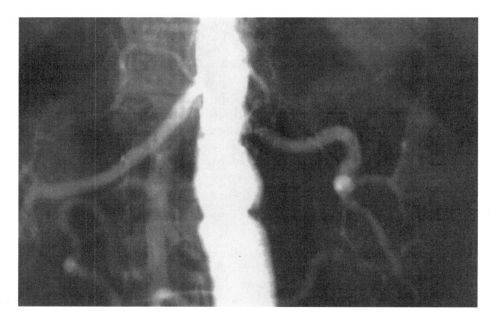

(A)

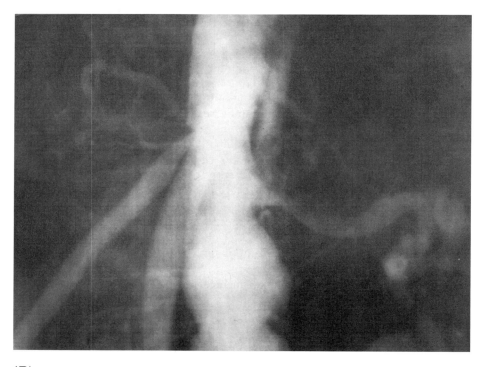

(B)

than 5% of a peripheral blood smear may indicate that significant cholesterol emboli have occurred (44). Large randomized trials are required to determine whether distal embolic protection during PTA and stenting actually has an impact on outcomes and on long-term preservation of renal function.

Late restenosis is a common problem after stenting using current technology. Restenosis is due to myointimal hyperplasia or progression of atherosclerotic disease. However, myointimal hyperplasia is more likely, as stent restenosis occurs within a relatively short time span. Some authors have claimed that most restenosis, if it occurs, will take place within the first year (31). However, others have found this not to be true (37). Stent restenosis rates range from 9.3 to 44% at 6 months–1 year (11,14,17,30,31,37,40,45) to 11.4–55% at 2 years (45,46). Leertouwer's metanalysis found a mean stent restenosis rate of 17% in a follow-up of 6–29 months (41). Primary assisted patency, during close surveillance, is approximately 80–100% (14,30,34,35,37) (Fig. 2). Lederman's review emphasizes the importance of vessel size in restenosis, with rates (at a mean of 303 days) of 36.0, 15.8, and 6.5% for vessels less than 4.5 mm, 4.5–6 mm, and larger than 6 mm, respectively (11). Stent restenosis may be reduced with such technological advances as drug-eluting stents, which are the subject of several ongoing trials.

3. Systemic Complications

With the knowledge that the majority of these patients have a diffuse form of atherosclerosis, it is not surprising that systemic complications occur. Myocardial infarction, stroke, sepsis, and emboli to other vessels all occur, but uncommonly in the percutaneous procedure. Emboli to other vessels, when they do occur, most commonly travel to the lower extremities, manifesting themselves as claudication, the blue toe syndrome, or frankly ischemic digits. Other sites of emboli have included the superior mesenteric artery.

Death has occurred as a result of transluminal procedures, but this is rare. Causes of death include massive hemorrhage from puncture sites; profound systemic complications such as massive myocardial infarction, stroke, or bowel infarction; and consequences of acute renal failure. Thirty-day mortality rates are as high as 3.8% (14,29,33,34). The mean mortality rate is 1% (41). A preoperative serum creatinine of more than 1.5 mg/dL is a strong independent risk factor of death in the years after stenting (33). This risk is five times higher than that of patients with creatinine below 1.5 mg/dL and most likely represents the severity of associated comorbidities (17). This is reinforced by studies showing that patients on hemodialysis with end-stage renal disease due to RAS have a poorer survival than patients with end-stage renal disease due to other causes (47).

B. Surgical Procedures

Surgical revascularization for renovascular hypertension dates back to 1952, when Wylie performed the first renal artery endarterectomy (48,49). Since that time, techniques of renal revascularization have evolved, along with the rest of vascular surgery. A wide vari-

---

Figure 1 A. A 55 year-old woman undergoing angiography for claudication. She also had two-drug hypertension. A left renal artery ostial stenosis was noted, and PTA was performed with a 6-mm balloon. B. After the PTA. A dissection is noted propagating proximally in the aorta. This dissection progressed up to the left subclavian artery. As this occurred prior to the advent of stents, this patient was managed on an aggressive oral antihypertensive regimen.

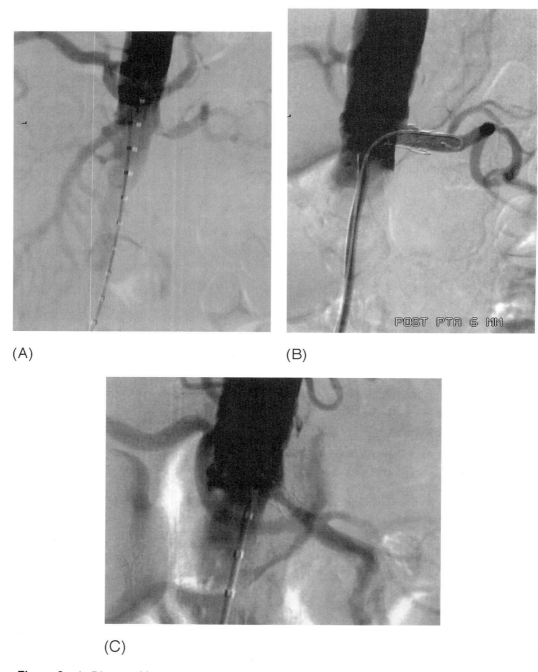

(A)

(B)

(C)

Figure 2   A. 74-year-old man with an occluded right renal artery and a stenosis of left renal artery. B. The same patient after successful placement of a 6-mm Palmaz stent. C. Restenosis noted 4 months after stent deployment. This was diagnosed by ultrasonography ordered in response to a new rise in serum creatinine. D. Successful reopening of stent restenosis with repeat balloon angioplasty.

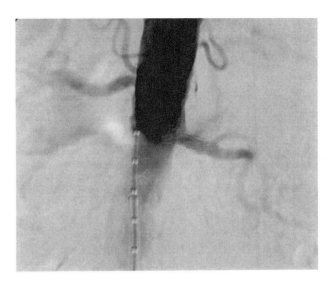

(D)

Figure 2 Continued.

ety of surgical approaches have been used in this setting based on the etiology of the RAS, patient comorbidities, the need for concomitant operations, and even regional geographic preferences. The occurrence of open surgical revascularization has declined, while percutaneous interventions have markedly risen. Based on charges submitted to Medicare from 1995 to 2001, open renovascular operations have declined by 45%, while stenting has increased over 350% (50). Nonetheless, surgical repair will continue to have a role, particularly in younger patients, after the failure of stenting and after complications encountered because of stenting. The durability of transaortic renal endarterectomy and aortorenal bypass has been well established. For good-risk patients and patients who require concomitant aortic reconstruction, these will remain the procedures of choice.

Overall complications range from 9.1 to 37.9% (9,10,12,17,29,35,40,48,51–56). Complications related to open renovascular repair can be categorized, analogously to percutaneous procedures, into renal-related and systemic (Table 2). Further, special consideration must be given to the type of operation performed and its attendant complications.

1. Renal-Related Complications

When all types of renal revascularization operations are examined collectively, the early revascularization failure rate is approximately 5% (57) (Fig. 3). The need for transient postoperative dialysis ranges from zero to 10.2% (52,58). Long-term permanent dialysis is significantly dependent on the degree of preoperative renal function. In a recent study, Tsoukas showed an outcome difference between the groups of patients with serum creatinine less than 2.0 mg/dL and those with creatinine greater than 2.0 mg/dL. Long-term dialysis for these two groups was 2.3 versus 12%, respectively (52).

Aortorenal Bypass. Aortorenal bypass can be performed with a variety of conduits. Autogenous vein, hypogastric artery, and prosthetic all have been used with essentially

Table 2 Approximate Cited Ranges of Complications After Open
Surgical Renal Revascularization

Overall	9.1–37.9%
Renal	
Distal intimal flap requiring repair	4–5
Artery occlusion	1–3.4
Transient worsening of renal function	4.6–43
requiring dialysis	≈5
Prolonged azotemia	1.5–12
Early graft failure	2.1–17.6
Late graft failure	1.8–18
Systemic	
Postoperative hemorrhage	1.5–3.4
Multisystem organ failure	4.6
Sepsis	<1
Respiratory failure or pneumonia	0.9–25
Stroke	0–3.3
Myocardial infarction	2–8.6
Distal emboli (eg: limbs or other organs)	2.2–6.9
Limb ischemia	4.5
Mortality overall	0–7.1
Mortality (isolated renal revascularization)	0–7.0
Mortality (with concomitant aortic repair)	1–9.2

similar long-term results (10,57). A key reason for the long-term success of these grafts is that 20% of the total cardiac output goes to the renal bed, which is also of low vascular resistance. Early graft failure occurs in approximately 5% of modern series at most and almost certainly represents technical problems of the graft (12,59). Examples include inadequate spatulation of the anastomosis, purse-stringing the anastomosis, uncorrected intimal flaps, and placement of an excessively long graft, leading to kinking (59). Bypass with saphenous vein can be complicated by aneurysmal degeneration. In Stanley's series of 100 consecutive saphenous aortorenal grafts, 6 of 74 grafts (8.1%) examined late had aneurysmal expansion (60). However, the large majority—in some series, all (59)—of these grafts with aneurysmal dilatation occurred in children, with this problem being very rare in the adult patient. Thus, this conduit is generally not considered an appropriate revascularization technique in children (60–62).

Late graft stenosis can be heralded by worsening of previously improved renal function or recurrence of hypertension. However, late graft stenosis can also be asymptomatic. Conversely, clinical deterioration can occur without graft failure or stenosis (51). Nonetheless, noted clinical deterioration of glomerular filtration rate or hypertension

Figure 3 A. MRA of a 55-year-old woman after thoraco-bi-iliac bypass. Note a graft-to–renal artery bypass arising from the main body of the aortic graft as well as a separate bypass from the right iliac limb to a second renal artery. B. MRA of the same patient approximately 6 months later. There is now occlusion of the bypass graft arising from the aortic graft to the main renal artery. C. Aortography confirms the MRA finding of the occluded renal bypass.

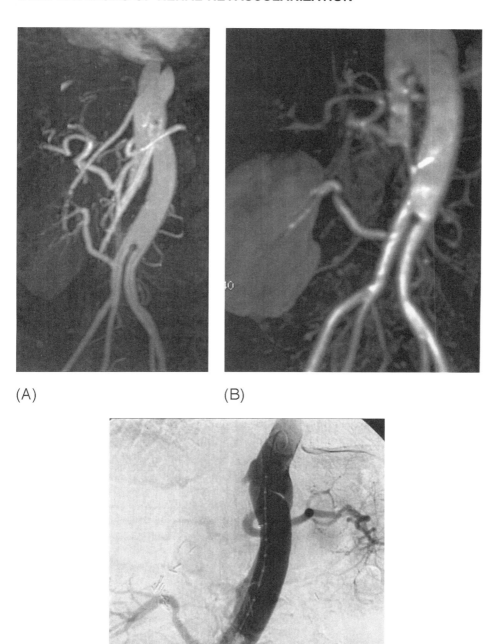

(A)

(B)

(C)

control should prompt investigation of the graft with duplex ultrasound, MRA, or angiography. Late graft stenosis occurs in 1.3–19% of grafts (9,52,53,59,60). Graft stenosis can often be successfully treated by PTA (Fig. 4).

Transaortic Renal Endarterectomy. Although endarterectomy has been described being performed through an arteriotomy of the renal artery itself, the preferred method now is through either a longitudinal or transverse aortotomy, in which a diffuse atherosclerotic plaque can potentially be excised from the renal arteries, the paravisceral aorta, and mesenteric arteries if necessary.

Endarterectomy can be performed on occluded arteries provided that there is reconstitution of the main renal artery (55). Additionally, endarterectomy has been successfully performed after restenosis of bilateral renal artery stenting (63). Conversion from endarterectomy to another procedure, such as direct reimplantation of the artery or bypass graft, occurs because of aortic or arterial fragility after endarterectomy. This conversion rate is approximately 6.5% (55). An intimal flap in the endpoint of the endarterectomized renal artery has been noted to occur in almost 50% of arteries when surveyed by duplex ultrasonography, but this manifests itself as a hemodynamic problem in only about 4% of vessels (48), as has been confirmed in other studies (55,64). When necessary, a transverse renal arteriotomy just distal to the flap is sufficient to resect the flap and restore normal renal flow.

Nonanatomic Renal Artery Bypass. Nonanatomical bypass for renovascular hypertension is becoming more common (17). This may be intuitive in light of studies showing that the mean age of patients is increasing, as is the prevalence of atherosclerosis of the diffuse type (9). These operations include bypass grafts arising from the hepatic, splenic, or mesenteric vessels as well as the iliac arteries. However, it is important to remember that these patients may have concomitant disease of the origins of their visceral vessels, precluding the possibility of splenorenal or hepatorenal bypasses. Advantages of iliorenal bypasses include the ability to avoid aortic cross-clamping and thus avoiding increases in afterload in patients with impaired cardiac function. Additionally, clamping of a diffusely calcified aorta can be obviated. Iliorenal bypasses can be performed with either an autogenous or a prosthetic conduit. A recent review of 323 renal artery revascularizations showed no difference in early or long-term patency between aortorenal and nonanatomic bypass (57), with 5-year patency of 88.7 versus 82.1%, respectively.

2. Systemic Complications

Other complications cited include many of those expected after a major intra-abdominal procedure, such as postoperative hemorrhage, multisystem organ failure, sepsis, respiratory failure, pneumonia, stroke, and myocardial infarction.

Thirty-day mortality ranges from zero to 7.9% for all procedures combined (9,48,51–53,55,57,58,64). There does not appear to be a consensus on whether there is a significant difference in mortality between those patients receiving isolated renal revascularization and those also receiving a concomitant aortic repair (10,12,57,58).

One recurrent significant risk factor for perioperative mortality is poor preoperative renal function. One study of 73 patients divided them into those with creatinine below 2.0 mg/dL and those with higher levels; these groups had surgery-related mortalities of 4.4 versus 14% respectively (52). Similar analyses of other series confirmed this difference, using 3.0 mg/dL as the dividing line (58). Hansen and colleagues found that 22 of 26 late deaths in a group of 200 patients followed over the long term (up to 58 months) were patients who had preoperative levels of serum creatinine greater than 2.0 mg/dL. This was

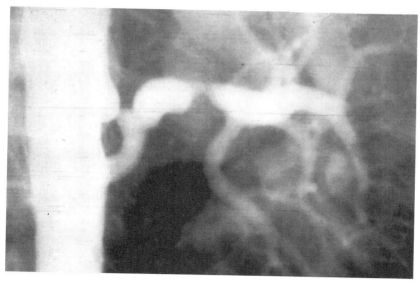

(A)

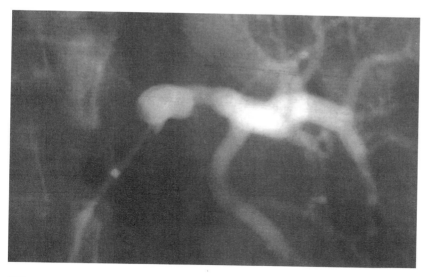

(B)

Figure 4 A. 58-year-old woman 6 months after placement of an aortorenal bypass using the hypogastric artery. A stenosis of the distal anastomosis is now evident. B. The same patient after successful PTA of the distal anastomotic stenosis.

the only preoperative risk factor statistically associated with mortality (53). Additionally, 20 of these 22 patients did not have a postoperative improvement in renal function.

The survival of such patients in general is poor and reflects the severe systemic comorbidities. Actuarial survival after renal revascularization ranges from 61 to 81% at 5 years (8,56,58,65,66). Cardiovascular causes of death, not surprisingly, are most common (53,58), followed by stroke, renal failure, and malignancy (8).

REFERENCES

1. Messina LM, Stanley JC. Renal artery fibrodysplasia and renovascular hypertension. In: Rutherford RB, eds. Vascular Surgery. Philadelphia: Saunders, 2000:1650–1664.
2. Upchurch GR Jr, Stanley JC. Renal artery occlusive disease. In: Greenfield LJ, Mulholland MW, Oldham KT, Zelenock GB, Lillemoe KD, eds. Surgery: Scientific Principles and Practice. Philadelphia: Lippincott Williams & Wilkins, 2001:1708–1724.
3. Tucker RM, Labarthe DR. Frequency of surgical treatment for hypertension in adults at the Mayo Clinic from 1973 through 1975. Mayo Clin Proc 1977; 52:549–555.
4. Nally JV Jr. Provocative captopril testing in the diagnosis of renovascular hypertension. Urol Clin North Am 1994; 21:227–234.
5. Xue F, Bettmann MA, Langdon DR, Wivell WA. Outcome and cost comparison of percutaneous transluminal renal angioplasty, renal arterial stent placement, and renal arterial bypass grafting. Radiology 1999; 212:378–384.
6. Hansen KJ, Wong JM. Aortorenal bypass for renovascular hypertension in adults. In: Stanley JC, Ernst CB, eds. Current Therapy in Vascular Surgery. St. Louis: Mosby, 2001:735–741.
7. Fatica RA, Port FK, Young EW. Incidence trends and mortality in end-stage renal disease attributed to renovascular disease in the United States. Am J Kidney Dis 2001; 37:1184–1190.
8. Steinbach F, Novick AC, Campbell S, Dykstra D. Long-term survival after surgical revascularization for atherosclerotic renal artery disease. J Urol 1997; 158:38–41.
9. Novick AC, Ziegelbaum M, Vidt DG, Gifford RW Jr, Pohl MA, Goormastic M. Trends in surgical revascularization for renal artery disease. Ten years' experience. JAMA 1987; 257:498–501.
10. Lawrie GM, Morris GC Jr, Glaeser DH, DeBakey ME. Renovascular reconstruction: factors affecting long-term prognosis in 919 patients followed up to 31 years. Am J Cardiol 1989; 63:1085–1092.
11. Lederman RJ, Mendelsohn FO, Santos R, Phillips HR, Stack RS, Crowley JJ. Primary renal artery stenting: Characteristics and outcomes after 363 procedures. Am Heart J 2001; 142:314–323.
12. Bredenberg CE, Sampson LN, Ray FS, Cormier RA, Heintz S, Eldrup-Jorgensen J. Changing patterns in surgery for chronic renal artery occlusive diseases. J Vasc Surg 1992; 15:1018–1023.
13. Hunt JC, Strong CG. Renovascular hypertension. Mechanisms, natural history and treatment. Am J Cardiol 1973; 32:562–574.
14. MacLeod M, Taylor AD, Baxter G, Harden P, Briggs D, Moss J, Semple PF, Connell JM, Dominiczak AF. Renal artery stenosis managed by Palmaz stent insertion: technical and clinical outcome. J Hypertens 1995; 13:1791–1795.
15. Textor SC, Wilcox CS. Renal artery stenosis: a common, treatable cause of renal failure? Annu Rev Med 2001; 52:421–442.
16. van Jaarsveld BC, Krijnen P, Pieterman H, Derkx FH, Deinum J, Postma CT, Dees A, Woittiez AJ, Bartelink AK, Man in 't Veld AJ, Schalekamp MA. The effect of balloon angioplasty on hypertension in atherosclerotic renal-artery stenosis. Dutch Renal Artery Stenosis Intervention Cooperative Study Group. N Engl J Med 2000; 342:1007–1014.
17. Safian RD, Textor SC. Renal-artery stenosis. N Engl J Med 2001; 344:431–442.
18. Messina LM, Zelenock GB, Yao KA, Stanley JC. Renal revascularization for recurrent

pulmonary edema in patients with poorly controlled hypertension and renal insufficiency: a distinct subgroup of patients with arteriosclerotic renal artery occlusive disease. J Vasc Surg 1992; 15:73–80.

19. Appel RG, Bleyer AJ, Reavis S, Hansen KJ. Renovascular disease in older patients beginning renal replacement therapy. Kidney Int 1995; 48:171–176.

20. IV. Patient characteristics at the start of ESRD: data from the HCFA medical evidence form. Am J Kidney Dis 1999; 34:S63–S73.

21. Hansen KJ, Edwards MS, Craven TE, Cherr GS, Jackson SA, Appel RG, Burke GL, Dean RH. Prevalence of renovascular disease in the elderly: a population-based study. J Vasc Surg 2002; 36:443–451.

22. Sacks D, Rundback JH, Martin LG. Renal angioplasty/stent placement and hypertension in the year 2000. J Vasc Interv Radiol 2000; 11:949–953.

23. Zierler RE. Duplex scanning for renal arterial occlusive disease. In: Stanley JC, Ernst CB, eds. Current Therapy in Vascular Surgery. St. Louis: Mosby, 2001:717–722.

24. Olin JW, Piedmonte MR, Young JR, DeAnna S, Grubb M, Childs MB. The utility of duplex ultrasound scanning of the renal arteries for diagnosing significant renal artery stenosis. Ann Intern Med 1995; 122:833–838.

25. Radermacher J, Chavan A, Bleck J, Vitzthum A, Stoess B, Gebel MJ, Galanski M, Koch KM, Haller H. Use of Doppler ultrasonography to predict the outcome of therapy for renal-artery stenosis. N Engl J Med 2001; 344:410–417.

26. Muller FB, Sealey JE, Case DB, Atlas SA, Pickering TG, Pecker MS, Preibisz JJ, Laragh JH. The captopril test for identifying renovascular disease in hypertensive patients. Am J Med 1986; 80:633–644.

27. Elliott WJ, Martin WB, Murphy MB. Comparison of two noninvasive screening tests for renovascular hypertension. Arch Intern Med 1993; 153:755–764.

28. Prince MR, Dong Q, Schoenberg SO. Magnetic resonance angiographic diagnosis of renovascular disease. In: Stanley JC, Ernst CB, eds. Current Therapy in Vascular Surgery. St. Louis: Mosby, 2001:723–728.

29. Libertino JA, Beckmann CF. Surgery and percutaneous angioplasty in the management of renovascular hypertension. Urol Clin North Am 1994; 21:235–243.

30. van de Ven PJ, Kaatee R, Beutler JJ, Beek FJ, Woittiez AJ, Buskens E, Koomans HA, Mali WP. Arterial stenting and balloon angioplasty in ostial atherosclerotic renovascular disease: a randomised trial. Lancet 1999; 353:282–286.

31. Blum U, Krumme B, Flugel P, Gabelmann A, Lehnert T, Buitrago-Tellez C, Schollmeyer P, Langer M. Treatment of ostial renal-artery stenoses with vascular endoprostheses after unsuccessful balloon angioplasty. N Engl J Med 1997; 336:459–465.

32. Canzanello VJ, Millan VG, Spiegel JE, Ponce PS, Kopelman RI, Madias NE. Percutaneous transluminal renal angioplasty in management of atherosclerotic renovascular hypertension: results in 100 patients. Hypertension 1989; 13:163–172.

33. Dorros G, Jaff M, Mathiak L, Dorros II, Lowe A, Murphy K, He T. Four-year follow-up of Palmaz-Schatz stent revascularization as treatment for atherosclerotic renal artery stenosis. Circulation 1998; 98:642–647.

34. Yutan E, Glickerman DJ, Caps MT, Hatsukami T, Harley JD, Kohler TR, Davies MG. Percutaneous transluminal revascularization for renal artery stenosis: Veterans Affairs Puget Sound Health Care System experience. J Vasc Surg 2001; 34:685–693.

35. Weibull H, Bergqvist D, Bergentz SE, Jonsson K, Hulthen L, Manhem P. Percutaneous transluminal renal angioplasty versus surgical reconstruction of atherosclerotic renal artery stenosis: a prospective randomized study. J Vasc Surg 1993; 18:841–850.

36. Plouin PF, Chatellier G, Darne B, Raynaud A. Blood pressure outcome of angioplasty in atherosclerotic renal artery stenosis: a randomized trial. Essai Multicentrique Medicaments vs Angioplastie (EMMA) Study Group. Hypertension 1998; 31:823–829.

37. Beutler JJ, Van Ampting JM, van de Ven PJ, Koomans HA, Beek FJ, Woittiez AJ, Mali WP.

Long-term effects of arterial stenting on kidney function for patients with ostial atherosclerotic renal artery stenosis and renal insufficiency. J Am Soc Nephrol 2001; 12:1475–1481.

38. Tuttle KR, Chouinard RF, Webber JT, Dahlstrom LR, Short RA, Henneberry KJ, Dunham LA, Raabe RD. Treatment of atherosclerotic ostial renal artery stenosis with the intravascular stent. Am J Kidney Dis 1998; 32:611–622.

39. Ramsay LE, Waller PC. Blood pressure response to percutaneous transluminal angioplasty for renovascular hypertension: an overview of published series. Br Med J 1990; 300:569–572.

40. Harden PN, MacLeod MJ, Rodger RS, Baxter GM, Connell JM, Dominiczak AF, Junor BJ, Briggs JD, Moss JG. Effect of renal-artery stenting on progression of renovascular renal failure. Lancet 1997; 349:1133–1136.

41. Leertouwer TC, Gussenhoven EJ, Bosch JL, van Jaarsveld BC, van Dijk LC, Deinum J, Man in 't Veld AJ. Stent placement for renal arterial stenosis: where do we stand? A meta-analysis. Radiology 2000; 216:78–85.

42. Stanson AW. Complications of transluminal angioplasty of renal arteries. In: Bernhard VM, Towne JB, eds. Complications in Vascular Surgery. Orlando, FL: Grune & Stratton, 1985:247–257.

43. Bush RL, Najibi S, MacDonald MJ, Lin PH, Chaikof EL, Martin LG, Lumsden AB. Endovascular revascularization of renal artery stenosis: technical and clinical results. J Vasc Surg 2001; 33:1041–1049.

44. Dejani H, Eisen TD, Finkelstein FO. Revascularization of renal artery stenosis in patients with renal insufficiency. Am J Kidney Dis 2000; 36:752–758.

45. Tullis MJ, Zierler RE, Glickerman DJ, Bergelin RO, Cantwell-Gab K, Strandness DE Jr. Results of percutaneous transluminal angioplasty for atherosclerotic renal artery stenosis: a follow-up study with duplex ultrasonography. J Vasc Surg 1997; 25:46–54.

46. Henry M, Amor M, Henry I, Ethevenot G, Tzvetanov K, Courvoisier A, Mentre B, Chati Z. Stents in the treatment of renal artery stenosis: long-term follow-up. J Endovasc Surg 1999; 6:42–51.

47. Mailloux LU, Napolitano B, Bellucci AG, Vernace M, Wilkes BM, Mossey RT. Renal vascular disease causing end-stage renal disease, incidence, clinical correlates, and outcomes: a 20-year clinical experience. Am J Kidney Dis 1994; 24:622–629.

48. Stoney RJ, Messina LM, Goldstone J, Reilly LM. Renal endarterectomy through the transected aorta: a new technique for combined aortorenal atherosclerosis—A preliminary report. J Vasc Surg 1989; 9:224–233.

49. Wylie EJ, Perloff DL, Stoney RJ. Autogenous tissue revascularization technics in surgery for renovascular hypertension. Ann Surg 1969; 170:416–428.

50. Rosenfield K. Renal Artery Disease—Rationale for Invasive Management and Consideration Regarding Distal Embolic Protection. Washington, D.C.: Transcatheter Cardiovascular Therapeutics, 2002.

51. Cambria RP, Brewster DC, L'Italien GJ, Gertler JP, Abbott WM, LaMuraglia GM, Moncure AC, Vignati J, Bazari H, Fang LT, Atamian S. Renal artery reconstruction for the preservation of renal function. J Vasc Surg 1996; 24:371–380.

52. Tsoukas AI, Hertzer NR, Mascha EJ, O'Hara PJ, Krajewski LP, Beven EG. Simultaneous aortic replacement and renal artery revascularization: the influence of preoperative renal function on early risk and late outcome. J Vasc Surg 2001; 34:1041–1049.

53. Hansen KJ, Starr SM, Sands RE, Burkart JM, Plonk GW Jr, Dean RH. Contemporary surgical management of renovascular disease. J Vasc Surg 1992; 16:319–330.

54. Libertino JA, Bosco PJ, Ying CY, Breslin DJ, Woods BO, Tsapatsaris NP, Swinton NW Jr. Renal revascularization to preserve and restore renal function. J Urol 1992; 147:1485–1487.

55. Clair DG, Belkin M, Whittemore AD, Mannick JA, Donaldson MC. Safety and efficacy of transaortic renal endarterectomy as an adjunct to aortic surgery. J Vasc Surg 1995; 21:926–933.

56. Chaikof EL, Smith RB III, Salam AA, Dodson TF, Lumsden AB, Kosinski AS, Coyle KA,

Allen RC. Ischemic nephropathy and concomitant aortic disease: a ten-year experience. J Vasc Surg 1994; 19:135–146.

57. Cambria RP, Brewster DC, L'Italien GJ, Moncure A, Darling RC Jr, Gertler JP, La Muraglia GM, Atamian S, Abbott WM. The durability of different reconstructive techniques for atherosclerotic renal artery disease. J Vasc Surg 1994; 20:76–85.

58. Hallett JW Jr, Fowl R, O'Brien PC, Bernatz PE, Pairolero PC, Cherry KJ Jr, Hollier LH. Renovascular operations in patients with chronic renal insufficiency: do the benefits justify the risks? J Vasc Surg 1987; 5:622–627.

59. Dean RH. Complications of renal revascularization. In: Bernhard VM, Towne JB, eds. Complications in Vascular Surgery. Orlando, FL: Grune & Stratton, 1985:229–246.

60. Stanley JC, Ernst CB, Fry WJ. Fate of 100 aortorenal vein grafts: characteristics of late graft expansion, aneurysmal dilatation, and stenosis. Surgery 1973; 74:931–944.

61. Berkowitz HD, O'Neill JA Jr. Renovascular hypertension in children. Surgical repair with special reference to the use of reinforced vein grafts. J Vasc Surg 1989; 9:46–55.

62. Stoney RJ, De Luccia N, Ehrenfeld WK, Wylie EJ. Aortorenal arterial autografts. Arch Surg 1981; 116:1416–1422.

63. Pak LK, Kerlan RK, Mully TW, Messina LM. Successful bilateral transaortic renal endarterectomy after failed renal artery angioplasty and stenting: a case report. J Vasc Surg 2002; 35:808–810.

64. Dougherty MJ, Hallett JW Jr, Naessens JM, Bower TC, Cherry KJ, Gloviczki P, James EM. Optimizing technical success of renal revascularization: the impact of intraoperative color-flow duplex ultrasonography. J Vasc Surg 1993; 17:849–856.

65. Wollenweber J, Sheps SG, Davis GD. Clinical course of atherosclerotic renovascular disease. Am J Cardiol 1968; 21:60–71.

66. Ernst CB, Stanley JC, Marshall FF, Fry WJ. Renal revascularization for arteriosclerotic renovascular hypertension: prognostic implications of focal renal arterial vs. overt generalized arteriosclerosis. Surgery 1973; 73:859–867.

14

The Diagnosis and Management of Aortic Bifurcation Graft Limb Occlusions

Mark T. Eginton and Robert A. Cambria

Medical College of Wisconsin, Milwaukee, Wisconsin, U.S.A.

Aortic bifurcation grafts remain among the most successful and durable procedures performed by vascular surgeons. Five-year patency rates in excess of 80% have been widely reported in grafts placed for aortoiliac occlusive disease (1,2), with even higher patency rates reported in grafts placed for aneurysmal disease (3). However, thrombosis of an aortic graft limb represents the most common complication following reconstruction of the abdominal aorta (4). This chapter focuses on the incidence, etiology, diagnosis, and treatment of graft limb thrombosis.

I. INCIDENCE

Patency of aortobifemoral bypass grafts in the perioperative period is excellent, with reported thrombosis of 2% or less (2). Patency rates decrease steadily over the follow-up period, with a limb occlusion rate of approximately 4% per year, resulting in 10-year patency from 66 to 78% (1,5,6). Table 1 illustrates not only the durability of these procedures but also the continued risk for graft limb thrombosis 5–10 years following implantation. Therefore thrombosis of an aortic graft limb continues to represent a common clinical problem in spite of a recent trend away from aortic reconstruction for aortoiliac occlusive disease (7).

The incidence of graft thrombosis is influenced by risk factors that range beyond the technical and anatomic considerations of the graft itself. Smoking has been demonstrated to be associated with failure of aortofemoral reconstruction (3), and the thrombosis rate has been correlated with the amount of smoke exposure (8,9). Tibial vessel occlusive disease, both alone and in tandem with profunda femoris occlusive disease, has been associated with aortic graft limb occlusion (10). As noted above, grafts placed for aneurysmal disease have higher patency rates than those placed for occlusive disease (11). All of these factors are likely related to more advanced atherosclerotic occlusive disease, resulting in compromised graft outflow over longer follow-up periods.

Table 1 Patency of Aortic Bifurcation Grafts

Author	Number of Grafts	Patency Rate (%)	Follow-up (years)
Najafi (12)	601	92	3.5
Malone (10)	180	82	5
		66	10
Martinez (1)	355	88	5
		78	10
Brewster (6)	464	88	5
		74	10
Nevelsteen (5)	869	74	10
		70	15

II. ETIOLOGY

Traditionally, aortic graft limb occlusions have been classified as those occurring early in the postoperative period or at later points during follow-up. Early thrombosis is defined as occurring within 30 days of the primary procedure. As noted above, early thrombosis is quite rare, occurring after 2% or less of aortic reconstructions (10,12), and early thromboses typically represents 10% or less of the cases in large series of thrombosed limbs (13) (Table 2). Conversely, the majority of graft limb occlusions occur later in the follow-up period, with the average interval from the primary procedure ranging from 28 to 60 months (4,14).

The etiology of graft occlusion, regardless of temporal relation to the original procedure, must fall into one of three generic categories: inadequate inflow, inadequate outflow, or problems within the graft itself. The most common problem is inadequate outflow, usually due to progression of distal disease over time. Table 2 details the preponderance of outflow occlusion as an etiology for graft limb failure in several series.

A. Early Failure

Early graft occlusions, occurring within 30 days of the primary procedure, are usually due to a technical error resulting in a mechanical problem within the graft or at one of the anastomoses or to a judgmental error resulting in inadequate inflow or outflow. There is no substitute for thoughtful preoperative planning and meticulous surgical technique in the prevention of early graft thrombosis. This includes high-resolution preoperative angiography to demonstrate the extent of occlusive disease in the entire abdominal aorta as well as the common, superficial, and deep femoral arteries. Appropriate oblique views must be obtained to delineate potential stenoses in the runoff vessels that could compromise flow and result in graft occlusion. If concern exists for aortic intraluminal thrombus or extensive calcification, which may complicate aortic cross-clamping, consideration should be given to preoperative computed tomography to assist in planning the operative approach.

Tailoring, flushing, tunneling, and suturing of the prosthetic graft are all potential sources of technical error that may result in early postoperative thrombosis. If the common trunk of the graft is left too long, the iliac limb may kink at its origin, resulting in a flow-limiting stenosis (Fig. 1). Thrombus that accumulates in the graft at the time of placement must be carefully evacuated prior to clamp release. External compression by the

Table 2 Timing and Causes of Aortic Graft Limb Occlusion

| Author | Number of limbs | Early graft occlusion | Interval to occlusion | Etiology of graft occlusion (% of series) | | | |
				Outflow occlusion	Inflow occlusion	Intragraft abnormality[a]	Indeterminate or systemic[b]
Brewster (4)	129	28 (22%)	33 months	89 (69)	1 (<1)	16 (12)	23 (18)
Bernhard (13)	50	3 (6%)	28 months	42 (84)	0	6 (12)	2 (4)
Erodes (14)	46	4 (9%)	60 months	36 (78)	3 (6.5)	4 (9)	3 (6.5)

[a] Includes pseudoaneurysms, kinks in graft, infection, and early thromboses not otherwise accounted for.
[b] Includes hypercoagulable states.

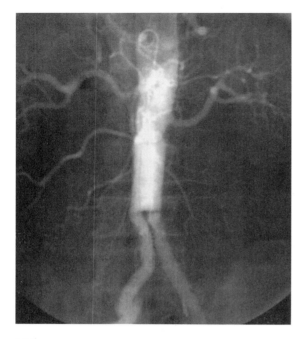

(A)

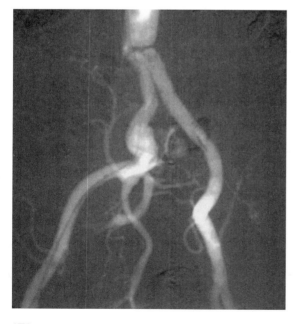

(B)

inguinal ligament has been described and can be avoided by careful examination of the tunnel into the retroperitoneum from the groin incision. Twisting of the graft limb as it is tunneled from the abdomen must be avoided and will obviously lead to decreased patency if unnoticed. Finally, improper placement of anastomotic sutures or creation of unfavorable anastomotic angles can lead to early thrombosis.

Infrequently, early graft occlusion may occur in the absence of an identifiable cause. Disorders of blood coagulation have been implicated in this process (14). Certainly, given the relatively high frequency of hypercoagulable states in patients with vascular disease, this must be a part of the differential diagnosis. Prosthetic grafts are thrombogenic by their nature, and some patients may be prone to thrombosis of these grafts even in the absence of a distinct flow-limiting lesion. Perioperative fluid shifts and alterations in blood pressure and coagulability may contribute to early graft thrombosis in this setting.

B. Late Failure

The vast majority of late graft failures are due to compromised outflow. This may be due to intimal hyperplasia at the distal anastomosis in the intermediate time periods, up to 2 or 3 years following the primary procedure. More commonly, gradual progression of atherosclerotic occlusive disease results in compromise of the outflow vessels and eventual thrombosis of the graft. This may take the form of superficial femoral artery occlusion where this vessel had been previously patent, progressive profunda femoris disease where this had been the primary outflow vessel, or occlusion of an infrainguinal bypass that had been contributing to graft outflow. As the flow through the graft becomes diminished, progressive deposition of luminal thrombus leads to thickening of the graft neointima. Eventually, flow is reduced to a point where thrombosis of the graft occurs.

Less common causes of late graft failure include thrombosis of an anastomotic pseudoaneurysm, infection of the bypass conduit, embolism from a more central source, or progression of aortic disease above the conduit, resulting in compromised inflow. Although problems with inflow can lead to unilateral limb thrombosis, this type of problem more commonly results in occlusion of the entire aortic reconstruction. With the increased utilization of intravascular therapy—including coronary angioplasty and stenting—access to the vascular space is frequently gained through previous aortic bifurcation grafts. In this instance, catheter disruption of graft pseudointima may lead to thrombosis of a graft that had otherwise been functioning well.

III. DIAGNOSIS AND EVALUATION

Acute occlusion of an aortic graft limb typically presents with the abrupt onset of lower extremity ischemic symptoms. The majority of patients will have limb-threatening ischemia with rest pain, requiring urgent intervention (4,15). Less frequently, patients may simply present complaining of decreased exercise tolerance, or with an occult limb occlusion. An absent femoral pulse usually confirms the diagnosis, and a diminution in high thigh pressure or ankle brachial index supports the presumptive diagnosis if there is

Figure 1 Anteroposterior (A) and left anterior oblique (B) views of an aortogram that demonstrates kinking of both graft limbs. This aortoiliac graft had been placed 6 years earlier for aneurysmal disease. Excessive graft length has resulted in limb kinking, which is a potential cause of graft limb occlusion.

doubt. As the diagnostic workup continues, heparin anticoagulation should be instituted to prevent thrombus propagation and maintain patency in the outflow vessels.

A minority of patients will present without detectable blood flow in the extremity and with a cadaveric foot. Further diagnostic evaluation is contraindicated in this situation, and the patient should be explored on an emergency basis, with restoration of inflow and evaluation of outflow performed intraoperatively. More commonly, patients will present with an ischemic but viable extremity. In this instance, angiography can provide important information to assist in planning reconstructive intervention and should be obtained.

The aortic anastomosis and more proximal aorta should be visualized using biplanar high-resolution images to exclude anastomotic abnormalities or compromised inflow. The contralateral iliac or femoral limb should be examined for intrinsic stenoses, anastomotic strictures, or distal emboli. Finally, the outflow vessels in the ischemic extremity should be visualized if possible, looking for occlusive disease distal to the groin that may need to be addressed. It should be noted that even if no outflow vessels can be visualized in the ischemic extremity, exploration of the groin frequently reveals a suitable profunda femoris vessel to provide outflow for the graft revision. Computed tomography can occasionally be useful, particularly when intraluminal aortic thrombus, anastomotic pseudoaneurysms, or graft infection is suspected.

Given the likelihood that operative intervention will be required to revise the graft, medical comorbidities should be evaluated, and their management optimized as the diagnostic studies are obtained. The approach to graft revision may be tailored based on these factors, avoiding abdominal exploration and "redo" aortic dissection in patients with prohibitive risk profiles.

IV. MANAGEMENT OF THE OCCLUDED LIMB

Intervention for graft limb occlusion should be individualized to the clinical scenario. Options in the management of these patients include observation without intervention, simple thrombectomy, thrombectomy with outflow reconstruction, thrombolysis, redo aortofemoral reconstruction, or extra-anatomic inflow reconstruction. Factors that influence decision making in this situation include but are not limited to the degree of extremity ischemia, adequacy of contralateral inflow, interval since original inflow reconstruction, interval since graft limb occlusion, angiographic findings, and the general medical condition of the patient. It is well recognized that reoperative intervention for aortic graft failure is technically demanding; therefore all of the above options should be considered, as each may have advantages or disadvantages in any given patient.

As noted above, a minority of patients with graft limb occlusion may have this found incidentally and be without symptoms or may present with a chronic history of decreased exercise tolerance in the absence of limb-threatening ischemia. While reintervention to relieve claudication may be warranted, nonoperative management is preferable in certain patients with significant comorbidity and in asymptomatic patients.

A. Restoration of Inflow

The majority of patients will be able to be treated by retrograde graft thrombectomy with outflow reconstruction. However, the surgeon must be prepared to find an alternate source of inflow or to perform more distal revascularization, as the situation dictates. With this in mind, the patient should be widely prepped and draped to include the entire chest, abdomen, both groins, and the involved lower extremity. General anesthesia is preferred, although, in extenuating circumstances, thrombectomy under local anesthesia may be possible.

The previous groin incision is reopened, and the thrombosed graft limb, common femoral artery, superficial femoral and profunda femoris arteries are dissected and isolated. Heparin should be administered to elevate the activated clotting time above 200–250 s if this drug had not already been initiated preoperatively. A transverse incision in the graft limb close to the femoral anastomosis allows for exploration of the runoff vessels. If necessary, thrombectomy catheters can be passed distally to retrieve thrombotic material and achieve back-bleeding. If the orifices of the runoff vessels are involved with occlusive disease, reconstruction to improve outflow is necessary (see below).

Thrombectomy catheters are then passed proximally. This should be done serially, inserting the catheter 5 cm initially, and then 10 cm, and so on. Thrombotic material is removed sequentially in this fashion to avoid pushing the thrombus over the bifurcation of the graft and causing an embolus in the contralateral limb. Pressure on the contralateral femoral pulse, occluding flow in the opposite limb while the thrombectomy is being performed, also serves to prevent embolism. Once the thrombotic material is cleared, pulsatile inflow should be restored. In early postoperative limb thrombosis, careful examination for technical defects within the graft or at the anastomoses should follow. If no cause for failure is identified, the graft can be closed and the patient managed with short-term anticoagulation.

In all cases of late graft limb occlusion or if any doubt exists as to the adequacy of inflow or the presence of residual thrombus or technical defect, further investigation is warranted after initial thrombectomy. Surgeons comfortable with angioscopy have advocated the use of this instrument for evaluation of the graft limb following thrombectomy (16). More commonly, retrograde injection of contrast material from the groin for angiographic analysis is performed. Intraluminal filling defects in the graft limb represent either residual thrombus or graft pseudointima. Specialized graft thrombectomy catheters are available and should be used in this situation. These catheters have wire loops instead of a balloon at the tip to scrape material from the wall of the graft. In the past, ring strippers have been used over an occlusion balloon more proximally (17), and this technique may still be useful in selected instances. However, the graft thrombectomy catheters have been quite effective in removing adherent thrombus (Fig. 2). Angiography to confirm adequate clearance of the graft limb should be obtained once inflow is restored.

If adequate inflow cannot be obtained with thrombectomy catheters, alternative sources of inflow must be considered; these include redo aortofemoral reconstruction or extra-anatomic reconstruction (cross-femoral or axillofemoral bypass). In the absence of stenotic lesions in the contralateral limb, a cross-femoral graft is frequently the best option. Primary and secondary 5-year patency rates of 54 and 84%, respectively, have been reported for femorofemoral crossover grafts used to treat aortic graft limb occlusion, with a limb salvage rate of 84% (18). Revision or replacement of the entire prosthesis is generally required for lesions at the proximal anastomosis or in the aorta above, precluding establishment of adequate inflow (Fig. 3). This was required in less than 3% of aortobifemoral bypass procedures reviewed by Szilagyi (19). In those patients with prohibitive risk profiles, axillobifemoral bypass is a viable alternative to aortic reoperation.

Thrombolytic agents have been used successfully to reestablish patency of a thrombosed aortofemoral graft limb. As in other situations where this type of treatment is

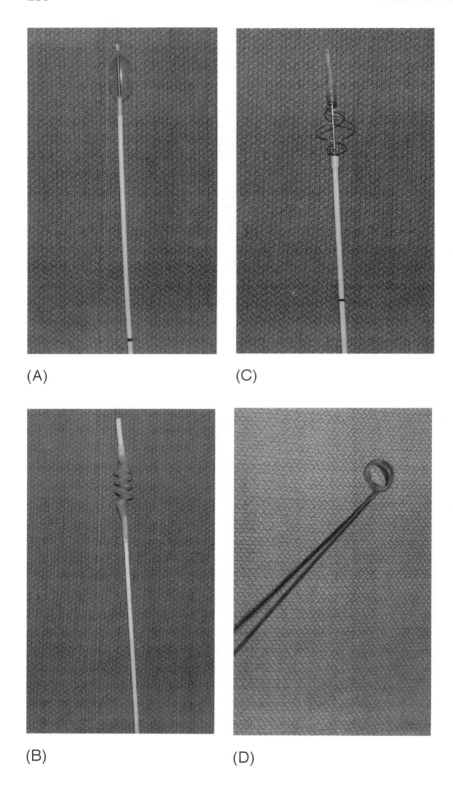

(A)

(C)

(B)

(D)

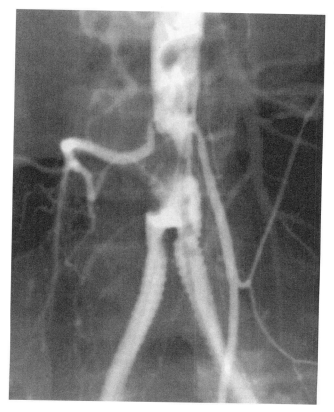

Figure 3 Adherent thrombus at the proximal anastomosis of an aortobifemoral bypass graft. This patient was referred after her aortic graft had occluded and had been treated with thrombolytic therapy. The intraluminal filling defect persisted and was treated by revision of her proximal anastomosis to the more proximal infrarenal aorta.

employed, thrombolytic agents require more time to restore inflow than direct operative thrombectomy; typically, additional procedures will be required to correct the underlying cause of graft limb occlusion. In one series of 19 patients (20), restoration of inflow was achieved in every case with urokinase, with an average infusion time of 32 h (range 12–60 h). Additional treatment was required in 16 cases, the majority of which required conventional surgical repair. Occasionally, focal stenoses above the inguinal ligament may be treatable with endovascular techniques (20,21). Because of the time required for thrombolysis, this approach should not be considered when the involved extremity is

Figure 2 The tools of the trade. (A.) Syntel balloon thrombectomy catheter. (B.) Fogarty adherent clot catheter for use in grafts or arteries. Wire spiral is covered with latex to minimize intimal injury. (C.) Fogarty graft thrombectomy catheter. Exposed wire hoops for use in removal of neointima and thrombus from luminal surface of prosthetic grafts. Not intended for use in native vessels. (D.) Endarterectomy loop. May be used coaxially with balloon occlusion catheter to facilitate removal of densely adherent thrombotic plug or graft neointima.

profoundly ischemic. Given that the majority of patients will require operative revision, many have argued effectively that operative thrombectomy is preferred in most instances (4,14). Thrombolytic therapy may be quite helpful in selected circumstances where the etiology of recurrent graft limb thrombosis remains elusive.

B. Outflow Revision

As noted above, the majority of late graft failures result from diminished outflow due to anastomotic stricture or progression of distal disease. Patency of graft limb thrombectomy in this instance is directly related to either correction or bypass of stenotic disease in the groin or lower extremity (Fig. 4). Preoperative angiography may identify significant femoropopliteal occlusive disease, but intraoperative evaluation of the femoral artery branches is mandatory to assure adequate graft outflow.

The profunda femoris (deep femoral) artery is the primary outflow vessel in the majority of patients with graft limb occlusion. The orifice of this vessel should be explored at the time of thrombectomy and should admit a 4-mm dilator. Additional assessment could include intraoperative angiography or gentle passage of embolectomy catheters. A

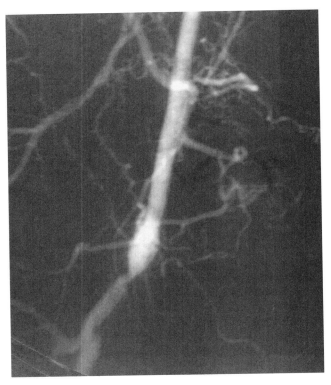

Figure 4 Right femoral anastomosis of an aortobifemoral graft 9 years following implantation. Stenosis at the origin of profunda femoris runoff ultimately resulted in occlusion of this graft limb. Thrombectomy with profundaplasty was performed, but the graft limb reoccluded within several months. Repeat thrombectomy with adjunctive femoropopliteal bypass resulted in continued patency of the graft limb.

profunda vessel length of 20–25 cm has been suggested to be adequate to support graft limb outflow. Stenosis at the origin of the profunda vessel should be treated with profundaplasty. Exposure of the vessel followed by longitudinal arteriotomy, endarterectomy, and patch angioplasty is usually possible and will provide adequate outflow in the majority of cases. While some authors have advocated the benefits of autogenous tissue patch angioplasty of the profunda vessel (22), the distal anastomosis can usually be fashioned to incorporate the profunda femoris angioplasty with equivalent results. Alternatively, a stenosis at the origin of the deep femoral artery can be bypassed by moving the distal anastomosis farther down this vessel (23).

In the absence of an adequate deep femoral artery, aortic graft limb outflow will require adjunctive bypass in the lower extremity. In this instance, either preoperative or intraoperative angiography is mandatory to identify a suitable target vessel in continuity with the infrageniculate arteries. Infrainguinal bypass was required in 10–15% of patients following aortic reconstruction in one series (24). While distal bypass is required in the minority of patients with initial graft limb occlusion, this rate increases in those who present with recurrent limb occlusion (4).

V. RESULTS

Morbidity and mortality following operations for occluded aortofemoral bypass limbs are low. Mortality rates ranging from 2 to 5% have been quoted in the literature (4,13,14). Local complications include groin wound complications, graft infection,

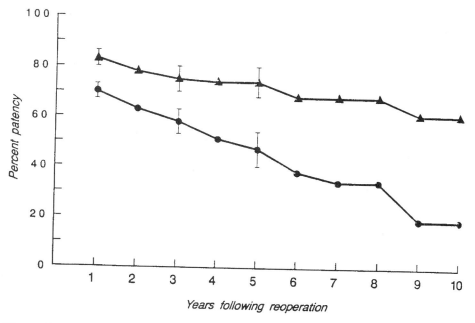

Figure 5 Primary (circles) and secondary (triangles) patency following graft limb thrombectomy in 110 patients. The utility of repeated thrombectomy for graft limb reocclusion is evidenced by the dramatic improvement in secondary patency. (Adapted from Ref. 4.)

pseudoaneurysm, and embolism to the ipsilateral or contralateral extremity. Systemic complications are typical of the vascular patient population, with cardiovascular events predominating. Taken together, complication rate for graft limb occlusion is on the order of 10–15%.

Operations to restore patency for an occluded aortic graft limb are quite successful. Primary patency rates following thrombectomy and outflow revision are 70 and 47% at 1 and 5 years, respectively (4). Repeat thrombectomy is valuable in the event of reocclusion, with 5-year patency rates approaching 75% following aggressive rethrombectomy with adjunctive procedures when necessary (Fig. 5). Many authors have emphasized the benefit of repeated operations for recurrent graft limb occlusion, with this type of diligence resulting in enhanced secondary patency.

VI. SUMMARY

Occlusion of an aortic graft limb represents the most common complication following reconstruction for aortoiliac occlusive disease. Perioperative failure represents a minority of these patients ($< 10\%$), and usually results from a technical or judgmental error. The vast majority of limb occlusions occur from 2 to 5 years following graft implantation and are associated with atherosclerotic deterioration of the outflow vessels. These patients typically present with limb-threatening ischemia or claudication, which is more severe than the symptoms that had prompted the original procedure. Preoperative imaging is desirable to rule out unsuspected inflow restriction and evaluate potential outflow stenoses. While thrombolytic therapy has been employed successfully, most patients go on to require operative intervention. Therefore direct operative thrombectomy with concomitant outflow revision represents the most expeditious and efficient way to deal with this problem. A minority of patients will require alternative inflow procedures or adjunctive distal bypass in the lower extremity. Aggressive management of limb occlusions with reexploration for recurrent thrombosis has resulted in a secondary 5-year patency approaching 75% after graft limb occlusion.

REFERENCES

1. Martinez BD, Hertzer NR, Beven EG. Influence of distal arterial occlusive disease on prognosis following aortobifemoral bypass. Surgery 1980; 88:795–805.
2. Poulias GE, Polemis L, Skoutas B, Doundoulakis N, Papaioannou K, Ershaid B, Sendekeya S. Bilateral aortofemoral bypass in the presence of aorto-iliac occlusive disease and factors determining results. J Cardiovasc Surg 1985; 26:527–538.
3. Wray R, DePalma RG, Hubay CH. Late occlusion of aortofemoral bypass grafts: influence of cigarette smoking. Surgery 1971; 70:969–973.
4. Brewster DC, Meier GH III, Darling RC, Moncure AC, LaMuraglia GM, Abbott WM. Reoperation for aortofemoral graft limb occlusion: optimal methods and long-term results. J Vasc Surg 1987; 5:363–374.
5. Nevelsteen A, Suy R, Daenen W, Boel A, Stalpaert G. Aortofemoral grafting: factors influencing late results. Surgery 1980; 88:642–653.
6. Brewster DC, Darling RC. Optimal methods of aortoiliac reconstruction. Surgery 1978; 84:739–748.
7. Brewster DC. Current controversies in the management of aortoiliac occlusive disease. J Vasc Surg 1997; 25:365–379.
8. Robicsek F, Daugherty HK, Mullen DC, Masters TN, Narbay D, Sanger PW. The effect of

continued cigarette smoking on the patency of synthetic vascular grafts in Leriche syndrome. J Throac Cardiovasc Surg 1975; 70:107–112.

9. Myers KA, King RB, Scott DF, Johnson N, Morris PJ. The effect of smoking on the late patency of arterial reconstructions in the legs. Br J Surg 1978; 65:267–271.

10. Malone JM, Moore WS, Goldstone J. The natural history of bilateral aortofemoral bypass grafts for ischemia of the lower extremities. Arch Surg 1975; 110:1300–1306.

11. Hallett JW, Marshall DM, Petterson TM, Gray DT, Bower TC, Cherry KJ, Gloviczki P, Pairolero PC. Graft related complications after abdominal aortic aneurysm repair: reassurance from a 36-year population-based experience. J Vasc Surg 1997; 25:277–286.

12. Najafi H, Dye WS, Javid H, Hunter JA, Goldin MD, Serry C, Julian OC. Late thrombosis affecting one limb of aortic bifurcation graft. Arch Surg 1975; 110:409–412.

13. Bernhard VM, Ray LI, Towne JB. The reoperation of choice for aortofemoral graft occlusion. Surgery 1977; 82:867–874.

14. Erodes LS, Bernhard VM, Berman SS. Aortofemoral graft occlusion: strategy and timing of reoperation. Cardiovasc Surg 1995; 3:277–283.

15. Lyons JH, Weismann RE. Surgical management of late closure of aortofemoral reconstruction grafts. N Engl J Med 1968; 278:1035–1037.

16. Towne JB, Bernhard VM. Technique of intraoperative endoscopic evaluation of occluded aorto-femoral grafts following thrombectomy. Surg Gynecol Obstet 1979; 148:87–89.

17. Ernst CB, Dougherty ME. Removal of a thrombotic plug from an occluded limb of an aorto-femoral graft. Arch Surg 1978; 113:301–302.

18. Nolan KD, Benjamin ME, Murphy TJ, Pearce WH, McCarthy WJ, Yao JST, Flinn WR. Femorofemoral bypass for aortofemoral graft limb occlusion: a ten-year experience. J Vasc Surg 1994; 19:851–857.

19. Szilagyi DE, Elliot JP, Smith RF, Reddy DJ, McPharlin M. A thirty-year survey of the reconstructive surgical treatment of aortoiliac occlusive disease. J Vasc Surg 1986; 3:421–436.

20. Enron B, Reigner B, Lescalie F, l'Hoste P, Peret M, Chevalier JM. In situ thrombolysis for late occlusion of suprafemoral prosthetic grafts. Ann Vasc Surg 1993; 7:270–274.

21. Mitchell SE, Kadir S, Kaufman SL, Chang R, Williams GM, Kan JS, White RI Jr. Percutaneous transluminal angioplasty of aortic graft stenoses. Radiology 1983; 149:439–444.

22. Malone JM, Goldstone J, Moore WS. Autogenous profundaplasty: the key to long-term patency in secondary repair of aortofemoral graft occlusion. Ann Surg 1978; 188:817–823.

23. Ouriel K, DeWeese JA, Ricotta JJ, Green RM. Revascularization of the distal profunda femoris artery in the reconstructive treatment of aortoiliac occlusive disease. J Vasc Surg 1987; 6:217–220.

24. Baird RJ, Feldman P, Miles JT, Madras PM, Gurry JF. Subsequent downstream repair after aorto-iliac and aorto-femoral bypass operations. Surgery 1977; 82:785–793.

15

Problems Related to Extra-Anatomic Bypass—Including Axillofemoral, Femorofemoral, Obturator, and Thoracofemoral Bypasses

Kyle Mueller and William H. Pearce

Northwestern University, Chicago, Illinois, U.S.A.

The novel concept of extra-anatomic bypass appeared more than four decades ago and this procedure has now become a widely used and accepted method of revascularization. It is mainly performed for patients who, due to comorbid conditions, are poor surgical risks for standard revascularization procedures or for those who have had a complication related to a previous bypass, such as an infected aortic graft or aortoduodenal fistula. The four types of extra-anatomic bypass commonly used include axillofemoral, femorofemoral, obturator, and thoracofemoral grafts. Because the majority of patients undergoing these procedures are poor surgical risks, any complication can be catastrophic. For this reason it is important that the vascular surgeon be aware of the complications associated with these procedures, so as to avoid complications when possible and to intervene in a timely manner when they do occur. This chapter reviews the diagnosis and management of complications commonly associated with extra-anatomic bypass procedures.

I. AXILLOFEMORAL BYPASS

The axillofemoral bypass graft was introduced by Blaisdell and colleagues in the early 1960s (1,2). It has become the procedure of choice for revascularization in patients with aortoiliac occlusion who are found to be at an unacceptably high surgical risk for transabdominal aortic bypass. Axillofemoral bypass is also an integral technique for the management of patients with an infected aortic graft or aortoenteric fistula. In their review of 916 axillofemoral grafts reported in the literature, Bunt and Moore found a 1.6% incidence of complications (15 of 916) (3). Over the past several decades, as the use of this technique has dramatically increased, a large number of studies and case reports dealing with the specific and unique complications seen with this type of extra-anatomic bypass have emerged. These include proximal anastomotic disruption, upper extremity thrombo-embolic events, graft infection, and several others, which are discussed in this chapter.

A. Proximal Anastomotic Disruption

Disruption of the axillary anastomosis was initially thought to be a sporadic occurrence, but a study by Taylor et al. reports that 5% of patients (10 of 202) undergoing axillofemoral bypass developed this serious complication (4). It occurs primarily in the early postoperative period, as demonstrated by the Taylor study, with disruption seen over a range of 1–46 days postoperatively. A study by White et al. demonstrates disruption at 13–30 days after the procedure (5). The causes of axillary anastomotic disruption include infection, technical error, and mechanical stress (6,7). The associated clinical findings include axillary pain, expanding hematoma causing brachial plexus injury, and pseudoaneurysm formation. Axillary anastomotic disruption is most commonly related to mechanical stress and, more specifically, to overexertion or extreme upper extremity movements. This complication related to exertional disruption has been reported by several authors and termed *axillary pullout syndrome* (5). Daar and Finch describe how full abduction of the upper extremity and maximal lateral flexion of the spine contralateral to the site of measurement can lead to an increase in the length of the axillofemoral graft pathway of 4–12 cm (8). Another contributing factor to disruption of the axillary anastomosis is the widespread use of an external ring–reinforced polytetrafluoroethylene (PTFE) graft, which is very inelastic compared to the previously used Dacron grafts.

The key to avoiding proximal anastomotic disruption is correct anatomical placement of the axillary anastomosis. Blaisdell and Hall (1), in their first report on this technique in 1963, clearly stated that the anastomosis should be placed medial to the pectoralis minor tendon on the first part of the axillary artery, a statement that they reemphasized in a 1985 study (9). This first part of the axillary artery has no branches, is less mobile, and should be the only site used for anastomosis. It is not necessary to divide the pectoralis minor muscle in order to expose the first part of the axillary artery; doing so only increases the risk of anastomotic complications. Another technical point is to perform the axillofemoral bypass procedure with the upper extremity abducted, which creates some redundancy in the graft, permitting the pathway length to increase as the arm goes through a full range of motion. Landry et al. described a lateral tunneled approach with an anterior anastomosis to the axillary artery (Fig. 1) (10). The management of axillary anastomotic disruption involves obtaining proximal control of the subclavian artery using a supraclavicular approach or balloon occlusion. Because simple repair of disruptions has been shown to lead to secondary disruption, repair should be performed by placing a new interposed graft with reanastomosis to the existing graft. In addition, wound cultures should be sent to make sure that infection was not a contributing factor to the disruption.

B. Upper Extremity Thromboembolic Events

Upper extremity thromboembolism is a rare complication of axillofemoral bypass that can occur early or late in the postoperative course; in the majority of cases, however, it is associated with axillofemoral graft occlusion. A 1995 study by McLafferty et al. found that upper extremity thromboembolism occurred in 2.7% of all patients after axillofemoral bypass and in 25% of patients with occluded grafts (11). These events occurred as early as 26 days and as late as 7 years postoperatively. Thrombosis of the donor axillary artery has been reported, but the incidence is very low (12). The common finding in several

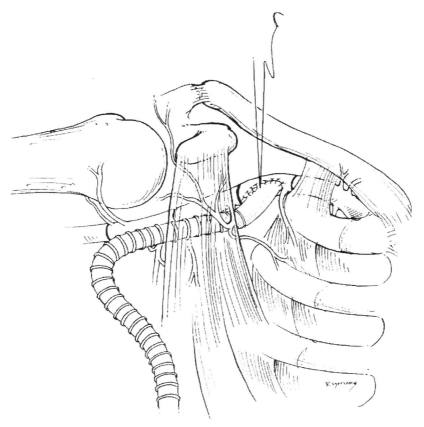

Figure 1 Alternative technique for the axillary anastomosis for an axillobifemoral bypass graft. This technique allows for redundancy along the course of the subclavian and axillary arteries for movement of the upper extremity. (From Ref. 10.)

cases of axillary artery thrombosis has been downward traction on the donor artery by the bypass graft, leading to a sharp angulation and subsequent thrombosis (13,14). Late severe ischemia of the upper extremity after axillofemoral bypass is rare, but there have been several reported cases of thromboembolic events after the procedure that caused severe ischemia, requiring amputation (15). If the site of the axillary anastomosis is appropriate, thrombosis seldom presents with upper extremity ischemia (Fig. 2). The first part of the axillary artery is devoid of significant branches, and all other areas proximal and distal to this segment have large collateral branches. If thrombosis occurs in a correctly placed axillary anastomosis, the collaterals will perfuse the arm; but if the anastomosis is placed in a segment with collaterals and thrombosis occurs, the collateral flow is interrupted and perfusion of the arm may be jeopardized. Management of axillary artery thrombosis should involve immediate exploration of the proximal anastomosis and repair of the axillary artery rather than anticoagulation or an attempt to reach the thrombosis from a distal approach.

In addition to thrombosis of the axillofemoral graft at the axillary anastomosis, there are reports of thrombosis occurring in the body of the graft due to compression from

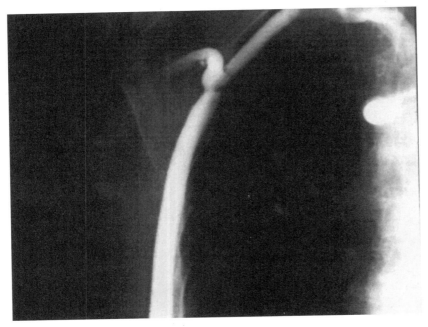

Figure 2 Axillopopliteal graft with excessive tension at the proximal anastomosis. Over time, the axillary-subclavian artery elongates to present with kinking and potential sources of distal embolization.

external body weight and kinking or twisting of the body of the graft, leading to graft occlusion. The effect of body-weight compression has been debated, as Jarowenko et al. found no hemodynamic changes after external body-weight compression, while Cavallaro et al. demonstrated changes in graft hemodynamics using ankle pressure index and pulse volume recording while patients were lying on the side of the bypass (16,17). Because the use of external ring–reinforced polytetrefluoroethylene (PTFE) grafts has increased, compression by body weight is seldom the cause of graft thrombosis. Redundancy in the graft has been shown to contribute to twisting or kinking of the body of the graft leading to stenosis and occlusion (Fig. 3). This is exaggerated in elderly patients who are in a seated position and may be developing mild kyphosis from degenerative changes of the spine. This complication demonstrates the balance required to provide some redundancy, allowing for increases in the length of the graft pathway for arm movement, yet avoiding excessive redundancy which could lead to thrombosis. Treatment is simply resection of the redundant graft with end to end anastomosis.

Distal embolization of the upper extremity following axillofemoral bypass is an extremely rare complication and primarily occurs after graft thrombosis. Bandyk et al. reported four episodes of distal embolic events and described the source of the emboli as the blind stump of the proximal graft limb that had remained patent (18). Embolization to the brachial artery can cause severe, limb-threatening ischemia. Management of this complication varies from brachial embolectomy to prophylactic detachment of the proximal graft and patch angioplasty of the axillary artery in patients who do not need immediate revision of their occluded bypass graft.

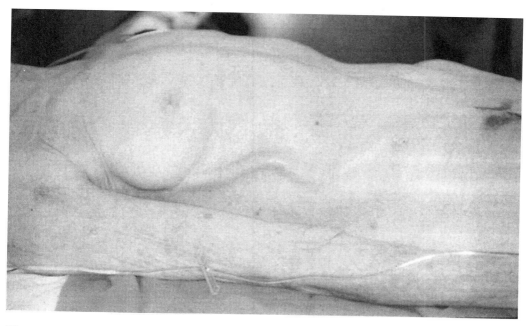

Figure 3 Lateral photograph of a tortuous axillofemoral bypass. Occasionally, such tortuosity is severe, producing flow-limiting lesions.

C. Axillofemoral Graft Infection

Infection of the axillofemoral graft is a rare but serious complication. In their review of 55 axillopopliteal bypass grafts, Ascher et al. found a 3.6% incidence of infection (19). Marston et al. demonstrated that infection of axillofemoral grafts is associated with a perioperative mortality rate of 22%, and 57% of survivors required amputation (20). Infection often occurs in the groin area, but midgraft infection has also been observed. Because of the excellent incorporation of PTFE graft by surrounding tissue, removal of the entire graft is seldom needed. Most graft infections can be managed with local debridement, systemic antibiotic therapy, and aggressive local wound care (Fig. 4A and B). If necessary, the infected segment can be removed and replaced with an interposed autogenous graft. Should the infection necessitate removal of the entire graft, an alternative reconstruction is a bypass from the descending thoracic aorta to the femoral artery, which is described further on in this chapter.

D. Perigraft Seroma

Perigraft seroma is a rare complication that has been reported to occur in various bypass procedures using Dacron or PTFE. A study by Buche et al. describes three cases of perigraft seroma in a total of 123 axillofemoral bypass grafts (21). The clinical findings of perigraft seroma are a nonpulsatile, painless mass overlying a graft, which must be distinguished from a pseudoaneurysm. The etiology of perigraft seroma is unclear, but its formation is related to inadequate incorporation of the graft by the surrounding connective tissue. Histologically, the seroma is confined within a pseudocapsule formed by a thin fibrous membrane. The pseudocapsule usually contains a clear, sterile serous

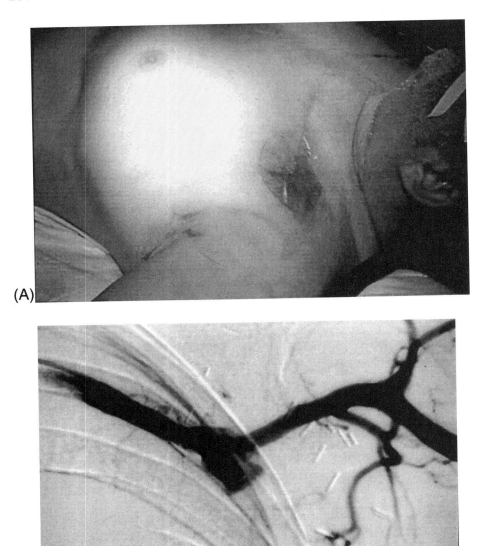

Figure 4   A. Infected axillofemoral bypass. The patient had previously undergone removal of the axillofemoral bypass with a stump of the graft material left. B. An arteriogram demonstrating the residual stump of the prosthetic material, which had become infected. The artery was repaired with an interposition vein graft.

fluid, but gelatinous material has been reported (22,23). A 1994 study by Ahn et al. reported the identification of a fibroblast growth inhibition factor from the sera of patients with perigraft seromas (24). Chronic perigraft seroma often becomes apparent at 4–8 weeks after graft implantation. Diagnosis can be made by duplex scan, computed tomography, or direct aspiration of the seroma. Some authors advocate observation of perigraft seromas, but standard treatment is excision with new graft replacement. Since perigraft seromas are often related to graft biofilm infections, special culture techniques are necessary for the diagnosis.

E. Structural Failure

The majority of axillofemoral bypasses are performed using external ring–reinforced PTFE grafts, which offer greater strength and durability than knitted Dacron. Despite this advantage, several authors have reported material failure of PTFE grafts, leading to graft disruption or pseudoaneurysm (25). We as well as other authors have observed disruption of PTFE grafts with suture lines remaining intact (26). According to White et al. (5), more than 40 such cases have been recorded, suggesting that this problem is not as rare as previously thought. Another serious complication related to the mechanical failure of PTFE grafts is the formation of pseudoaneurysms in the body of the bypass graft. There have been documented cases of pseudoaneurysms developing in axillofemoral grafts after direct trauma, but a 1993 report by Piazza et al. describes a nonanastomotic pseudoaneurysm occurring without any trauma (27). Another report describes multiple aneurysms in an axillofemoral graft with coagulopathy (28). The management of such complications from structural failure includes prompt surgical exploration with replacement of the affected portion of the graft using a short segment interposed graft.

II. FEMOROFEMORAL GRAFT

Since the technique was introduced by Oudot and Beaconfield and Freeman and Leeds in the early 1950s and popularized by Vetto in the 1960s, the femorofemoral graft has been shown to have good long-term patency and is now considered a permanent reconstructive procedure (29–31). The femorofemoral graft is an acceptable alternative bypass to aortofemoral reconstruction when unilateral iliac artery occlusion is present; it has also been used for the management of aortofemoral graft limb occlusion (32). Initially the procedure was reserved for high-risk older patients, but it is now probably the procedure of choice in the young adult when donor iliac arterial occlusive disease is minimal and avoidance of sexual dysfunction is important.

Early complications of femorofemoral bypass grafts are similar to those associated with other bypass procedures; they include hemorrhage, thrombosis, hematoma, and local wound complications. A complication unique to femorofemoral bypass is penile swelling or scrotal hematoma related to the tunneling of the graft. These result from attempting to pass the graft retrofascially with disruption of the venous plexus in Retzius's space. As in the case of axillofemoral bypass, the graft pathway is extremely important for femorofemoral bypass. Kinking of the graft at the proximal or distal anastamosis, leading to stenosis or thrombosis, can occur if care is not taken in aligning the graft with both the donor and the recipient arteries. To avoid this complication, the graft should be placed in the subcutaneous tunnel first. Then the arteriotomies and subsequent anastomoses are made based on the angle of the graft with the donor and recipient arteries and on whether the anastomosis is to be constructed in a C or S manner.

Late complications include the formation of anastomotic aneurysm, distal embolization, and development of the steal phenomenon. With the increased use of PTFE grafts, it is now uncommon to encounter an anastomotic aneurysm in femorofemoral grafts. Thrombosis in a femorofemoral graft and distal embolization to the superficial femoral or popliteal artery have been reported (33). Donor limb steal has been observed, especially when the graft is performed for intermittent claudication. The decrease of donor limb ankle pressure seen in our series was caused by either unrecognized iliac disease or multilevel disease (34). For patients with intermittent claudication, ankle pressure of the donor limb must be evaluated by treadmill exercise testing. A decrease in ankle pressure after exercise of the donor limb increases the likelihood of the steal phenomenon if a femorofemoral graft is performed. Other hemodynamic tests—such as duplex scanning and intra-arterial pressure measurement of the femoral artery—may also help to detect hemodynamically significant iliac artery disease. When, after femorofemoral bypass, a large femoral/brachial pressure gradient correlating to steal is measured, one alternative treatment is percutaneous transluminal angioplasty of the common iliac artery (35). Treatment of superficial groin infections after femorofemoral bypass involves systemic antibiotics and local wound care. Infection of the femorofemoral bypass is a serious complication, as demonstrated by a 1995 study by de Virgilio et al. describing a mortality rate of 20% and an amputation rate of 10% (36). Treatment requires prompt graft removal and reconstitution of blood flow by another route.

III. OBTURATOR BYPASS

Obturator bypass is often performed in patients with an infected groin or dense scar tissue as a result of multiple groin dissections or postradiation changes. The procedure first described by Shaw and Baue is now regarded as acceptable for bypass (37).

Complications of the procedure include injury to the obturator artery, obturator nerve, or the genitourinary tract. The original description of the procedure called for passing the tunneling device from above after identification of the obturator foramen. Such a maneuver may be difficult and injury to the obturator nerve or artery during dissection is a real possibility. Injury to the obturator nerve is manifest by pain radiating from the groin to the medial aspect of the knee. Paresthesia and hyperesthesia may also occur. Motor dysfunction produces a wide-based gait that results from adductor muscle weakness.

Electromyography or obturator nerve blocks are useful to establish the diagnosis (38). Injury of the obturator artery may result in a retroperitoneal hematoma or excessive blood loss. The urological complications that have been reported are perforation of the bladder and transection of the ipsilateral ureter (39). We have observed bladder injury in 1 of 14 patients who underwent this procedure. This patient had a history of pelvic surgery followed by radiation therapy and should not have been considered for this type of bypass.

To simplify this procedure, we favor passing the tunneling device from below (40,41). After an incision is made just below the adductor longus tendon in the midthigh, the tunnel is created below the adductor longus and magnus muscles with the leg abducted and externally rotated. Next, a large DeBakey clamp is passed upward from below and directed toward the obturator foramen. At this time the operator's hand is placed over the obturator foramen and the membrane penetrated. The graft then is drawn from above into the thigh to be anastomosed to the popliteal artery.

One of the interesting complications of obturator bypass is interval gangrene of the thigh. Unless there are sufficient collateral pathways connecting the popliteal and tibial trunks with the profunda femoris, proximal myonecrosis may occur because the obturator graft bypasses the profunda femoris artery at the groin. This complication can be avoided by including the profunda femoris artery in the reconstruction.

IV. THORACOFEMORAL BYPASS

Extra-anatomic bypass from the descending thoracic aorta to the femoral artery was first introduced by Blaisdell and coworkers in 1961 (42). Since its development, the procedure has been used by many surgeons for various indications. We use this type of bypass in patients for the following reasons: (a) conversion of existing or recently failed axillopop-liteal or axillofemoral bypasses originally placed for septic abdominal aortic indications (infected aortic grafts or aortoduodenal fistulas), (b) avoidance of redissection of the retroperitoneum in patients after many other complex operations or infections, or (c) multiple failed aortofemoral bypasses. In each instance the infrarenal abdominal aorta is relatively inaccessible to reoperation (43). The procedure is rather simple and the descending thoracic aorta is approached through a posterolateral thoracotomy. The graft is then tunneled in a transdiaphragmatic retroperitoneal anterior axillary line to the left femoral artery. A femorofemoral bypass is then added to complete the revascularization. The technique has not been widely used; therefore the incidence of complications is unknown. In our series the 4-year patency rate of the thoracic aorta to femoral artery bypass was 100%, with a single graft failing at 49 months (44). There were 5 total complications in 21 patients, including a fracture of the spleen during tunneling requiring splenectomy and a bladder injury with retrofascial tunneling during the femorofemoral bypass portion of the procedure. The remaining complications were a minor vein injury during tunneling and reoperation for persistent thoracic bleeding in another patient. Another patient developed a late complication of thoracic aorta infection from an ascending groin infection after two failed lower extremity bypass procedures. A recent study by Passman et al. describes a 5-year primary patency rate for bypass procedures from the descending thoracic aorta to the iliofemoral artery of 79%, supporting a more widespread use of this durable procedure for primary revascularization (45).

V. CONCLUSION

Extra-anatomic bypass grafts are useful and often provide an effective means to restore blood flow in special conditions and in a unique population of patients. Although some of these grafts may be considered temporary, enough data have now been accumulated to demonstrate that femorofemoral grafts may be considered permanent reconstructions and the other grafts to be more durable than anticipated. Similarly, the frequent use of external ring-reinforced PTFE grafts may provide patients with a much better patency rate and fewer graft complications than previously reported. Extra-anatomic bypass represents an advance in techniques in vascular surgery. With the rather low incidence of complications and an aging population, these procedures should remain viable and important alternate surgical techniques for revascularization.

REFERENCES

1. Blaisdell FW, Hall AD. Axillary-femoral artery bypass for lower extremity ischemia. Surgery 1963; 54:563–568.
2. Louw JH. Splenic to femoral and axillary to femoral bypass grafts in diffuse arteriosclerotic occlusive disease. Lancet 1963; 1:401–402.
3. Bunt TJ, Moore W. Optimal proximal anastomosis/tunnel for axillofemoral grafts. J Vasc Surg 1986; 3:673–676.
4. Taylor LM Jr, Park TC, Edwards JM, Yeager RA, McConnell DC, Moneta GA, Porer JM, McConnell DC, Moneta GA, Porter JM. Acute disruption of polytetrafluoroethylene grafts adjacent to axillary anastomoses: a complication of axillogemoral grafting. J Vasc Surg 1994; 20:520–526.
5. White GH, Donayre CE, Williams RA, White RA, Stabile BE, Wilson SE. Exertional disruption of axillofemoral graft anastomosis—"The axillary pull-out syndrome". Arch Surg 1990; 125:625–627.
6. Yeager RA, Taylor LM Jr. Axillary artery anastomosis to avoid axillofemoral bypass disruption. Semin Vasc Surg 2000; 13:74–76.
7. Sullivan LP, Davidson PG, D'Anna JA, Sithian N. Disruption of the proximal anastomosis of axillofemoral grafts: Two case reports. J Vasc Surg 1989; 10:190–192.
8. Darr AS, Finch DRA. Graft avulsion: An unreported complication of axillofemoral bypass grafts. Br J Surg 1978; 65:442–446.
9. Blaisdell FW. Late axillary thrombosis in patients with occluded axillary-femoral bypass grafts. J Vasc Surg 1985; 2:925.
10. Landry GJ, Moneta GL, Taylor LM, Porter JM. Axillobifemoral bypass. Ann Vasc Surg 2000; 14:296–305.
11. McLafferty RB, Taylor LM Jr, Moneta GL, Yeager RA, Edwards JM, Porter JM. Upper extremity thromboembolism caused by occlusion of axillofemoral grafts. Am J Surg 1995; 169:492–495.
12. Kempczinski R, Penn I. Upper extremity complication of axillofemoral grafts. Am J Surg 1978; 136:209–211.
13. Rashleigh-Belcher HJC, Newcombe JF. Axillary artery thrombosis: A complication of axillofemoral bypass grafts. Surgery 1987; 101:373–375.
14. Farina C, Schultz RD, Feldhaus RJ. Late upper limb acute ischemia in a patient with an occluded axillofemoral bypass graft. J Cardiovasc Surg 1990; 31:178–181.
15. Hartman AR, Fried KS, Khalil I, Riles TS. Late axillary artery thrombosis in patients with occluded axillary-femoral bypass grafts. J Vasc Surg 1985; 2:285–287.
16. Jarowenko MV, Buchbinder D, Shah DM. Effect of external pressure on axillo-femoral bypass grafts. Arch Surg 1981; 193:274–276.
17. Cavallaro A, Sclacca V, di Marzo LD, Bove S, Mingoli A. The effect of body weight compression on axillo-femoral bypass patency. J Cardiovasc Surg 1988; 29:476–479.
18. Bandyk DF, Thiele BG, Radke HM. Upper extremity embolus secondary to axillofemoral bypass grafts. Arch Surg 1983; 118:673–676.
19. Ascher E, Veith FJ, Gupta S. Axillopopliteal bypass grafting: Indications, late results, and determinants of long-term patency. J Vasc Surg 1989; 10:285–291.
20. Marston WA, Risley GL, Criado E, Burnham SJ, Keagy BA. Management of failed and infected axillofemoral grafts. J Vasc Surg 1994; 20:357–365.
21. Buche M, Schoevaerdts JC, Jaumin P, Ponlot R, Chalant CH. Perigraft seroma following axillofemoral bypass: Report of three cases. Ann Vasc Surg 1986; 1:374–377.
22. Blumberg RM, Gelfand ML, Dale WA. Perigraft seromas complicating arterial grafts. J Cardiovasc Surg 1983; 24:372.
23. Borreor E, Doscher W. Chronic perigraft seromas in PTFE grafts. J Cardiovasc Surg 1988; 29:46–49.

24. Ahn SS, Williams DE, Thye DA, Cheng KQ, Lee DA. The isolation of a fibroblast growth inhibitor associated with perigraft seroma. J Vasc Surg 1994; 20:202–208.

25. Friedman SG, Long KC, Scher LA. Axillofemoral bypass graft fracture. Ann Vasc Surg 1996; 10:490–492.

26. Brophy CM, Quist WC, Kwolek C, LoGerfo FW. Disruption of proximal axillobifemoral bypass graft anastomosis. J Vasc Surg 1992; 15:218–220.

27. Piazza D, Ameli FM, von Schroeder HP, Lossing A. Nonanastomotic pseudoaneurysm of expanded polytetrafluoroethylene axillofemoral bypass graft. J Vasc Surg 1993; 17:777–779.

28. Okadome SMK, Onohara T, Yamamura S, et al. Recurrent multiple aneurysms in an axillofemoral graft with coagulopathy. Acta Chir Scand 1990; 156:571–573.

29. Oudot J, Beaconfield P. Thrombosis of the aortic bifurcation treated by resection and homograft replacement. Arch Surg 1953; 66:365–374.

30. Freeman NE, Leeds FH. Operations of large arteries: Application of recent advances. Calif Med 1952; 77:229–233.

31. Vetto RM. The femoro-femoral shunt: An appraisal. Am J Surg 1966; 112:162.

32. Nolan KD, Benjamin ME, Murphy TJ, Pearce WH, McCarthy WJ, Yao JST, Flinn WR. Femorofemoral bypass for aortofemoral graft limb occlusion: A ten year experience. J Vasc Surg 1994; 19:851–857.

33. Seeger JM, Kwab-Gatt CS, Lazarus HM, Albo D. Embolic and occlusive complications from thrombosed femorofemoral grafts. J Cardiovasc Surg 1980; 21:547–558.

34. Harris JP, Flinn WR, Rudo ND, Bergan JJ, Yao JS. Assessment of donor limb hemodynamics in femorofemoral bypass for claudication. Surgery 1981; 90:764–773.

35. Gupta SK, Veith FJ, Kram HB, Wengerter KA. Significance and management of inflow gradients unexpectedly generated after femorofemoral, femoropopliteal, and femoroinfrapopliteal bypass grafting. J Vasc Surg 1990; 12:278–283.

36. de Virgilio C, Cherry KJ Jr, Gloviczki P, Naessens J, Bower T, Hallett J, Pairolero P. Infected lower extremity extra-anatomic bypass grafts: Management of a serious complication in high-risk patients. Ann Vasc Surg 1995; 9:459–466.

37. Shaw RS, Baue AE. Management of sepsis complicating arterial reconstructive procedures. Surgery 1962; 53:75–76.

38. Sheiner NM, Sigman H, Stilman A. An unusual complication of obturator foramen arterial bypass. J Caardiovasc Surg 1969; 10:324.

39. Pearce WH, Ricco JB, Yao JST. Modified technique of obturator bypass in failed or infected grafts. Ann Surg 1983; 197:344–347.

40. Pearce WH, McCarthy WJ, Flinn WR, Yao JST. Obturator foramen bypass. In: Bergan JJ, Yao JST, eds. Techniques in Arterial Surgery. Orlando, FL: Saunders, 1990:367–371.

41. Rudich M, Gutierrez IZ, Gage AA. Obturator foramen bypass in the management of infected vascular prostheses. Am J Surg 1979; 137:657–660.

42. Blaisdell FW, DeMattei GA, Gauder PJ. Extraperitoneal thoracic aorta to femoral bypass graft as replacement for an infected aortic bifurcation prosthesis. Am J Surg 1961; 102:583–585.

43. McCarthy WJ, Rubin JR, Flinn WR, Williams LR, Bergan JJ, Yao JS. Descending thoracic aorta-to-femoral artery bypass. Arch Surg 1986; 121:681–688.

44. McCarthy WJ, Mesh CL, McMillan WD, Flinn WR, Pearce WH, Yao JST. Descending thoracic aorta-to-femoral artery bypass: Ten years' experience with a durable procedure. J Vasc Surg 1993; 17:336–347.

45. Passman MA, Farber MA, Criado E, Marston WA, Burnham SJ, Keagy BA. Descending thoracic aorta to iliofemoral artery bypass grafting: A role for primary revascularization for aortoiliac occlusive disease. J Vasc Surg 1999; 29:249–258.

16

Vascular Graft Infections: Epidemiology, Microbiology, Pathogenesis, and Prevention

John M. Draus, Jr.
University of Louisville School of Medicine, Louisville, Kentucky, U.S.A.

Thomas M. Bergamini
University of Louisville School of Medicine and Surgical Care Associates, Louisville, Kentucky, U.S.A.

The development of biomaterials to replace or bypass diseased arterial segments has revolutionized the management of arterial disease. Although the search for the ideal conduit continues, present-day grafts have proven to be durable alternatives with acceptable patency for the treatment of both aneurysmal and occlusive disease in the peripheral circulation. Their usage has allowed successful revascularization operations in numerous patients who otherwise would have suffered loss of life or limb. Vascular surgical graft infection is among the most feared complications that the vascular surgeon faces, often resulting in prolonged hospitalization, multiple operations, and removal of the graft with resulting organ failure, amputation, and death. This chapter focuses on the epidemiology of vascular graft infection, reviews the most common pathogens, explores the theories of pathogenesis, and suggests practical strategies for the prevention of this ominous complication.

I. EPIDEMIOLOGY

Infection of a vascular prosthesis is a relatively uncommon complication of vascular surgery. The reported incidence of infection involving synthetic vascular grafts ranges from 1 to 6% with an average of 2.1% (Table 1). This variability can be partially explained by differences in duration of postoperative follow-up, type of graft material and method of construction, use of antibiotic prophylaxis, and virulence of the infecting pathogens. The actual incidence may be higher, since many graft infections do not become clinically evident until years after implantation. The indication for intervention and the implantation site have been shown to influence the incidence of vascular graft infection. Infection is

Table 1 Incidence of Vascular Graft Infections

Study	Number of cases	Number of infections (%)
Hoffert et al., 1965 (1)	201	12 (6.0)
Lindenauer et al., 1967 (2)	890	12 (1.3)
Conn et al., 1970 (3)	435	22 (5.1)
Szilagyi et al., 1972 (4)	3,397	40 (1.2)
Goldstone and Moore, 1974 (5)	566	27 (4.8)
Jameison et al., 1975 (6)	664	15 (2.3)
Liekweg and Greenfield, 1976 (7)	859	22 (2.6)
Yasher et al., 1978 (8)	590	32 (5.4)
Edwards et al., 1987 (9)	2,614	24 (0.92)
Fletcher et al., 1991 (10)	322	11 (3.4)
Total	10,538	217 (2.1)

most common in grafts placed in the inguinal region or in superficial locations, possibly associated with increased bacterial colonization and contamination with the patient's skin flora at this site (10).

Vascular graft infections are commonly associated with operative events that lead to bacterial contamination of the graft and patient characteristics that impair host defenses (Table 2). Greater than 90% of vascular patients have one or more risk factors for the development of a graft infection at the time of their operation. Graft infection is more likely to occur after emergent procedures, such as the repair of a ruptured abdominal aortic aneurysm. Breaks in sterile surgical technique and improper sterilization of grafts or instruments are obvious sources of contamination. Prolonged preoperative hospitalization increases the patient's risk of becoming colonized by more virulent bacterial species, which are frequently resistant to conventional antibiotic therapy. Infected skin ulcers, gangrenous toes, and other remote infection sites represent potential sources of graft sepsis. Operative time greater than 4 h has been linked to intraoperative bacterial seeding. Concomitant biliary, bowel, or urological procedures introduce additional sources of potential contamination that may jeopardize the clean vascular bed into which the graft is placed. Infection rates after reoperative vascular procedures for hematoma or graft thrombosis reflect the frequency of arterial wall and wound colonization. Bile fistula, anastomosis breakdown, and other postoperative complications often result in colonization of the vascular graft. Patients with impaired immune function due to malnutrition, malignancy, or autoimmune disease will have more difficulty fighting infection. Similarly, the administration of medications such as steroids or immunosuppressive chemotherapy will alter the patient's immunological competence.

Infection of a vascular graft is an ominous complication whose outcome is often worse than the natural history of the vascular problem that led to implantation. Despite aggressive antibiotic administration and surgical treatment, overall mortality rates remain between 10 and 50% and overall amputation rates between 15 and 60% (9–11). Infected aortic grafts have the highest mortality rates (40–75%) due to hemorrhage, sepsis, and complications of multiple operative procedures (7,11,12). When systemic sepsis is the presenting symptom, the prognosis is particularly grim. In contrast, femoropopliteal graft infections have a lower mortality (10–25%) (7,12). However, the amputation rate approaches 80% in some studies,

Table 2 Risk Factors for Graft Infection

Contamination of the graft
Emergency surgery
Prolonged preoperative hospital stay
Remote infection
Faulty sterile technique
Extended operating time
Simultaneous gastrointestinal procedure
Reoperative vascular procedure
Postoperative superficial wound infection

Altered host defenses
Local factors
    Biomaterial properties
    Bacterial adherence
    Slime production
    Biofilm proliferation
    Macrophage suppression
    Cytokine production
    Fibroblast inhibition
    Collagen hyperplasia
Systemic factors
    Malnutrition
    Malignancy
    Diabetes mellitus
    Autoimmune disease
    Chronic renal failure
    Leukopenia
    Chemotherapy
    Corticosteroid administration

especially when infected grafts present with sepsis or anastomotic bleeding (13). Although prosthetic vascular graft infection is uncommon, the threat of amputation, loss of organ function, or death from this complication justifies the concern of the vascular surgeon and the use of aggressive prophylaxis.

II. BACTERIOLOGY

Virtually any micro-organism is capable of infecting a synthetic graft. Initial studies considered graft infection to be an early complication of vascular surgery and regarded *Staphylococcus aureus* as the most prevalent pathogen (4,7,14,15). Refinements in arterial grafting techniques, prosthetic materials, and antibiotic usage have influenced the frequency and nature of graft infections. Since the 1970s, coagulase-negative staphylococci, gram-negative bacteria, and polymicrobial infections have become significant (Table 3). Surgeons have become cognizant of the possibility of microbiological sampling errors, especially in late-appearing infections, when low numbers of bacteria are present (16). Gram-negative bacteria—such as *Escherichia coli* and *Pseudomonas*, *Klebsiella*, *Proteus*, and *Enterobacter* species—are particularly virulent. The incidence of anastomotic dehis-

Table 3 Bacteriology of Prosthetic Vascular Graft Infections: Data from 1305 Collected Cases

Pathogen	Number of Cases (%)						
	AEF 397	AI 86	AF 460	FD 251	TA 55	ICS 56	Total 1305
Staphylococcus aureus	16 (4)	7 (8)	124 (27)	70 (28)	12 (22)	28 (50)	257 (19)
Staphylococcus epidermidis	8 (2)	22 (26)	120 (26)	28 (11)	14 (25)	11 (20)	203 (16)
Streptococcus species	75 (19)	3 (3)	46 (10)	28 (11)	1 (2)	—	153 (12)
Escherichia coli	71 (18)	18 (21)	55 (12)	18 (7)	1 (2)	—	163 (12)
Pseudomonas species	12 (3)	8 (9)	28 (6)	40 (16)	8 (14)	—	96 (7)
Klebsiella species	20 (5)	4 (5)	23 (5)	5 (2)	1 (2)	6 (10)	59 (5)
Enterococcus species	32 (8)	8 (9)	9 (2)	18 (7)	2 (4)	—	69 (5)
Bacteroides species	32 (8)	1 (1)	14 (3)	5 (2)	—	—	52 (4)
Proteus species	16 (4)	1 (1)	18 (4)	18 (7)	1 (2)	—	54 (4)
Enterobacter species	20 (5)	8 (9)	9 (2)	5 (2)	—	—	42 (3)
Candida species	12 (3)	—	5 (1)	3 (1)	2 (4)	—	22 (2)
Serratia species	4 (1)	—	5 (1)	5 (2)	—	—	14 (1)
Other species	12 (3)	3 (3)	18 (4)	15 (2)	—	—	48 (4)
No growth culture	71 (18)	11 (13)	9 (2)	5 (2)	9 (16)	11 (20)	116 (9)

Abbreviations: AEF = aortoenteric fistula or erosion; AI = aortoiliac, aortofemoral, or aortic tube graft; AF = aortobifemoral or iliofemoral graft; FD = femoropopliteal, femorotibial, axillofemoral, or femorofemoral graft; TA = thoracic aorta graft; ICS = innominate, carotid, or subclavian bypass graft or carotid patch following endarterectomy.

cence and artery rupture is high and is due to the organisms' ability to produce destructive endotoxins (e.g., elastase and alkaline protease) that act to compromise the structural integrity of the vessel wall. (17,18). Fungal infections due to *Candida*, *Mycobacterium*, and *Aspergillus* species are rare and are typically seen in patients with previously established fungal infections or severe immunosuppression.

Early-appearing graft infections occur within the first 4 months following vascular bypass surgery and are associated with virulent pathogens. Patients present with classic signs of graft sepsis, such as fever, leukocytosis, and bacteremia. The pathogens are easily identified by cultures of blood or perigraft tissues. *S. aureus* continues to be the most prevalent pathogen. Coagulase-positive strains produce hemolysis and toxins to leukocytes that provoke an intense local and systemic host response and permit early recognition of the infectious complications. Gram-negative bacteria are also implicated in early graft infection. *Pseudomonas aeruginosa* infection is most commonly associated with anastomotic bleeding. Graft healing complications, such as graft-enteric erosion or fistula, typically involve infection with gram-negative enteric bacteria and can develop in both the early and late postoperative periods.

Late-appearing infections are most frequently the result of graft colonization by *Staphylococcus epidermidis* or other coagulase-negative staphylococci (19,20). These indolent infections manifest themselves months to years after implantation and have replaced early graft infections as the most common presentation in vascular patients (19,21). Coagulase-negative staphylococci, organisms of low-virulence are normal inhabitants of the skin flora. Bacteria are sequestered on prosthetic surfaces and survive within an adherent biofilm (22). This bacteria-laden surface biofilm is composed of coalescing microcolonies enclosed in an extracellular nutrient glycocalyx produced by the organisms (23). Initially, the bacterial biofilm creates a symbiotic infection that is localized to the prosthetic surface. Signs of graft sepsis (e.g., fever, leukocytosis) are absent. If the bacterial biofilm is recognized by host defenses, local inflammation of the perigraft tissue and adjacent artery ensues. Gram's stain of perigraft fluid shows only white blood cells, and routine cultures of blood and perigraft tissue or fluid are sterile. Bacterial biofilm infections present as a wound-healing complication, such as anastomotic aneurysm, perigraft abscess, graft–enteric fistula, or graft–cutaneous sinus tract.

III. PATHOGENESIS

A. Bacterial Seeding of Biomaterial Surfaces

Any process that exposes the prosthetic conduit to microorganisms via direct, lymphatic, or hematogenous routes can result in graft colonization and subsequent infection. Biomaterial surfaces can become seeded with bacteria or fungi during the implantation procedure, during postoperative wound-healing complications, or at any time thereafter during occurrences of transient bacteremia.

Direct contamination of the vascular graft during arterial reconstruction results from breaks in aseptic technique by the operative team. Improper sterilization of grafts and surgical instruments are obvious sources of contamination. Contact with the skin and epidermal appendages exposes the prosthetic graft to the patient's endogenous flora. It is not surprising that an increased incidence of graft infections is observed when grafts are placed in superficial locations (e.g., femoral, popliteal, and axillary anastomoses), where skin contact is likely. Intestinal bag effluents and injury to or opening of the intestinal or urinary tract are other sources of endogenous flora that can compromise graft placement. Diseased artery walls (e.g., atherosclerotic plaque or aneurysmal thrombus) are a frequently unrecognized source of bacteria, especially coagulase-negative staphylococci. Infected lymph nodes and lymph channels are other important sources of direct contamination. Transection of the lymphatics proximal to a septic focus bathes the implanted graft in a bacterial inoculum that has been shown to contribute to the development of acute graft infection in canine models (24). Femoral anastomoses are particularly vulnerable to this type of contamination, especially when ischemic foot ulcers or gangrene is present in the lower extremity. A concomitantly performed surgical procedure (e.g., gastrointestinal or biliary tract) provides additional sources of potential contamination to the prosthetic graft.

The risk of prosthetic vascular graft contamination via a direct route continues into the postoperative period. If the surgical wound does not promptly develop a fibrin seal following the revascularization, the underlying graft is susceptible to direct extension from initially trivial superficial wound problems. With persistent wound drainage, a septic focus can develop in ischemic or injured tissues and progress by deep extension to involve the vascular prosthesis (25). Hematomas and lymphoceles create an area of dead space around the graft that is favorable to bacterial growth, unfavorable to host defenses, and inhibitory to graft incorporation by perigraft tissues. Patients that undergo graft revision for failed revascularization are repeatedly exposed to potential sources of graft infection. These patients commonly harbor bacteria within scar tissue and lymphoceles and on the surfaces of previously implanted prosthetic grafts and suture materials. In explanted prosthetic material, micro-organisms were cultured from 90% of grafts associated with anastomotic aneurysm and from 69% of thrombosed grafts (26). Furthermore, multiple operations cause additional trauma to the tissues and increase the risk of poor wound healing.

Bacterial seeding of the graft via a hematogenous route is an uncommon but potentially important mechanism of graft infection. Experimentally, a single intravenous infusion of 107 colony-forming units (CFUs) of *S. aureus* produces positive graft cultures in 100% of animals up to 1 month following graft placement (27). During the perioperative period, hematogenous seeding of the graft may occur via transient bacteremias from sources such as intravenous catheters, an infected urinary tract, or remote tissue infection (e.g., pneumonia or infected foot ulcers). Experimentally, parenteral antibiotic therapy reduces the incidence of graft infection from bacteremia and is the basis of culture-specific antibiotic therapy in patients with known infection at remote sites. The susceptibility of graft to contamination from hematogenous sources is influenced by the integrity of the cellular lining that covers biomaterial surfaces. The risk of contamination is highest immediately after implantation and gradually decreases as the luminal pseudointimal lining develops and matures over time (28). The graft remains susceptible to hematogenous seeding long after implantation; infection from bacteremia has been documented beyond 1 year after implantation. Transient bacteremia in an immunocompromised patient may account for graft infections occurring years after the original revascularization.

B. Microcolony Formation and Bacterial Biofilms

Once micro-organisms seed the prosthetic surface, the ability of bacteria to produce a vascular graft infection depends on adhesion, colonization, and biofilm formation. The biomaterial infection persists because of the failure of the host immune system to kill adherent bacteria and the surrounding inflammation and cellular damage that inhibits tissue incorporation.

The physical properties and chemical composition of the vascular conduit significantly influence the ability of bacteria to adhere to the biomaterial surface. Autogenous grafts, such as the saphenous vein, have the lowest susceptibility to infection. In the absence of immediate postoperative infection, these grafts exhibit long-term patency and represent the best natural replacement for the original conduit. The two most common synthetic materials used are external velour-knitted Dacron and expanded polytetrafluoroethylene (ePTFE). Dacron is composed of multiple interlocking strands. The porous nature of the material favors bacterial sequestration. Bacterial strains have been shown to have greater affinity for Dacron than for ePTFE (22,29,30). The extrusion process in the manufacturing of ePTFE significantly decreases the porosity of the graft material. ePTFE is the material of choice when prosthetic graft is used in patients at risk for bacteremia.

Bacterial adherence to the vascular prosthesis depends on the cell wall and the growth characteristics of the bacteria species. Bacteria adhere by means of a mass of tangled fibers of polysaccharides that extend from the bacterial cell surface and form a felt-like "glycocalyx" surrounding an individual cell or colony of cells (31). In a competitive natural environment, the glycocalyx influences the selection and protection of a particular kind of bacteria from all others in the population. The prevalence of staphylococcal graft infections can be partially explained by the increased adherence of gram-positive bacteria to prosthetic surfaces. Under experimental conditions, *Staphylococcus* species have been shown to adhere to synthetic vascular graft materials in as high as 1000 times greater number than do gram-negative bacteria (32). Similarly, *S. aureus* has been demonstrated to adhere to suture material in as high as 1000 times greater number than *E. coli* (33). The adherence of staphylococci is postulated to be enhanced by specific capsular adhesions that potentiate micro-organism attachment and colonization. Antibodies to these specific cell surface glycoproteins have been developed, and their application to graft surfaces can inhibit adherence of adhesin-producing strains.

The pathogenesis of late-appearing graft infections is the result of prosthesis colonization by low-virulence microorganisms. Some strains of coagulase-negative staphylococci, such as *S. epidermidis*, adhere to the graft surface and survive in a bacteria-laden biofilm. Unlike *S. aureus* and gram-negative bacteria, *S. epidermidis* grows only within the biofilm, does not produce toxins or products capable of producing tissue autolysis, and does not invade the surrounding tissues in the presence of host defenses (25). The surface biofilm is a complex structure composed of coalescing microcolonies enclosed in an extracellular nutrient glycocalyx that is produced by the organisms (23). The biofilm plays an important role in promoting persistence of the infection by protecting it from host defense mechanisms, entrapping nutrients from the environment, and resisting antimicrobial penetration (21,34,35).

C. Activation of the Immune System

Graft infection is a complex process involving activation of the host immune system by coinflammatory stimuli produced by both the micro-organisms and the vascular biomaterials. The inflammatory process attempts to localize the infection but results in microvascular disruption, cellular death, tissue necrosis, and neutrophils at the interface between the surrounding tissues and the biomaterial surface. The virulence of the infecting pathogen determines the extent of perigraft inflammation and tissue injury, but even indolent infections can produce tissue autolysis that results in vessel wall or anastomotic disruption and hemorrhage. The clinical effects of graft infection manifest themselves as a broad spectrum of signs including graft sepsis, localized perigraft abscess, anastomotic pseudoaneurysm, graft cutaneous sinus tract, or graft-enteric erosion or fistula (aortoduodenal fistula).

Biomaterial infection is characterized by a lack of normal tissue incorporation. The monocyte, or tissue macrophage, is crucial for directing this activity via specific growth factors and enzymes (36). Using a mouse model of *S. epidermidis* vascular graft infection, we have shown that vascular graft infection does suppress the expression of local macrophage Ia, which is associated with a local elevation of the proinflammatory cytokines and a lack of normal healing (37,38). The overproduction of tumor necrosis factor alpha (TNF-α) and interleukin 1 (IL-1) has been shown to cause tissue damage. TNF-α is a major monocyte product that enhances the expression of neutrophil complement receptor. The release of IL-1 has been shown to correlate with the extent of fibrous capsule formation. Moreover, TNF-α and IL-1 are known to stimulate collagenases, which would favor nonhealing. These two cytokines may mediate the local tissue damage associated with chronic bacterial biofilm infections. Persistent growth of *S. epidermidis* in the biomaterial's surface biofilm results in a chronic inflammatory process and cellular damage to the surrounding tissues, inhibiting incorporation of the perigraft tissue into the biomaterial and resulting in the formation of a perigraft cavity and abscess. This process is mediated by the host's immune response, producing autolysis of the periprosthetic tissues. The immune response results in poor graft incorporation, with surrounding tissue inflammation and a perigraft cavity containing an exudate of many polymorphonuclear leukocytes (39–41). Further progression of the inflammation in the perigraft tissues can result in a graft–cutaneous sinus tract or graft–enteric fistula, depending on the site of the graft. The chronic inflammation mediated by the host's immune system can also result in an adjacent arteritis, producing a decreased anastomotic tensile strength and subsequent pseudoaneurysm formation.

In the mouse model of subcutaneous vascular graft infection, we have shown that biomaterial infection is associated with fibroblast inhibition that is independent of proinflammatory cytokines (42). The mediators of fibroblast inhibition using this mouse model were bacterial cell products. Effective removal of this inhibitor of fibroblast proliferation has been reported by plasmapheresis and also by removal of the implanted biomaterial. In our rabbit model of vascular graft aortic infection, we have shown that the perigraft fluid as well as serum from animals with infected grafts as compared to sterile grafts inhibits fibroblast proliferation.

The prosthetic graft materials invoke a foreign-body reaction that produces an acidic, ischemic microenvironment conductive to bacterial biofilm proliferation. Unlike autogenous grafts, implanted synthetic biomaterials never develop vascular connections with the surrounding tissue. This prevents host immune defenses and antibiotics from exerting their maximal effect on infecting organisms. Furthermore, a complete cellular pseudointima never develops on the luminal surfaces of biomaterials. Possible mechanisms include a lack of fibroblast hyperplasia and collagen production. Failure of prosthetic grafts to develop a protective endothelial lining renders them susceptible to late infection by bacterial seeding.

IV. PREVENTION

The prevention of prosthetic graft infection is a critical concept in vascular surgery. Prophylactic measures must be taken preoperatively, intraoperatively, and postoperatively to help reduce the risk of this dreaded complication.

A. Preoperative Measures

A prolonged preoperative hospital stay should be avoided so as to reduce the patient's risk of becoming colonized with nosocomial bacterial strains that are resistant to commonly used antibiotics. Within 5 days of admission to a hospital, a patient's skin flora may already have become resistant to several antibiotics (43). Preoperative angiography should be performed more than 1 week or less than 24 h prior to graft implantation. When transfemoral angiography is completed between 1 and 7 days before surgery, the incidence of wound infection has been shown to increase (44).

Since the patient's own flora is the primary source of graft contamination, special consideration should be given to skin preparation. Preoperative bathing with an antiseptic soap may help reduce the number of bacterial colonies present (45,46). Shaving the skin increases the incidence of wound infections when compared the use of a depilatory cream (46). If shaving is preferred, it should be delayed until the patient's arrival in the operative suite. Prior to the incision, the skin should be thoroughly cleansed with povidone-iodine, chlorhexidine, or both (46,47).

The standard administration of prophylactic antibiotics has been shown to decrease the occurrence of wound infections that potentially lead to vascular graft infections (26). The choice of antibiotic should be determined by local bacterial prevalence and sensitivities, remembering that *S. aureus*, *S. epidermidis*, and gram-negative organisms are the most prevalent pathogens. The first dose of the antibiotic should be administered prior to the skin incision; subsequent doses should be given at regular intervals during the operation to maintain tissue levels above the minimal bactericidal concentration for expected pathogens. Alterations in the dosing regimen may be required during the procedure based on the antibiotic's elimination and volume of distribution. It may become necessary to increase the dosage or frequency of administration when the operative time exceeds 4 h or if the patient experiences extreme changes in blood volume, fluid administration, or renal perfusion. Cefazolin sodium, 1 g given intravenously 1 h before surgery; 1 g given every 2–3 h during surgery; and then 1 g given every 8 h postoperatively for three doses will achieve excellent tissue levels in the majority of patients undergoing prosthetic graft implantation. When methicillin-resistant *S. aureus* is cultured on the patient's skin or is a known pathogen in hospitalized patients, a single dose of vancomycin hydrochloride, 1 g given intravenously may be added 1 h before surgery. For patients with allergies to penicillin or the cephalosporins, parenteral vancomycin (1 g) plus gentamicin (1.5 mg/kg), administered 1 h before surgery and then repeated every 8–12 h for three additional doses is also an appropriate prophylactic antibiotic regimen. Patients undergoing vascular graft implantation who have coexisting infections of the leg or another remote site should be placed on culture-specific antibiotics. Some vascular centers continue prophylactic antibiotics for 3–5 days in patients considered to be at high risk for transient bacteremia or until all central intravenous catheters have been removed. However, there is no solid evidence to substantiate the continued administration of prophylactic antibiotics for more than two or three postoperative doses.

B.   Intraoperative Measures

The importance of sound judgment and meticulous surgical technique is illustrated by the observation that up to 60% of vascular graft infections are associated with a preventable operative complication (5,6,48). When feasible, autologous vein should be used because it is associated with a reduced risk of infection and with less serious consequences should infection occur (49,50). Reconstructive procedures should avoid the groin region if possible, because groin wounds are the most prone to infection. The use of iodine-impregnated plastic drapes or antibiotic-soaked towels protects the graft from contact with potentially contaminating sources outside the operative field. Gentle handling of tissues, meticulous hemostasis to prevent hematoma formation, and closure of the incision in multiple layers to eliminate dead space are important technical caveats for reducing the risk of wound-healing problems and subsequent infections. The application of topical antibiotics prior to wound closure may offer some benefit by increasing the antibiotic concentration in the tissues surrounding the graft.

Simultaneous gastrointestinal procedures are best avoided during vascular graft implantation to prevent contamination with enteric pathogens. If an inadvertent enterotomy should occur during celiotomy, the patient's incision should be closed and the arterial reconstruction rescheduled for a second operation in a few days, with planned implantation of an antibiotic-impregnated prosthesis. One possible exception to the admonition against simultaneous gastrointestinal procedures is cholecystectomy for asymptomatic cholelithiasis, which can be safely performed in patients undergoing aortic graft implantation. An 18% incidence of postoperative acute cholecystitis has been reported in patients with cholelithiasis after elective repair of an abdominal aortic aneurysm (51). The risk of aortic graft infection after concomitant cholecystectomy remains low, but an increased complication rate has been reported in a large retrospective study of the

Mayo Clinic experience. The surgeon should proceed with gallbladder removal only after the aortic graft has been implanted and the retroperitoneum completely closed.

C. Postoperative Measures

The patient's urinary catheter and intravenous lines should be removed as soon as possible to eliminate potential sources of bacteremia. Early recognition and aggressive treatment of postoperative wound infections are essential in minimizing the risk of extension to the underlying graft. Patients with prosthetic vascular grafts should be fully educated as to the potential risks of bacteremia following interventional procedures. Hematogenous seeding is a continuing risk for as long as the graft remains in place. Antibiotic prophylaxis is recommended prior to dental work, angiography, cystoscopy, and colonoscopy to prevent bacterial colonization and subsequent late graft infection.

REFERENCES

1. Hoffert PW, Gensler S, Haimovici H. Infection complicating arterial grafts. Arch Surg 1965; 90:427–435.
2. Lindenauer SM, Fry WS, Schaub G, Wild D. The use of antibiotics in the prevention of vascular graft infections. Surgery 1967; 62:487–492.
3. Conn JH, Hardy JD, Chavez CM, Fain WR. Infected arterial grafts: Experience in 22 cases with emphasis on unusual bacteria and techniques. Ann Surg 1970; 171:704–712.
4. Szilagyi DE, Smith RE, Elliott JP, Vrandecic MP. Infection in arterial reconstruction with synthetic grafts. Ann Surg 1972; 176:321–333.
5. Goldstone J, Moore WS. Infection in vascular prostheses: Clinical manifestations and surgical management. Am J Surg 1974; 128:225–233.
6. Jamieson GC, DeWeese JA, Rob CG. Infected arterial grafts. Ann Surg 1975; 181:850–852.
7. Liekweg WG, Greenfield LJ. Vascular prosthetic infections: Collected experience and results of treatment. Surgery 1977; 81:335–342.
8. Yashar JJ, Wevman AK, Burnard RJ, Yashar J. Survival and limb salvage in patients with infected arterial prostheses. Am J Surg 1978; 135:499–504.
9. Edwards WH, Martin RS, Jenkins JM, Edwards WH, Mulherin JL. Primary graft infections. J Vasc Surg 1987; 6:235–239.
10. Fletcher JP, Dryden M, Sorrell TC. Infection of vascular prostheses. Aust NZ J Surg 1991; 61:432–435.
11. Seeger JM, Back MR, Albright JL, Carlton LM, Harward TRS, Kubulis MS, Flynn TC, Huber TS. Influence of patient characteristics and treatment options on outcome of patients with prosthetic aortic graft infection. Ann Vasc Surg 1999; 13:413–420.
12. Bunt TJ. Synthetic vascular graft infections: I. Graft infections. Surgery 1983; 93:733–746.
13. O'Brien T, Collin J. Prosthetic vascular graft infection. Br J Surg 1992; 79:1262–1267.
14. Javid H, Julian OC, Dye WS, Hunter JA. Complications of abdominal aortic grafts. Arch Surg 1962; 85:650–662.
15. Fry WS, Lindenauer SM. Infection complicating the use of plastic arterial implants. Arch Surg 1967; 94:600–609.
16. Kwaan JHM, Connolly JE. Successful management of prosthetic graft infection with continuous povidone-iodine irrigation. Arch Surg 1981; 116:716–720.
17. Calligaro KD, Westcott CJ, Buckley RM, Savarese RP, DeLaurentis DA. Infrainguinal anastomotic arterial graft infections treated by selective graft preservation. Ann Surg 1992; 216:74–79.
18. Calligaro KD, Veith FJ, Gupta SK, Ascer E, Dietzek AM, Franco CD, Wengerter KR. A

modified method of management of prosthetic graft infections involving an anastomosis to the common femoral artery. J Vasc Surg 1990; 11:485–492.

19. Bandyk DF, Berni GA, Thiele BL, Towne JB. Aortofemoral graft infection due to *Staphylococcus epidermidis*. Arch Surg 1984; 119:102–108.

20. Santini C, Baiocchi P, Venditti M, Brandimarte C, Tarasi A, Rizzo L, Speziale F, Fiorani P, Serra P. Aorto-femoral graft infections: A clinical and microbiological analysis. J Infect 1993; 27:17–26.

21. Dougherty SH, Simmons RL. Infections in bionic man: the pathobiology of infection in prosthetic devices. Curr Probl Surg 1982; 119:268–319.

22. Bergamini TM, Bandyk DF, Govostis D, Keabnick HW, Towne JB. Infection of vascular prosthesis caused by bacterial biofilms. J Vasc Surg 1988; 7:21–30.

23. Schmitt DD, Bandyk DF, Pequet AJ, Malangoni MA, Towne JB. Mucin production by *Staphylococcus epidermidis*: A virulence factor promoting adherence to vascular grafts. Arch Surg 1986; 121:89–95.

24. Rubin JR, Malone JM, Goldstone J. The role of the lymphatic system in acute arterial prosthetic graft infections. J Vasc Surg 1985; 2:92–98.

25. Bergamini TM. Vascular prosthesis infection caused by bacterial biofilms. Semin Vasc Surg 1990; 3:101–109.

26. Bandyk DF. Vascular graft infections: epidemiology, microbiology, pathogenesis and prevention. In: Bernhard VM, Towne JB, eds. Complications in Vascular Surgery. St. Louis: Quality Medical Publishing, 1991:223–234.

27. Roon AJ, Malone JM, Moore WS, Bean B, Campagna G. Bacteremic infectability: A function of vascular graft material and design. J Surg Res 1977; 22:489–498.

28. Malone JM, Moore WS, Campagna G, Bean B. Bacteremic infectability of vascular grafts: The influence of pseudointimal integrity and duration of graft function. Surgery 1975; 78:211–216.

29. Schmitt DD, Bandyk DF, Pequet AJ, Towne JB. Bacterial adherence to vascular prostheses: A determinant of graft infectivity. J Vasc Surg 1986; 3:732–740.

30. Sugarman B. In vitro adherence of bacteria to prosthetic vascular grafts. Infection 1982; 10: 9–12.

31. Costerton JW, Geesey GG, Cheng K-J. How bacteria stick. Sci Am 1978; 238:86–95.

32. Bergamini TM, Bandyk DF, Govostis D, Vetsch R, Towne JB. Identification of *Staphylococcus epidermidis* vascular graft infections: A comparison of culture techniques. J Vasc Surg 1989; 9:665–670.

33. Chih-Chang C, Williams DF. Effects of physical configuration and chemical structure of materials on bacterial adhesion. Am J Surg 1984; 174:197–204.

34. McAuley CE, Steed DL, Webster MW. Bacteria presence in aortic thrombus at elective aneurysm resection: Is it clinically significant? Am J Surg 1984; 147:322–324.

35. Costerton JW, Irvin RT, Cheng K-J. The bacterial glycocalyx in nature and disease. Annu Rev Microbiol 1981; 35:299–334.

36. Ziegler-Heitbrock HW, Strobel M, Kieper D, Fingerle G, Schlunck T, Petersmann I, Ellwart J, Blumenstein M, Haas JG. Differential expression of cytokines in human blood monocyte subpopulations. Blood 1992; 79:503–511.

37. Henke PK, Bergamini TM, Garrison JR, Brittian KR, Peyton JR, Lam TM. *Staphylococcus epidermidis* graft infection is associated with locally suppressed MHC-II and elevated MAC-1 expression. Arch Surg 1997; 132:894–902.

38. Henke PK, Bergamini TM, Brittian KR, Polk HC Jr. Prostaglandin E2 modulates monocyte MCH-II(Ia) suppression in biomaterial infection. J Surg Res 1997; 69:372–378.

39. Steenfoos HH, Hunt TK, Scheuenstuhl H, Goodson WH. Selective effects of tumor necrosis factor-alpha on wound healing in rats. Surgery 1989; 106:171–176.

40. Knighton DR, Fiegel VD. The macrophage: Effector cell wound repair. Perspect Shock Res 1989; 21:217–226.

41. Barbul A. Immune aspects of wound repair. Clin Plast Surg 1990; 17:433–442.

42. Henke PK, Bergamini TM, Watson AL, Brittian KR, Powell DW, Peyton JC. Bacterial products primarily mediate fibroblast inhibition in biomaterial infection. J Surg Res 1998; 74:17–22.

43. Levy M, Schmitt DD, Edmistone CE. Sequential analysis of staphylococcal colonization of body surfaces of patients undergoing vascular surgery. J Clin Microbiol 1990; 28:664–669.

44. Landreneau MD, Raju S. Infections after elective bypass surgery for lower limb ischemia: The influence of pre-operative transcutaneous arteriography. Surgery 1981; 90:956–961.

45. Cruse PJ, Foord R. A five-year prospective study of 23,649 surgical wounds. Arch Surg 1973; 107:206–209.

46. Cruse PJ, Foord R. A ten-year prospective study of 62939 wounds. The epidemiology of wound infection. Surg Clin North Am 1980; 60:27–40.

47. Berry AR, Watt B, Goldacre MJ, Thomson JWW, McNair TJ. A comparison of the use of povidone-iodine and chlorhexidine in the prophylaxis of postoperative wound infection. J Hosp Infect 1982; 3:55–63.

48. Lorentzen JE, Nielsen OM, Arendrup H, Kimose HH, Bille S, Anderson J, Jensen CH, Jacobsen F, Roder OC. Vascular graft infection: An analysis of sixty-two graft infections in 2411 consecutively implanted synthetic vascular grafts. Surgery 1985; 98:81–86.

49. Johnson JA, Cogbill TH, Strutt PJ, Gundersen AL. Wound complications after infra-inguinal bypass: Classification, predisposing factors, and management. Arch Surg 1988; 123:859–862.

50. Newington D, Houghton PWJ, Baird RN, Horrocks M. Groin wound infections after arterial surgery. Br J Surg 1991; 78:617–619.

51. Calligaro KE, Veith FJ. Surgery of the infected aortic graft. In: Bergan JJ, Yao JST, eds. Aortic Surgery. Philadelphia: Saunders, 1989:485–496.

17

Aortic Graft Infections

G. Patrick Clagett

University of Texas Southwestern Medical Center, Dallas, Texas, U.S.A.

Aortic graft infections are among the most challenging and taxing problems encountered by vascular surgeons. Patients with these infections are often elderly, frail, and severely ill with multiple medical comorbidities; they are poorly equipped to tolerate the extensive, complex operations usually required to treat the problem. Complete resection and excision of all infected graft material and debridement of vascular structures are usually necessary to eradicate infection. Immediate restoration of flow to critical vascular beds by alternate anatomical routes or with in situ replacements that minimize the risk of recurrent infection challenge the skill and ingenuity of the vascular surgeon. Despite a great deal of progress in the treatment of aortic graft infections, morbidity and mortality remain higher than in any other vascular condition (1–3).

I. PATHOGENESIS

Vascular grafts are foreign bodies that can be primarily infected by contamination at the time of placement or secondarily infected after implantation by hematogenous, lymphatic, or contiguous spread. The overall incidence of clinically overt graft infection varies according to anatomical site. Aortic grafts confined to the abdominal or thoracic cavity rarely become infected; the incidence ranges from 0.5 to 2% (2). The incidence is higher, from 2 to 6%, when distal anastomotic sites are at the femoral level (4).

Several features of the femoral area predispose to infectious complications. The groin is difficult to clean and incisions placed in the groin are prone to infection and healing problems. Groin incisions that extend obliquely across the inguinal crease tend to gape, and in obese patients they lie buried in moist skin folds. Furthermore, superficial inguinal lymph nodes are usually transected during exposure of the common femoral artery; if they are not ligated, they will bathe a vascular graft in lymphatic fluid that may contain bacteria. Potential sources of graft contamination in this circumstance include open, infected ischemic ulcers of a lower extremity, gangrenous toes, and wounds in any other area drained by the inguinal lymphatics, such as the perineum and perianal area. Another factor implicating the groin wound in the etiology of vascular graft infections is transient local ischemia during placement of the graft, which may render the wound more susceptible to infection.

The majority of vascular graft infections are initiated at the time of operation (2,3,5). Although direct proof of this is difficult to obtain, the prevalence of *Staphylococcus epidermidis* among offending organisms suggests that skin contamination with the patient's own flora is an important mechanism (6,7). *S. epidermidis* can often be cultured from the gloves of the surgical team, and grafts may be contaminated by this source during placement (8). The presence of *S. aureus* and other nosocomially acquired bacteria is also common and points to other environmental sources of contamination. These include intestinal flora when the gastrointestinal tract is entered or when operations such as cholecystectomy are performed at the time of vascular reconstruction. Laminated thrombus lining the walls of aneurysms has been implicated as a source of contamination and, when cultured, yields bacteria in about 10% of specimens (9,10). *S. epidermidis* is the most common isolate. Postoperative sources of aortic graft infection include wound complications, urinary tract infections, and invasive line sepsis. Early and late hematogenous seeding of grafts can occur during transient bacteremia associated with remote infections or dental procedures (11).

Although bacteria cause most aortic graft infections, other, less common microorganisms such as fungi, mycoplasmas, and mycobacteria have been encountered. *S. epidermidis* is the most common pathogen reported in modern series and outnumbers *S. aureus* infections two to one. Gram-negative and polymicrobial infections are increasingly being encountered but remain less prevalent than gram-positive infections. In many instances, negative cultures are reported despite convincing local evidence of infection, including nonincorporated graft material surrounded by grossly purulent fluid (12). These cases are most likely caused by *S. epidermidis* or other low-virulence organisms that are exposed to perioperative antibiotics at the time of sampling and require fastidious microbiological techniques for growth. Sonication of graft material, growth in tryptic soy broth, and prolonged incubation for several days have been reported to increase the yield of cultures positive for *S. epidermidis* (13).

Methicillin-resistant *S. aureus* (MRSA) has emerged as a serious and prevalent pathogen in some recent series tracking the epidemiology of vascular infections (14). These microorganisms can infect native arteries, destroy vascular tissue, and be difficult to eradicate (15). MRSA appear to be particularly virulent, leading to poor outcomes. In one recent series of 55 MRSA graft infections, 55% of patients died or underwent amputation (14).

The presence of a foreign body, such as an implanted device, increases the risk of infection. Early investigations documented that it takes only 10^2 *S. aureus* organisms to cause an abscess at the site of a suture but 10^6 organisms to cause an infection in normal skin. The vulnerability of foreign materials to infection involves physicochemical properties of the material, impairment of host defenses, and special properties of the bacteria themselves that facilitate their growth in the presence of a biomaterial (16). The biological reaction to an implanted vascular graft comprises an acute inflammatory response in the early stages that progresses to formation of a fibrous capsule or tissue ingrowth. Neutrophils rapidly become associated with any implanted biomaterial in vivo, become prematurely activated by contact with the material, and rapidly lose the capacity to become activated in response to subsequent stimuli, such as the presence of bacteria. Neutrophils in contact with biomaterials rapidly lose their ability to produce superoxide and other reactive oxygen species and become relatively impotent in their microbicidal activity (17,18). Thus the biomaterial acts as a massive "decoy" that prevents the neutrophils from responding normally to bacteria in the microenvironment. In addition, neutrophil products released in these circumstances may promote dysfunction of new neutrophils entering the microenvironment (19).

Vascular graft materials may vary in their susceptibility to infection by different micro-organisms. Highly textured or rough-surfaced biomaterials, such as textiles made of Dacron (woven or knitted), are more prone to bacterial adherence than smooth-surfaced biomaterials, such as expanded polytetrafluoroethylene (ePTFE) or polyurethane (20). In vivo, the adherence of platelets, plasma proteins, and other blood constituents and varying conditions of shear may dramatically alter the responses of different biomaterials to micro-organisms, and all biomaterials remain susceptible to infection (21,22).

The principal organism responsible for infections of all implanted medical devices, including vascular grafts, is *S. epidermidis*. This organism is a ubiquitous skin commensal with of relatively slow growth and low virulence. It causes chronic infections with local manifestations and little or no systemic toxicity. Pivotal in the pathogenesis of *Staphylococcus epidermidis* infection is the production of multilayered biofilms composed of exopolysaccharides, usually referred to as "slime." The elaboration of biofilms takes place following the adherence of *S. epidermidis* to biomaterials and usually occurs when organisms adhere to one another in microcolonies (23). Adherence of organisms to both polymer surfaces and each other (cell–cell adhesion) is mediated by capsular polysaccharide adhesins (23,24). Mutant bacteria that do not produce adhesins lack cell–cell adhesions and do not produce biofilms (25). Once elaborated, biofilms form a protective shield that allows continued bacterial growth in relatively hostile environments. Bacterial nutrients and metabolic wastes freely traverse the polysaccharide biofilm, but antibiotics do not. Biofilms also alter inflammatory changes, impair host defenses, and promote tenacious adherence of microbial colonies to the biomaterial (26). *S. epidermidis* infections tend to be persistent and refractory to antibiotics; therefore the implant must be removed to clear the infection.

Once established, bacterial infection spreads throughout a vascular graft and eventually involves anastomotic sites. The eventual destruction of vascular tissue leads to the formation of an anastomotic false aneurysm. The first manifestation of a vascular graft infection is often an anastomotic false aneurysm or its most frequent complication, graft thrombosis. When the false aneurysm involves the aortic anastomosis, rupture into the duodenum may occur and produce an aortoduodenal fistula with catastrophic hemorrhage. Although all micro-organisms producing vascular graft infections are associated with false aneurysms, they vary in their propensity to destroy vascular tissue. Gram-negative organisms—such as *Pseudomonas aeruginosa*, *Proteus* species, and *Escherichia coli*—are particularly notorious for their ability to digest vascular tissue (27). These organisms elaborate elastase and alkaline protease, which break down elastin, collagen, fibronectin, and fibrin. In addition to causing vascular disruption and the formation of false aneurysms, many bacteria produce substances that are highly thrombogenic and can induce thrombosis that may be the first manifestation of a vascular graft infection.

Aortic stent grafts would appear to be uniquely predisposed to infection. Tissue ingrowth from surrounding tissues is generally absent (28), and lack of tissue incorporation into prosthetic interstices is widely acknowledged to be a permissive condition for prosthetic infections. In addition, stent grafts are usually surrounded by luminal thrombus, which may harbor micro-organisms. Despite these theoretical considerations, acute aortic stent graft infections have been reported infrequently. Environmental sources of infection from gloved hands and the operating field are reduced because most commercial stent grafts are jacketed in sterile packages until deployed. In cases of acute stent graft infection, bacteremia was clearly documented (29). Infection may emerge as a significant problem on longer follow-up. In one series with a mean follow-up of 49 months, the incidence of infection of stent grafts requiring removal was an alarming 3.3% (30).

II. CLINICAL PRESENTATION

The clinical presentation of aortic graft infections can be protean and subtle, making the diagnosis difficult. The tempo and severity of the clinical manifestations often depend on the micro-organism. A patient whose infection is caused by a virulent organism—such as *S. aureus*, *P. aeruginosa*, and *E. coli*—presents with systemic signs of sepsis. As an example, a patient with a vascular graft who has persistent fever, chills, and an elevated white blood cell count with a left shift should be suspected of having a vascular graft infection. Virulent micro-organisms also tend to cause earlier manifestations of infection, with the interval between implantation of the graft and diagnosis of infection being months. Very early graft infections, diagnosed within weeks of implantation, are often associated with wound complications that involve vascular grafts by contiguous spread.

In contrast, patients with graft infection caused by a low-virulence organism, such as *S. epidermidis*, present later, often years after placement (7). Systemic signs and symptoms are usually mild or absent. These patients most often present with local manifestations, such as a chronic groin sinus that discharges small amounts of purulent material, a chronic wound infection with exposed graft, femoral anastomotic false aneurysm, or aortofemoral bypass limb thrombosis. They may have low-grade fever and mild constitutional symptoms, but overt signs of sepsis are absent. The white blood cell count is usually normal or only mildly elevated, but the erythrocyte sedimentation rate is often elevated. A patient presenting with a femoral anastomotic false aneurysm or limb thrombosis who has an elevated erythrocyte sedimentation rate should be suspected of having a graft infection.

Patients presenting with massive gastrointestinal hemorrhage from an aortoduodenal or aortoenteric fistula have frequently had lesser episodes of bleeding hours to days before the major episode. These are often referred to as "herald" or "sentinel" episodes of bleeding and offer a window of opportunity for the diagnosis and management prior to the onset of exsanguinating hemorrhage. Any patient with an aortic graft who has an episode of upper or lower gastrointestinal bleeding should be suspected of having an underlying aortoenteric fistula, and an expeditious workup is important. Chronic gastrointestinal bleeding can also occur in patients with an aortoenteric fistula but is more often associated with an enteric erosion. This condition, often referred to as a "graft–enteric erosion," differs from aortoenteric fistula in that the body or limb of the aortic graft erodes into bowel and the aortic suture line is not involved. This produces chronic bleeding from the eroded bowel mucosa, analogous to bleeding from an ulcer, and patients may present with chronic anemia. The diagnosis should be suspected in a patient with an aortic graft who has anemia, stool positive for occult blood, and fever.

Hydroureteronephrosis may also be the first manifestation of an aortic graft infection. This can develop if the ureter becomes obstructed as a result of perigraft inflammation and may be bilateral or unilateral, depending on the extent of infection.

III. DIAGNOSIS

Because the manifestations of aortic graft infections are so varied and subtle and the consequences of a missed diagnosis may be lethal, imaging tests are important (31). The types of imaging and other diagnostic tests used are based on the clinical presentation. Computed tomography (CT) has been the mainstay of diagnostic imaging for a suspected aortic graft infection. CT findings suggestive of infection include ectopic gas, periprosthetic fluid, loss of tissue planes, perigraft inflammatory changes, thickening of adjacent bowel, hydroureteronephrosis, and anastomotic false aneurysm (32). These findings are most specific and useful for late infections. During the immediate perioperative period following implantation, perigraft fluid, air, and inflammatory changes may persist for 2–3 months. After 3 months, postoperative hematoma and gas should resolve and tissue planes return to normal (33).

Magnetic resonance imaging (MRI) has provided an alternative to CT for cross-sectional imaging. In addition to demonstrating the same features seen on CT (periprosthetic air, fluid, and structural abnormalities), MRI is particularly helpful in assessing periprosthetic inflammatory changes. These changes are high intensity signals on T2-weighted images in the tissues surrounding the prosthesis and accurately portray tissue edema (34). Such images can be particularly helpful in assessing the extent of infection, which may determine the operative approach. For example, in a patient with an infection localized to a single distal limb of an aortobifemoral bypass, removal of the entire prosthesis may not be required for adequate treatment of the infection.

Radionuclide scanning has also been used in the diagnosis of vascular prosthetic infections. Scintigraphy with the use of autologous white blood cells labeled with indium 111 ([111]I) is the most common technique currently used, although the use of white cells labeled with gallium 67, technetium, and other isotopes has been reported (35,36). In addition, scintigraphy based on labeled human immunoglobulin G has been used and may be more sensitive than scintigraphy with white cells (37). A problem with all scintigraphic methods in diagnosing vascular graft infections is the lack of specificity caused by uptake in other organs or tissues that may be contiguous. In addition, faint or no uptake in the presence of limited or low-virulence infection can result in false-negative results. Scintigraphy is most helpful when occult prosthetic infection is suspected. An example would be a patient with an aortic graft presenting with a fever of unknown origin or a complex of other nonspecific symptoms in whom white blood cell scintigraphy identifies the graft as the source.

Arteriography is of limited usefulness in the diagnosis of vascular graft infection but it may, on occasion, demonstrate an aortic false aneurysm or even leakage of contrast into the bowel lumen, which is pathognomonic for an aortoenteric fistula. Arteriography is helpful in planning reconstruction after removal of the prosthesis and is most useful in late infection, when the vascular anatomy may have been altered by progressive occlusive disease. CT angiography may replace conventional angiography and provide additional information obtained by conventional cross-sectional CT imaging.

In patients presenting with gastrointestinal bleeding and suspected aortoenteric fistula, complete upper gastrointestinal endoscopy with visualization of the third and fourth portions of the duodenum, the most common sites of fistula, is necessary. Even if this study is incomplete, with inability to visualize the distal duodenum or the finding of gastrointestinal lesions such as chronic peptic ulcer that are not actively bleeding, an aortoenteric fistula may still be present. Continued unexplained bleeding mandates operative exploration to rule out aortoenteric fistula. At the time of operation, the duodenum, proximal jejunum, and any other bowel in contact with an aortic graft must be dissected free to make or exclude this diagnosis.

IV. PREVENTION OF AORTIC GRAFT INFECTIONS

The benefit of short-term antibiotic prophylaxis in preventing wound infections after vascular surgery has been demonstrated in randomized trials (38–40). Most often, a first-generation cephalosporin is administered intravenously shortly before operation, during operation if blood loss is extensive or the operation is prolonged, and 2 h after operation. Some evidence suggests that a more prolonged course for up to 4–5 days after operation or until all invasive lines are removed may provide additional protection (41). In circumstances where patients have infected lower extremity ischemic lesions, culture-specific antibiotics should be administered perioperatively. Also, the use of more specific prophylactic antibiotic therapy should be considered in hospital settings where certain organisms are prevalent, especially when exposure is increased by prolonged preoperative hospitalization.

Attention to intraoperative factors is also important in preventing aortic graft infections. Reoperations and emergency operations are especially prone to wound infections and present additional risks. Meticulous attention to hemostasis and avoidance of wound hematomas and seromas that can become secondarily infected are important surgical goals that are often difficult to achieve in patients anticoagulated during the operation who are also being treated with antiplatelet agents. If possible, these agents should be discontinued one week prior to operation. Ligation and control of femoral lymphatics are also important technical features in preventing aortic graft infections. Electrocautery of lymphatic tissue leads to coagulation necrosis of lymphatic vessels but does not prevent extravasation of lymph fluid. Fibrin glue applied to groin wounds has been shown to decrease lymph drainage and groin would complications (42).

Patients undergoing aortic operations are prone to intraoperative hypothermia; this condition has been shown to impair neutrophil function and increase the incidence of postoperative wound infection (43). Maintenance of normal body temperature should be the goal during major vascular operations. Additional procedures on the gastrointestinal or biliary tract that may result in intraoperative contamination of an aortic graft should be avoided unless the additional procedure is deemed necessary to avoid life-threatening postoperative complications. Hematogenous seeding of a vascular graft is a continuing risk for as long as the graft is in place. Dental work, procedures on the gastrointestinal and genitourinary tracts, and angiographic procedures should be carried out under the protection of prophylactic antibiotics.

V. TREATMENT

The primary goals of treatment are to save life and limb, and these are best accomplished by eradicating infection and maintaining adequate circulation to portions of the body perfused by the infected aortic graft. Secondary goals include minimizing morbidity, restorating of normal function, and maintaining of long-term function without the need for reintervention and risk of amputation.

These goals are best achieved by the removal of all infected graft material and vascular tissues combined with appropriate arterial reconstruction. The currently favored methods

Table 1 Aortic Graft Infections[a]

	References	Number of patients	Percent mortality (range)	Percent major amputation (range)	Percent aortic or anastomotic disruption	Percent reinfection	Percent 5-year primary patency
Extra-anatomic bypass	44–57	582	20.3 (5.0–40.6)	12.1 (0–15.6)	8.4	12.0	60.3 (30–80)
In situ superficial femoral-popliteal vein replacement	58–61	66	10.6 (6.7–20.0)	6.1 (4.9–10.0)	0	1.5	84
In situ allograft replacement	62–70	379	23.2 (8.3–6.4)	1.8 (0–3.0)	8.1	7.1	?
In situ prosthetic replacement	71–75	102	11.8 (4.0–21.7)	0	0	15.5	?

[a] Pooled data from major series reported since 1985.

of arterial reconstruction for aortic graft infection include extra-anatomic bypass (44–57) and in situ replacement using autogenous superficial femoral popliteal veins (58–61), arterial allografts (62–70), or vascular prostheses often treated or soaked in antibiotic solutions (71–75). Pooled outcome data from contemporary series reported since 1985 are presented in Table 1. Direct comparisons in attempting to judge the relative success of these approaches is difficult from these data because of the heterogeneity of patients with varying severity of illness and comorbidities among reported series. All of these approaches are valid and have utility depending upon patient-specific characteristics and circumstances. *It is a mistake to think that a single surgical approach is applicable to all patients with this condition.* These complicated patients with varying levels of illness severity require individualized attention.

VI. EXTRA-ANATOMIC BYPASS

Extra-anatomic bypass usually involving axillofemoral bypass is an excellent choice for infected aortoiliac reconstructions in which femoral sites are free of sepsis and the arterial runoff is good. It is also possibly less of a physiological insult in comparison to other procedures, particularly when the operations can be staged with extra-anatomic bypass preceding removal of the infected aortic prosthesis by a period of days (45). This approach has the advantage of preserving lower extremity blood flow during removal of the aortic prosthesis, thus minimizing lower extremity ischemia time.

Unfortunately, extra-anatomic bypasses have limited durability in patients with multilevel occlusive disease and poor runoff. Most patients with infected aortic grafts have aortobifemoral bypasses, and extra-anatomic bypass in such patients usually requires bilateral axillofemoral procedures with distal anastomoses to diseased and small, deep femoral or popliteal arteries. These are disadvantaged reconstructions with poor long-term patency despite the use of antithrombotic agents. They are prone to sudden thrombotic occlusion without warning and amputation rates are high, even with thrombectomy and multiple revisions. In one large series, one-third of patients required major amputation during long-term follow-up (46). In addition, reinfection of extra-anatomic bypass grafts occurs in 10–20% of patients, and this condition is often lethal. A final problem with extra-anatomic bypass is continuing infection at the site of aortic closure or the aortic "stump." Although an infrequent occurrence (less than 10%), aortic stump blowout is almost always fatal.

VII. IN SITU REPLACEMENT WITH SUPERFICIAL FEMOROPOPLITEAL VEINS

Dissatisfaction with the long-term patency of extra-anatomic bypass led to the development of in situ autogenous vein reconstruction (58–60). Early experiences were with greater saphenous veins, but this procedure rapidly evolved to the use of superficial femoropopliteal veins because of their large caliber and superior patency (58). This procedure has been referred to as creation of a "neoaortoiliac" system (NAIS) procedure. This reconstruction is most applicable in patients with extensive occlusive disease and poor runoff, a circumstance where an autogenous venous reconstruction would have better patency than a prosthetic graft bypass. The situation is analogous to the superior patency of vein grafts in comparison to prosthetic conduits in the performance of femoropopliteal and distal bypasses. This advantage has been realized in excellent 5-year cumulative patency rates for NAIS reconstructions of 85% for primary patency and 100% for secondary/assisted patency (60). Long-term amputation rates have been reported to be correspondingly low.

Although the technical details of the NAIS procedure have been previously published (60,76,77), some features merit emphasis. Duplex ultrasound imaging of the lower extremity's deep and superficial veins is essential in preoperative planning. Duplex vein mapping allows preoperative determination of diameter and length of available superficial femoropopliteal veins. Important findings that may alter the operative plan include deep venous thrombosis involving the superficial femoropopliteal veins, recanalization changes, and congenital absence or unusually small superficial femoropopliteal veins. In our experience, these findings are fortunately limited to one side. In situations where the superficial femoropopliteal vein is incomplete, absent, or unusually small (less than 4–5 mm in diameter), a dominant deep femoral vein is often present. This large vein courses posteriorly through the thigh to connect with the popliteal vein and can be used as a venous autograft for the NAIS procedure. Duplex vein mapping of the greater saphenous vein will also give information that may be useful if concomitant femoropopliteal/distal or visceral/renal reconstruction is required.

In order to minimize body exposure and lower extremity ischemia, the operation is sequenced as follows: (a) dissect superficial femoropopliteal veins and leave in situ until needed; (b) isolate femoral vessels; (c) enter abdomen and obtain aortic control; (d) remove infected aortic graft, and (e) perform reconstruction with superficial femoropopliteal veins. In the initial phases of the operation, it is useful to use two surgical teams to dissect the veins and isolate the femoral vessels.

The sartorius muscle is reflected medially and posteriorly and the subsartorial canal is opened in the midthigh. The saphenous nerve is vulnerable during this dissection, and excessive traction or unplanned division of this nerve can result in annoying postoperative medial leg neuralgia. Care must be taken in mobilizing the branches of the superficial femoral artery, especially around the adductor hiatus. These branches may represent important collaterals to distal arterial beds. Interruption of these when the superficial femoral artery is occluded may result in critical and unanticipated distal ischemia after completion of the proximal reconstruction.

The superficial femoropopliteal vein has multiple large and small branches. The larger ones are doubly ligated with 2-0 and 3-0 silk. Very large side branches are suture-ligated. The importance of secure branch ligature cannot be overemphasized. A "popped" tie can result in exsanguinating hemorrhage. The walls of the superficial femoropopliteal vein tend to be thin and tenuous near the origins of side branches. Torn branches can be frustrating to repair and require tedious closure with 7-0 polypropylene sutures. It is best to avoid this with careful and patient dissection of all branches. In addition, placement of branch ligatures should be close and contiguous to the vein wall. This is different from dissection of the greater saphenous vein, where emphasis is placed on securing ligatures slightly away from the vein wall so as not to constrict the vein. The superficial femoropopliteal vein is large and can easily tolerate close ligatures, which are helpful in preventing tears from the thin wall near the branch origins.

Dissection is carried proximally to where the superficial femoral vein joins the deep femoral vein to form the common femoral vein. The deep femoral vein is readily identified as a large-caliber vessel penetrating deep through the fascia on the floor of Hunter's canal. The dissection is then carried distally with division of the adductor tendons to open the adductor hiatus. The distal dissection is carried to the level of the knee and, if necessary, the dissection can be continued below the knee for an additional few centimeters of autograft.

The next portion of the operation involves isolation of the femoral vessels and distal limbs of the aortobifemoral bypass graft. In most patients, this can be accomplished by extending the vein harvest incision along the lateral border of the sartorius muscle to its attachment site at the anterosuperior iliac spine. In thin patients, the entire common femoral artery can be exposed by reflecting the sartorius medially. On occasion, dissection medial to the sartorius is helpful to complete this exposure. This approach obviates the need to dissect through the old femoral incisions.

The abdomen is then entered through the old incision or through a left flank retroperitoneal approach. The latter is particularly helpful in avoiding tedious adhesions and facilitates obtaining aortic control. This approach also facilitates suprarenal or supraceliac control if the proximal anastomosis is close to the renal arteries. The vein grafts are then prepared and the lengths required are determined by measuring the distance from the proximal anastomosis to the femoral levels on both sides. The proximal superficial femoral vein is divided flush with the deep femoral vein and oversewn with 5-0 polypropylene continuous sutures. This allows unimpeded flow from the deep femoral to the common femoral vein and minimizes the possibility of thrombus forming in a residual venous culde-sac of the superficial femoral vein. The vein graft usually has three to four large valves that are easily identified and ablated using a valvulotome or directly excised by temporarily everting the vein graft. The nonreversed configuration will allow placement of the larger end of the vein at the proximal aortic anastomosis.

Following systemic heparinization, cross clamps are placed on the proximal aorta and the distal limbs of the aortic graft. The body of the graft is removed and the femoral limbs are left in place while the proximal anastomosis to the superficial femoral vein is performed. Leaving the femoral limbs in place during this period cuts down on blood loss that typically occurs when the femoral limbs are extracted from their tunnels.

Several configurations using superficial femoral popliteal vein grafts are possible and allow flexibility in performing the NAIS reconstruction (Fig. 1). The proximal end of the superficial femoral vein is frequently (1.5 cm in diameter and can easily be anastomosed to a normal aorta. Standard, continuous polypropylene (4-0) suture technique is used, taking care to make slightly more advancement on the aorta than the venous autograft because of the greater circumference of the aorta (Fig. 2). Larger aortas and greater size mismatches are often encountered and require different anastomotic techniques. Plication of the distal aorta may be performed to reduce the diameter of the aorta at the anastomosis (Fig. 3). Both superficial femoral popliteal vein grafts can be joined together in a "pantaloon" configuration (Fig. 4). This technique essentially doubles the circumference of the vein graft's proximal anastomosis. Another technique to increase circumference is shown in Figure 5.

Following completion of the proximal anastomosis, the old graft limbs are carefully removed. Most often, superficial femoral popliteal vein grafts are placed in the old tunnels because it is difficult to fashion new tunnels through the scarred retroperitoneum. The superficial femoral popliteal vein grafts are often larger than the tunnels; when this occurs, careful proximal and distal finger dilation can be useful to prevent luminal compromise of the vein graft. Care must be taken when pulling vein grafts through the tunnels, as side branch ligatures may become dislodged. To avoid this problem, vein grafts are passed nondistended.

Following operation, antibiotic coverage is continued for 5–7 days. Antibiotics are modified as culture results isolate organisms sensitive to specific antibiotics. In patients

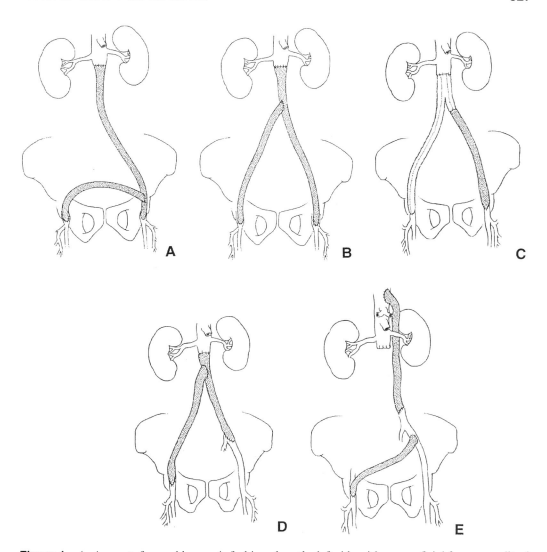

Figure 1 A. An aortofemoral bypass is fashioned on the left side with a superficial femoropopliteal vein graft. Another vein graft is used to cross over to the right femoral region. B. Instead of a crossover femoral bypass, the right limb is connected to the aorta-left femoral bypass using an end-to-side anastomosis. In both A and B, a shorter length of superficial femoropopliteal vein graft is required for the right side. C. In this example, infection was limited to the femoral region and the distal aortofemoral limb was replaced with a superficial femoropopliteal vein graft. Care must be taken to prevent cross contamination and the vein graft routed lateral to the infected area or via a transobturator route. D. In this circumstance, an aortic–left common iliac bypass is fashioned from one-third to one-half of a superficial femoropopliteal vein graft and the right limb is fashioned from the remainder of the vein graft. This technique permits the harvesting of only a single femoro-popliteal vein graft. E. In some circumstances, it is easier to approach the paraceliac aorta via a retroperitoneal approach and to use this area for the proximal anastomosis, as shown in this figure. Although the distal anastomosis is to the common iliac artery in this case, an additional length superficial femoropopliteal vein graft can be harvested, if necessary, to reach the femoral area.

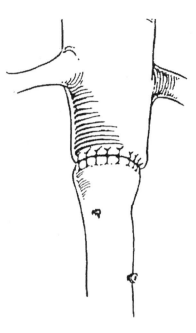

Figure 2   When the aorta is of normal size, the proximal end of the superficial femoropopliteal vein graft is anastomosed end to end.

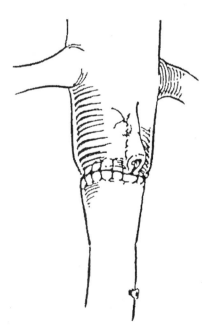

Figure 3   Simple plication of a portion of the aorta can be performed to allow comfortable end-to-end anastomosis when the aorta is either larger than normal or the vein graft is of comparatively small size.

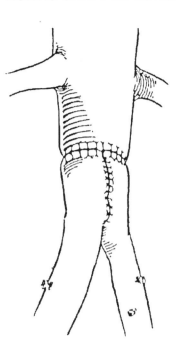

Figure 4 In this example, two superficial femoropopliteal vein grafts are joined together ("pantaloon" technique) and sewn end to end to the aorta. This effectively doubles the circumstance of the vein graft and is used to accommodate very large aortas.

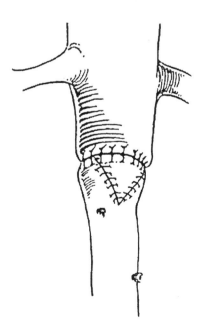

Figure 5 In this case, a wedge-shaped portion of vein is incorporated into the proximal end to increase the circumstance of the superficial femoropopliteal vein graft.

who are severely immunocompromised, prolonged antibiotic therapy for 4–6 weeks may sometimes be necessary. Intermittent pneumatic compression plus low-dose subcutaneous heparin (5000 U q 8–12 h) are used for prophylaxis of venous thromboembolism. Most patients develop venous thrombosis in the residual popliteal vein segment or "stump." Aggressive prophylaxis may prevent propagation into calf veins. Full anticoagulation for this limited venous thrombosis is unnecessary, since—because of the absence of the superficial femoral popliteal vein—proximal extension and pulmonary embolism are unlikely. Patients are seen every 3 months on an outpatient basis for the first year following operation. Noninvasive vascular testing includes ankle/brachial pressure indices and complete graft duplex examination. Surveillance is directed at detecting vein graft and anastomotic stenoses as well as progression of distal disease.

The principal disadvantage of the NAIS reconstruction is that it is a technically demanding, a long procedure. The mean operative time is approximately 8 h. The lower extremity ischemic time is longer than with other approaches but can be minimized by using a two-team approach and carefully sequencing the procedure to shorten aortic cross-clamp time.

Acute venous hypertension following harvest of the superficial femoral popliteal vein can contribute to the development of lower extremity compartment syndromes. Leg fasciotomy is required in approximately 25% of patients. Preexisting lower extremity ischemia, prolonged aortic cross-clamp times, and absence of the ipsilateral saphenous vein are risk factors for the development of a compartment syndrome. Prophylactic four-compartment fasciotomy should be considered when these risk factors are present.

Long-term lower extremity venous morbidity is also a potential drawback to harvesting the superficial femoral popliteal veins. However, venous morbidity has been surprisingly infrequent and mild (59,60). Approximately 30% of patients will have transient lower extremity swelling that requires compression stockings. This usually resolves within a period of weeks to months after operation; then compression stockings are no longer necessary. The benign course following removal of the superficial femoral popliteal vein is due to several compensating mechanisms (78). First, the junction of the deep and common femoral veins is carefully preserved after disconnecting the proximal superficial femoral vein, thus allowing unimpeded drainage via the deep venous system. Second, there are other anatomical collateral connections between the remaining distal popliteal vein and the deep venous system; many of these collaterals enlarge to accommodate the increase in volume flow following removal of the superficial femoral popliteal vein. Finally, the valves in the tibial veins and collateral circuits remain functional, such that distal venous reflux does not occur.

A final concern is that the placement of superfemoral popliteal veins in an infected field might lead to reinfection and disruption. This has been rare and experience with this approach has documented that these vein grafts resist gram-positive, gram-negative, and fungal infections. Long-term aneurysmal degeneration has been studied up to 10 years after placement of these vein grafts, and the incidence of this problem has been <1%.

VIII. IN SITU REPLACEMENT WITH ALLOGRAFT AND ANTIBIOTIC-TREATED PROSTHETIC GRAFTS

In situ allograft replacement with varying degrees of success has been reported. Most authors prefer to use cryopreserved rather than fresh allografts because they increase the availability of suitable conduits for emergency use, blood compatibility can be matched, and long-term storage allows the allografts to be judged relatively safe from viral transmission by observing outcomes in recipients of organs from the same donor (69,70). In addition, in contrast to refrigerated or freshly implanted allografts, cryopreserved arterial allografts may be relatively inert immunologically. Optimal cryopreservation methods for arterial allografts are not well delineated (68). Current cryopreservation protocols usually recommend rate-controlled freezing and storage at very low temperatures in liquid nitrogen vapor, mainly as a means of achieving long-term preservation of functional endothelium and smooth muscle cells. However, preservation of cellular viability may be unnecessary for performance as a large-caliber replacement graft, and viable endothelial and smooth muscle cells may elicit immune responses that could be deleterious. In addition, some authors feel that current cryopreservation protocols result in making arterial allografts brittle and predisposed to graft dilation and rupture (69).

Degenerative changes in allografts are the major drawback of this technique. Numerous studies on arterial allograft rejection have identified the sequence of events in arterial wall immune injury and response that progressively leads to graft dilation and rupture. Acute and delayed allograft disruption has been reported and is a distinct limitation of using allografts in infected fields (64,70,79).

Technical refinements in the use of cryopreserved allografts have been reported to reduce the incidence of early and late complications (69). These include use of allografts of appropriate length to prevent tension at anastomoses, careful through-and-through ligature of side branches (simple ligation of side branches may lead to rupture at these sites), and circumferential anastomotic reinforcement with allograft strips. In addition, aggressive retroperitoneal drainage and prolonged antibiotic and antifungal therapy has been recommended to prevent infection of allografts (69).

Replacement of the infected aortic graft with a new synthetic graft has also been reported (71–75). Most often, the new aortic graft is soaked in an antibiotic solution prior to implantation. It is recommended that a gelatin-sealed polyester graft be soaked in a rifampin solution of 60 mg/mL for this purpose (74,75). This approach is most often successful with limited infections of low virulence following aggressive debridement of all infected vascular and surrounding tissues to create a clean field. Despite this, the potential for reinfection is a serious drawback, and patients treated in this manner require close and vigilant follow-up with frequent imaging studies such as CT scanning or MRI. They are also usually treated with lifelong oral antibiotics.

In situ prosthetic and allograft reconstructions may have their greatest utility in very ill and unstable patients and also in those with actively bleeding aortoenteric fistulas. Expeditious in situ replacement in such cases may be lifesaving. Under these circumstances, the procedure may be used as a "bridge" procedure, with definitive reconstruction (extra-anatomic or NAIS) carried out at a later date, when the patient has been rendered fit for such a reconstruction.

IX. ALTERNATIVE APPROACHES TO REMOVING THE ENTIRE AORTIC GRAFT

Conservative approaches that do not involve removal of the infected aortic graft have also been reported (80–83). These are based on aggressive drainage and debridement of infected tissues; intensive, culture-specific antibiotic therapy; meticulous wound care to achieve coverage of exposed prosthetic material; and coverage of exposed prosthetic material with muscle flaps. The most appropriate use of these conservative approaches is when infection is extracavitary and limited in extent, systemic signs of sepsis are absent, the infecting organisms are of low virulence, and anastomotic sites are uninvolved (83). As with in situ prosthetic replacement, these patients need close follow-up and indefinite oral antibiotic treatment. A conservative approach may be the only option in some frail and desperately ill patients who would not be able to tolerate aortic graft removal.

With infections that involve only one limb of an aortobifemoral bypass graft, resection of the limb is usually performed (13,84–87). Revascularization is often carried out via obturator bypass or other reconstructions performed in clean fields. Autogenous superficial femoropopliteal or greater saphenous vein grafts have also been used for this purpose (87). It is important that the extent of infection be assessed with imaging studies as well as direct visual inspection. In the case of unilateral femoral infection of an aortofemoral bypass, the general approach is to begin the operation by inspection of the intraabdominal portion of the prosthesis. If the infection grossly involves the main body of the bifurcated prosthesis, complete removal is necessary. If the suspected limb is well incorporated and free of gross infection, division of the limb, closure of the tunnel, and obturator or other extra-anatomic bypass is performed. The final portion of this operation is to remove the infected limb from below, taking care to prevent cross-contamination of other freshly placed incisions that have been closed.

X. CONCLUSIONS

There are multiple operative management strategies that are appropriate for the treatment of infected aortic grafts. All have advantages and disadvantages that must be taken into account in dealing with individual patients. Extra-anatomic bypass is a relatively straightforward procedure, can be staged, and may be physiologically less stressful than others. However, thrombectomy and revision are often required and long-term patency is only fair. The long-term amputation rates are high and anticoagulation is often used to maintain patency. In addition, reinfection of the prosthetic extra-anatomic bypass and aortic stump blowout are of concern. In situ replacement with superficial femoropopliteal vein grafts provides the best long-term patency and durability. Amputation rates are low and indefinite antithrombotic and antibiotic therapies are unnecessary. However, the procedure is long and complex; it can be associated with significant lower extremity ischemia times. Leg fasciotomy is also necessary in about one-quarter of these patients. In situ allograft replacement is expeditious, but reinfection, allograft aneurysmal and occlusive deterioration, and limited availability make this option less attractive. In situ prosthetic replacement is also expeditious, but its use is limited to low-grade, nonvirulent infections involving only part of the prosthesis. In addition, antibiotic therapy of indefinite duration is usually required and the potential for reinfection is always present. All of these management options are appropriate in specific circumstances; their judicious use will lead to improved outcomes.

REFERENCES

1. Balas P. An overview of aortofemoral graft infection. Eur J Vasc Endovasc Surg 1997; 14(suppl A):3–4.
2. Kearney RA, Eisen HJ, Wolf JE. Nonvalvular infections of the cardiovascular system. Ann Intern Med 1994; 121:219–230.

3. O'Brien T, Collin J. Prosthetic vascular graft infection. Br J Surg 1992; 79:1262–1267.

4. Lorentzen JE, Nielsen OM, Arendrup H, et al. Vascular graft infection: An analysis of sixty-two graft infections in 2411 consecutively implanted synthetic vascular grafts. Surgery 1985; 98:81–86.

5. Seabrook GR. Pathobiology of graft infections. Semin Vasc Surg 1990; 3:81–88.

6. Bandyk DF, Berni GA, Thiele BL, Towne JB. Aortofemoral graft infection due to *Staphylococcus epidermidis*. Arch Surg 1984; 119:102–108.

7. Jones L, Braithwaite BD, Davies B, Heather BP, Earnshaw JJ. Mechanism of late prosthetic vascular graft infection. Cardiovasc Surg 1997; 5:486–489.

8. Zdanowski Z, Danielsson G, Jonung T, Norgren L, Ribbe E, Thorne J, Kamme C, Schalen C. Intraoperative contamination of synthetic vascular grafts. Effect of glove change before graft implantation. A prospective randomized study. Eur J Vasc Endovasc Surg 2000; 19:283–287.

9. Schwartz JA, Powell TW, Burnham SJ, Johnson G Jr. Culture of abdominal aortic aneurysm contents. Arch Surg 1987; 122:777–780.

10. Ernst CB, Campbell HC, Daugherty ME, et al. Incidence and significance of intra-operative bacterial cultures during abdominal aortic aneurysmectomy. Ann Surg 1977; 185:626–633.

11. Häyrinen-Immonen R, Ikonen TS, Lepantalo M, Lindgren L, Lindqvist C. Oral health of patients scheduled for elective abdominal aortic correction with prosthesis. Eur J Vasc Endovasc Surg 2000; 19:294–298.

12. Padberg FT Jr, Smith SM, Eng RHK. Accuracy of disincorporation for identification of vascular graft infection. Arch Surg 1995; 130:183–187.

13. Bandyk DF, Bergamini TM, Kinney EV, Seabrook GR, Towne JB. In situ replacement of vascular prostheses infected by bacterial biofilms. J Vasc Surg 1991; 13:575–583.

14. Naylor AR, Hayes PD, Darke S, on behalf of the Joint Vascular Research Group. A prospective audit of complex wound and graft infections in Great Britain and Ireland: The emergence of MRSA. Eur J Vasc Endovasc Surg 2001; 21:289–294.

15. Nasim A, Thompson MM, Naylor AR, Bell PRF, London NJM. The impact of MRSA on vascular surgery. Eur J Vasc Endovasc Surg 2001; 22:211–214.

16. Merritt K, Hitchins VM, Neale AR. Tissue colonization from implantable biomaterials with low numbers of bacteria. J Biomed Mater Res 1999; 44:261–265.

17. Kaplan SS, Basford RE, Jeong MH, Simmons RL. Mechanisms of biomaterial-induced superoxide release by neutrophils. J Biomed Mater Res 1994; 28:377–386.

18. Kaplan SS, Basford RE, Jeong MH, Simmons RL. Biomaterial-neutrophil interactions: Dysregulation of oxidative functions of fresh neutrophils induced by prior neutrophil-biomaterial interaction. B Biomed Mater Res 1996; 30:67–75.

19. Kaplan SS, Heine RP, Simmons RL. Defensins impair phagocytic killing by neutrophils in biomaterial-related infection. Infect Immun 1999; 67:1640–1645.

20. Brunstedt MR, Sapatnekar S, Rubin KR, Kieswetter KM, Ziats NP, Merritt K, Anderson JM. Bacterial/blood/material interactions: I. Injected and preseeded slime-forming *Staphylococcus epidermidis* in flowing blood with biomaterials. J Biomed Mater Res 1995; 29:455–466.

21. Wang I, Anderson JM, Jacobs MR, Marchant RE. Adhesion of *Staphylococcus epidermidis* to biomedical polymers: contributions of surface thermodynamics and hemodynamic shear conditions. J Biomed Mater Res 1995; 29:485–493.

22. Shive MS, Hasan SM, Anderson JM. Shear stress effects on bacterial adhesion, leukocyte adhesion, and leukocyte oxidative capacity on a polyetherurethane. J Biomed Mater Res 1999; 46:511–519.

23. Veenstra GC, Cremers FFM, van Dijk H, Fleer A. Ultrastructural organization and regulation of a biomaterial adhesion of *Staphylococcus epidermidis*. J Bacteriol 1996; 178:537–541.

24. Mack D, Riedewald J, Rohde H, et al. Essential functional role of the polysaccharide intercellular adhesion of *Staphylococcus epidermidis* in hemagglutination. Infect Immun 1999; 67:1004–1008.

25. Rupp ME, Ulphani JS, Fey PD, Bartscht K, Mack D. Characterization of the importance of

polysaccharide intercellular adhesin/hemagglutinin of *Staphylococcus epidermidis* in the pathogenesis of biomaterial-based infection in a mouse foreign body infection model. Infect Immun 199; 67:2627–2632.

26. Henke PK, Bergamini TM, Watson AL, Brittian KR, Powell DW, Peyton JC. Bacterial products primarily mediate fibroblast inhibition in biomaterial infection. J Surg Res 1998; 74:17–22.

27. Geary KJ, Tomkiewicz ZM, Harrison HN, et al. Differential effects of a gram-negative and a gram-positive infection on autogenous and prosthetic grafts. J Vasc Surg 1990; 11:339–347.

28. McArthur C, Teodorescu V, Eisen L, et al. Histopathologic analysis of endovascular stent grafts from patients with aortic aneurysms: Does healing occur? J Vasc Surg 2001; 33:733–738.

29. Jackson MR, Joiner DR, Clagett GP. Excision and autogenous revascularization of an infected aortic stent graft resulting from a urinary tract Infection. J Vasc Surg 2002; 36:622–624.

30. Schlensak C, Doenst T, Hauer M, et al. Serious complications that require surgical interventions after endoluminal stent-graft placement for the treatment of infrarenal aortic aneurysms. J Vasc Surg 2001; 34:198–203.

31. Modrall JG, Clagett GP. The role of imaging techniques in evaluating possible graft infections. Semin Vasc Surg 1999; 12:339–347.

32. Low RN, Wall SD, Jeffrey RB, et al. Aortoenteric fistula and perigraft infection: evaluation with CT. Radiology 1990; 175:157–162.

33. Qvafordt PG, Reilly LM, Mark AS, et al. Computerized tomographic assessment of graft incorporation after reconstruction. Am J Surg 1985; 150:227–231.

34. Auffermann W, Olofsson PA, Rabahie GN, et al. Incorporation versus infection of retroperitoneal aortic grafts: MR imaging features. Radiology 1989; 172:359–362.

35. Brunner MC, Mitchell RS, Baldwin JC, et al. Prosthetic graft infection: Limitations of indium white blood cell scanning. J Vasc Surg 1986; 3:42–48.

36. Fiorani P, Speziale F, Rizzo L, et al. Detection of aortic graft infection with leukocytes labeled with technetium 99m-hexametazime. J Vasc Surg 1993; 17:87–96.

37. LaMuraglia GM, Fischman AJ, Strauss HW, et al. Utility of the indium 111–labeled human immunoglobulin G scan for the detection of focal vascular graft infection. J Vasc Surg 1989; 10:20–28.

38. Kaiser A, Kaiser B, Clayson KR, Mulherin JL, et al. Antibiotic prophylaxis in vascular surgery. Ann Surg 1978; 188:283–288.

39. Pitt HA, Postier RG, MacGowan WAL, et al. Prophylactic antibiotics in vascular surgery: Topical, systemic, or both? Ann Surg 1980; 192:356–364.

40. Hasselgren P, Ivarsson L, Risberg B, Seeman T. Effects of prophylactic antibiotics in vascular surgery: A prospective, randomized, double-blind study. Ann Surg 1984; 200:86–92.

41. Hall JC, Christiansen KJ, Goodman M, et al. Duration of antimicrobial prophylaxis in vascular surgery. Am J Surg 1998; 175:87–90.

42. Giovannacci L, Renggli JC, Eugster T, et al. Reduction of groin lymphatic complications by application of fibrin glue: Preliminary results of a randomized study. Ann Vasc Surg 2001; 15:182–185.

43. Kurz A, Sessler DL, Lenhardt R. Study of Wound Infection and Temperature Group. Perioperative normothermia to reduce the incidence of surgical wound infection and shorten hospitalization. N Engl J Med 1996; 334:1209–1215.

44. O'Hara PJ, Hertzer NR, Beven EG, Krajewski LP. Surgical management of infected abdominal aortic grafts: Review of a 25-year experience. J Vasc Surg 1986; 2:725–731.

45. Reilly LM, Stoney RJ, Goldstone J, Ehrenfeld WK. Improved management of aortic graft infection: The influence of operation sequence and staging. Vasc Surg 1987; 5:421–431.

46. Quinones-Baldrich WJ, Hernandez JJ, Moore WS. Long-term results following surgical management of aortic graft infection. Arch Surg 1991; 126:507–511.

47. Ricotta JJ, Faggioli GL, Stella A, et al. Total excision and extra-anatomic bypass for aortic graft infection. Am J Surg 1991; 162:145–149.

48. Leather RP, Darling RC III, Chang BB, Shah DM. Retroperitoneal in-line aortic bypass for treatment of infected infrarenal aortic grafts. Surg Gynecol Obstet 1992; 175:491–494.

49. Olah A, Vogt M, Laske A, Carrell T, Bauer E, Turina M. Axillo-femoral bypass and simultaneous removal of the aorto-femoral vascular infection site: Is the procedure safe? Eur J Vasc Surg 1992; 6:252–254.

50. Bacourt F, Koskas F, and the French University Association for Research in Surgery. Axillobifemoral bypass and aortic exclusion for vascular septic lesions: A multicenter retrospective study of 98 cases. Ann Vasc Surg 1992; 6:119–126.

51. Lehnert T, Gruber HP, Maeder N, Allenberg JR. Management of primary aortic graft infection by extra-anatomic bypass reconstruction. Eur J Vasc Surg,, 307–701.

52. Sharp WJ, Hoballah JJ, Mohan CR, et al. The management of the infected aortic prosthesis: A current decade of experience. J Vasc Surg 1994; 19:844–850.

53. Kuestner LM, Reilly LM, Jicha DL, Ehrenfeld WK, Goldstone J, Stoney RJ. Secondary aortoenteric fistula: Contemporary outcome with use of extraanatomic bypass and infected graft excision. J Vasc Surg 1995; 21:184–196.

54. Hannon RJ, Wolfe JHN, Mansfield AO. Aortic prosthetic infection: 50 patients treated by radical or local surgery. Br J Surg 1996; 83:654–658.

55. Schmitt DD, Seabrook GR, Bandyk DF, Towne JB. Graft excision and extra-anatomic revascularization: The treatment of choice for the septic aortic prosthesis. J Cardiovasc Surg 1990; 31:327–332.

56. Bunt TJ. Vascular graft infections: A personal experience. Cardiovasc Surg 1993; 1:489–492.

57. Yeager RA, Taylor LM, Moneta GL, Edwards JM, Nicoloff AD, McConnell DB, Porter JM. Improved results with conventional management of infrarenal aortic infection. J Vasc Surg 1999; 30:76–83.

58. Clagett GP, Bowers BL, Lopez-Viego MA, Rossi MB, Valentine RJ, Myers SI, Chervu A. Creation of a neo-aortoiliac system from lower extremity deep and superficial veins. Ann Surg 1993; 218:239–249.

59. Nevelsteen A, Lacroix H, Suy R. Autogenous reconstruction with the lower extremity deep veins: An alternative treatment of prosthetic infection after reconstructive surgery for aortoiliac disease. J Vasc Surg 1995; 22:129–134.

60. Clagett GP, Valentine RJ, Hagino RT. Autogenous aortoiliac/femoral reconstruction from superficial femoral-popliteal veins: Feasibility and durability. J Vasc Surg 1997; 25:255–270.

61. Gorden LL, Hagino RT, Jackson MR, Modrall JG, Valentine RJ, Clagett GP. Complex aortofemoral prosthetic infections—The role of autogenous superficial femoropopliteal vein reconstruction. Arch Surg 1999; 134:615–621.

62. Kieffer E, Bahnini A, Koskas F, Ruotolo C, LeBlevec D, Plissonnier D. In situ allograft replacement of infected infrarenal aortic prosthetic grafts: results in forty-three patients. J Vasc Surg 1993; 17:349–356.

63. Vogt PR, Pfammatter T, Schlumph R, et al. In situ repair of aortobronchial, aortoesophageal, and aortoenteric fistulae with cryopreserved aortic homografts. J Vasc Surg 1997; 26:11–17.

64. Ruotolo C, Plissonnier D, Bahnini A, Koskas F, Kieffer E. In situ arterial allografts: a new treatment for aortic prosthetic infection. Eur J Vasc Endovasc Surg 1997; 14(suppl A):102–107.

65. Nevelsteen A, Feryn T, Lacroix H, Suy R, Goffin Y. Experience with cryopreserved arterial allografts in the treatment of prosthetic graft infections. Cardiovasc Surg 1998; 4:378–383.

66. Chiesa R, Astore S, Piccolo G, Melissano G, et al. Fresh and cryopreserved arterial homografts in the treatment of prosthetic graft infections: Experience of the Italian Collaborative Vascular Homograft Group. Ann Vasc Surg 1998; 12:457–462.

67. Verhelst R, Lacroix V, Vraux H, Lavigne JP, Vandamme H, Limet R, Nevelsteen A, Bellens B, Vasseur MA, Wozniak B, Goffin Y. Use of cryopreserved arterial homografts for management of infected prosthetic grafts: a multicentric study. Ann Vasc Surg 2000; 14:602–607.

68. Leseche G, Castier Y, Petit MD, Bertrand P, Kitzis M, Mussot S, Besnard M, Cerceau O.

Long-term results of cryopreserved arterial allograft reconstruction in infected prosthetic grafts and mycotic aneurysms of the abdominal aorta. J Vasc Surg 2001; 34:616–622.

69. Vogt PR, Brunner-LaRocca HP, Lachat M, Ruef C, Turina MI. Technical details with the use of cryopreserved arterial allografts for aortic infection: Influence on early and midterm mortality. J Vasc Surg 2002; 35:80–86.

70. Noel AA, Gloviczki P, Cherry KJ Jr, Safi H, Goldstone J, Morasch MD, Johansen KH, members of the United States Cryopreserved Aortic Allograft Registry. Abdominal aortic reconstruction in infected fields: Early results of the United States Cryopreserved Aortic Allograft Registry. J Vasc Surg 2002; 35:847–852.

71. Walker WE, Cooley DA, Duncan JM, Hallman GL, Ott DA, Reul GJ. The management of aortoduodenal fistula by in situ replacement of the infected abdominal aortic graft. Ann Surg 1987; 205:727–732.

72. Speziale F, Rizzo L, Sbarigia E, et al. Bacterial and clinical criteria relating to the outcome of patients undergoing in situ replacement of infected abdominal aortic grafts. Eur J Vasc Endovasc Surg 1997; 13:127–133.

73. Hayes PD, Nasim A, London NJM, Sayers RD, Barrie WW, Bell PRF, Naylor AR. In situ replacement of infected aortic grafts with rifampicin-bonded prostheses: The Leicester experience (1992 to 1998). J Vasc Surg 1999; 30:92–98.

74. Young RM, Cherry KJ Jr, Davis PM, Gloviczki P, Bower TC, Panneton JM, Hallett JW Jr. The results of in situ prosthetic replacement for infected aortic grafts. Am J Surg 1999; 178:136–140.

75. Bandyk DF, Novotney ML, Back MR, et al. Expanded application of in situ replacement for prosthetic graft infection. J Vasc Surg 2001; 34:411–420.

76. Clagett GP. Treatment of aortic graft infection. In: Ernst CB Stanley JC, eds. Current Therapy in Vascular Surgery. 4th ed. Philadelphia: Mosby–Year Book, 2001:422–428.

77. Seidel SA, Modrall JG, Jackson MR, Valentine RJ, Clagett GP. The superficial femoral-popliteal vein graft: A reliable conduit for large caliber arterial and venous reconstructions. Perspect Vasc Surg Endovasc Ther 2001; 14(1):57–80.

78. Wells JK, Hagino RT, Bargmann KM, Jackson MR, Valentine RJ, Kakish HB, Clagett GP. Venous morbidity after superficial femoral-popliteal vein harvest. J Vasc Surg 1999; 29:282–291.

79. Koskas F, Plissonnier D, Bahnini A, Ruotolo C, Kieffer E. In situ arterial allografting for aortoiliac graft infection: A 6-year experience. Cardiovasc Surg 1996; 4:495–499.

80. Calligaro KD, Veith FJ, Schwartz ML, et al. Selective preservation of infected prosthetic arterial grafts. Analysis of a 20-year experience with 120 extracavitary-infected grafts. Ann Surg 1994; 220:461–471.

81. Morris GE, Friend PJ, Vassallo DJ, Farrington M, Leapman S, Quick CRG. Antibiotic irrigation and conservative surgery for major aortic graft infection. J Vasc Surg 1994; 20:88–95.

82. Belair M, Soulez G, Oliva VL, et al. Aortic graft infection: The value of percutaneous drainage. Am J Radiol 1998; 171:119–124.

83. Calligaro KD, Veith FJ. Graft preserving methods for managing aortofemoral prosthetic graft infection. Eur J Vasc Endovasc Surg 1997; 14(suppl A):38–42.

84. Becquemin JP, Qvarfordt P, Kron J, et al. Aortic graft infection: Is there a place for partial graft removal? Eur J Vasc Endovasc Surg 1997; 14(suppl A):53–58.

85. Miller JH. Partial replacement of an infected arterial graft by a new prosthetic polytetrafluoroethylene segment: A new therapeutic option. J Vasc Surg 1993; 17:546–558.

86. Towne JB, Seabrook GR, Bandyk D, Freischlag JA, Edmiston CE. In situ replacement of arterial prosthesis infected by bacterial biofilms: Long-term follow-up. J Vasc Surg 1994; 19:226–235.

87. Sladen JG, Chen JC, Reid JDS. An aggressive local approach to vascular graft infection. Am J Surg 1998; 176:222–225.

18

Detection and Management of Failing Autogenous Grafts

Jonathan B. Towne

Medical College of Wisconsin, Milwaukee, Wisconsin, U.S.A.

A significant decline in primary patency of autogenous grafts invariably occurs over time because of the development of fibrointimal hyperplasia of the vein conduit or anastomotic sites and the progression of atherosclerotic disease of the native arteries. The incidence of lesions that threaten the long-term patency of both in situ and reversed saphenous vein bypasses ranges from 20 to 26% (1–3). Anatomical and hemodynamic alternations that require revision will develop in approximately 5% of vein bypasses per year; the majority of these will occur with the first 2 years after bypass (4). The failure to detect and correct lesions that threaten bypass patency before graft thrombosis significantly decreases long-term patency of the autogenous graft. The long-term patency for revisions of autogenous grafts after thrombosis is dismal. The 3-year patency rate of revision of thrombosed in situ and reversed saphenous vein grafts ranges from 22 to 47% in recent reports (1,5,6).

By contrast, the result of revision on hemodynamically failing but patent conduits are excellent: secondary patency rates are equivalent to those for bypasses that never undergo revision (1). Secondary procedures on patent grafts normalize the hemodynamics at the revision site and are associated with a low incidence of restenosis; long-term patency rates range from 80 to 93% (1,7–9). The excellent durability of secondary procedures on the patent but hemodynamically abnormal bypass coupled with the dismal results of revision of the thrombosed bypass underscores the significant impact of monitoring graft hemodynamics with a surveillance protocol and elective bypass revision. This chapter discusses the definition and detection of autogenous graft failure by intraoperative and postoperative surveillance and details the surgical principles and results of management of the failing autogenous graft.

I. ETIOLOGY OF AUTOGENOUS GRAFT FAILURE

The etiology of autogenous graft failure differs according to the time of occurrence. Perioperatively (up to 30 days), autogenous graft failure most commonly is caused by technical errors, an inadequate inflow or outflow artery, or an inadequate vein. From 30 days to 2 years postoperatively, stenosis of the vein conduit or the anastomotic sites caused by fibrointimal hyperplasia is the most common cause of graft failure. Autogenous graft failure occurring more than 2 years postoperatively is likely a result of atherosclerotic disease progression of the inflow or outflow artery. Lesions associated with a diameter-reducing stenosis of the graft or native artery, regardless of the cause, can be identified reliably by abnormal graft hemodynamics. Occasionally autogenous graft thrombosis occurs despite normal hemodynamics because of thromboembolism, anastomotic pseudo-aneurysm formation, aneurysmal degeneration of the conduit, infection, or a hypercoagu-lable state.

II. PERIOPERATIVE FAILURE

Perioperative failure of the autogenous graft is related to technical errors and the quality of the arterial and venous systems used for bypass. Technical errors in constructing the proximal and distal anastomoses and preparing the conduit can occur. Dissecting and clamping the inflow and outflow arteries can raise intimal flaps, which can create luminal stenoses and/or thromboses. Errors in performing the proximal and distal anastomoses can result in suture line bleeding, pseudoaneurysm formation, or suture line stricture. Likewise, proximal occlusive disease in the aortoiliac segment can cause graft failure. Technical imperfections of the vein conduit include luminal thrombus, platelet aggregates, graft torsion, kinking of the graft, graft entrapment, inadequate ligation of venous branches, and vein injury from dissection or valve ablation.

The quality of the vein and artery used for the bypass is important for success of the autogenous graft. A poor-quality vein (i.e., one with sclerotic segments, varicosities, or a small diameter) can predispose to technical errors in handling the venous conduit and result in graft thrombosis. Sclerotic vein segments can have a thrombogenic flow surface and can also result in significant luminal stenosis, both of which can result in graft failure. Veins less than 2 mm in diameter are inadequate for long bypasses with both the in situ and reverse techniques. Inadequate arterial outflow caused by florid tibial and pedal occlusive disease can cause high outflow resistance, resulting in low graft flow and subsequent graft failure.

III. POSTOPERATIVE FAILURE

Beyond the perioperative period, the two main disease processes that result in autogenous graft failure are fibrointimal hyperplasia of the vein conduit or anastomotic sites and the progression of atherosclerotic disease of the inflow or outflow vessel. From 1 to 24 months postoperatively, fibrointimal hyperplasia is the most common cause of vein graft stenosis; the incidence is 5% per year. Approximately half of the lesions causing hemodynamic failure are located in the vein conduit itself. The remaining sites involve the proximal or distal anastomosis or the adjacent inflow or outflow artery. Lesions such as anastomotic stenoses, valve leaflet fibrosis, and focal or extensive fibrotic stenoses of the vein result in significant diameter-reducing stenosis with time. Beyond 2 years, the incidence of significant graft stenoses decreases to 1–3% per year (10). During this time interval, atherosclerotic disease progression is the most common cause of late graft failure. Atherosclerosis can progress in the native arterial inflow and outflow vessels, resulting in significant diameter-reducing stenosis and a decrease in blood flow. Atherosclerosis also can develop in the vein bypass itself, resulting in aneurysmal dilatation or stenosis of the vein graft and native arteries, which yields hemodynamic abnormalities that can be detected and corrected during post-operative surveillance (11,12).

IV. GRAFT SURVEILLANCE PROTOCOL

The ideal autogenous graft surveillance protocol should be noninvasive, associated with minimal complications, and highly accurate and reliable in identifying graft lesions that threaten patency. Based on the time course of occurrence of graft failure, surveillance of the autogenous grafts should be most frequent during the perioperative period and the first 2 years postoperatively. The graft surveillance techniques should be applicable intraoper-atively, immediately postoperatively, and throughout the postoperative follow-up period. The results should be reproducible and correlate with one another on serial examinations. Follow-up of autogenous grafts based on the recurrence of symptoms of limb ischemia is inadequate in identifying grafts at risk for thrombosis. In studies of the in situ saphenous vein bypass, Bandyk and associates (7,10) have documented that only one-third of patients had recurrence of symptoms despite noninvasive vascular laboratory studies indicating hemodynamic graft failure. In a study of reverse saphenous vein grafts, Minh Chau et al. (2) documented that only 29% of limbs with low graft flow velocities (less than 45 cm/s) had recurrence of symptoms alone. This would result in up to two-thirds of patients with autogenous grafts at risk for thrombosis not being identified. Clinical and hemodynamic assessment with use of noninvasive vascular laboratory testing is essential for the post-operative surveillance protocol. Graft failure is indicated by the following:

Recurrence of symptoms of limb ischemia
Low peak systolic graft flow velocity (<45 cm/s)
Decrease of flow velocity >30 cm/s
Ankle/brachial index >0.15 on serial examinations

Surveillance protocols for autogenous grafts include hemodynamic monitoring of the arterial systolic pressure of the limb and the blood-flow velocities of the venous conduit and native arteries. Ankle systolic pressure measurements correlate with the clinical symptoms of limb ischemia and are predictive of healing of ulcers or amputation sites, but they are unable to localize the obstructive lesion to the inflow conduit or outflow. Also, because of the high rate of lower limb bypass required by diabetic patients, the presence of incompres-sible calf vessels makes measurement of ankle pressures impossible. Analysis of blood-flow velocity with the use of a duplex scanner can evaluate the venous conduit, anastomotic sites, and adjacent arteries for hemodynamic abnormalities of flow. Unlike limb pressures, the duplex scan can reliably identify the location and anatomy of the lesions by ultrasound and quantitate the severity of flow disturbance and stenosis. Systolic pressure measurement and analysis of blood-flow velocity are complementary tests that can aid in the prediction of recurrence of symptoms or graft thromboses, both should be used during postoperative surveillance of the autogenous graft (10,13) (Table 1).

Hemodynamic surveillance should be used intraoperatively, perioperatively, and dur-ing the postoperative follow-up period for both in situ and reversed autogenous grafts (1,2,7,10). B-mode imaging has been used to assess completed arterial reconstructions, and intravascular defects can be detected by this method. Advances in technology have provided instrumentation that combines the advantages of Doppler spectral analysis for hemody-namic assessment and B-mode imaging to determine vessel wall integrity. The further

Table 1 Duplex Scan Classification of Severity of Stenosis

Classification	Velocity Waveform Analysis
<20% DR	No increase in peak systolic velocity compared with adjacent proximal segment spectral broadening during systole
20–50% DR	>30% increase in peak systolic velocity compared with adjacent proximal segment; spectral broadening during systole and diastole
50–75 % DR	>100% increase peak systolic velocity (Vp > 125 cm/s) compared with adjacent proximal segment, end-diastolic velocity <100 cm/s: spectral broadening during systole and diastole
>75% DR	>100% increase in peak systolic velocity (Vp > 125 cm/s) compared with adjacent proximal segment end-diastolic velocity >100 cm/s: spectral broadening during systole and diastole

Abbreviations: DR, diameter reduction; Vp, velocity peak.

addition of color-coded imaging greatly facilitates vessel imaging, making this the ideal method for intraoperative evaluation of arterial reconstructions.

V. TECHNIQUE

Duplex examinations use color coding to display velocity spectra within the B-mode image (14). Intraoperative techniques are identical, whether gray-scale or color-coded imaging is employed, although color allows for more rapid vessel identification and interrogation. This technique can be used for cerebrovascular; peripheral arterial, and visceral vessels and requires a high-frequency transducer, because it is applied directly to the reconstructed vessel. The duplex scan is performed and recorded on videotape after closure of the arteriotomy and restoration of blood flow. A sterile plastic sleeve is filled at one end with acoustic gel or saline before the transducer is placed inside. The vascular technologist is present to make necessary adjustments in Doppler angle assignment, sample volume placement, and color parameters in order to obtain the optimal image and accurate spectral display.

The examination begins with the location of patient arteriovenous fistulas (AVFs). With the duplex probe placed on the proximal graft, the distal graft is occluded with finger pressure. Persistence of forward flow anywhere along the conduit indicates an AVF between the point of the probe and the point of finger occlusion. The duplex probe then is passed down the length of the graft and the persistence of forward flow proximal to the AVF is noted. Once past the fistula, the forward flow diminishes. When the fistulas are ligated, there should be no forward flow with distal finger pressure occlusion. The proximal and distal anastomoses, the inflow and outflow arteries, and the flow along the entire graft conduit—especially at the valve incision sites—are then evaluated. Anatomical and technical defects are identified and quantitated according to the extent of spectral broadening and increase of peak systolic frequency. Mild to moderate flow disturbances are associated with spectral broadening during systole and peak systolic velocity (Va > 125 cm/s). Severe flow disturbances are associated with spectral broadening during systole and diastole and peak systolic velocity greater than 125 cm/s and end diastolic velocity > 100 cm/s. With the in situ technique, partial valve lysis is associated with severe flow disturbances just distal to the valve site. Sclerotic vein segments, graft torsion, platelet aggregates, and anastomotic stenosis are often associated with severe flow disturbances at the site and just distal to the abnormal graft segment. The location, length, and severity of stenosis can be identified precisely with intraoperative spectral analysis.

Postoperative graft surveillance should be performed before hospital discharge using limb blood pressure measurement and duplex scanning. Systolic pressure measurements are obtained by measuring the ankle/brachial index (ABI); duplex scanning of proximal and distal anastomoses, inflow and outflow arteries, and the entire autogenous conduit can be performed. Velocity waveform analysis can be performed by placing the sample volume in the center of the vessel lumen at the desired Doppler beam angle. Calculation of the graft flow velocities at designated sites with normal arterial flow patterns, where the vessel diameter does not vary, is necessary for reliable and reproducible results from one examination to the next. Flow velocity should be measured with the patient in the supine position, limbs slightly rotated externally, and the knee bent and at rest.

Vein graft lesions detected in this time period include arteriovenous fistulas, residual intact valve leaflets, and graft or anastomotic stenosis. Arteriovenous fistulas are recognized by proximally located high diastolic flows, increased flow turbulence at the site, and decreased or absent diastolic flow distal to the site of the fistula. Stenotic lesions of the graft conduit or anastomotic site are identified by increases in spectral broadening and peak systolic and diastolic velocities at or just distal to the site. In addition to identifying hemodynamically significant lesions predisposing to early graft failure, early duplex scanning provides a baseline for subsequent graft surveillance studies. Serial evaluations with postoperative hemodynamic surveillance should be performed at 6 weeks postoperatively, every 3 months for the first year, and every 6 months thereafter. Each examination should include limb pressure measurements and determination of peak systolic flow velocities at the middle and distal graft; the results should be compared with prior studies. Autogenous grafts that exhibit abnormal hemodynamics (low graft flow velocities, >50% graft stenoses, significant decrease in peak systolic frequency on serial examinations greater than 30 cm/s, or decrease in ABI greater than 0.15) should be evaluated by complete duplex scanning of the entire graft and by arteriography.

More recently, studies have been conducted to determine whether ongoing surveillance needs to be done for the life of the conduit. In the long-term evaluation of 462 saphenous vein in situ bypasses performed over a 13-year period, 30% of the grafts required at least one revision (11). Even grafts that have exhibited good hemodynamics for up to 24 months are at risk for developing abnormalities that could lead to graft failure. Of the initial graft revisions in this study, 18% occurred after 24 months. Because of the increasing incidence of atherosclerosis in the inflow and outflow vessels with long-term follow-up, a greater percentage of revisions involve inflow and outflow vessels as opposed to the conduit itself. Of the revisions performed after 24 months, 68% were to the conduit, compared with 85% in the earlier time period.

As the follow-up becomes longer, degenerative changes can develop in the conduit itself. Previous work from our institution has demonstrated that more than 50% of vein bypass conduits followed for at least 5 years demonstrated evidence of atherosclerotic degeneration (12). Often these changes represent areas of intimal thickening, but in the significant portion the disease has progressed to form focal point stenosis caused by atherosclerosis. The likelihood of developing graft-threatening lesions is even greater in conduits that have previously been revised or have hemodynamic abnormalities, but some conduits that have been free of abnormalities for the first 2 years will go on to require revision. By recognizing that conduits which have previously required revision are more prone to develop secondary degenerative processes, the surveillance of these conduits can be more focused.

Other authors have suggested that if the conduit has normal hemodynamics in the early perioperative period, the chances that problems may arise are such that further surveillance may not be warranted (15). Our study reveals that of the 67 graft revisions performed after 24 months, 37 were to previously revised conduits, but 30 were to vein grafts that had required no previous revision (11). Conduits that are hemodynamically normal beyond 2 years evolved lesions at a rate significant enough to warrant ongoing surveillance. The average incidence of primary graft failure was 10% of the number of grafts remaining patent at each yearly time interval beyond 24 months. If vascular surgeons want to optimize long-term graft patency, surveillance must continue for the life of the conduit. Other authors whose series consist of primarily reverse vein bypasses have drawn similar conclusions (16).

The failure to identify and revise a graft with a hemodynamically significant lesion before thrombosis is associated with poor patency. Long-term patency rates are improved markedly for autogenous grafts revised while patent, compared with long-term patency rates for revision of thrombosed bypass conduits. The secondary patency rates for bypasses patent at the time of revision are equivalent to those for bypasses that never undergo revision. Revision of the thrombosed reversed or in situ saphenous vein bypass uniformly results in poor long-term patency. In a study of 109 autogenous grafts, Whittemore et al. (17) reported that revision of the patent but failing autogenous graft yielded an 85% 5-year patency rate, compared with a 37% 5-year patency rate for revision of the thrombosed bypass. In a study of 95 bypasses that underwent revision, Bergamini et al. (1) found a significant decline in the secondary patency for bypasses thrombosed at the time of revision (47%) compared with that for bypasses patent at the time of revision (93%)(Fig. 1).

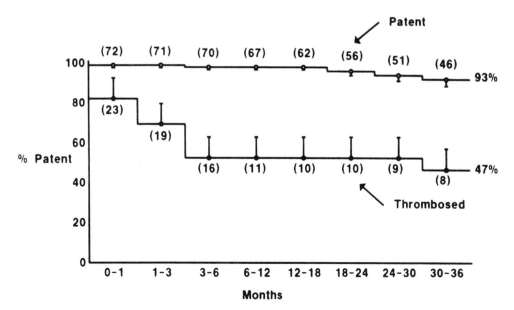

Figure 1 Secondary patency of in situ saphenous vein bypasses that were patent at time of revision (open circles) was significantly higher ($p < 0.0000005$) than that of bypasses that were thrombosed at time of revision (closed circles).

Table 2 Incidence of Technical Errors with In Situ Saphenous Vein Bypass: First Half of Series vs. Later Half [a]

Technical error	1981–1985	1986–1990
Valvulotome injury	20	9
Anastomotic stenosis	5	0
Bypass torsion	4	0
Residual valve leaflet	4	0
Total[b]	33 (18%)	9 (5%)

[a] In the first half of the series (1981–1985), there were 179 cases; in the second half (1986–1990), there were 182 cases.
[b] Total number of technical errors for the first half compared with the second half is significantly different $p = 0.0001 (z^2$ analysis).

Compulsive bypass surveillance can identify the failing autogenous graft and permit elective revision, a practice that has significant impact on long-term patency.

The superior long-term patency rates of both in situ and reversed autogenous grafts also were related directly to improved surgical technique and the experience of the vascular surgeon (1,18,19). Increasing surgical experience was associated with a significant decrease in the number of technical errors encountered with vein preparation (1) (Table 2). Increasing surgical experience was also associated with a significant improvement in the secondary patency rate (92%) compared with the secondary patency rate of the first half of the series (80%) at 3 years (Fig. 2). Taylor et al. (19) have also attributed the recent improvement in long-term patency of reversed autogenous grafts to improvements in surgical technique and

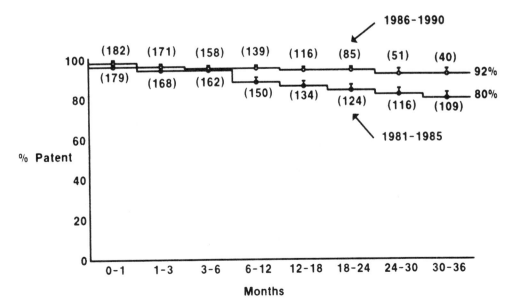

Figure 2 Secondary patency of in situ saphenous vein bypasses performed by the more experienced surgeon from 1986 to 1990 (open circles) was significantly higher ($p < 0.02$) than that of bypasses in the earlier years from 1981 to 1985 (closed circles).

increasing surgical experience. Long-term patency rates of the in situ and reversed autogenous grafts are improved with careful operative technique, meticulous postoperative graft surveillance, and increasing surgical experience.

VI. LONG-TERM CHANGES IN AUTOGENOUS GRAFTS

Autogenous grafts that are in place for a long time are vulnerable to the same atherosclerotic changes as the native arteries, although in overall timing they take less time to develop. In a study of 72 lower extremity vein grafts that functioned and were patent from 4.6 to 21.6 years, the median being 6.6 years, we found that only 43% were normal (12). In addition, nearly 1 in 5 grafts harbored a lesion that was felt to pose a threat to continued graft patency.

Atherosclerotic degeneration of saphenous vein grafts was first described in 1947 when a femoral interposition graft that had been in place for 22 years was removed and found to contain atheromatous plaques. In 1973, Szilagyi et al. reported their experience with a lower extremity saphenous vein graft that had been monitored with arteriography (20). They described eight different morphological findings in grafts of varying ages. Several of these were related to surgical technique, including suture stenosis caused by tying side branches too closely, long venous side branch stumps, and traumatic stenosis caused by clamps. They also described the changes that occur, including intimal thickening, myointimal hyperplasia at valve sites, atherosclerotic irregularity, and aneurysmal dilatation. In our study, autogenous grafts were examined at least 4.6 years after construction. The early post-operative changes that Szilagyi et al. described were not detectable. However, we did find three distinct atherosclerotic abnormalities: wall plaque, aneurysmal dilatation, and discrete stenosis.

The most prevalent finding was wall plaque, which was present in all of the abnormal grafts, although this was frequently overshadowed by more impressive stenosis or aneurysms. Typically, plaques were several centimeters long, multicentric, echogenic, and slightly raised from the normal wall. These are mild forms of atherosclerotic degeneration. In the series of Szilagyi et al., atherosclerotic changes developed at approximately 45 months. Atkinson et al. looked at coronary artery saphenous vein grafts during autopsy and found atherosclerotic changes in 21% of the grafts that had been placed an average of 62 months (21). However, when DeWeese and Rob monitored long-term grafts with the use of arteriography, they noted atherosclerotic changes in only 3 of 18 patients studied after 5 years, and two grafts did not develop changes until after 10 years (22). We use color duplex ultrasonography to study the grafts and have been able to visualize changes in the arterial wall, such as thickening and wall plaque, that are not necessarily seen on contrast arteriography, which defines only the column of flowing blood.

VII. EFFECT OF SITE OF DISTAL ANASTOMOSIS

In contrast to the patency for in situ saphenous vein bypass, the long-term patency for the reversed vein graft was significantly decreased for infrapopliteal bypasses, long bypasses performed with vein less than 3 mm in diameter, and reversed vein grafts in diabetic patients. Taylor and coworkers (19) reported a significant decline in primary patency for autogenous reversed grafts to the infrapopliteal arteries (69%) compared with that for below-knee popliteal arteries (80%). The secondary patency for infrapopliteal arteries (77%) was also decreased compared with that for below-knee popliteal artery grafts (86%). Rutherford et al. (23) also showed a decrease in the cumulative patency rate at 3 years for reversed vein grafts (63%) compared with that for in situ (88%) vein bypasses to the tibial outflow artery.

VIII. EFFECT OF VEIN GRAFT DIAMETER AND DIABETES MELLITUS

The long-term patency of reversed autogenous grafts with vein diameters less than 3 mm is decreased significantly compared with that for reversed autogenous grafts with greater vein diameters (24). The in situ autogenous graft is less affected by vein size (1,18), but 2 mm is the lowest diameter of usable vein.

Long-term patency and limb salvage are adversely affected by the presence of diabetes in patients with reversed autogenous grafts (9,19,25). On the other hand, in situ autogenous graft long-term patency and limb salvage are not significantly different for the diabetic patient compared with those for the nondiabetic patient (1).

IX. OPERATIVE MANAGEMENT OF THE PATENT BUT FAILING AUTOGENOUS GRAFT

The goals of intraoperative modification or postoperative revision of the patent but failing autogenous graft should be correction of the anatomic abnormality, restoration of normal hemodynamics of the autogenous graft, and maintenance of long-term bypass patency. The principles and techniques of treatment of a graft stenosis are the same for the in situ and reversed saphenous vein grafts. Graft revisions require a clear understanding of the cause, location, and extent of the lesion (7). Secondary procedures require meticulous dissection and technical precision. Regional and general anesthesia is preferred over local anesthesia to perform the revision with minimal patient discomfort. The use of scalpel dissection is essential to expose the autogenous graft without vein injury. After dissection of the abnormal segment of the autogenous graft, intraoperative spectral analysis can be performed to confirm the precise location and extent of the lesion. After exposure and control of bleeding points, the patients are heparinized systemically. Secondary procedures on the distal graft, distal anastomotic site, or native outflow artery are enhanced by the use of a pneumatic tourniquet as a substitute for vascular clamps for proximal and distal control in the scarred tissue planes (26). The limb is exsanguinated by leg elevation and the use of an elastic wrap before inflation of the tourniquet (40 to 50 mmHg above brachial systolic pressure). The secondary procedure can then be performed without the necessity to dissect the proximal and distal conduits circumferentially for control and without the need to work around the vascular clamps. Just before completion of the revision, the tourniquet should be deflated to confirm the presence of back-bleeding from the distal conduit. Intraoperative spectral analysis and arteriography are performed routinely to document the restoration of normal graft hemodynamics and anatomic configuration.

A. Modification of the Failing Autogenous Graft During the Primary Procedure

During the placement of the primary in situ or reversed autogenous graft, intraoperative modification of the venous conduit is performed to correct technical errors or a poor-quality vein. The key to successful treatment is recognition and correction of the lesion before graft thrombosis occurs. The intraoperative occurrence of the low-flow state can be caused by problems with the inflow artery, vein conduit, anastomotic site, or out flow artery. Significant stenosis of the inflow artery can be identified by intraoperative measurement of the systolic pressure by insertion of an 18- to 20-gauge needle in the common femoral artery connected to the arterial line monitor. A significant gradient (greater than 20 mmHg) at rest or after injection of 20 mg of papaverine between the inflow artery pressure and the brachial systolic pressure confirms the presence of a poor inflow artery. Improved inflow can be achieved by a proximal aortic bypass, extra-anatomic bypass, or intraoperative balloon angioplasty if a short segmental lesion is present.

The low-flow state caused by lesions of the vein conduit or anastomotic sites can be detected by complete survey of the graft from the proximal to the distal anastomosis with high-frequency spectral analysis. Technical errors or poor-quality vein segments are associated uniformly with increased peak systolic frequency and spectral broadening. Anastomotic stenoses are caused by technical errors, such as missing the endothelium, incorporation of adventitial tissue in the intraluminal flow surface, poorly placed stitches resulting in suture line stricture or bleeding, and intimal flaps or raised plaques. The distal anastomotic stricture usually involves the toe of the end-to-side anastomosis. This is best corrected by reconstructing the entire anastomosis. Endarterectomy of the native artery to correct intimal flaps or atherosclerotic plaques is sometimes necessary. With the reversed vein graft, meticulous technique is mandatory in anastomosing the large end of the reversed vein to the smaller outflow artery.

Intraoperative modification of the venous conduit for both in situ and reversed autogenous grafts is performed to correct a poor-quality vein or technical error. Sclerotic veins have been treated by vein patching of the sclerotic segment or resection of sclerotic segment and replacement with a translocated vein segment from another source. If the endothelium of the sclerotic segment is abnormal and an alternate vein source of adequate diameter and quality is available, resection and replacement of the sclerotic vein segment is preferred. Varicosities of the vein are treated with plication of the wall or a partial resection and vein patch angioplasty. Small-diameter vein segment or previously used segments of vein in the leg should be replaced with an alternate source of vein. The translocated vein segments used for interposition replacement should be of good quality, with a thin wall, a diameter greater than 2 mm, and a glistening endothelial flow surface. Intraoperative modification caused by technical failure of the in situ bypass is most commonly performed for retained valve leaflets or AVFs. The retained valve leaflet can be incised simply by reinserting the valvulotome through a side branch or directly into the vein conduit via an 18-gauge needle puncture hole. Sclerotic valves prompt valve excision under direct vision through a longitudinal venotomy. The venotomy is closed primarily if it this technically achievable without creating luminal stenosis or, if this is not possible, with a vein patch. Arteriovenous fistulas are treated simply by ligation. Injured segments of vein during dissection are repaired simply with lateral venorrhaphy, vein patch angioplasty, resection and primary anastomosis, or resection and interposition grafting. The key to the treatment of this technical problem is to resect all abnormal endothelium and injured vein wall and then reconstruct the bypass graft without creating luminal stenosis or increased tension on the anastomosis. Vein conduit torsion is best treated by transecting the conduit, untwisting it, and performing a primary reanastomosis. Minor kinks or twists of less the 90 degrees in the bypass are treated with vein patch angioplasty across the twisted segment. Graft entrapment is detected by the presence of normal graft velocities with the knee flexed, but the development of a low-flow state with absence of diastolic flow with the knee extended is seen in patients who spend significant amounts of time in wheelchairs. Treatment of this complication includes a myotomy of the tendons and muscles in which the vein bypass is entrapped. The formation of platelet aggregates along the endothelial flow surface caused by heparin-induced platelet aggregation should be treated with reversal of the heparin, low-molecular-weight dextran drip, removal of the platelet aggregates by means of longitudinal venotomy, and subsequent primary or vein patch closure of the venotomy. Intraoperative thrombosis of the vein graft without the presence of a poor inflow artery, technical errors, or poor-quality vein should prompt a search for evidence of a hypercoagulable state (antithrombin III deficiency, heparin-induce platelet aggregation, abnormal plasminogen) or a poor outflow artery. Conduits with a poor outflow artery have a low-flow state and an absence of diastolic forward flow caused by high outflow resistance (27). The best management is a translocated vein sequential graft or jump graft from the vein bypass to an alternate outflow artery, if available, to increase the outflow and decrease the resistance. Following the secondary graft procedures, intraoperative pulsed Doppler spectral analysis and arteriography should be repeated to make sure that there is normalization of the bypassed hemodynamic and anatomical abnormalities.

X. SECONDARY PROCEDURES FOR REVISION OF THE FAILING AUTOGENOUS GRAFT

During postoperative surveillance, operative management of the failing but patent autogenous graft depends on the anatomy and location of the lesion. Stenoses of the graft conduit are secondary to fibrointimal hyperplasia at the anastomotic sites, valve sites or areas of intraoperative vein injury. The areas of graft stenosis can vary from focal to extensive, affecting a long segment of the graft conduit (Fig. 3). Focal stenosis in the in situ saphenous vein bypass occurs at fibrotic valve sites. The formation of lesions caused by fibrointimal hyperplasia usually is associated with technical errors or injury in preparing the venous conduit for bypass. If focal stenosis develops in the vein conduit, sufficient length usually is present to permit resection of the lesion and primary end-to-end anastomosis to restore bypass patency. The amount of redundant graft is less for reversed autogenous grafts, making reanastomosis an infrequent option. If there is inadequate vein length or the stenosis is immediately adjacent to an anastomotic site, the focal stenosis is treated by a longitudinal venotomy across the length of the stenosis and vein patch angioplasty reconstruction. Stenoses of the proximal and distal anastomoses are treated with a vein patch angioplasty extending distally onto the native artery. A third treatment option for focal graft stenosis is percutaneous transluminal angioplasty (PTA). PTA is especially suitable for treatment of focal stenosis in high-risk patients or in the native arteries proximal or distal to the graft.

More extensive lesions include long sclerotic vein segments, multiple stenotic lesions, and fibrointimal hyperplasia or atherosclerosis involving a long segment of the distal anastomosis or outflow artery. Long or multiple stenotic lesions of the vein conduit are treated by vein patch angioplasty or resection and interposition of a translocated vein segment if an alternate, good-quality vein of similar diameter is available. Long stenotic lesions of the distal anastomosis are treated with vein patch angioplasty across the stenotic segment. Extensive lesions of the distal vein conduit and outflow artery are treated with a jump graft (extension of the graft to the same outflow artery) or a sequential graft (translocated vein segment to a different outflow artery) using translocated vein (greater saphenous, lesser saphenous, cephalic). The technical success of secondary procedures is evaluated by intraoperative spectral analysis and angiography to ensure achievement of normal graft hemodynamics and anatomic reconstruction.

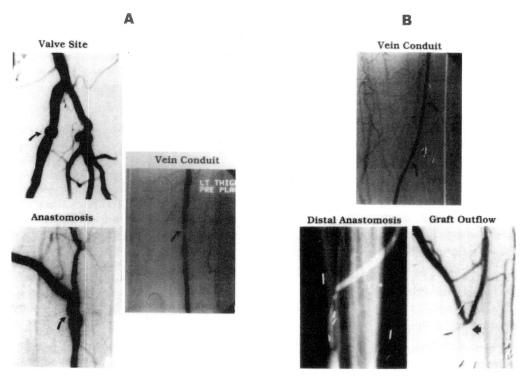

Figure 3   A. Focal stenotic lesions of the failing autogenous graft detected during postoperative surveillance were caused by fibrointimal hyperplasia. Valve site stenosis was treated by excision and end-to-end reanastomosis. Vein conduit stenosis was treated with percutaneous balloon angioplasty. Anastomotic stenosis was treated by vein patch angioplasty. B. Extensive stenotic lesions of the failing autogenous graft detected during postoperative surveillance. Segmental stenotic lesions of the vein conduit and distal anastomosis caused by fibrointimal hyperplasia were treated with resection and interposition translocated vein graft. Extensive disease of the outflow artery caused by progression of atherosclerotic disease was treated with sequential jump grafting to the more distal outflow artery site.

XI.   PERIOPERATIVE RESULTS OF MANAGEMENT OF THE PATENT BUT FAILING AUTOGENOUS GRAFT

The early patency (30 days) of the autogenous graft is excellent if intraoperative normal hemodynamics and arteriography are achieved with the revascularization procedure (20). In a study of in situ saphenous vein bypasses, the 30-day patency for the 83 bypasses in the series with normal intraoperative hemodynamics was 100%. Initially, 77 of the 83 in situ saphenous vein grafts had normal intraoperative hemodynamics with peak systolic velocity of greater than 40 cm/s and biphasic (hyperemic flow) waveform. Six (7%) of the bypasses had low peak systolic blood flow velocity (less than 40 cm/s) and an absence of hyperemic flow, a predictor of early failure of the in situ bypass (29). Correction of the underlying causes (AVF, intact valve leaflet, poor-quality vein segment) resulted in early bypass patency with normal hemodynamics after modification in these six bypasses. The short-term patency was dependent on intraoperative identification and correction of the lesions causing flow abnormalities (28). The determination of normal intraoperative hemodynamics of the autogenous graft is a highly accurate predictor of early patency following lower extremity revascularization. The primary and secondary patencies for both in situ and reversed autogenous grafts are decreased when intraoperative modification of the vein conduit is required to complete the lower extremity arterial reconstruction (1,19).

XII. FACTORS THAT AFFECT THE LONG-TERM PATENCY RATE OF AUTOGENOUS GRAFTS

The use of postoperative surveillance protocol of in situ and reversed autogenous grafts allows the study of the pathophysiology of autogenous graft failure and also the analysis of factors that adversely affect long-term patency. The determinant factors that significantly affect long-term patency for both the in situ and reversed saphenous vein grafts are modification of the venous conduit at the initial operation to correct a poor-quality vein with patch angioplasty or vein interposition, technical error caused by injury to the vein during valve ablation, failure to revise the bypass before thrombosis during the surveillance period, and experience of the vascular surgeon in placing the autogenous graft. The long-term patency of autogenous grafts is decreased significantly when the ipsilateral saphenous vein is not adequate and requires some modification. In a recent large series of reversed saphenous vein grafts, Taylor and colleagues (19) found that the ipsilateral greater saphenous vein was inadequate in 45% of the cases. The ipsilateral saphenous vein was inadequate because the vein was removed previously, the available vein was to short, the available vein was to small or the vein contained sclerotic segments. Techniques practiced in performing the reversed vein graft in patients with inadequate ipsilateral saphenous vein were to use a more distal inflow artery, performed a venovenous anastomosis after removal of the abnormal segment, or use another source of vein—contralateral greater saphenous vein, cephalic vein, or lesser saphenous vein. The primary patency of the reversed vein grafts that had inadequate ipsilateral saphenous vein was 68%, a significant decrease compared with the 80% primary patency of those grafts that had adequate ipsilateral saphenous veins. The secondary patency of the grafts with inadequate veins requiring a modification technique was 77%, which also was decreased compared with the 84% patency of the reversed vein grafts with nonmodified conduits. Similarly, in a recent large series of in situ saphenous vein bypasses (1), the primary and secondary patency rates also were decreased significantly for those bypassed veins undergoing modification at the time of bypass. The need to modify the vein conduit because of a technical failure or inadequate vein was associated with a significant increase in the incidence of late-appearing bypass stenosis and revision. The bypass stenoses were most commonly caused by the occurrence and progression of fibrointimal hyperplasia resulting from the injurious effects of the bypass modification (Fig. 4). The primary (50%) and secondary (72%) patencies of the in situ saphenous vein bypasses that required modification were decreased significantly compared with the primary (70%) and secondary (84%) patency rates of bypasses that did not undergo modification at the time of the bypass procedure. This increase in incidence of graft stenoses, bypass revision, and decline in primary and secondary patencies was believed to be caused by the occurrence of fibrointimal hyperplasia associated with the injurious effects of the bypass modification. The long-term patency of these conduits is dependent on the meticulous postoperative surveillance protocol identifying correctable lesions before thrombosis, permitting elective revision of patent conduits. Reversed and in situ autogenous grafts

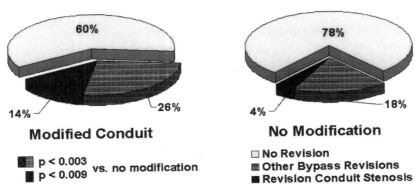

Modified Conduit   **No Modification**

■ p < 0.003
■ p < 0.009 vs. no modification

☐ No Revision
▨ Other Bypass Revisions
■ Revision Conduit Stenosis

Figure 4 Modification to correct an inadequate vein or technical failure during the in situ saphenous vein bypass procedure was associated with a significant increase in number of bypasses in which graft stenoses developed and that required revision during the postoperative surveillance period. Late-appearing stenoses occurred in 12 of 86 modified conduits (14%) compared with only 12 of 269 in situ bypasses (4.5%) not undergoing modification at the time initial modification. During the post-operative surveillance period, revision of the bypasses with modified conduits (34 of 86, 40%) was significantly more frequent than that of bypasses with no modification of conduits (60 of 269, 22%).

that have modified conduits mandate close postoperative surveillance to identify the development of lesions that threaten graft patency.

For the in situ saphenous vein bypasses, severe atherosclerotic disease of the common femoral artery was associated with a decline in primary patency but did not significantly alter secondary patency (1). Severe disease of the common femoral artery necessitated endarterectomy, replacement with an interposition prosthetic or vein graft, or closure with a patch angioplasty in order to perform the proximal anastomosis. Bypasses originating from a reconstructed inflow artery had a significant increase in the number of revisions performed to correct anastomotic or outflow artery stenosis compared to bypasses with no recon-struction of the inflow artery (Fig. 5). With postoperative surveillance and elective revision, the secondary patency was not decreased significantly for the bypasses originating from a reconstructed inflow artery.

Long-term patency of the failing autogenous graft can be maintained if revision is performed before graft thrombosis occurs. Attempts to treat focal short-segment stenoses of the autogenous vein conduit by total excision of the short segment of diseased vein and primary end-to-end reanastomosis were highly successful, with no occurrence of late re-stenosis or bypass failure. The treatment of graft stenosis with vein patch angioplasty also resulted in excellent long-term patency (greater than 80%) (7,17) but was associated with an increased incidence of late restenosis at the revision site itself. In a recent study Bandyk et al. (7) demonstrated that 8 of 31 stenotic lesions (24%) treated by vein patch angioplasty re-sulted in restenosis; most occurred more than 3 months after the secondary procedure. PTA of focal vein graft stenosis also was associated with early bypass patency (8); however, recurrent stenosis did occur in at least half of the cases (6,7,30,31). Because of the high incidence of recurrent graft stenosis, PTA should be used primarily for high-risk patients with a failing autogenous graft caused by focal lesion or for the management of athero-sclerotic lesions in the native arteries. Restenosis of vein patch angioplasty or PTA site was

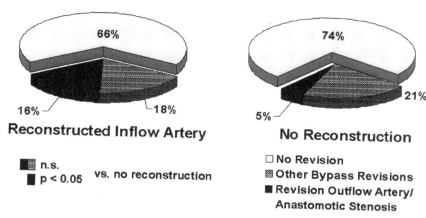

Reconstructed Inflow Artery   **No Reconstruction**

■ n.s.
■ p < 0.05   vs. no reconstruction

☐ No Revision
▦ Other Bypass Revisions
■ Revision Outflow Artery/
   Anastomotic Stenosis

Figure 5 In situ saphenous vein bypass revision performed to correct anastomotic or outflow artery stenosis was significantly more frequent for grafts with reconstructed inflow arteries (7 of 44, 16%) than for bypasses originating from nonreconstructed inflow arteries (14 of 312, 4.5%). Revision of graft stenosis was not significantly different for bypasses with reconstruction of the inflow arteries (15 of 44, 34%) and those without (78 of 310, 25%).

best treated by resection of the diseased, stenotic segment of vein and replacement with a translocated interposition vein graft.

Secondary procedures used to treat extensive lesions of the graft, distal anastomosis, or outflow artery also result in maintenance of long-term patency. In a recent study by Bandyk et al. (7), recurrent stenosis and graft failure occurred less frequently after resection and interposition grafting compared with a sequential or jump graft procedure. Only 1 of 17 of the interposition grafts had a recurrent stenosis or jump graft failure. However, 11 of 21 sequential or jump grafting procedures were associated with recurrent stenosis or autogenous graft failure. The difference in patency was partially explained by the fact that the interposition grafts were placed for fibrointimal hyperplasia of a graft that was resectable and reconstructible, but the sequential or jump grafts were placed primarily for progression of atherosclerotic disease of the outflow artery. The bypass of the failing graft caused by progression of atherosclerotic disease of the outflow arteries with sequential or jump grafting was the least durable procedure in 5 of 21 grafts that eventually failed.

Graft revision uniformly resulted in the restoration of normal hemodynamics of the autogenous graft. The ABIs and the peak systolic velocities returned to comparable levels that were present for the graft before the occurrence of the graft stenosis. The ABI was usually in the range of 0.6 before the secondary procedure and increased to greater than 0.9 following revision in 85% of the lower extremities. The peak systolic velocity was less than 45cm/s in 845 of the autogenous grafts in this series and uniformly increased to a level comparable to the initial postoperative studies (5,7).

XIII. CONCLUSION

Long-term patency of the autogenous vein graft hinges on the detection and correction of the failing bypass before thrombosis. The development of fibrointimal hyperplasia of the graft or progression of atherosclerosis of the native arteries can result in diameter-reducing stenoses that threaten bypass patency. The need for intraoperative reconstruction of the inflow artery or for modification of the vein conduit during a bypass procedure because of a technical error or poor-quality vein significantly increases the risk of late-appearing stenoses and the need for bypass revision. The long-term patency of the autogenous vein grafts that develop hemodynamically significant lesions (low graft flow velocity, >75% stenosis) and threaten bypass *patency* is dependent on the identification and correction of the lesions before thrombosis. The secondary patency rates for the revision of the *patent* but hemodynamically failing autogenous graft have been equal to those of bypasses that do not undergo revisions of the *thrombosed* autogenous graft has been uniformly poor (1,5). The success of graft revision is dependent on excision of the lesion, use of autogenous tissue for reconstruction, restoration of normal hemodynamics, and continued postoperative surveillance. Secondary procedures to cored the failing graft result in excellent long-term patency greater than 85% at 5 years (7,12). Secondary procedures should restore normal graft and hemodynamics with the excision of the pathoanatomical lesion and the use of normal autogenous tissue for reconstruction.

REFERENCES

1. Bergamini TM, Towne JB, Bandy DF, et al. Experience with in situ saphenous vein bypasses from 1981–1989: determinant factors of long-term patency. J Vasc Surg 1991; 13:137–147.
2. Minh-Chau L, Friedman EI, Figg-Hoblyn L, et al. Decreased graft flow is a reliable predictor of impending failure of reversed vein grafts. J Vasc Technol 1988; 12:133.
3. Sladen JG, Gilmour JL. Vein graft stenosis. Am J Surg 1981; 141:549.
4. Bandyk DF, Kaebnick HW, Stewart GW, et al. Durability of the in situ vein arterial bypass: a comparison of primary and secondary patency. J Vasc Surg 1987; 5:526.
5. Belkin M, Donaldson MC, Whittemore AD, et al. Observations on the use of thrombolytic agents fro thrombotic occlusion of infrainguinal vein grafts. J Vasc Surg 1990; 11:299.
6. Cohen JR, Mannick JA, Couch NP, et al. Recognition and management of impending vein-graft failure. Arch Surg 1986; 121:758.
7. Bandyk DF, Bergamini TM, Towne JB, et al. Durability of vein graft revision: the outcome of secondary procedures. J Vasc Surg 1991; 13:200–210.
8. Berkowitz HD, Hobbs CL, Roberts B, et al. Value of routine vascular laboratory studies to identify vein graft stenosis. Surgery 1081; 90:971.
9. Veith FJ, Weiser RK, Gupta SK, et al. Diagnosis and management of failing lower extremity arterial reconstructions prior to graft occlusion. J Cardiovasc Surg 1984; 25:381.
10. Bandyk DF, Schmitt DD, Seabrook GR, et al. Monitoring patency of in situ saphenous vein bypasses: the impact of a surveillance protocol and elective revision. J Vasc Surg 1989; 9:286.
11. Erickson CA, Towne JB, Seabrook GR, et al. Ongoing vascular laboratory surveillance is essential to maximize long-term in situ saphenous vein bypass patency. J Vasc Surg 1996; 23:18–27.
12. Reifsnyder T, Towne JB, et al. Biologic characteristics of long-term autogenous vein grafts—A dynamic evaluation. J Vasc Surg 1993; 71:207–217.
13. Green RM, McNamara J, Ouriel K, et al. Comparison of infrainguinal graft surveillance techniques. J Vasc Surg 1990; 11:207.
14. Cato R, Bandyk DF, et al. Duplex scanning after carotid reconstruction: A comparison of interoperative and postoperative results. J Vasc Tech 1991; 15:61–65.
15. Mills JL, Bandyk DF, Gahton V, Esses GE. The origin of infrainguinal vein graft stenosis: A prospective study based on duplex surveillance. J Vasc Surg 1995; 21:16–25.
16. Passman MA, Monetta GL, Naylor ME, Taylor LM, et al. Do normal early color flow duplex surveillance examination results of infrainguinal vein graft preclude the need for late graft revision. J Vasc Surg 1995; 22:476–484.

17. Whittemore AD, Clowes AW, Couch NP, et al. Secondary femoropopliteal reconstruction. Ann Surg 1981; 193:35.
18. Leather RP, Shah DM, Chang BB, et al. Resurrection of the in situ saphenous vein bypass 1000 cases later. Ann Surg 1988, 208–435.
19. Taylor LM, Edwards JM, Porter JM. Present status of reversed vein bypass grafting: five-year results of a modern series. J Vasc Surg 1990; 11:193.
20. Szilagyi DE, Elliott JB, et al. Biologic fate of autogenous vein implants as arterial substitutes. Ann Surg 1973; 178:775–784.
21. Atkinson JB, Forman MB, et al. Morphologic changes in long-term saphenous vein bypass grafts. Chest 1985; 88:341–348.
22. DeWeise JA, Rob CG. Autogenous venous grafts ten years later. Surgery 1978; 82:775–784.
23. Rutherford RB, Jones DN, Bergentz SE, et al. Factors affecting the patency of infrainguinal bypass. J Vasc Surg 1988; 8:236.
24. Wengerter KR, Veith FJ, Gupta SK, et al. Influence of vein size (diameter) on infrapopliteal reversed vein graft patency. J Vasc Surg 1990; 11:525.
25. Cutler BS, Thompson JE, Kleinsasser JG, et al. Autogenous saphenous vein femoropopliteal bypass: analysis of 298 cases. Surgery 1976; 79:325.
26. Bernhard VM, Boren CH, Towne JB. Pneumatic tourniquet as a substitute for vascular clamps in distal bypass surgery. Surgery 1980; 87:709.
27. Bandyk DF. Postoperative surveillance of infrainguinal bypass. Surg Clin North Am 1990; 70:71.
28. Schmitt DD, Seabrook GR, Bandyk DF, et al. Early patency of in situ saphenous vein bypasses as determined by intraoperative velocity waveform analysis. Ann Vasc Surg 1990; 4:270.
29. Bandyk DF, Kaebnick HW, Bergamini TM, et al. Hemodynamics of in situ saphenous vein arterial bypass. Arch Surg 1988; 123:477.
30. Greenspan B, Pillari G, Schulman ML, et al. Percutaneous transluminal angioplasty of stenotic, deep vein arterial bypass grafts. Arch Surg 1985; 120:492.
31. Sheridan J, Thompson J, Gazzard S, et al. The role of transluminal angioplasty in the management of femoro-distal graft stenosis. Br J Radiol Suppl 1989; 62:564.

19

An Approach to Treatment of Infrainguinal Graft Occlusions

Lloyd M. Taylor, Jr., Gregory J. Landry, and Gregory L. Moneta

Oregon Health & Science University, Portland, Oregon, U.S.A.

Management of patients with infrainguinal bypass graft occlusions is an inevitable part of all vascular surgery practices. Included within this category are a wide-ranging group of clinical scenarios. Graft occlusions may occur in the immediate postoperative period or years later. The occlusion may result in acute, severe limb-threatening ischemia, or be completely asymptomatic and discovered by accident at the time of examinations for other causes. Despite their fabled objectivity, most surgeons have considerable emotional/ego involvement in their work—their natural response to graft occlusions is nearly always to try to restore patency to the existing system by the most efficient method possible. In the opinion of the authors, this is rarely if ever the correct response.

This chapter describes the approach to graft occlusions followed by the vascular surgery service at Oregon Health & Sciences University. Due to the referral nature of this practice, we have treated more than 20 cases of infrainguinal graft occlusions per year for the past 17 years. This large clinical volume combined with the experience of others reported in the literature has allowed the development of an approach to graft occlusions that, in the opinion of the authors, results in maximal patient survival, limb salvage, and long-term graft patency. The following discussion is divided into (a) treatment of acute postoperative occlusions and (b) treatment of those that occur after the immediate postoperative period, because the management of these two clinical scenarios differs somewhat. Before discussing the treatment of graft occlusions, a few remarks regarding prevention are in order.

I. PREVENTION OF POSTOPERATIVE GRAFT OCCLUSION

A. The Decision to Operate

A very large percentage of the patients presenting to our service for treatment of infrainguinal bypass graft occlusions were originally operated on for claudication. For fortunate patients, bypass graft occlusion results in a return to the original symptomatic state, but this is not always the case. A disturbingly large number of patients with graft occlusions develop more severe ischemia than was present at the time of the original operation. Thus patients who had a very low likelihood of ever developing limb-threatening ischemia from their original disease process are suddenly placed into this category as a complication of treatment, which, in retrospect, they (and their surgeons) naturally wish they had never undertaken. This disturbing and dangerous tendency is especially true when the original bypass graft was placed using prosthetic material (1).

It is not overstating the case to say that the best way to avoid progression to limb-threatening ischemia in a patient with claudication is to not operate for the claudication, especially using a prosthetic graft. Surgery for claudication should be approached very cautiously and only when fully informed patients clearly understand that the most significant risk to their limb is probably from the treatment and not from the disease.

B. Arteriography

It is axiomatic that successful bypass grafting requires unobstructed arterial inflow and a site of distal anastomosis to a distal vessel of the best possible quality with the best possible unobstructed outflow bed. The sites of proximal and distal anastomosis are best chosen using high-quality arteriography. In our practice, more than half of the patients referred for bypass grafting with previously obtained arteriograms undergo repeat arteriography prior to surgery so as to better delineate anastomotic sites. Intraoperative "exploration" is unreliable for choosing anastomotic sites. Widely patent vessels that are perfectly suitable for anastomosis may be deceptively calcified and needlessly rejected; pliable, apparently suitable arteries may be severely diseased intraluminally.

C. Conduit

The most effective means of preventing postoperative bypass graft occlusion is to construct the bypass conduit from autogenous vein. Intact, good-quality greater saphenous vein is the best available conduit, but lesser saphenous, arm, and deep leg veins are all satisfactory and are all superior to prosthetic grafts, even when multiple segments must be anastomosed together to form conduits of adequate length. Two techniques are of great assistance in maximizing the number of grafts that can be placed using autogenous vein. The first is the use of duplex scan vein mapping to identify which autogenous veins are the most likely adequate conduits. The second is using multiple operative teams to facilitate the multiple steps required in complex "redo" bypass surgery. A single operative team of surgeon and an assistant (faculty attending and resident in our practice) can nearly always complete a first-time tibial bypass using intact ipsilateral greater saphenous vein within 3–4 h. Make the operation a redo, with a need to harvest three segments of vein from both arms to create a conduit of adequate length, and the time required may exceed twice that—really not an acceptable length operation for an elderly patient with multisystem comorbidities. In this dilemma lies the origin of many a prosthetic graft. On the other hand, two or three operating teams working simultaneously can easily complete such complex operations within the same time required for first-time surgery. In our opinion, the advantages of using autogenous conduit are sufficiently great that surgeons who are unable to muster the necessary manpower for multiple operating teams should seriously consider referring complex redo cases to medical center services that can.

D. Confirmation of Technical Success

Adequacy of inflow, conduit, proximal and distal anastomoses, and outflow vessels should be confirmed by objective means prior to closing wounds and/or leaving the operating room. At a minimum, improved ankle continuous-wave Doppler signals that respond appropriately to temporary graft occlusion and release should be confirmed. Intraoperative duplex scanning or operative completion arteriography are more cumbersome but provide more detailed and anatomical information. Abnormalities should be explained and corrected before leaving the operating room.

E. Pharmacological Management

All patients with atherosclerotic disease should be on regular aspirin therapy or its equivalent. This should be continued perioperatively. The authors add perioperative heparin anticoagulation and postoperative warfarin for patients with documented hypercoagulable disorders. The most common of these is the presence of anticardiolipin antibodies, which may be found in as many as one-third of patients requiring redo bypass surgery (2). Perioperative heparin therapy results in an increased incidence of postoperative wound hematomas requiring reoperation for drainage. This is a reasonable exchange for improved graft patency.

F. Postoperative Graft Surveillance

Stenotic lesions develop in 20–30% of autogenous vein grafts, the majority within the first postoperative year (3). These lesions can be reliably detected by duplex scanning. If uncorrected, at least 50% of such stenoses will result in graft occlusion within 12 months of their detection (4). Vein grafts in which stenoses are detected and corrected have excellent long-term patency (5). The authors obtain duplex scans of autogenous vein grafts every 3 months for the first postoperative year and every 6 months thereafter. The majority of detected lesions are repaired surgically; a few with especially favorable characteristics can be treated by balloon angioplasty. Duplex scanning has not been shown to be useful in preventing stenoses of prosthetic infrainguinal grafts.

G. Other Factors

A recent review from our service identified continued cigarette smoking and poor compliance with postoperative graft surveillance as the most important modifiable risk factors associated with graft occlusion (6). The message seems clear. Patients need support and counseling, especially about the importance of smoking cessation, and this must be repeated and reinforced at every visit. The importance of the graft surveillance studies must be emphasized clearly. Patients who fail to keep appointments should be contacted; the risk incurred by missing surveillance examinations must be explained.

II. TREATMENT OF ACUTE POSTOPERATIVE GRAFT OCCLUSIONS

For the purpose of this chapter, acute postoperative graft occlusions are those that occur prior to the patient's discharge from the hospital during which the bypass procedure was performed. During this interval, occlusions are usually detected promptly and can be treated immediately with a reasonable expectation that patency can be restored and that long-term patency will be acceptable, which is almost never true once the patient has been discharged.

A. Initial Management

Acute postoperative graft occlusions result in the return of ankle brachial pressure indices (ABI) to preoperative levels or below and recurrence of preoperative ischemic symptoms. If the indication for the bypass was claudication, there may be no symptoms in a bed-confined hospital patient. Any decrease in ABI from immediate postoperative values must be explained. In some patients, emergency duplex scanning or arteriography may be necessary to determine whether grafts are occluded or patent, with another explanation (proximal stenosis, graft stenosis, runoff occlusion, etc.) for the reduced ABI. Once diagnosed, the most appropriate response to immediate postoperative graft occlusions is full heparinization followed by an immediate return to the operating room. Of course there may be compelling reasons not to follow this course. Patients' conditions may change markedly postoperatively. Myocardial infarction, pneumonia, or other acute conditions may preclude early reoperation, and other conditions—such as gastrointestinal bleeding—may preclude anticoagulation. If immediate reoperation is contraindicated, it is extremely unlikely that the original bypass conduit can be salvaged. This may be a reasonable and appropriate price for delay when dictated by patient condition.

B. Conduct of the Operation

In addition to the operated extremity, the surgical field should include a source of additional vein conduit sufficient to replace or to extend the original graft. The patient should be placed on an operating table that will accommodate fluoroscopy of the extremity's entire arterial tree, from the aortic bifurcation to the toes. Full heparin anticoagulation should be maintained until the cause of the graft occlusion has been determined and corrected. It is helpful to monitor the dose of heparin using the activated clotting time (ACT).

The first step is to open the incisions over the proximal and distal anastomoses and determine the cause of the occlusion. A normal pulse in the inflow artery/proximal graft rules out inflow obstruction as the cause. Liquid blood in the hood of the distal anastomosis similarly rules out distal obstruction. Hard thrombus in either location points to a cause at the site where it is found. In the absence of a problem with the proximal or distal arteries/anastomoses, a problem with the vein graft must be assumed.

Catheter thrombectomy is difficult in the immediate postoperative period. The venous valves, whether lysed for in situ grafts or reversed, trap adjacent thrombus, which is highly resistant to removal by balloon catheter and can serve as the nidus for further thrombosis. The authors prefer to open and/or detach the distal vein graft anastomosis. If the occlusion is very fresh, the thrombus is often ejected from the graft simply by the incoming arterial pressure. Intraoperative arteriography can then be performed to locate the site of the obstruction that produced the occlusion. If the graft remains obstructed after the distal anastomosis is detached, it is best to extract it from the tunnel and express the remaining thrombus by gentle digital pressure. The graft can then be inspected for sclerotic/stenotic segments. If none are discovered and this is confirmed by intraoperative arteriography, extrinsic compression in the tunnel can be assumed to be the cause of the occlusion. Retunneling and reanastomosis of the distal end of the graft will solve the problem.

Sclerotic/stenotic segments of vein must be excised and replaced. Unsuspected or undetected proximal or distal occlusive disease must be repaired or bypassed by graft extension. Technically unsatisfactory anastomoses should never be the cause of graft occlusion; they should have been detected by the measures used to ensure technical success at the time of the first operation.

Regardless of the cause of the graft occlusion and the method chosen for its correction, operative completion arteriography should conclude operations performed to correct acute graft occlusions. Once the final reconstruction has been proven to be technically perfect, the authors prefer to continue heparin anticoagulation for several days postoperatively to prevent early rethrombosis due to the highly thrombogenic inner surface of the graft from which thrombus has been removed. An increased incidence of wound hematomas requiring drainage is an inescapable result of this approach.

C. Rethrombosis

Bypass grafts that reocclude after the operative steps described above have been taken will not remain patent after another operation in which the thrombus is reremoved (1). If a different operation (different anastomotic sites, new conduit) is possible, it is acceptable to proceed with this taking the patient's condition into account. If not, there is little to be gained from repeated and increasingly futile attempts to make a flawed system work.

III. TREATMENT OF LATE GRAFT OCCLUSIONS

Four courses of action are possible in response to graft occlusions that occur following hospital discharge. These include no treatment, percutaneous endovascular treatment (lytic therapy with correction of stenoses by angioplasty and/or stenting), operative graft thrombectomy with correction of stenoses, and reoperation with a new graft. The factors that govern decision making among these options include the severity of ischemia that exists following graft occlusion, the patient's need for a patent graft, and the likelihood that the planned intervention will remain patent. Three easily quantitated objective factors are relevant to the long term outcome of graft occlusion treatment. These are patient survival, limb salvage, and graft patency. Other factors are also very important, but some are subjective and inherently difficult to quantitate and some are important only transiently. These include patient inconvenience, pain, physical impairment, and long-term functional status.

A. Severity of Ischemia

Bypass grafts performed for mild to moderate claudication may become occluded and not produce any symptoms in sedentary patients, particularly if years have passed and the patient's activity level, for which the surgery was originally performed, has declined. Most grafts performed for severe claudication and/or limb-threatening ischemia produce clear-cut ischemic symptoms when occlusion occurs. Initially the degree of ischemia that is present may be severe, with no detectable circulation and neuromuscular impairment in the distal extremity. These prominent symptoms may lead to a mistaken impression that the limb is acutely threatened and that a true emergency exists, in which case revascularization would have to be accomplished within a few hours to avoid amputation. Experienced vascular surgeons recognize that this is rarely the case, as first demonstrated by Blaisdell (7). For most patients with acute graft occlusions, the initial severe symptoms improve rapidly and adequate neuromuscular function returns, allowing for a deliberate, elective approach to treatment. The authors treat acute bypass graft occlusions with hospitalization, bed rest, and anticoagulation with intravenous unfractionated heparin. Only when ischemic symptoms fail to respond to these measures is urgent or emergent revascularization considered. Thankfully such patients are rare.

B. No Treatment

When the initial indication for bypass grafting was claudication, no treatment is frequently an option for the management of graft occlusion. Patients may not wish to have further invasive treatment for claudication symptoms that have lessened in importance since the time of the bypass. No treatment is a particularly attractive option if the initial operation was performed using prosthetic conduit and sources of autogenous vein are limited. Some patients with diabetes may have required bypass grafting for relatively mild occlusive disease in order to assist with the healing of neuropathic/infectious ulcers. Once the ulcers have healed, graft occlusion may be well tolerated. Obviously, decisions for no treatment must be individualized. It is reasonable to assume that the ischemic symptoms existing at the time of graft occlusion are the most severe that will occur. Some spontaneous improvement can be anticipated in nearly all patients. It is reasonable to observe patients for this improvement and to postpone the decision about repeat revascularization if the absolute need for revascularization is not initially clear.

C. Percutaneous Treatment

Infusion of thrombolytic agents into thrombosed bypass grafts frequently results in restoration of patency and resolution of ischemic symptoms. This fact is extraordinarily seductive. The bypass graft is thrombosed, and the leg is ischemic; lytic therapy is applied, the graft is patent, and the leg is no longer ischemic. Patients are much relieved, emergency surgery is avoided, and—perhaps most seductive—the surgeon's ego is assuaged. What was lost has been regained and the graft is once again patent. Add to this the potential to reveal by lysis the stenosis that led to the thrombosis and to correct this by percutaneous means—for example angioplasty and stenting—and there is a possibility that this clinical catastrophe can be efficiently and effectively managed by a single trip to the interventional suite, with hospitalization required at most overnight if at all.

Since thrombolytic treatment for thrombosed infrainguinal grafts was first described in 1981, a mass of evidence has accumulated that this ideal scenario rarely if ever occurs. There have been many advances in thrombolytic therapy: better drugs, improved technology, more rational dosing, etc. Each has resulted in increases in the percentage of patients in whom lysis can be accomplished and in the speed and safety with which it can be done. Despite these advances, lytic therapy remains dangerous. No large series is free of occasional deaths from intracerebral hemorrhage, and less lethal bleeding complications remain common. The main problem with the lytic approach to graft occlusion, however, has to do with disappointing long-term patency. Multiple series accumulated over the past two decades, examples of which are summarized in Table 1, indicate that fewer than half of the grafts to which patency has been restored by lysis remain patent for as long as 1 year, with or without adjunctive correction of underlying stenoses. A single prospective randomized clinical trial (the STILE study) compared lytic therapy to best surgery for infrainguinal graft occlusion. This study was stopped because of superiority of the surgical group, even though many operations were thrombectomies, or far from ideal surgery (8).

Proponents of lytic therapy acknowledge this flaw but point out that at least lysis relieves the acute ischemia, so that more definitive elective treatments can be carried out in

Table 1 Results of Lytic Therapy for Infrainguinal Bypass Graft Occlusion

Author and year (ref)	n	Initial success (%)	Mortality	Long-term patency[a]
Graor, 1985 (13)	24	15 (62%)	0	not given
Graor, 1988 (14)	33	29 (88%)	0	20%
Gardiner, 1989 (15)	72	50 (69%)	1.4%	18%/75%[b]
Belkin, 1990 (16)	35	22 (60%)	0	37%
Faggioli, 1994 (17)	51	23 (45%)	1.9%	39%
Comerota, 1996 (8)	78	37 (47%)	6%[c]	27%

[a] Long-term patency = patency by life table at 1 year postthrombolysis.
[b] Patency of grafts in which stenosis was not corrected/patency in those with corrected stenosis.
[c] Mortality at 1 year postlysis.

appropriate patients. If the acute ischemia of graft occlusion were truly immediately limb-threatening, this would be an advantage indeed. But in fact this is rarely the case. Nearly all patients with graft occlusion can be managed by hospitalization, bed rest, anticoagulation, elective arteriography, and revascularization without incurring the considerable expense and risk of an initial episode of lytic therapy.

The authors reserve lytic therapy for graft occlusions that occur in patients known to have no further possibilities for reconstruction or for those with documented hypercoagulable states who have previously had graft thromboses in the absence of stenosis. In actual practice, such patients are rare.

D. Graft Thrombectomy

Effective thrombectomy of vein grafts using balloon catheters is very difficult. The reasons include the varying caliber of the vein, the fact that most autogenous graft thromboses result from fixed stenoses, and the tendency of thrombus to adhere very tightly to the inflamed intimal surface. In contrast, thrombectomy of prosthetic grafts is usually easily accomplished. Unfortunately numerous studies—examples of which are listed in Table 2—have shown that thrombectomy is rarely if ever followed by durable long-term patency. Even when the culprit stenoses are discovered and corrected at the time of thrombectomy, all studies have shown disappointing patency. Despite these facts, the temptation to restore patency to the existing system through the use of thrombectomy with revision when appropriate is strong. It is best resisted. The authors do not use thrombectomy to treat infrainguinal graft thrombosis that occurs after the immediate postoperative period. Available information indicates that patient survival, limb salvage, and long-term recon-

Table 2 Results of Thrombectomy for Infrainguinal Bypass Graft Occlusions

Author and year (ref)	n	Initial success	Mortality	Long-term patency[a]
Ascer, 1987 (18)	128	Not given	5.6%	20–40%[b]
Graor, 1988 (13)	38	42%	5%	18%
Lombardi, 2000 (19)	21	Not given	3%	47%

[a] Long-term patency = patency at 1 year.
[b] Difference in patency depending on site of distal anastomosis.

struction patency are best maximized by elective reoperation with a new autogenous vein graft.

E. Elective Reoperation with a New Autogeneous Vein Graft

Patients with infrainguinal graft thrombosis have varying degrees of ischemia, some of which is acute. The authors decide whether emergency hospitalization is needed based upon three patient factors: the presence of ischemic rest pain, absent ankle Doppler signals, and neuromuscular dysfunction. Any of these is an indication for immediate hospitalization, bed rest, and heparin anticoagulation. Patients with lesser degrees of ischemia can be scheduled for elective hospitalization.

Once hospitalized and anticoagulated, most patients find that their ischemic symptoms improve rapidly. Return of adible ankle Doppler signals within a day or two is common. During this time, patients can be carefully assessed for surgery and medically evaluated and stabilized. Duplex scan vein mapping can be performed to accurately delineate available sources of autogenous conduit.

The authors prefer to delay arteriography for an interval of at least 2–3 days from the time of the acute graft occlusion. This allows initial ischemic vasospasm to resolve and full collateral development. Arteriograms performed immediately after acute occlusions are frequently noninformative; those performed after an appropriate interval are much more likely to reveal satisfactory distal bypass targets.

Once the arteriogram has been obtained, it is possible to plan in detailed fashion an operation to revascularize the ischemic limb using autogenous vein. The need to use arm vein conduits arises frequently, as does the need for anastomosis of multiple venous segments to create conduits of adequate length. The common femoral artery has frequently been seriously compromised by a combination of disease and multiple previous surgeries. Common femoral excision and interposition prosthetic grafting is an excellent and durable solution for this problem (9).

These reoperative procedures are frequently extensive, involving multiple operative sites and extremities and difficult redissections of previously operated areas. This type of operation is ideally suited to a multiple operative team approach. Indeed, some of the more extensive procedures cannot be accomplished within reasonable time limits without multiple operating teams.

Table 3 Results of Treatment of Infrainguinal Graft Occlusions with Reoperation with New Autogenous Vein Grafting

Author and Year (ref)	n	Initial Success	Mortality	Long-Term Patency[a]
Brewster, 1983 (11)	19	NA[b]	NA	63%[c]
Ascer, 1987 (18)	27	100%	NA	39–48%[d]
Edwards, 1990 (20)	103	98%	NA	62%/71%[e]
DeFrang, 1994 (10)	85	100%	3.5%	80%
Biancari, 2000 (21)	30	100%	6%	44%

[a] Long term patency = patency at 3 years.
[b] NA = not available.
[c] Five-year patency.
[d] Two-thirds of patients had prosthetic grafts.
[e] Primary/secondary patency at 3 years.

As seen from the examples listed in Table 3, the results achieved in this difficult patient population compare very favorably in terms of morbidity, mortality, and patency with those reported for thrombolysis and/or thrombectomy (Tables 1 and 2). This is true even in patients presenting after failure of more than two previous attempts at bypass grafting. DeFrang and coauthors were able to achieve 80% primary patency and 70% limb salvage at 3 years using repeat autogenous vein grafting in this highly selected patient group (10).

Other vascular surgery units with extensive experience in the management of occluded infrainguinal graft have reached the same conclusion regarding optimal management. Veith and coworkers from Montefiore in New York (11) and Brewster and colleagues from Boston (12) have also found that reoperation with a new autogenous vein graft is the treatment with the best outcome.

IV. CONCLUSIONS

Based upon the data summarized in Tables 1, 2, and 3 and a considerable personal practice experience, the authors have developed an approach to lower extremity graft occlusion that first emphasizes prevention. Indications for surgery should be conservative. The vast majority of claudicants are best managed nonoperatively. Surgery requires careful planning. Detailed arteriography is necessary. Autogenous vein is always the best conduit. The technical result of surgery should be objectively confirmed in the operating room. Postoperative duplex surveillance with correction of detected lesions maximizes patency.

Immediate postoperative occlusions are best managed by immediate reoperation, with a systematic approach to the detection of the underlying cause and its correction. Intraoperative imaging is essential for these procedures.

Despite the temptation to restore the patency to bypass grafts that occlude after the immediate postoperative period, the long-term patency results achieved do not justify this approach to the treatment of occlusions. The great majority of such patients are best managed by hospitalization and heparin anticoagulation, followed by elective arteriography and elective reoperation using a new autogenous vein bypass.

REFERENCES

1. Robinson KD, Sato DT, Gregory RT, Gayle RG, DeMasi RJ, Parent FN III, Wheeler JR. Long-term outcome after early infrainguinal graft failure. J Vasc Surg 1997; 26:425–438.
2. Taylor LM Jr, Chitwood RW, Dalman RL, Sexton G, Goodnight SH, Porter JM. Antiphospholipid antibodies in vascular surgery patients: a cross-sectional Study. Ann Surg 1994; 220:544–551.
3. Passman MA, Moneta GL, Nehler MR, Taylor LM Jr, Edwards JM, Yeager RA, McConnell DB, Porter JM. Do normal early color flow duplex surveillance examinations of infrainguinal vein grafts preclude the need for late graft revision? J Vasc Surg 1995; 22:476–484.
4. Mattos MA, Van Bemmelen PS, Hodgson KJ, Ramsey DE, Barkmeier LD, Sumner DS. Does correction of stenoses identified with color duplex scanning improve infrainguinal graft patency? J Vasc Surg 1993; 17:54–66.
5. Nehler MR, Moneta GL, Yeager RA, Edwards JM, Taylor LM Jr, Porter JM. Results of surgical revision of threatened reversed infrainguinal vein grafts. J Vasc Surg 1994; 20:558–565.
6. Giswold MA, Moneta GL, Landry GL, Yeager RA, Edwards JM, Taylor LM Jr. Modifiable risk factors associated with infrainguinal vein graft occlusion. J Vasc Surg 2003; 37:47–53.
7. Blaisdell FW, Steele M, Allen R. Management of acute lower extremity arterial ischemia due to embolism and thrombosis. Surgery 1978; 84:822–834.

8. Comerota AJ, Weaver FA, Hosking JD, Froehlich J, Folander H, Sussman B, Rosenfield K. Results of a prospective randomized trial of surgery versus thrombolysis for occluded lower extremity bypass grafts. Am J Surg 1996; 172:105–112.

9. Nehler MR, Taylor LM Jr, Lee RW, Moneta GL, Porter JM. Interposition grafting for reoperation on the common femoral artery. J Vasc Surg 1998; 28:37–44.

10. DeFrang RD, Edward JM, Moneta GL, Yeager RA, Taylor LM Jr, Porter JM. Repeat leg bypass following multiple prior bypass failures. J Vasc Surg 1994; 19:258–278.

11. Veith FJ, Ascer E, Gupta SK, et al. Management of the occluded and failing PTFE graft. Acta Chir Scand 1987; 538:117–124.

12. Brewster DC, LaSalle AJ, Robinson JG, et al. Femoropopliteal graft failures: Clinical consequences and success of secondary procedures. Arch Surg 1983; 118:1043–1047.

13. Graor RA, Risius B, Denny KM, Young JR, Beven EG, Hertzer NR, Ruschhaupt WF III, O'Hara PJ, Geisinger MA, Zelch MG. Local thrombolysis in the treatment of thrombosed arteries, bypass grafts, and arteriovenous fistulas. J Vasc Surg 1985; 2:406–414.

14. Graor RA, Risuis G, Young JR, Lucas FV, Beven EG, Hertzer NR, Krajewski LP, O'Hara PJ, Olin J, Ruschhaupt WE. Thrombolysis of peripheral arterial bypass grafts: Surgical thrombectomy compared with thrombolysis. J Vasc Surg 1988; 7:347–355.

15. Gardiner GA, Harrington DP, Koltun W, Whittemore A, Mannick JA, Levin DC. Salvage of occluded arterial bypass grafts by means of thrombolysis. J Vasc Surg 1989; 9:426–431.

16. Belkin M, Donaldson MC, Whittemore AD, Polak JF, Grassi CJ, Harrington DP, Mannick JA. Observations on the use of thrombolytic agents for thrombotic occlusion of infrainguinal vein grafts. J Vasc Surg 1990; 11:289–296.

17. Faggioli GL, Peer RM, Pedrini L, Di Paola MD, Upson JA, D'Addato M, Ricotta JJ. Failure of thrombolytic therapy to improve long-term vascular patency. J Vasc Surg 1994; 19:289–297.

18. Ascer E, Collier P, Gupta SK, Veith FJ. Reoperation for polytetrafluoroethylene bypass failure: The importance of distal outflow site and operative technique in determining outcome. J Vasc Surg 1987; 5:298–310.

19. Lombardi JV, Dougherty MJ, Calligaro KD, Compbell FJ, Schindler N, Raviola C. Predictors of outcome when reoperating for early infrainguinal bypass occlusion. Ann Vasc Surg 2000; 14:350–355.

20. Edwards JM, Taylor LM Jr, Porter JM. Treatment of failed lower extremity bypass grafts with new autogenous vein grafting. J Vasc Surg 1990; 11:132–145.

21. Biancari F, Railo M, Lundin J, Alback A, Kantonen I, Lehtola A, Lepantalo M. Redo bypass surgery to the infrapopliteal arteries for critical leg ischaemia. Eur J Vasc Endovasc Surg 2000; 21:137–142.

20

Wound Complications Following Vascular Reconstructive Surgery

David R. Lorelli

St. John Hospital and Medical Center, Detroit, Michigan, U.S.A.

Jonathan B. Towne

Medical College of Wisconsin, Milwaukee, Wisconsin, U.S.A.

I. INTRODUCTION

Wound healing problems are the most frustrating and dangerous possible complications associated with vascular reconstructive surgery. Wound healing complications are related to age, advanced atherosclerotic disease, tissue ischemia, lengthy incisions, and the multiple comorbid medical conditions that routinely exist in the vascular patient population. However, the significance of wound complications in patients undergoing vascular reconstruction has received only minor emphasis in the literature. Fortunately, most wound complications are superficial and are not limb-nor graft-threatening, causing only inconvenience and additional expense to the patient. In the most severe cases, wound have the potential to involve the underlying graft, either prosthetic or autogenous, which may often lead to hemorrhage or graft occlusion with resultant loss of life or limb. This chapter reviews the classification, incidence, and etiological factors responsible for wound complications in different anatomical locations as well as methods of prevention and treatment, including alternative operative techniques, that may have a favorable impact upon the frequency of wound complications following vascular reconstructive surgery.

II. CLASSIFICATION SCHEMES

Two classification schemes for wound complications have been proposed over the past 30 years. The original clinical classification of infection was put forth by Szilagyi and associates (1) in a review of over 3300 arterial reconstructions over a 20-year period. Wounds were classified into three grades in accordance with the depth of involvement.

Grade I infections involved the dermis only. Infections extending into the subcutaneous region without graft involvement were classified as grade II. The most serious infections, or grade III, involved the arterial graft itself. This classification scheme had significant practical implications as the management strategies were more complex and the risk of limb or life loss significant with grade III infections.

A second scheme to classify wound complications following infrainguinal arterial bypass grafting was proposed by Johnson et al. (2) in 1988. They further divided Szilagyi grade II wound complications into two groups based on the presence or absence of culture-proven wound infection. Erythema or seroma formation without wound edge separation encompassed class 1 wounds. Class 2 wounds were those with ischemic necrosis of the wound edge without infection. Class 3 wounds included ischemic necrosis of the wound edge with overt infection. Open, infected wounds with exposed graft comprised class 4 wounds.

Wound complications following vascular reconstruction and following saphenous vein harvest for coronary artery bypass account for the vast majority of wound problems faced by the vascular surgeon. Wound healing is a complex process. Many factors contribute to this process and any alteration in one or more of these factors can influence the success of primary wound healing.

III. ETIOLOGICAL FACTORS

A. Preoperative Factors

Wound healing is a complex sequence of events with a multitude of factors, which may influence its ultimate outcome. Optimization of the preoperative factors affecting wound healing provides the best foundation for a successful outcome. Probably no other condition has been investigated as much as diabetes in its relation to wound healing. Poorly controlled diabetics may have defects in leukocyte chemotaxis and phagocytosis, which reduces the ability to heal wounds and fight infection (3). This defect can be improved with appropriate insulin therapy that maintains blood glucose at normal levels (4). Despite some conflicting data, numerous studies have demonstrated diabetes to be a risk factor for wound complications (5–11). Careful control of blood glucose may help to lessen the impact of diabetes on wound healing.

Patients with chronic renal insufficiency or end-stage renal disease are at high risk for wound healing difficulties (12,13). This is likely due to a significant association with uremia, diabetes, anemia, malnutrition, and altered immune function, resulting in rates of perioperative wound complications are as high as 29–54% (14–16). In patients with end-stage renal disease undergoing infrainguinal arterial bypass, the amputation rate—despite a functioning graft—due to wound complications or progressive necrosis is 14% (13). Because of concern about this devastating problem, some have advocated anatomical tunneling of all infrainguinal grafts in renal patients with the avoidance of an in situ bypass (12).

Treatment with anti-inflammatory steroids or other immunosuppressive agents can hinder wound healing. This is likely mediated through a reduction in transforming growth factor beta (TGF-β), which can be countered by administration of vitamin A (17). Anemia may also play an important role. Taylor et al. studied the effects on wound healing in rats with compensated oligemia. They found that the effect of anemia on wound healing is more pronounced in skin than in muscle tissue and that this is due to a specific increase in collagen turnover, with the increase in reabsorption exceeding that in synthesis (18). In addition, malnutrition correlates with an increased incidence of wound complications. In a study of 79 patients undergoing a variety of vascular surgical operations, Casey et al. correlated the immune and nutritional status of patients with the development of significant wound complications (11). A comprehensive nutritional assessment—including anthropometric measurements, serological testing, neutrophil functional analysis, and cutaneous assessment of delayed hypersensitivity—was performed on all patients. Those patients with albumin levels less than 3 g/dL or those with serum transferrin levels below 150 mg/dL had significantly more wound complications than the rest of the cohort. It is certainly advisable for any elective procedure to optimize a patient's nutritional status in order to reduce operative morbidity and mortality. To evaluate the multiple factors that predisposed to wound infections in our series, we evaluated 126 consecutive patients who underwent in situ bypass, and found that early graft revision (<4 days) and the presence of a lymph leak significantly increased the risk for post-operative wound infection (19). However, factors such as age, race, diabetes, duration of operation, and presence of gangrene or ulceration did not significantly influence the incidence of infectious complications in that series. Wengrovitz and coworkers retrospectively studied 163 subcutaneous saphenous vein bypasses and found on regression analysis that chronic steroid use, ipsilateral ulceration, and pedal bypasses predicted an increased incidence of wound infection (6). They also identified female gender, diabetes, use of continuous incisions, and procedures for limb salvage as factors associated with wound complications in their group of patients.

The natural history of graft infection depends partly on the timing of presentation, which has a widely variable interval between implantation and recognition of the infection. Multiple studies have indicated that wound and graft infections tend to occur early. In Lorentzen's study, 85% of graft infections occurred in the first 30 days (20). Likewise, Liekweg et al. reported that 85% of groin wound infections in their series presented within 5 weeks of the initial operation (21). However, graft infection may not become clinically evident for months to years after placement. Early graft infections are usually easily identified due to associated wound complications and signs of systemic inflammation. Graft infections that are present in a delayed fashion, on the other hand, usually do not present with signs of sepsis and are associated with more nonspecific symptoms.

Morbidity and mortality associated with graft infection depends not only on the timing of presentation but also on microbiology, graft location, and method of treatment. Unrecognized or inadequately treated infrainguinal graft infection has a mortality rate ranging from 0 to 22% and results in amputation in between 8 and 53% of cases, with one series reporting an amputation rate of 79% (1,22,23).

B. Intraoperative Management

The conduct of the operation itself has a significant impact on primary wound healing and the incidence of wound complications. Meticulous sterile technique begins at the scrub sink and does not end until the dressings are applied. During this variable length of time, the surgeon must not only concentrate on the procedure at hand but also be ever vigilant toward issues that may ultimately influence the balance of wound healing. There is no doubt that the stakes are high when it comes to managing the risk of infection in vascular surgery, especially with the use of prosthetic material. As an adjunct to meticulous surgical technique, the administration of prophylactic antibiotics has helped to limit the incidence of wound infections. Multiple retrospective studies have demonstrated this efficacy. In addition, two prospective, randomized, and blinded studies have also shown that the use of cephalosporins results in a highly significant decrease in infection rates compared to placebo (24,25). Another intraoperative concern is maintaining normothermia. All anesthetics tend to cause hypothermia by decreasing heat production and causing vaso-dilatation (26). Evidence suggests that intraoperative normothermia may decrease wound infection rates by as much as two-thirds (27). High ambient room temperature and forced-air warming seem to be the two most efficacious methods for maintaining normal body temperature (28).

Avoiding the creation of skin flaps is paramount to avoid eventual ischemia of the undermined skin (5,29). This is especially important in harvesting the saphenous vein in the thigh because of its unpredictable and deep location (30). Routine preoperative vein map-ping to evaluate the quality of vein and determine its exact location helps to avoid large dissection flaps (25). Intraoperative ultrasound can also aid in determining saphenous vein location. Lack of adequate hemostasis can also lead to considerable problems, especially if large potential dead spaces are created due to poorly placed saphenectomy incisions. If any question remains in regards to adequate hemostasis following saphenectomy for cor-onary artery bypass, the wound should be closed only after heparin reversal. The type of conduit used for lower extremity bypasses can influence the incidence of postoperative wound problems. Prospective, randomized data have shown autogenous vein to be su-perior to prosthetic grafts when considering long-term patency for infrapopliteal bypasses (31). Additionally, the use of autologous tissue may reduce the potential for graft in-fection. Johnson et al. (2) noted a statistically significant difference in the incidence of wound complications when comparing PTFE bypasses (43%) to autogenous vein (27%) grafts. Lorentzen et al. reviewed over 2400 arterial synthetic reconstructions over a 4-year period with an incidence of graft infection of 2.6%. However, local wound complications such as infection, necrosis, and hematoma were predisposing factors in half of these cases (20).

There is no incision longer than that required for saphenous vein harvesting, and studies have demonstrated that a reduced morbidity can be achieved with the use of in-terrupted incisions rather than a continuous incision. Schwartz et al. analyzed 93 patients for wound complications after in situ bypass with an overall incidence of 33%. However, only 20.5% of patients with interrupted incisions developed wound problems compared to 42.5% of patients with a continuous incision. This proved to be a significant difference (32). Likewise, a review of 163 autogenous bypass grafts by Wengrovitz et al. revealed a wound complication incidence of 27.7% for a continuous incision versus 9.6% for in-terrupted incisions with an overall incidence of 17% (6). Prospective, randomized, multi-center data comparing reversed and in situ grafts revealed no difference in the incidence of wound complications in 125 patients (33).

No general consensus exists in regards to the best method of skin closure. Often the choice is guided by surgeon preference. The only prospective, randomized data are from Angelini et al., in which they compared the outcome of saphenectomy incisions in 113 patients undergoing coronary artery bypass grafting (34). Four different skin closure techniques were used, including continuous nylon vertical mattress suture, continuous subcuticular absorbable suture, skin staples, and adhesive sutureless skin closure. Two independent observers evaluated all wounds at 5, 10, and 45 days after operation. The incidence of established wound infection was 4.5% overall; however, no patient developed an infection in wounds closed with a continuous subcuticular absorbable suture. In addi-tion, this method of skin closure produced the best cosmetic results and therefore should be the method of choice for closure of saphenectomy wounds.

C. Postoperative Care

Routine postoperative principals of wound care certainly apply to vascular patients. Sterile operative dressings should be left untouched for at least 48 h to allow for wound epithelialization. Any part of a wound that drains serous fluid should continue to be cleansed daily and dressed with sterile technique. Some would also advocate prophylactic antibiotic coverage in addition. All groin wounds, especially those in obese patients, should continue to have wound dressings to avoid direct skin-to-skin contact from a large pannus. Another aspect unique to vascular surgery is managing lower limb edema following distal arterial bypass grafting. This is a common problem occurring in 40–100% of patients after bypass (35,36). Up to a 40% increase in leg volume has been shown to occur in the subcutaneous tissue via computed tomography (CT) and magnetic resonance imaging (MRI) (37). The control of this dependent edema is important in minimizing wound complications following distal bypass (10). The etiology of this edema is incompletely understood but is likely due to a multitude of factors, which may contribute to edema formation to varying degrees in different patients. These include deep venous thrombosis, lymphatic disruption, increased capillary filtration, and the generation of oxygen-derived free radicals during reperfusion (37). While the use of antioxidants and lymphatic-sparing incisions has been advocated, the best results are achieved with leg elevation and compressive stockings to reduce postoperative leg edema (37).

IV. IMPACT

Wound complications have a significant impact on the overall outcome of patients undergoing lower extremity bypass surgery. A recent review of 112 consecutive infrainguinal bypass grafts by Nicoloff et al. from Portland was performed to determine how often an ideal result is actually achieved with bypass surgery for limb salvage (38). An ideal result was defined as an uncomplicated operation, elimination of ischemia, prompt wound healing, and rapid return to premorbid functional status without recurrence or repeat surgery for wound complications or to maintain graft patency. While clinically important palliation was frequently achieved (5-year graft patency and limb salvage of 77 and 87%), ideal results occurred in only 14% of patients. Wound complications occurred in 24% of patients, with operative and ischemic wounds requiring a mean of 4.2 months to heal. This—along with other operative complications, graft patency, limb salvage, survival, functional status, recurrent ischemia, and the need for repeat operations—contributed significantly to the low number of ideal results in this study. Additionally, the data underscore the point that all patients undergoing infrainguinal bypass require ongoing surveillance and treatment to achieve optimal results. Indeed, another study, which was a prospective evaluation of 119 patients with 156 infrainguinal incisions, revealed that distal wound complications incurred additional expense related to reoperation, extended hospitalization or rehospitalization, and rehabilitation or visiting nurse services (39).

V. ANATOMICAL CONSIDERATIONS AND INCIDENCE

A. Cervical Incisions

Differing anatomical areas in vascular reconstructive surgery carry very different concerns and implications for wound complications. Cervical incisions for carotid endarterectomy rarely develop problems with wound healing. This is likely due to an exceptional blood supply in this area and the clean nature of the case. Thompson et al. noted an incidence of wound infection of 0.09% in 1140 carotid endarterectomies (40). Infected wounds should be incised and drained, along with consideration given to replacing any prosthetic patch with an autogenous vein if the vascular reconstruction is involved in the infection.

B. Abdominal Approach

There is much debate as well as conflicting data about the best method with which to approach abdominal aortoiliac procedures (41–43). Those favoring the retroperitoneal approach claim this to be a more physiological route and thus preferable to the more widely applied midline approach (41–43). However, the only prospective, randomized study, by Cambria et al., enrolled 59 transperitoneal and 54 retroperitoneal approaches to elective aortic reconstructions (44). A multitude of parameters were evaluated, including incidence of wound complications, cross-clamp times, crystalloid and transfusion requirements, respiratory morbidity, return of gastrointestinal function, and duration of hospital stay. They were unable to demonstrate an advantage for the retroperitoneal approach in regard to any of these factors; thus it should not be adopted as a preferred technique for routine aortic reconstruction.

C. Groin Incisions

Access to the common femoral, superficial femoral, and profunda femoris arteries is a mainstay in vascular reconstruction. These vessels often provide outflow for aortoiliac procedures and are universally used to provide inflow for lower extremity bypasses. Incisions in this area can be hazardous given its proximity to the perineum and the potential for direct contamination from both urine and stool. This part of the body tends to remain moist from lack of hygiene and contact from an overlying pannus. Studies have shown value to preoperative cleansing and the use of a povidone-iodine surgical scrub to reduce the incidence of wound infections (7,19). Patients and surgeons must be vigilant in regard to wound hygiene to avoid problems before they arise. Kent et al. noted a 10% incidence of wound complications in 77 isolated groin incisions (39).

Another unique aspect of groin wounds is the propensity for development of lymphatic complications due to the rich lymphatic network of the femoral triangle. These are uncommon but potentially serious complications of femoral reconstruction, particularly if a vascular prosthesis is involved. A review of the Henry Ford Hospital experience by Tyndall et al. identified 41 lymphatic complications (28 lymphocutaneous fistulas and 13 lymphoceles) in 2679 arterial reconstructions over a 15-year period, for an incidence of 1.2% per incision (40). Interestingly, the incidence varied with the type of procedure and whether the procedure was a reoperation. Aortobifemoral bypass for aneurysmal disease in a previously operated groin had the highest incidence (8.1%) of lymphatic complications, followed by an isolated femoral procedure in a previously operated groin (5.3%). The lowest frequency was found in patients undergoing a femoropopliteal/tibial bypass for the first time (0.5%). Aggressive treatment of lymphatic fistulas provided the best results. There were no wound or graft infections in patients treated with operation; in them, resolution of the fistula occurred 2 1/2 times sooner than in those treated conservatively. Length of hospital stay, time to resolution, and incidence of wound complications did not vary between those treated operatively or with aspiration and in those with lymphoceles treated conservatively. A similar incidence of lymphatic complications with improved outcomes with operative therapy has been shown in other studies (46).

Drainage of the leg wound, especially the groin, early in the postoperative period is often the result of divided lymphatics that have not sealed. These complications, a common problem in patients who have undergone kidney transplantation, are presumably caused by an increase in lymph drainage from placement of the donor kidney in the lower quadrant. The problems caused by a lymph leak were documented in a series of 126 consecutive patients reported by Reifsnyder et al., who underwent in situ bypasses of the lower extremity (19). Risk-factor analysis demonstrated that the development of a postoperative lymph leak was significantly related to the subsequent wound infection. Rubin et al. demonstrated, in an animal model, that lymphatics contaminated with bacteria resulted in positive blood and graft cultures (47). Experimentally, transection of lymphatics at the graft site in the presence of a distal infection leads to significantly more graft infections than does lymphatic ligation and exclusion. Lymphatic bacterial transport contributed to the graft infection both from direct seeding and from transmission of bacteria to the blood, leading to seeding of the graft.

Because of the relationship of lymph leak with subsequent significant wound infections, these patients should be treated aggressively. Our initial plan is to paint the wound with povidone-iodine (Betadine) and apply a tight compressive dressing. Antibiotics, usually cephalosporins, are given and the patient is placed on bed rest. If the wound continues to drain for greater than 72 h, the patient should be returned to the operating room and the wound explored. The offending lymphatic can often be identified and suture-ligated. A subcutaneous drain, well separated from the arterial prosthesis, is then brought out through a separate stab hole. Placement of the drain allows the skin incision to heal. This technique is generally successful in controlling the wound drainage and, more importantly, prevents secondary infection of the lymphatic cavity.

1. Lymphocele

Patients who develop lymphoceles following groin surgery are followed expectantly. If the lymphoceles increase in size with time, they should be operatively explored and treated as noted above with regard to the leaking wound. Likewise, if they communicate with the groin wound and begin to leak, they should also be explored. Small to moderate-size lymphoceles that are away from the incision and do not involve the graft can be followed. Many times these will resolve slowly over time. Lymphoceles also can be treated operatively if they become large or uncomfortable for the patient; a lymphocele that distends the groin wound should be treated operatively as well. The injection of isosulfan blue into the foot prior to the operation helps to identify the lymphatic channels that feed the lymphocele. The use of duplex ultrasound can clearly identify the lymphocele and determine whether it is adjacent to the prosthesis. Lymphoceles that are in close proximity to the vascular prosthesis are best drained surgically in order to prevent any possible secondary infection of the vascular graft. When the lymphocele is well separated from the vascular prosthesis, sclerotherapy using powdered tetracycline can be used. Powdered tetracycline is mixed with sterile saline and injected into the lymphocele; this will often sclerose the lymphocele (48). The most important factor in dealing with lymphatic problems of the groin is prevention, which may be achieved by doing meticulous dissection with ligation of any lymphatic channels noted during vascular exposure. In particular, if a lymph node is inadvertently bisected during the dissection, both halves should be suture-ligated.

With the number of endovascular aortic stent graft procedures increasing over the last few years, wound problems with the femoral cutdown have been scrutinized. Oblique groin incisions have become a popular method of femoral access (49). In a study of 98 consecutive stent graft patients, infectious and lymphatic complications developed in 5 of 176 groin incisions (2.8%) (43). This compares favorably with the results of other studies employing the standard vertical incision for both endovascular and conventional procedures and is thus advocated as the preferred technique for femoral access (19,39,50,51).

D. Lower Extremity Incisions

Lower leg incisions account for a significant proportion of wound complications; they and tend to be the most difficult to heal and take the longest to do so. These wounds also cause additional anxiety to those using the in situ technique, in which even superficial wounds may place the underlying subcutaneous graft at risk for exposure and infection. Multiple studies have shown an incidence of wound complications for lower extremity bypass in the range of 13–44% (19,39,52,53). Independent predictors of subsequent wound problems include obesity (39) age, early graft revision, and lymph leak as well as ipsilateral limb ulcer and pedal bypasses. Of the deep grade III infections that involve the bypass graft, the best results to achieve limb salvage are found with aggressive therapy involving surgical debridement and soft tissue or muscle flap coverage in order to preserve the bypass graft (19,54).

With this in mind, many have investigated the usefulness of the endoscope in performing lower extremity bypasses. Two relatively small, retrospective studies have compared conventional saphenectomy to endoscopic saphenous vein harvest in the performance of reversed vein bypasses. Illig et al. showed a difference in all wound complications (21 and 51%) between endoscopic and conventional techniques (55). Serious wound problems (Szilagyi class II or III) also differed (25 and 14%) between the two groups. No difference existed in the short-term (30-day) graft patency, or the average length of stay for all patients. Robbins et al. found no difference in wound complications or short-term patency. In addition, endoscopic vein harvest was associated with an increased operative time but a shorter length of hospital stay (56).

Endovascular assisted in situ bypass grafting has been advocated to lessen the incidence of operative wound problems. This technique utilizes a coaxial catheter embolization system for intraoperative coil embolization of the vein's side branches. This obviates the need for one long or multiple short incisions for vein preparation. A prospective, randomized trial of 97 in situ bypasses by van Dijk et al. revealed significantly less overall wound complications in the endovascular-assisted group (34%) compared to the conventional group (72%) (57). However, the number of Szilagyi grade III wounds was equal in both groups. While 1-year patency rates were similar, 14% of the endovascular-assisted group had to have skin incisions performed for technical failure. which included branch ligation due to inability to cannulate side branches or because the greater saphenous vein was too small in diameter to accept the coaxial catheter. In addition, 20 of the 47 endovascular-assisted patients required postoperative intervention for retained arteriovenous fistulas, while only 4 of the 50 conventional patients required such an intervention. A report by Cikrit et al. found similar results in regard to wound complication rates and an increased number of retained arteriovenous fistulas in the endovascular-assisted patients (58).

Over half a million coronary artery bypass graft (CABG) procedures are performed in the United States each year. This produces a significant number of saphenectomy wounds, many of which lead to evaluation by vascular surgeons because of wound breakdown.

While the potential for exposure of an underlying bypass graft does not exist in these patients, wound problems still pose a significant morbidity for a large number of patients, which may result in prolonged length of stay, increased hospital cost, additional surgical procedures, and possibly limb loss. The reported incidence of saphenectomy problems after CABG ranges from 1 to 35% (58–61). One of the largest series, by Paletta et al., retrospectively reviewed 3525 CABG procedures over a 10-year period, finding wound complications in 145 patients (4.1%), 23 of whom (0.65%) required additional surgical interventions, including 11 vascular bypass procedures and 5 amputations (62).

Endoscopic vein harvesting has been used to help reduce the incidence of wound complications. The data in the published literature are mixed in regards to the usefulness of endoscopic vein harvesting for CABG. The results of three prospective studies have been published within the last 5 years. The first, by Allen et al., is a prospective, randomized trial of 112 patients undergoing elective CABG. They found a significant reduction in leg wound complications (4 vs. 19%) between the endoscopic and traditional technique, with a 5.6% conversion rate to an open saphenectomy harvest (63). Hayward et al. prospectively randomized 100 patients to endoscopic or open vein harvest. No significant difference in wound complications or length of hospital stay between the two groups was noted (64). Another prospective study of 60 patients compared endoscopic harvest to the skin bridge harvesting technique (65). While harvesting times were shorter with the endoscopic approach, this group had a wound complication rate of 32%, which compared to only 3% in the skin bridge group. Even excluding wound hematomas, the endoscopic group still had a wound complication rate of 13%.

VI. WOUND INFECTION

Once wound complications have occurred, they must be treated in an appropriate and timely manner in order to prevent further morbidity. A multitude of treatment modalities exist for wound care; however, basic surgical principles of wound care take precedence and all other modalities are likely to fail if these principles are not upheld. The most important of these is operative debridement of all devitalized tissue. Necrotic tissue provides an excellent nidus for further infection and will significantly hinder any other attempts at wound healing by other modalities. In order for a wound to heal, viable tissue is needed in order to foster an environment for the development of granulation tissue. In the most severe cases, soft tissue or muscle flap coverage may be necessary in order to provide even viable tissue to promote healing and, in some instances, to provide soft tissue coverage for an underlying vascular graft (54,66). All wounds should be appropriately dressed to protect them while healing, and wound care applications or changes should be performed in a clean or sterile fashion depending on the particular wound. The use of antibiotics is an adjunctive measure to the treatment of wound infection, especially after vascular bypass operations in which perfusion has been improved dramatically. Any localized collection or abscess needs open drainage.

The wound care market has been expanding significantly in recent years. Most health care companies have some sort of wound care product on the market and available for use by any physician, nurse, or wound care specialist. Wound care ointments include papain-urea debriding ointment for the removal of necrotic tissue, which can also be combined with a chlorophyllin copper complex to aid in deodorizing. Other gels include iodine-containing hydrophilic beads for the reduction of microbial load and exudate absorption. While not strictly a wound complication, many of the patients undergoing lower extremity bypass have nonhealing diabetic ulcers. The treatment of these hard-to-heal wounds has been assisted by the use of becaplermin, a recombinant human platelet-derived growth factor for topical administration. The biological activity of this agent includes promoting the chemotactic recruitment and proliferation of cells involved in wound repair and promoting the formation of granulation tissue.

Treatment options also include different mechanical devices. A subatmospheric pressure dressing has been approved for wound treatment in the United States since 1995. These dressings use negative pressure to create a suction force that promotes wound healing in two ways. First, it enables wound drainage by removing excess interstitial fluid. Second, it transmits mechanical forces to the surrounding tissues, with resultant deformation of the extracellular matrix and cells. This encourages rapid ingrowth of granulation tissue, allowing wounds to close more quickly than with other forms of therapy (67,68). This method of wound treatment has been extensively studied in animal models and been shown to create an environment that promotes wound healing by increasing blood flow levels and rates of granulation tissue formation while also decreasing bacterial counts (69).

Given that tissue hypoxia is a major component in wound complications, theoretically hyperbaric oxygen therapy (HBO), which transiently increases the partial pressure of oxygen in the plasma, should aid in wound healing. However, the published data on the benefit of HBO in wound healing are inconclusive. Most studies are small, retrospective, and nonrandomized, with several potential sources of bias (70). Indeed, Ciaravino et al. reviewed 54 patients with lower extremity wounds, all of whom underwent HBO therapy for an average of 30 treatments (71). The average cost for the HBO treatments alone was $14,000. A total of 80% of patients showed no improvement, 11% showed some improvement, and none were completely healed. Complications of HBO occurred in 63% of patients; most commonly barotrauma to the ears occurred in 43%, as a result of which the vast majority required myringotomy tubes. Other complications included cardiac arrhythmias, stroke, and seizure. Without strong prospective, randomized, placebo-controlled data, it is difficult to justify any benefit to HBO therapy in the treatment of wound problems given the current data, the cost and the incidence of complications.

In conclusion, wound complications following vascular surgery constitute a significant problem that, if not addressed in a timely and appropriate manner, may lead to significant morbidity and mortality with compromise of any underlying vascular graft. The treatment must be aggressive, with prompt exploration of wounds, wound debridement, and coverage of exposed vascular structures with viable autogenous tissue is the cornerstone of effective treatment. Delay results in an increase of limb loss and mortality secondary to graft complication of anastomotic bleeding and thrombosis.

REFERENCES

1. Szilagyi DE, Smith RF, Elliott JP, Vrandecic MP. Infection in arterial reconstruction with synthetic grafts. Ann Surg 1972; 176:321–333.
2. Johnson JA, Cogbill TH, Strutt PJ, Gundersen AL. Wound complications after infrainguinal bypass. Arch Surg 1988; 123:859–862.
3. Goodson WH III, Hunt TK. Wound healing in experimental diabetes mellitus: importance of early insulin therapy. Surg Forum 1978; 29:95–98.
4. Bagdade JD, Root RK, Bulger RJ. Impaired leukocyte function in patients with poorly controlled diabetes. Diabetes 1974; 23:9–15.
5. Utley JR, Thomason ME, Wallace DJ, Mutch DW, Staton L, Brown V, Wilde CM, Bell MS.

Preoperative correlates of impaired wound healing after saphenous vein excision. J Thorac Cardiovasc Surg 1989; 98:147–149.

6. Wengrovitz M, Atnip RG, Gifford RR, Neumyer MM, Heitjian DF, Thiele BL. Wound complications of autogenous subcutaneous infrainguinal arterial bypass surgery: predisposing factors and management. J Vasc Surg 1990; 11:156–163.

7. Cruse PJ, Foord R. A prospective study of 23,649 surgical wounds. Arch Surg 1973; 107:206–210.

8. Verta MJ, Gross WS, van Bellen B, Yao JS, Bergan JJ. Forefoot perfusion pressure and minor amputation for gangrene. Surg 1976; 80:729–734.

9. Edwards WH, Martin RS, Jenkins JM, Edwards WH Sr, Mulherin JL. Primary graft infections. J Vasc Surg 1987; 6:235–239.

10. Robison JG, Ross JP, Brothers TE, Elliott BM. Distal wound complications following pedal bypass: analysis of risk factors. Ann Vasc Surg 1995; 9:53–59.

11. Casey J, Flinn WR, Yao JS, Fahey V, Pawlowski J, Bergan JJ. Correlation of immune and nutritional status with wound complications in patients undergoing vascular operations. Surg 1983; 93:822–827.

12. Blankensteijn JD, Gertier JP, Peterson MJ, Brewster DC, Cambria RP, LaMuraglia GM, Abbott WM. Avoiding infrainguinal bypass wound complications in patients with chronic renal insufficiency: the role of the anatomic plane. Eur J Vasc Endovasc Surg 1996; 11:98–104.

13. Dovgan PS, Shepard AD, Nypaver TJ. Critical limb ischemia in patients with end stage renal disease: do long-term results justify an aggressive surgical approach? Perspect Vasc Surg 1999; 12:81–92.

14. Johnson BL, Glickman MH, Bandyk DF, Esses GE. Failure of foot salvage in patients with end-stage renal disease after surgical revascularization. J Vasc Surg 1995; 22:280–286.

15. Wasserman RJ, Saroyan RM, Rice JC, Kerstein MD. Infrainguinal revascularization for limb salvage in patients with end stage renal disease. S Med J 1991; 84:190–192.

16. Simsir SA, Cabellon A, Kohlman-Trigoboff D, Smith BM. Factors influencing limb salvage and survival after amputation and revascularization in patients with end stage renal disease. Am J Surg 1995; 170:113–117.

17. Hunt TK, Hopf HW. Wound healing and infection: what surgeons and anesthesiologists can do. Surg Clin North Am 1997; 77:587–606.

18. Taylor DE, Whamond JS, Penhallow JE. Effects of hemorrhage on wound strength and fibroblast function. Br J Surg 1987; 74:316–319.

19. Reifsnyder T, Bandyk D, Seabrook G, Kinney E, Towne JB. Wound complications of the in situ saphenous vein bypass technique. J Vasc Surg 1992; 15:843–850.

20. Lorentzen JE, Nielson OM, Arendrup H, Kimose HH, Bille S, Andersen J, Jensen CH, Jacobsen F, Roder OC. Vascular graft infection: an analysis of sixty-two graft infections in 2411 consecutively implanted synthetic vascular grafts. Surgery 1985; 98:81–86.

21. Liekweg WG Jr, Greenfield LJ. Vascular prosthetic infections: collected experience and results of treatment. Surgery 1977; 81:335–342.

22. Calligaro KD, Westcott CJ, Buckley RM, Savarese RP, DeLaurentis DA. Infrainguinal anastomotic arterial graft infections treated by selective graft preservation. Ann Surg 1992; 216:74–79.

23. Kilta MJ, Goodson SF, Bishara RA, Meyer JP, Schuler JJ, Flanigan DP. Mortality and limb loss with infected infrainguinal bypass. J Vasc Surg 1987; 5:566–571.

24. Kaiser AB, Clayson KR, Mulherin JL Jr, Roach AC, Allen TR, Edwards WH, Dale WA. Antibiotic prophylaxis in vascular surgery. Ann Surg 1978; 188:283–289.

25. Pitt HA, Postier RG, MacGowan WA, Frank LW, Surmak AJ, Sitzman JV, Bouchier-Hayes D. Prophylactic antibiotics in vascular surgery: topical, systemic, or both? Ann Surg 1980; 192:356–364.

26. Matsukawa T, Sessler DI, Sessler AM, Schroeder M, Ozaki M, Kurz A, Cheng C. Heat flow and distribution during induction of general anesthesia. Anesthesiology 1995; 82:662–673.

27. Kurz A, Sessler DI, Lenhardt R. Perioperative normothermia to reduce the incidence of surgical wound infection and shorten hospitalization. N Engl J Med 1996; 334:1209–1215.

28. Kurz A, Kurz M, Poeschl G, Faryniak B, Redl G, Hackl W. Forced air warming maintains intra-operative normothermia better than circulating water mattresses. Anesth Analg 1993; 77:89–95.

29. DeLaria GA, Hunter JA, Goldin MD, Serry C, Javid H, Najafi H. Leg wound complications associated with coronary revascularization. J Thorac Cardiovasc Surg 1981; 81:403–407.

30. Ruoff BA, Cranley JJ, Hannan LA, Aseffa N, Karkow WS, Stedje KG, Cranley RD. Real-time duplex ultrasound mapping of the greater saphenous vein before in situ infrainguinal revascularization. J Vasc Surg 1987; 6:107–113.

31. Veith FJ, Gupta SK, Ascer E, White-Flores S, Samson RH, Scher LA, Towne JB, Bernhard VM, Bonier P, Flinn WR, Astelford P, Yao JS, Bergan JJ. Six-year prospective multicenter randomized comparison of autologous saphenous vein and expanded polytetrafluoroethylene grafts in infrainguinal arterial reconstructions. J Vasc Surg 1986; 3:104–114.

32. Schwartz ME, Harrington EB, Schanzer H. Wound complications after in situ bypass. J Vasc Surg 1988; 7:802–807.

33. Wengerter KR, Veith FJ, Gupta SK, Goldsmith J, Farrell E, Harris PL, Moore D, Shanik G. Prospective randomized multicenter comparison of in situ and reversed vein infrapopliteal bypasses. J Vasc Surg 1991; 13:189–199.

34. Angelini GD, Butchart EG, Armistead SH, Breckenridge IM. Comparative study of leg wound skin closure in coronary artery bypass graft operations. Thorax 1984; 39:942–945.

35. AbuRahma AF, Wooddruff BA, Lucente FC. Edema after femoropopliteal bypass surgery: lymphatic and venous theories of causation. J Vasc Surg 1990; 11:461–467.

36. Eickhoff JH, Engell HC. Local regulation of blood flow and the occurrence of edema after arterial reconstruction of the lower limbs. Ann Surg 1982; 195:474–478.

37. Soong CV, Barros D'Sa AA. Lower limb oedema following distal arterial bypass grafting. Eur J Vasc Endovasc Surg 1998; 16:465–471.

38. Nicoloff AD, Taylor LM, McLafferty RB, Moneta GL, Porter JM. Patient recovery after infrainguinal bypass grafting for limb salvage. J Vasc Surg 1998; 27:256–266.

39. Kent CK, Bartek S, Kuntz KM, Anninos E, Skillman JJ. Prospective study of wound complications in continuous infrainguinal incisions after lower limb arterial reconstruction: incidence, risk factors, and cost. Surgery 1996; 119:378–383.

40. Thompson JE. Complications of carotid endarterectomy and their prevention. World J Surg 1979; 3:155–165.

41. Sicard GA, Freeman MB, VanderWoude JC, Anderson CB. Comparison between the transabdominal and retroperitoneal approach for reconstruction of the infrarenal abdominal aorta. J Vasc Surg 1987; 5:19–27.

42. Honig MP, Mason RA, Giron F. Wound complications of the retroperitoneal approach to the aorta and iliac vessels. J Vasc Surg 1992; 15:28–34.

43. Leather RP, Shah DM, Kaufmann JL, Fitzgerald KM, Chang BB, Feustel PJ. Comparative analysis of retroperitoneal and transperitoneal aortic replacement for aneurysm. Surg Gynecol Obstet 1989; 168:387–393.

44. Cambria RP, Brewster DC, Abbott WM, Freehan M, Megerman J, LaMuraglia G, Wilson R, Wilson D, Teplick R, Davison JK. Transperitoneal versus retroperitoneal approach for aortic reconstruction: a randomized prospective study. J Vasc Surg 1990; 11:314–325.

45. Tyndall SH, Shepard AD, Wilczewski JM, Reddy DJ, Elliott JP, Ernst CB. Groin lymphatic complications after arterial reconstruction. J Vasc Surg 1994; 19:858–864.

46. Roberts JR, Walters GK, Zenilman ME, Jones CE. Groin lymphorrhea complicating revascularization involving the femoral vessels. Am J Surg 1993; 165:341–344.

47. Rubin JR, Malone JM, Goldstone J. The role of lymphatic system in acute arterial prosthetic graft infections. J Vasc Surg 1985; 2:92–98.

48. Cannon L, Walker AJ. Sclerotherapy of a wound lymphocele using tetracycline. European J Vasc Endovas Surg 1997; 14(6):505.

49. Caiati JM, Kaplan D, Gitlitz D, Hollier LH, Marin ML. The value of the oblique groin incision for femoral artery access during endovascular procedures. Ann Vasc Surg 2000; 14:248–253.

50. Moore WS, Rutherford RB. Transfemoral endovascular repair of abdominal aortic aneurysm: results of the North American EVT phase I trial. J Vasc Surg 1996; 23:543–553.
51. Chuter TA, Reilly LM, Stoney RJ, Messina LM. Femoral artery exposure for endovascular aneurysm repair through oblique incisions. J Endovasc Surg 1998; 5:259–260.
52. Dalman RL, Abbruzzese T, Bushnik T, Harris EJ. Open saphenectomy complications following lower extremity revascularization. Cardiovasc Surg 2000; 8:51–57.
53. Treiman GS, Copland S, Yellin AE, Lawrence PF, McNamara RM, Treiman RL. Wound infections involving infrainguinal autogenous vein grafts: a current evaluation of factors determining successful graft preservation. J Vasc Surg 2001; 33:948–958.
54. Tukiainen E, Biancari F, Lepantalo M. Deep infection of infrapopliteal autogenous vein grafts— Immediate use of muscle flaps in leg salvage. J Vasc Surg 1998; 28:611–616.
55. Illig KA, Rhodes JM, Sternbach Y, Shortell CK, Davies MG, Green RM. Reduction in wound morbidity rates following endoscopic saphenous vein harvest. Ann Vasc Surg 2001; 15:104–109.
56. Robbins MR, Hutchinson SA, Helmer SD. Endoscopic saphenous vein harvest in infrainguinal bypass surgery. Am J Surg 1998; 176:586–590.
57. van Dijk LC, van Urk H, du Bois NA, Yo TI, Koning J, Jansen WB, Wittens CH. A new "closed" in situ vein bypass technique results in a reduced wound complication rate. Eur J Vasc Endovasc Surg 1995; 10:162–167.
58. Cikrit DF, Fiore NF, Dalsing MC, Lalka SG, Sawchuk AP, Ladd AP, Dodson S. A comparison of endovascular assisted and conventional in situ bypass grafts. Ann Vasc Surg 1995; 9:37–43.
59. Galbraith GF, Pica-Furey W. A retrospective comparative study of open and endoscopic saphenous vein harvesting. J Endovasc Ther 2000; 7:460–468.
60. L'Ecuyer PB, Murphy D, Little JR, Fraser VJ. The epidemiology of chest and leg wound infections following cardiothoracic surgery. Clin Infec Dis 1996; 22:424–429.
61. Slaughter MS, Olson MM, Lee JT Jr, Ward HB. A fifteen-year wound surveillance study after coronary artery bypass. Ann Thorac Surg 1993; 56:1063–1068.
62. Paletta CE, Huang DB, Fiore AC, Swartz MT, Rilloraza FL, Gardner JE. Major leg wound complications after saphenous vein harvest for coronary revascularization. Ann Thorac Surg 2000; 70:492–497.
63. Allen KB, Griffith GL, Heimansohn DA, Robison RJ, Matheny RG, Schier JJ, Fitzgerald EB, Shaar CJ. Endoscopic versus traditional saphenous vein harvesting: a prospective, randomized trial. Ann Thorac Surg 1998; 66:26–32.
64. Hayward TZ III, Hey LA, Newman LL, Duhaylongsod FG, Hayward KA, Lowe JE, Smith PK. Endoscopic versus open saphenous vein harvest: the effect on postoperative outcomes. Ann Thorac Surg 1999; 68:2107–2111.
65. Horvath KD, Gray D, Benton L, Hill J, Swanstrom LL. Operative outcomes of minimally invasive vein harvest. Am J Surg 1998; 175:391–395.
66. Patterson MA, Cambria RA, Seabrook GR, Towne JB. Rotational Myoplasty: Treatment Techniques for Covering Exposed or Infected Vascular Structures Associated with Complicated Inguinal Wounds [abstr]. Milwaukee, WI: Medical College of Wisconsin, 2002.
67. Evans D, Land L. Topical negative pressure for treating chronic wounds: a systematic review. Br J Plastic Surg 2001; 54:238–242.
68. Argenta LC, Morykwas MJ. Vacuum-assisted closure: a new method for wound control and treatment: clinical experience. Ann Plast Surg 1997; 38:563–577.
69. Morykwas MJ, Argenta LC, Shelton-Brown EI, McGuirt W. Vacuum-assisted closure: a new method for wound control and treatment: animal studies and basic foundation. Ann Plast Surg 1997; 38:553–562.
70. Wunderlich RP, Peters EJ, Lavery LA. Systemic hyperbaric oxygen therapy: lower extremity wound healing and the diabetic foot. Diabetes Care 2000; 23:1551–1555.
71. Ciaravino ME, Friedell ML, Kammerlocher TC. Is hyperbaric oxygen a useful adjunct in the management of problem lower extremity wounds? Ann Vasc Surg 1996; 10:558–562.

21

Complications in the Management of the Diabetic Foot

Gary R. Seabrook

Medical College of Wisconsin, Milwaukee, Wisconsin, U.S.A.

In 2000, the prevalence of diabetes in the United States was estimated to be 17 million, with 5.9 million of these cases undiagnosed. Of all American citizens over the age of 20, some 8.6% have diabetes mellitus; but in the age group over 65 years, 20.1% have the diagnosis. It is estimated that 60–70% of people with diabetes have some form of neuropathy, leading in large part to impaired sensation of the extremities. In combination with peripheral vascular disease, these nervous system changes place the feet of diabetic patients at significant risk for injury and tissue loss. From 1997 to 1999, the Centers for Disease Control recorded 82,000 nontraumatic lower extremity amputations performed on patients with diabetes mellitus. It is estimated that $44 billion is spent annually in direct medical expenses for the treatment of diabetes in the United States and that indirect costs—including long-term disability, time lost from work, and premature mortality—account for another $54 billion spent in association with this disease process (1). Aside from the financial costs associated with diabetes, there are significant physical and emotional costs associated with the possibility of lower extremity limb loss. Because of this significant health care risk, complications in the management of the diabetic foot require particular attention.

For patients with diabetes mellitus, foot ulcers and foot infections are themselves complications of the disease process. The triad of atherosclerotic vascular disease, peripheral neuropathy, and a propensity to develop polymicrobial infection places the patient with diabetes at constant risk for injury to the integument, soft tissue infection, osteomyelitis, chronic ulceration, derangement of the skeletal architecture, and amputation. Mechanical trauma that would result in only a trivial injury to an individual with a normal arterial system plagues the patient with diabetes with the risk of cellulitis, ulcerating wounds, necrotizing infection, systemic sepsis, gangrene, and in some cases death. The severity of the patient's diabetes, duration of the disease process, precision of glucose control, or daily insulin requirements are not good predictors of which patients will be at greater risk for foot complications. Every patient with diabetes is advised to be compulsive about wearing well-fitting footwear and inspecting the feet on a daily basis to detect any sign of minor injury or neurotrophic trauma. Minor abrasions or a superficial blister that would immediately be recognized by a patient with normal peripheral sensation can easily be ignored by a diabetic patient because the pain is not appreciated; or, owing to visual impairment related to diabetic retinopathy, the patient may simply be unable to see the soft tissue defect.

Because the etiology of diabetic foot wounds is so closely related to microangiopathy and the resulting chronic ischemia to the muscles, nerves, and bones of the foot, the treatment of these lesions falls within the diagnostic and therapeutic purview of the vascular surgeon. Even though many of the clinical presentations do not require arterial revascularization, the expertise of a vascular specialist is appropriate in their management.

The chronic metabolic derangement of hyperglycemia from inappropriate insulin secretion results in the common pathway of inadequate perfusion to the surface tissues, intrinsic muscles, neural tissue, and osseous structures of the foot. The most obvious clinical presentation of this chronic ischemia is tissue breakdown in a spectrum beginning with superficial loss of the dermis and progressing to bullae, full-thickness skin loss, a penetrating ulcer, destruction of underlying bone, or gangrene. Vascular occlusive disease in diabetic patients results in arterial obliteration primarily in the vessels at the level of the tibia, forefoot, and digits. It is not uncommon for the diabetic population to have normal aortoiliac segments and even a patent femoral popliteal system, although arterial wall calcification may be present at these levels. Not only does the distribution of the occlusive process follow a unique pattern in the diabetic patient but there is a difference in the structure of the blood vessel that is different from atherosclerotic changes due to cardiovascular risk factors such as hypertension, hypercholesterolemia, and cigarette smoking. Arterial wall abnormalities are associated with calcification adjacent to the internal elastic lamina. At the arteriolar level, histopathology reveals thickening of intima at the basement membrane. The changes in the capillary walls may reveal a patchy distribution, with normal capillaries interspersed with those that are diseased. Because these findings are present in patients who may not yet have been diagnosed with clinical diabetes, it suggests that the thickening of the basement membrane may be due to a genetic predisposition rather than simply altered glucose metabolism (2).

While surface injuries from arterial insufficiency may be obvious, ischemic injury to sensory and motor nerves results in more subtle insults. The lack of normal sensation allows direct trauma to the foot to go unnoticed. It is not uncommon to hear that the patient has walked for an entire day with a pebble in his or her shoe or even a nail protruding through the soul of a shoe or boot into the foot. Were the patient to have a normal sensory system, a foreign or penetrating object or would be promptly recognized and removed. Even poorly fitting shoes may cause significant trauma to the foot. If a patient has normal sensation, improperly fitting shoes are accommodated by subtle changes in weight and posture so as to offload the irritating focus and prevent injury. In addition to sensory denervation to the integument of the foot, diabetic neuropathy deprives the intrinsic muscles of the foot of normal motor innervation. This leads to disruption of the fine balance of the flexor and extensor mechanisms that provide for the usual precise motor function that results in a normal gait. The neuropathic dennervation of the intrinsic muscles leads to abnormalities in the foot architecture characterized and by extensor subluxation of the toes, protruding plantar prominence of the metatarsal heads, proximal migration of the metatarsal fat pads, and dominance of the action of the toe flexors over the extensors. With dislocation of the metatarsophalangeal joint, the metatarsal heads are no longer protected by the mechanical levers of the phalanx bones and the full weight of the patient's body becomes focused along a narrow strike point during ambulation. Because conventional footwear is designed for normal foot anatomy, the patient's shoes may actually play a role in provoking physical trauma to the surface of the foot. An ulceration will begin with local inflammation, frequently followed by the formation of a callus, within which a foreign body or bacteria may be sequestered. This closed-space environment provides a medium for bacterial growth resulting in abscess formation within the dermis or, in more serious cases, penetrating into the underlying a soft tissue. With further trauma, the callus breaks down, exposing the tissue defect. Because the etiology of the process frequently relates to abnormal forces applied to the underlying bone, the first presentation may involve not only tissue loss but also injury from osteomyelitis of the underlying phalanx or metatarsal (Fig. 1).

When chronic neuropathy leads to failure of the ligamentous structures between the metatarsal and tarsal bones, there is eventual collapse of the ankle mechanism. This orthopedic defect, termed *Charcot foot*, manifests initially as loss of the plantar arch; however, in the absence of protection from the intrinsic musculature, the disorganized tarsal bones may erode though the plantar surface of the foot (Fig. 2).

Polymicrobial infection completes the triad that plagues the foot of the diabetic patient. Infections in diabetic patients pose a more serious risk to the patient's limb because they occur in tissue that is poorly perfused and because the clinical signs of the infection may not be recognized in a timely fashion due to masking by the peripheral neuropathy. When there is a break in the integument, and invasive infection may spread rapidly because the inflammatory process is not perceived. The hyperglycemic state enhances the environment for an infection to flourish. Intracellular bactericidal activity of leukocytes is diminished in the hyperglycemic state. Tissue glycosylation further impairs wound healing by increasing the activity of collagenases, thereby reducing the structural collagen content at the site of injury and disrupting the normal reparative mechanisms. Dysfunctional phagocytes further enhance an environment conducive to a synergistic microbial

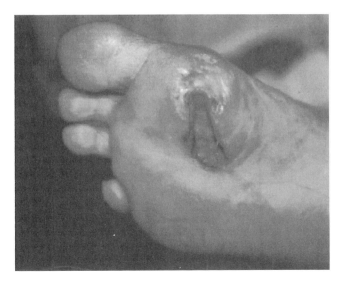

Figure 1   Neurotrophic ulcer on plantar surface of first metatarsal head with exposed bone involved with osteomyelitis.

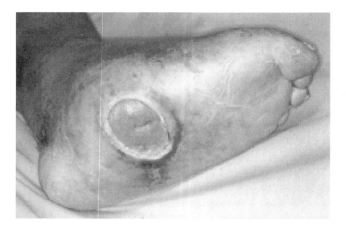

Figure 2   Charcot foot with large plantar ulcer at site of collapsed forefoot.

infection. Polymicrobial infections with aerobes and anaerobes result in increased potential for tissue destruction. The combined virulence of multiple organisms in the wound
exceeds the individual destructive capabilities of any of the microbes acting alone.
"Synergistic virulence" results in the rapid progression of foot infections, and dictates
in the need for broad-spectrum antimicrobial therapy in their treatment. The microbial
populations recovered in culture from diabetic foot infections includes Gram negative and
positive aerobes, and gram-negative and positive anaerobes. (Table 1). Peptostreptococci
are recovered in significant frequency from deep soft tissue cultures obtained from patients
with diabetic foot infections, with only *Bacteroides* species being recovered more frequently from anerobic cultures. *Peptostreptococcus magnus* has been identified as the
single most common clinical isolate from this bacterial group in diabetic foot infections.
These bacteria produce a potent collagenase that is responsible for skin and subcutaneous
tissue destruction, and this enzymatic activity results in the rapid progress of tissue destruction associated with diabetic foot infections. The ability to destroy tissue and proliferate in an anaerobic environment further enhances the ability of these organisms to
invade the deep anatomical spaces of the foot (3).

I. ANTIBIOTIC THERAPY

For patients with serious diabetic foot infections, surgical intervention to drain abscess
cavities, remove devitalized tissue, and excise any septic focus is the primary treatment
objective. Antibiotics serve as adjunctive therapy to eradicate micro-organisms in the soft
tissue adjacent to the site of the infection. Antibiotics do not kill bacteria in the soft tissue
that have already been devitalized, nor are they effective in reaching infected material
without adequate arterial perfusion. Bacteria that have collected in the ascending lymphatic system may be effectively eradicated by antibiotic therapy.

The pathobiology of infections in patients with diabetes must be considered in pre-
scribing antibiotic therapy for associated soft tissue infections. In addition to a significant
microbial presence, there may be injury to the microenvironment already contaminated with
foreign bodies or tissue debris. Secondary host factors, including tissue ischemia and a

Table 1 Microbial Organisms Identified in Culture from Diabetic Foot Infections–Prevalence of Isolate Recovered in a Population of 246 Patients

	Prevalence
Gram-negative aerobes	
Proteus species	60%
Escherichia coli	30%
Klebsiella species	25%
Pseudomonas aeruginosa	30%
Pseudomonas species	45%
Morganella morganii	10%
Enterobacter species	20%
Acinetobacter species	< 5%
Citrobacter species	< 5%
Gram-positive aerobes	
Enterococcus faecalis	40%
Enterococcus faecium	5%
Staphylococcus aureus	30%
Staphylococcus epidermidis	50%
Streptococcus milleri group	35%
Streptococcus agalactiae	10%
Micrococcus species	20%
Corynebacterium species	10%
Miscellaneous coagulase-negative staphylococci	25%
Gram-negative anaerobes	
Bacteroides fragilis group	70%
Bacteroides fragilis	45%
Porphyromonas species	5%
Fusobacterium species	25%
Prevotella species	15%
Veillonella parvula	< 5%
Bifidobacterium species	< 5%
Gram-positive anaerobes	
Peptostreptococcus manus	50%
Peptostreptococcus species	35%
Actinomyces species	5%
Propionibacterium	< 10%
Clostridium perfringens	< 10%
Clostridium species	< 5%

Source: Ref. 13.

compromised immune system, further complicate the environment in which antimicrobial activity must occur. In this milieu, the infection has the potential to be enhanced by microbial synergism, where the cooperative interaction of two or more bacterial species produces a result not achieved by the individual bacterial alone. In mixed soft tissue infections, several major microbial populations flourish. Anaerobes including Enterobacteriaceae, *Staphylococcus*, *Streptococcus*, and *Enterococcus* coexist with anaerobes including *Bacteroides*, *Fusobacterium*, *Peptostreptococcus*, and *Clostridium*, creating a population that contribute to microbial synergism. In the presence of this virulent microenvironment, there is both local and systemic anergy, further disrupting anatomical integrity of the soft tissue and creating a host for further bacterial proliferation. Conditions contributing to microbial proliferation include metabolic abnormalities, not the least of which is hyperglycemia. The immune system, which may already be compromised, is further suppressed in the presence of a synergistic infection.

The selection of antibiotic therapy must take into account this unique collection of conditions occurring in the foot of the diabetic patient. For this reason, antibiotics that would be appropriate for any subset of the identified infecting bacteria may be inadequate in this synergistic, polymicrobial infection. Because these infections tend to be invasive, destructive to the soft tissue, and rapid in their progression, even empirical antibiotic therapy must utilize a broad-spectrum regimen.

Semisynthetic penicillins with a beta-lactamase inhibitor provide a suitable broad-spectrum antibiotic regimen for patients presenting with diabetic foot infections. *Pseudomonas*, *Enterobacter*, and *Serratia* all possess a gene for inducible beta-lactamase production, which quickly hydrolyzes the beta-lactam ring of common penicillins including ampicillin, amoxicillin, ticarcillin, piperacillin, rendering them inert and ineffective. Adding the beta-lactamase inhibitor to the penicillin substrate results in a therapeutic compound that prevents the beta-lactamase from degrading the beta-lactam agent, which can then go on to inhibit cell wall synthesis in the micro-organism. Beta-lactamase inhibitors include clavulanic acid, sulbactam, and tazobactam. With the use of these agents, there is the risk of inducing of beta-lactamase activity within the infection; when new beta-lactam antibiotics are introduced into clinical use, some previously unrecognized beta-lactamases with the capacity to destroy the activity of the compound are identified.

Quinolones are ideal compounds for the treatment of diabetic foot infections. They act by inhibiting DNA gyrase, the enzyme that mediates supercoiling of the bacterial DNA into compacted domains capable of fitting within the confines of the bacterial wall. Inhibition of DNA gyrase causes relaxation of the supercoiled DNA, thereby terminating chromosomal replication, interfering with bacterial cell division, and blocking gene expression. The antimicrobial spectrum of these agents varies greatly depending on the specific generation of the drug. Second-generation quinolones (e.g., ciprofloxacin) exhibit excellent gram-negative facultative activity but are not effective alone in treating diabetic foot infections because they demonstrate little activity against the gram-negative anaerobic populations. Therefore these agents typically require the addition of an antianaerobic compound to provide effective coverage against the anaerobic microbial flora encountered in the diabetic foot. Fourth-generation quinolones, in which a fluorine atom is added to the bicyclic aromatic core, provide excellent aerobic and anaerobic coverage against both gram-positive and gram-negative microbial pathogens. This therapy is attractive because a single agent with a pharmacokinetic profile that often allows for once-a-day dosing may be employed effectively in treating these infections. Because tissue penetration is excellent, patients may be started on an intravenous dosing schedule while hospitalized and then discharged home on an oral formulation of the drug.

Traditional empirical therapy for polymicrobial infections has utilized prescription of an aminoglycoside, which functions by inhibiting the synthesis of bacterial cell proteins. Noteworthy are the significant potentially toxic side effects associated with this class of drugs. In the diabetic patient, the most serious complication is antibiotic-introduced nephrotoxicity, which is particularly hazardous in a patient population already likely to have impaired renal function due to diabetic nephrosclerosis. Despite potentially increased safety by careful pharmacokinetic dosing, the risk of renal failure in diabetic patients precludes the use of aminoglycosides for the treatment of foot infections.

Although vancomycin is particularly effective against gram-positive bacteria through its inhibition of cell-wall synthesis, the increasing amount of bacterial resistance that has developed due to its extensive use in the hospital setting dictates that it should be administered only in carefully selected patients (4). This drug should not be utilized as part of an empirical therapeutic regimen. It does remain as an appropriate antibiotic for methicillin-resistant *Staphylococcus aureus*. With the emergence of vancomycin-resistant *Enterococcus* (VRE), linezolid has become an appropriate therapy (5). As with vancomycin, this agent should be used with considerable discretion in an effort to control the emergence of new resistant organisms, particularly in the nosocomial setting (6).

II. WOUND CARE

Equally important to antibiotic therapy as an adjunct to effective control of a diabetic foot infection is appropriate care of the wound. Any break in the integument represents a wound that may require attention both to control the infection and to promote effective healing. Wound care is provided by removing the devitalized tissue, enhancing the normal reparative functions of the skin, and providing protection against further insult from mechanical or bacterial forces. Factors that impede wound healing include pressure, a dry environment, the presence of necrotic tissue, ischemia, and inadequate nutrition.

Foot wounds should be protected from extrinsic pressure, with the realization that neurotrophic trauma may, in fact, have been the initial etiology of the wound. Any wound should be covered with a clean, bulky dressing. Gauze pads should be inserted between the toes and a protective pad placed over the heel. In a compromised limb, the weight of the foot against the bed sheets and mattress may provide an impediment to wound healing or even cause further tissue injury.

A moist wound environment is one of the most important factors to promote healing of a soft tissue defect. While it is true that a warm, moist milieu is also advantageous for bacterial proliferation, effective wound treatment requires an environment conducive to tissue repair and epithelialization. Simply covering a wound is helpful in that it protects the site of wound healing from external trauma, and a wound dressing in that capacity mimics the function of the epidermis. Initial research supporting this concept demonstrated that experimentally induced blister wounds healed more rapidly when the blister roofs were left intact (7). This concept of a "biological dressing" leads to the recommendation of an occlusive dressing to both protect the wound and provide a constant degree of moisture. This may best be provided by hydrocolloid dressings (Replicare, Smith & Nephew; Thinsite and Transorbent, B. Braun Medical), which contain hydrophilic colloidal particles comprising gelatin or pectin formulated in an adhesive mass. Fluid in the wound is absorbed by capillary action, which occurs with slow swelling of the particles. Although the absorptive capacity of the hydrocolloid is significant, dressing changes may be required more frequently in the early phases of wound healing, when more exudate is being produced. Although hydrocolloid dressings are occlusive, skin maceration is prevented because of the absorptive qualities of the hydrophilic particles. The pliable nature of the hydrocolloid dressing allows it to conform to the irregular surfaces adjacent to a foot wound. When a hydrocolloid dressing is removed, a viscous, gel-like material is evident, the result of decomposition of the adhesive mass. The clinician is cautioned not to confuse this material with a purulent infection.

In the absence of an occlusive dressing, hydrogels (SoloSite, Smith & Nephew; Curasol, Healthpoint) may be used to create a moist environment. These agents, which contain a significant percentage of water, have a complex lattice that traps a dispersion medium, typically a cross-linked polymer. Because they possess high specific heat, these dressings feel cool to the touch and are perceived as soothing by the patient. Lidocaine gel may be incorporated with a hydrogel dressing to provide further analgesia for treatment of a sensitive wound. Although clearly superior to a simple saline-soaked gauze dressing, use of a hydrogel requires vigilant observation of the wound to prevent desiccation.

During the early inflammatory phase of wound healing, the coagulation cascade is activated to deposit fibrin, which is polymerized to stabilize the wound. In the normal course of wound healing, inflammation is followed by a process of granulation, in which a loose matrix infiltrated by macrophages, fibroblasts, and capillary endothelial cells appears in the open wound. Collagen, fibronectin, and hyaluronic acid add substance to the wound. When this granulation process deviates from its natural balance, there may be a proliferation of exudative materials, including tenacious fibrin strands that are actually counterproductive to wound closure. In such a case, which is more likely to occur when the wound edges are not in close proximity, debridement is required. The goal of debridement is to remove devitalized exudative products and expose healthy granulation tissue to allow epithelial cell migration. For the removal of gross material, mechanical debridement with scissors or scalpel is appropriate. As a rule, this is a painless procedure and should be performed whenever there is evidence of fibrinous exudate or devitalized tissue on the surface of a wound. Fibrin, an important constituent the initial phase of wound healing, can become counterproductive if a mechanical barrier develops over the wound surface. An alternative to mechanical debridement is the use of an enzymatic agent for chemical debridement. Proteolytic products (Collagenase Santyl, Smith & Nephew) contain a collagenase that breaks down necrotic tissue without destroying the viable granulation surface. Another product (Accuzyme, Healthpoint) uses papain (derived from the *Carica papaya*) combined with urea, which is effective in breaking protein cross links of wound debris. As the urea disrupts cross links, the proteins on the wound surface unfold and thereby become susceptible to the enzymatic effect of the papain. When the proteins are digested into small peptide fragments, the material can be washed from the wound surface. Wound gels are also employed to rid a wound surface of excess fibrin deposition. One product (Panafil, Healthpoint) contains a chlororphyllin copper complex that inhibits fibrin formation while enhancing the structural integrity of the collagen matrix of the granulation surface. The chlorophyll in the product is also an effective agent to reduce odor emitted from the wound surface. Silver compounds have been proven effective in augmenting wound healing, primarily by their bactericidal activity in reducing microbial colonization on a granulating wound. Silver sulfadiazine cream is particularly effective in controlling the growth of *Pseudomonas* on the wound surface.

Wounds with a clean, granulated surface and well-perfused epithelial margins may benefit from the use of growth factors administered topically. Belcaplermin (Regranex, Ortho-McNeil) is a recombinant human platelet-derived growth factor that, when applied in daily to the surface of diabetic foot wounds, has demonstrated an increased incidence of complete healing in a shorter period of time (8). The product requires refrigeration and is expensive, but the cost may be justified when the patient requires a shorter period of wound therapy and returns more promptly to a functional status.

Wound closure may also be enhanced with mechanical maneuvers. The application of a subatmospheric pressure dressing to a foot wound provides a number of features that promotes wound closure. A foam sponge placed on the surface of an open wound and connected by plastic tubing to a vacuum pump (Vacuum Assisted Closure, Kinetic Concepts, Inc.) is effective in promoting the formation of granulation tissue (Fig. 3A and B). The vacuum dressing augments wound contracture through the application of a constant, localized negative pressure. The apparatus is also effective in removing interstitial wound fluid and necrotic debris and thereby decreasing the buildup of devitalized exudative products that act to impede wound closure. In addition to the mechanical benefits of this process, the dressing provides a closed, moist wound-healing environment. Because the dressing is usually left in place for a 48-h period, wound care is simplified, allowing more efficient use of resources in the outpatient setting (9–11).

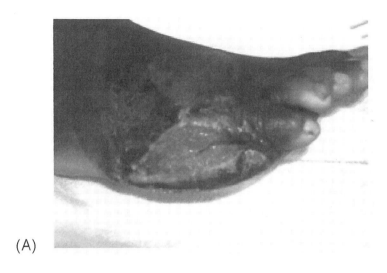

(A)

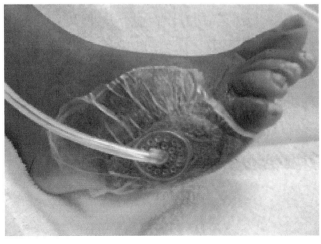

(B)

Figure 3 (A) Foot ulcer covered with granulation tissue; (B) Foot ulcer treated with vacuum closure device. Ulcer is covered with foam sponge secured with occlusive dressing incorporated with vacuum pump tubing.

III. CASE MANAGEMENT

A. Disordered Architecture—No Infection

The feet of patients with diabetic peripheral neuropathy will be at risk for complications from their disordered foot architecture. In some cases, the sensory deficit will lead to neurotrophic ulceration; while these lesions result in disruption of the skin envelope, they do not always represent a clinical infection. In the case of a superficial wound and in the absence of swelling, erythema, and purulent discharge or wound exudate, the patient does not require treatment for a soft tissue infection. The abnormal configuration of the foot skeleton requires adaptive footwear to offload abnormal strike points and weight-bearing surfaces that can result in continued soft tissue trauma.

A typical presentation involves superficial ulceration between the digits (Fig. 4). These lesions frequently occur due to simple compression of the toes within the toe box of the shoe. Diabetic patients are particularly at risk for developing these lesions when they are outfitted with new shoes. Their neuropathy will not allow them to notice that the shoes do not fit properly or to appreciate where the stiff fabric of the shoe is creating abnormal contact with the foot. Even this type of minor trauma, which would quickly be obvious to a person with normal sensation, will go unrecognized and lead to tissue breakdown. Diabetic patients must be cautioned to inspect their feet daily and, when using new footwear, more than once a day in order to prevent this complication. When a superficial ulcer forms, the offending pressure must be relieved. The wound should be treated with a hydrocolloid dressing to provide a proper wound-healing environment. In the presence of a normal arterial perfusion pressure, new epithelialization should occur.

B. Chronic Neurotrophic Ulcer—Callus—Sinus Tract

The patient with diabetic neuropathy may have a chronic callus, usually occurring over the first or fifth metatarsal head. This is likely to be due to pressure resulting from an abnormal gait due to the lack of normal sensation of the foot striking the floor. In the absence of protection of the skin surface, a thickened layer of epidermis forms a callus at the site. Eventually this thickened area of cornified skin becomes vulnerable to bacterial invasion, either from breakdown at the interface of the callus and the normal skin or due

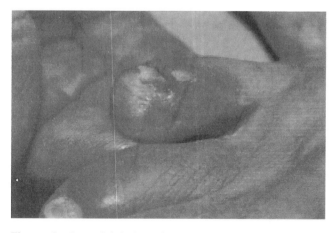

Figure 4 Superficial ulceration created from pressure of toes compacted in poorly fitting shoe.

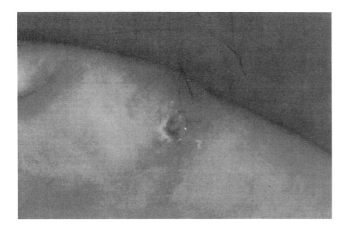

Figure 5 Chronic callus with subcutaneous abscess and sinus tract.

to some trivial injury to the foot. As the callus separates from the normal tissue, a space forms that may sequester fluid, leading to chronic drainage (Fig. 5). Reduction of the callus and the use of corrective footwear may eliminate the source of the abnormal pressure and allow soft tissue healing. If the space beneath the callus is not well drained, conditions exist for the formation of an abscess. Because of the neuropathy, it is unlikely that the patient will sense of the normal inflammatory response. Recognition of the problem may be prompted by the drainage of foul smelling fluid or swelling and erythema associated with the infection. This condition represents a surgical emergency. The wound should be explored under regional anesthesia and broad-spectrum antibiotics prescribed. In the operating room, the callus should be unroofed and the wound widely debrided. Usually the amount of underlying soft tissue destruction will be more extensive than might be anticipated from the initial appearance of the wound (Fig. 6). After surgical debridement, the wound should be treated with hydrogel dressings. The site should be inspected at

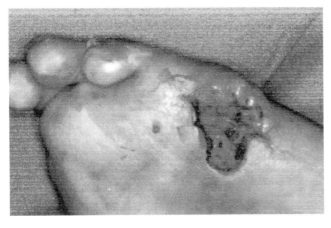

Figure 6 Site of chronic callus after surgical debridement.

least every 12 h to determine that all of the infection has been drained. The presence of purulent fluid entering the wound when pressure is applied to the margins dictates that the patient should be returned to the operating room for more extensive drainage. With adequate arterial perfusion and a proper wound-healing environment, these wounds will usually close by secondary intention. When the wound has completely healed and the foot has a stable configuration, the patient should be referred for a custom orthotic with a total-contact insert to prevent further soft tissue injury.

C. Web Space Infection

A soft tissue ulcer and/or associated gangrene occurring in the web space of the patient with diabetes must be treated as a potentially serious, deep soft tissue infection (Fig. 7). Even though the patient may report that the condition has been present for only a short time, there may be a considerable amount of tissue necrosis beneath the surface of the wound. Radiographs of the foot should be obtained to detect the presence of gas tracking into the plantar space (Fig. 8). This type of wound requires urgent exploration in the operating room, and broad-spectrum antibiotics should be administered. Commonly, the infection will have extended to the joint space between the phalanx and the metatarsal and will usually involve the soft tissue of both of the toes adjacent to the web space. It will not be uncommon for the process to have extended to adjacent metatarsophalangeal joints, where chronic neuropathy and altered foot architecture will have allowed disruption of the planes normally separating these structures. The involved toes should be amputated and the adjacent metatarsal heads resected so that no cartilaginous surface remains exposed. The cartilage has no blood supply and will not allow granulation or wound healing.

It is not uncommon for the bacterial contamination to extend along the tracks of the tendinous attachments to the phalanxes, creating a plantar space infection. This area must be opened to allow resection of the devitalized tissue and permit drainage, which is usually are accomplished by opening the plantar space below the level of the metatarsals. However, at times the infection may be so extensive that the entire tract must be opened,

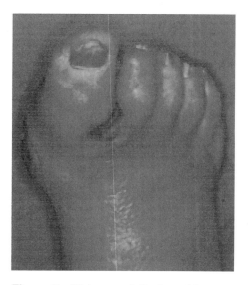

Figure 7   Web space infection with gangrene and invasive soft tissue infection.

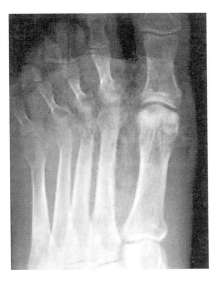

Figure 8   Radiograph of foot with severe soft tissue infection. Gas permeates the tissue and tracks into the plantar space.

onto both of the plantar and dorsal surfaces (Fig. 9). This creates a wedged defect in the foot. If there is viable tissue to form an adequate walking surface, and the soft tissue can be resected back to healthy margins, foot amputation should not proceed. After all of the infection has cleared, it is possible to reapproximate the defect and allow the remainder of the wound to heal by secondary intention (Fig. 10). This preserves a viable limb, providing a better alternative than below-knee amputation and lifetime use of a prosthesis.

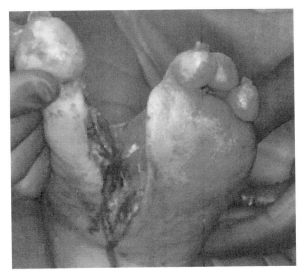

Figure 9   Surgical excision of complex soft tissue infection extending through the foot. The second metatarsal has been resected.

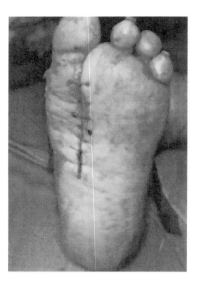

Figure 10 Following resolution of the infection, plantar surface is reconstructed to create a walking surface.

D. Maggots

On occasion a patient will present for evaluation with an open foot wound infested with maggots (Fig. 11). Such a condition obviously represents an aspect of poor personal hygiene, because the surface of the wound at some time would have been contaminated by the larvae, usually transmitted by a housefly. The maggots themselves are not actually harmful to the patient and, conversely, may be effective in cleansing the wound (12). However, their presence is usually untenable in a hospital situation, since they have not been prescribed as part of a medical application and are perceived as representing active wound contamination. Simple cleansing techniques are usually ineffective in removing the

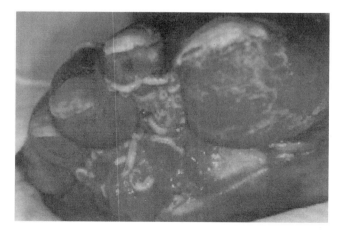

Figure 11 Maggots on surface of a chronic foot ulcer with gangrene.

creatures. However, they are rendered lifeless by the application of a topical spray anesthetic and can then be removed using simple surgical instruments.

E.   Tissue Loss and Gangrene

A diabetic foot infection may result from an ischemic site in one toe. Although one might think this due to neglect, in fact a polymicrobial infection in a diabetic patient can proceed very rapidly and destructively. At the time of presentation, there is not only dermal gangrene but also necrotic changes to the underlying soft tissue and frequently disintegration of the bone (Fig. 12 A and B). An infection of this magnitude represents a true surgical emergency as the patient is at risk for ascending infection and limb loss. Immediate

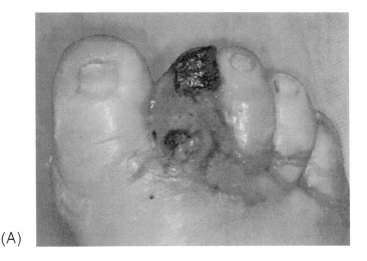

(A)

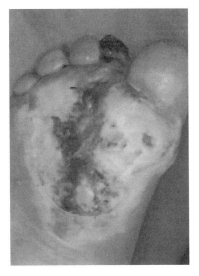

(B)

Figure 12   (A) Diabetic foot infection with extensive tissue loss and destruction of the second digit; (B) Gangrene and soft tissue infection involves the plantar surface over the second metatarsal.

operative intervention should be undertaken. Usually a general anesthetic is preferred if not contraindicated for cardiac or respiratory comorbidities, so that the scope of the resection will not be hindered by a limited regional anesthetic block. The surgeon and patient must be prepared to consider ankle disarticulation if the infection extends through the plantar space to the level of the ankle joint. However, it is possible that the infection will have been identified early enough that a local resection can be accomplished. The surgical incision should follow the margins of the devitalized tissue. Any exposed bone should be removed, and, with use of a bone rongeur, the metatarsals should be resected deep to the surface of the soft tissue plane. Exposed tendons should be divided and allowed to retract. The goal of the initial operation is to resect all infected material; attempts to preserve marginal anatomic structures for future reconstruction should be avoided. Scraping the soft tissue with a surgical curette is an effective method to differentiate viable from dead tissue. This maneuver will remove fragments of soft tissue that are unlikely to survive. At the conclusion of the surgical excision, the wound should be irrigated with saline solution (Fig. 13). A power irrigating system using up to 3L of fluid may be employed. The wound should then be treated with hydrogel dressings and inspected frequently for evidence of residual infection.

In the presence of a normal blood supply, granulation tissue should form on the surface of the wound after a week to 10 days (Fig. 14). When there is an extensive area of exposed soft tissue, a split-thickness skin graft is effective in providing wound closure (Fig. 15). If there is a suspicion of surface bacterial colonization, quantitative cultures can be obtained to avoid the complication of placing a skin graft on an infected surface. Colony counts of less than 10^5 micro-organisms per cubic centimeter are usually considered acceptable to proceed with skin grafting.

F.   Failed Transmetatarsal Amputation

A diabetic foot infection may lead to loss of all of the digits on a patient's foot, requiring open transmetatarsal amputation. It is not uncommon for this more extensive degree of tissue loss to be associated with poor arterial perfusion of the distal foot. Following the normal principles of treating a surgical infection, all of the devitalized tissue is debrided.

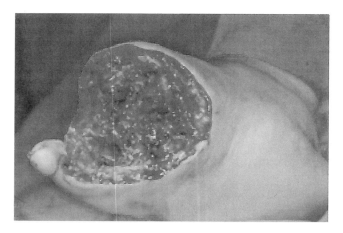

Figure 13   Forefoot immediately following wide debridement of extensive diabetic foot infection.

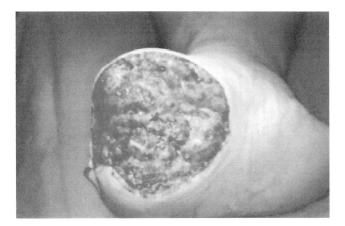

Figure 14 Surgical wound after 5 days with further debridement and amputation of the residual fifth digit.

Once it is evident that the wound is clean, the metatarsal bones are further resected and a plantar flap is fashioned to provide soft tissue coverage to the terminal aspect of the foot. Although at the time of the procedure the tissue may appear viable, there may be evidence of inadequate wound healing several days or sometimes even weeks after the procedure. This may be manifest by separation of the wound margins, wound edge necrosis, or even recurrent infection (Fig. 16). Such a patient should be returned to the operating room for debridement of the wound, which is a good candidate for vacuum-assisted closure. The vacuum-assisted closure device is effective in promoting granulation tissue, removing wound exudate, promoting wound edge contracture, and providing a proper environment for secondary wound closure (Fig. 17). Frequently diabetic patients facing this clinical problem are not candidates for arterial revascularization due to the lack of target vessels in the lower aspect of the extremity, following the typical pattern of distal small vessel disease

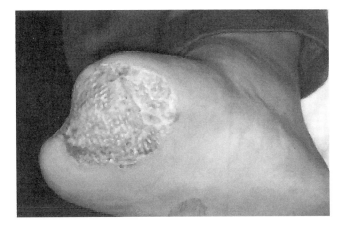

Figure 15 Wound after split thickness skin grafting. Wound edges have contracted.

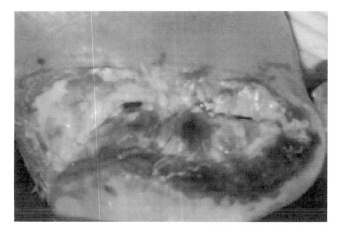

Figure 16 Transmetatarsal amputation on foot with chronic ischemia with wound edge necrosis and fibrinous exudate covering the wound surface.

in this population. Although the patient may require several months of wound care and often more than one return visit to the operating room, persistence will frequently result in limb salvage.

G. Ascending Infection

The most serious diabetic foot complication involves an ascending infection originating with involvement of a significant part of the foot. This surgical emergency requires urgent attention. Frequently these infections cause a necrotizing fasciitis that quickly spreads up the leg and can result in a true life-threatening condition. Patients should be moved promptly to the operating room and informed consent should be obtained for the possibility of open below-knee amputation. In the diabetic population, it is not unusual for these patients to be

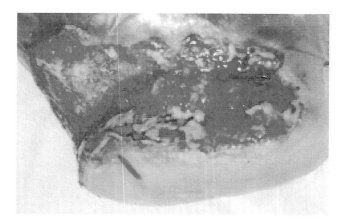

Figure 17 Transmetatarsal wound after treatment with vacuum dressing. Granulation tissue covers wound surface. Viable wound edges have contracted.

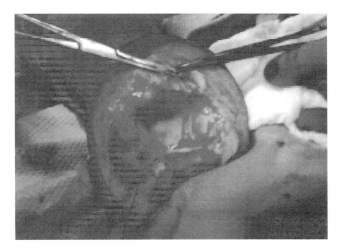

Figure 18 Ankle disarticulation for severe foot infection. Surgical clamps control the anterior and posterior tibial vessels.

metabolically unstable, with significant hyperglycemia and electrolyte abnormalities. When it is evident that there is no hope of salvaging the patient's foot, the surgeon should proceed to perform an ankle disarticulation. This procedure can be executed expeditiously with an incision that courses just distal to the lateral and medial malleoli, dividing the Achilles tendon posteriorly, and completing the incision across the dorsum of the foot. From this approach, the ankle joint space is easily entered and the foot can be removed without dividing any bone, requiring the incision of a minimal amount of soft tissue with a relatively limited blood supply (Fig. 18). Usually the infection will have been confined to the foot, and after a few days of antibiotic therapy, the residual soft tissue contamination will have been eradicated and the patient may be returned to the operating room for formal below-knee amputation. On occasion, however, there will be evidence of continued purulent drainage

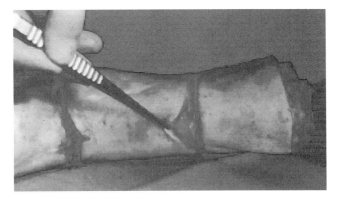

Figure 19 Level of ascending soft tissue infection is demonstrated with sequential transverse incisions.

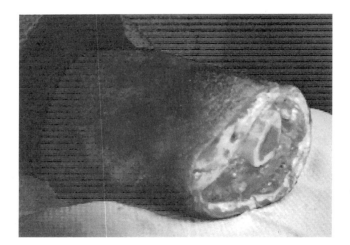

Figure 20   Guillotine amputation.

from the ankle disarticulation site. To determine the level of involvement, sequential transverse incisions should be performed above the level of the ankle until there is evidence of viable tissue free of infection (Fig. 19). At this level a guillotine amputation should be performed (Fig. 20). Secondary closure is performed when the patient is clinically stable and the wound free of residual infection.

REFERENCES

1. Centers for Disease Control and Prevention. National diabetes fact sheet: General information and national estimates on diabetes in the United States, 2000. Atlanta, GA: U.S. Department of Health and Human Services, Centers for Disease Control and Prevention, 2002.
2. Siperstein MD, Unger RH, Madison LL. Studies of muscle capillary basement membranes in normal subjects, diabetics and prediabetic patients. J Clin Invest 1968; 47:1973.
3. Krepel CJ, Gohr CM, Edmiston CE. Anaerobic pathogenesis: Collagenase production by *Peptostreptococcus magnus* and its relationship to site of infection. J Infect Dis 1991; 163:1148.
4. Centers for Disease Control and Prevention. *Staphylococcus aureus* resistant to vancomycin— United States, 2002. MMWR 2002; 51:557–565.
5. Murray BE. Drug therapy—Resistant enterococcal infections. N Engl J Med 2000; 342(10): 710–721.
6. Wilson P, Andrews JA, Charlesworth R, Walesby R, Singer M, Farrell DJ, Robbins M. Linezolid resistance in clinical isolates of *Staphylococcus aureus*. J Antimicrob Chemother 2003; 51:186–188.
7. Winter GD. Formation of scab and the rate of epithelialization on superficial wounds in the skin of the domestic pig. Nature 1962; 193:292–294.
8. Glover JL, Weingarten MS, Buchbinder DS, Poucher RL, Deitrick GA III, Fylling CP. A 4-year outcome-based retrospective study of wound healing and limb salvage in patients with chronic wounds. Adv Wound Care 1997; 10(1):33–38.
9. Argenta LC, Morykwas MJ. Vacuum assisted closure: a new method for wound control and treatment: Clinical experience. Ann Plast Surg 1997; 38(6):563–577.
10. DeFranzo AJ, Argenta LC, Marks MW, Molnar JA, David LR, Webb LX, Ward WG,

Teasdall RG. The use of vacuum-assisted closure therapy for the treatment of lower-extremity wounds with exposed bone. Plast Reconst Surg 2001; 108(5):1184–1191.

11. Kloth LC. 5 questions and answers about negative pressure wound therapy. Adv Skin Wound Care 2002; 15(5):226–229.

12. Sherman RA. Maggot versus conservative debridement therapy for the treatment of pressue ulcers. Wound Repair Regeneration 2002; 10(4):208–214.

13. Bacterial Isolate Reference Bank, Surgical Microbiology Research Laboratory. Department of Surgery. Milwaukee: Medical College of Wisconsin, 2002.

22

Complications of Lower Extremity Amputation

Kenneth E. McIntyre, Jr.

University of Nevada School of Medicine, Las Vegas, Nevada, U.S.A.

I. INTRODUCTION

Lower extremity amputation is one of the oldest and most commonly performed surgical procedures and yet has undergone very few modifications since its inception. Despite advances in limb-salvage surgery, lower extremity amputation is still commonly required as an end result of the progression of arterial occlusive disease or failed arterial reconstruction. Furthermore, the increasing prevalence of diabetes has led to the appearance of more patients with foot complications leading to eventual lower extremity amputation. In 1993, some 98,000 lower extremity amputations were performed in nonfederal acute care hospitals (1).

Since lower extremity amputation is an ablative procedure and often regarded as a "simple" one it is often delegated to interns in surgical training programs who may perform the operation without appropriate supervision. According to one Veterans Administration (VA) study, 75% of amputations were performed with a resident as the primary surgeon (2). Despite the fact that the procedure itself is not technically difficult, complications can and do occur. Moreover, a high surgical mortality rate is associated with major lower extremity amputation; this is often underappreciated by patients as well as physicians unfamiliar with amputation surgery. The most common chronic ailments leading to lower extremity amputation are diabetes mellitus and peripheral arterial occlusive disease (PAOD) (2–5). In a recent review of amputations performed at VA hospitals over a 10-year period, diabetes accounted for 62.9% and PAOD for 23.6% (2).

The complications and impressive operative mortality seen with lower extremity amputation are a reflection of the medical comorbidities of this high-risk group of patients. This chapter identifies and discusses the complications that may commonly be encountered following major (above-knee or below-knee) lower extremity amputation.

II. MORTALITY

One of the most striking characteristics of lower extremity amputation is the associated high operative mortality rate. Selection bias in this elderly group of patients with co-morbid diseases accounts for the high operative mortality (Table 1). The most common chronic illness in the amputee population is diabetes, accounting for more than half of the nontraumatic amputations performed yearly (2–5). For example, amputation rather than revascularization may be selected as the appropriate alternative in an elderly patient who does not ambulate because of chronic pain or hemiplegia from prior stroke. An operative mortality rate of 4–16% for below-knee and 12–40% for above-knee amputations has been well documented (3,5–7). The cause of death is almost always related to the significant cardiovascular disease that is always present in patients with limb-threatening ischemia of the lower extremity (3,5,8). Fully two-thirds of perioperative amputation deaths occur as a consequence of myocardial infarction, congestive heart failure, or stroke (3). Even with the associated high operative mortality, extensive preoperative cardiac evaluations are usually unnecessary unless there is also severe ventricular dysfunction, unstable angina, or recent myocardial infarction.

III. WOUND HEALING FAILURE

The most worrisome complication following amputation at any level is failure of the amputation stump to heal primarily. Healing failure results in prolonged hospitalization and delayed rehabilitation; it may even require amputation revision to a more proximal level. Primary healing occurs in direct relation to the level of amputation—i.e., the more proximal the level of amputation, the higher the rate of primary healing. However, the rehabilitation potential of an amputee with a healed below-knee amputation stump far exceeds that of one with an above-knee stump (9–11). For this reason, below-knee amputations should always be considered as a first alternative in patients who require major lower extremity amputation (Table 2).

When the amputation level is selected based on a physical examination alone, primary healing can be anticipated in 80–85% of below-knee and 85–90% of above-knee amputations (3,12). Failure of the suture line to heal primarily may be attributed to stump infection, hematoma, or poor nutritional state prior to amputation. However, as a general rule, the amputation site will heal primarily as long as there is enough blood flow to ensure

Table 1 Preexisting Disease in Patients Undergoing Lower Extremity Amputation

Disease	Percent
Diabetes mellitus	60–82
Ischemic heart disease	26–77
Cerebrovascular disease	20–25
Hypertension	15–70
Chronic obstructive pulmonary disease	5–20
Smoking	50–100
Renal failure	10

Source: Data from Refs. 3, 4, 7, 10, 11, 19, 33, and 37.

Table 2 Complications Occurring After Lower
Extremity Amputation

Complication	Percent
Failure to heal	3–28
Infection	12–28
Flexion contracture	1–3
Stump pain/phantom limb pain	5–30
Deep vein thrombosis	5–40

Source: Data from Refs. 3, 5, 7, 8, 12, 13, 19, 22,
28, 29, 33, 35, and 36.

healing at the skin level selected for amputation. Most commonly, failure of the amputation site to heal primarily often occurs when an inappropriate level for amputation is chosen without regard to skin perfusion at that level. For this reason, several preoperative tests have been developed to accurately assess the skin perfusion at any given level, thereby improving the rate of primary healing. These tests range in scope from determining Doppler-derived systolic ankle pressures to predicting skin blood flow using nuclear isotopes (3,13).

Doppler-derived systolic ankle pressures >30 mmHg predict below-knee amputation in 94% of patients (3,13). This test can easily be performed at the bedside and is highly reproducible. More involved preoperative tests can be performed using laser Doppler velocimetry, determining the washout of isotopic agents (Xenon 133) from the skin (14), or recording the transcutaneous P_{O_2} value at a selected amputation level. The accuracy of these tests in predicting successful amputation healing varies between 92 and 100% (3, 13,14). One must be aware, however, that systemic as well as local factors in the region selected for amputation level testing may reduce the reliability of the technetium P_{O_2} test. Oxygen content and cardiac output are systemic factors and local edema and/or cellulitis local factors that may adversely influence the reliability of the technetium P_{O_2} test (15).

Eneroth and Persson examined the risk factors for failure of wound healing in 177 consecutive patients undergoing amputation for ischemia. Absence of gangrene as well as a hemoglobin level >12 g predicted a higher rate of failure. In this review, age, sex diabetes, level of amputation, previous vascular surgery, smoking, preoperative blood pressure, serum creatinine, erythrocyte sedimentation rate, blood glucose, and fever had no correlation with ability of the amputation wound to heal (16).

Low serum albumin (<3.5 g) or total lymphocyte counts <1500/mm3 were both shown by Dickhaut et al. to adversely affect the healing ability of the amputee (17). The preoperative hematocrit may also have an effect on wound healing of amputation stumps. Hansen et al. documented a higher incidence of wound complications following below-knee amputation when the hematocrit was ≥40% (18). It has generally been accepted that patients with diabetes are more prone to wound complications. However, there is really no compelling scientific evidence that a difference in healing between those amputees with or without diabetes exists (7,19,20).

Finally, the specific technique used for below-knee amputations does not matter as long as standard surgical principles are utilized—i.e., meticulous technique, care not to leave devitalized tissue, strict hemostasis, and atraumatic tissue approximation without undue tension. Ruckley et al. compared the results of skew flaps versus long posterior flaps in a multicenter trial examining the outcomes after below-knee amputation. They found no significant difference in outcomes based on each surgical technique employed (21).

IV. INFECTION

Infectious gangrene alone rather than ischemia accounts for a significant number of amputations each year, especially among patients afflicted with diabetes mellitus. Unfortunately, when infection occurs in an amputation stump, revision of the stump to a higher level is often required. The incidence of infection in amputation stumps ranges from 12 to 28% and is correlated directly with the indication for amputation (7,19,20,22). When the amputation is performed following an unsalvageable foot infection, it is not surprising that the incidence of stump infection is four times greater than that when no foot infection exists (3). In the case of infectious gangrene of the foot, deep muscle as well as the lymphatics that drain the leg are filled with bacteria (23). Performing amputation with primary closure in this setting will often lead to infection of the stump and the need for subsequent revision. McIntyre et al. were the first to describe the benefit of two-stage amputation for infectious gangrene (20). This retrospective review documented a lower incidence of stump infection and need for revision in a group that underwent ankle guillotine amputation followed by definitive amputation at the below-knee level than in a group that underwent definitive below-knee amputation in one stage. In a related study, Desai et al. documented similar outcomes (24). In a prospective study designed to assess the benefit of two-stage amputation, Fisher et al. confirmed the benefits of two-stage amputation (23).

The use of prophylactic antibiotics was also found to be of benefit in reducing the risk of infection in the amputation stump. Sonne-Holm et al. compared preoperative cefoxitin to placebo in patients undergoing amputation for ischemia (25). They reported a wound infection rate of 16.9% in the antibiotic group compared to 38.7% in the placebo group. Norlin et al. employed prophylactic cefotaxime in 19 patients prior to amputation and compared it to placebo. They reported similar beneficial results, with 83% achieving healing in the antibiotic group compared to only 59% in the placebo group (26).

Rubin et al. documented an increased incidence of infection in the stump after below-knee amputation when a thrombosed prosthetic graft was left in place during the amputation procedure (27). When a thrombosed prosthetic graft is encountered during amputation, this complication can be avoided by retracting it the graft, carefully, transecting and allowing it to retract well away from the stump closure. A segment of the most distal remaining graft should be taken and sent for bacterial culture to ensure that no portion of retained graft is infected at the time of amputation.

V. PHANTOM LIMB PAIN

Chronic stump pain that occurs following lower extremity amputation can be difficult to treat. The incidence of chronic stump pain or phantom limb pain following major lower extremity amputation is between 5 and 30 (22,28). The etiology of chronic pain in the amputation stump is often unclear but may pose a significant problem that limits rehabilitation. The patient who develop, phantom limb pain following amputation may be so debilitated that he or she will not be able to walk with a prosthesis despite successful healing of the amputation stump. Phantom limb pain must be differentiated from a "phantom sensation," which is a feeling that the amputated limb is still present. True phantom limb pain is often described as "burning, aching, squeezing, and knife-like" often resembling the pain that the patient may have experienced prior to the amputation (3, 28,29). Phantom pain is persistent and can be exacerbated by proximal or remote stimuli. Moreover, phantom limb pain can be improved by changing the somatic input (28–30). Any stump pain that persists beyond 6 months following the amputation will be extraordinarily difficult to treat and will likely never resolve (30). Although there is no consensus on the best treatment for phantom limb pain, tricyclic antidepressants have been used successfully (28–30).

VI. FLEXION CONTRACTURES

Although it is not uncommon for flexion contractures to occur following lower extremity amputation, proper postoperative care will almost always avoid this problem. Unless careful attention is directed to prevention, flexion contractures following lower extremity amputation can be directly responsible for failure of rehabilitation. Flexion contractures should not be regarded as an insignificant problem, because without proper attention, successful rehabilitation cannot occur despite an otherwise well-healed amputation stump. Flexion contractures are due to disuse of a joint, because of major lower extremity amputation, and are more common in elderly amputees. The incidence of flexion contractures ranges from 1 to 3% and is more common in patients above 80 years of age and in those who have had a prior stroke on the same side as the amputation (3,7,19,31). The unopposed muscles responsible for hip and knee flexion after above-knee and below-knee amputation, respectively, cause these contractures. Strengthening and range-of-motion exercises directed by physical therapy preoperatively help to prepare the amputee for the physical requirements he or she will face following successful amputation. At the time of surgery, placing the below-knee amputation stump in a well-padded protective rigid dressing with the knee in slight flexion will help prevent flexion contractures of the knee (7,19,31). The above-knee amputee will tend to develop flexion contractures of the hip joint. Placing the patient in a prone position at regular intervals during the day will help to prevent flexion contractures of the hip. Standard daily physical therapy with range-of-motion exercises will also help to strengthen the patient and reduce the incidence of flexion contractures.

VII. INABILITY TO AMBULATE

Failure to ambulate with a prosthetic limb following an otherwise successful lower extremity amputation is attributable to several factors. First and most important is the patient's preamputation ambulatory status (3,5,7,32,33). Clearly, if a patient who is unable to walk undergoes lower extremity amputation, one cannot realistically expect that he or she will be able to walk following a successful lower amputation. All too often, patients who have been crippled by stroke or are disabled from severe arthritis require amputation and cannot successfully be rehabilitated, since they were unable to walk prior to the amputation. In addition, any cognitive impairment will have a negative influence on the ability to successfully complete rehabilitation. Similarly, if the preamputation medical condition is severe (e.g., congestive heart failure), the amputee will not usually be able to successfully rehabilitate, since more energy is needed to ambulate with a prothetic leg (5,32,33). That is, the amputee with limited cardiac reserve may not be able to generate the cardiac energy required to ambulate with a prosthetic leg. In these circumstances, it is really the patient's preamputation physical condition that determines his or her ability to achieve ambulation following lower extremity amputation. It is important to advise the patient undergoing amputation of the potential to fail rehabilitation based on the significance of comorbid illnesses.

VIII. DEEP VENOUS THROMBOSIS/PULMONARY EMBOLISM

The risk of deep venous thrombosis (DVT) and/or pulmonary embolism following lower extremity, amputation is not insignificant. However, DVT is often overlooked because swelling and pain, symptoms of DVT, often accompany lower extremity amputation. Of even greater concern is that DVT involving major veins may produce no symptoms. Therefore a high index of suspicion is needed to diagnose and treat DVT while reducing the risk of pulmonary embolism. Amputees are at increased risk over the conventional postoperative patient for several reasons. First, prolonged bed rest prior to and following amputation poses the risk of stasis. Second, vascular surgery patients are known to have an increased risk of hypercoagulability (34). Third, there is interruption (endothelial injury) of the major veins during the normal amputation procedure. It should come as no surprise, therefore, that the incidence of DVT occurring after lower extremity amputation varies between 5 and 40% (22,35). Yeager et al., in a prospective review of patients undergoing lower extremity amputations, reported no difference in the incidence of DVT between those who underwent above-knee versus below-knee amputations (35). Moreover, if DVT was present, it was diagnosed in the majority of patients (67%) preoperatively. If routine duplex venous scans is performed on amputees in the perioperative period, the incidence may well be higher. Fortunately, the risk of pulmonary embolism is significantly less than the risk of DVT. The incidence of pulmonary embolism following lower extremity amputation ranges between 1 and 5% (3). Certainly, if DVT is detected preoperatively, conventional intravenous heparin therapy should be used for several days prior to amputation to allow for some stability of the thrombus on the vein wall.

IX. LONG-TERM OUTLOOK

For elderly patients who have required lower extremity amputation as a consequence of diabetes and/or peripheral arterial disease, the long-term prognosis is not good. The mean survival of a lower extremity amputee is between 2 and 5 years (36). In patients with diabetes, the outlook for contralateral limb loss is even worse. Following a lower extremity amputation, 28–51% of the patients with diabetes will require amputation of the remaining leg within 5 years (37). A 5-year mortality rate of between 39 and 68% can be anticipated following lower extremity amputation in the patient with diabetes (37).

X. SUMMARY AND RECOMMENDATIONS

Lower extremity amputation is associated with a significant risk of perioperative mortality and complications. Those patients who undergo amputation have significant comorbid medical conditions that contribute to the risk of mortality and complications. Patients with diabetes and PAOD make up the greatest cohort of patients who undergo amputation of the lower extremity, and these risk factors are often responsible for the complications that may occur. Appropriate preoperative planning may help to reduce the complication rate. If an amputation is required to treat infectious gangrene, two-stage amputation should be performed to reduce the risk of stump infection, which may require revision to a higher level. When amputation is performed for ischemia, prophylactic antibiotics help to reduce the perioperative infection rate. Healing at the below-knee level should be the goal for any amputation that occurs above the ankle. If there is doubt whether an amputation will heal at a given level, several tests are available to evaluate skin perfusion. Appropriate preoperative physical therapy will help with rehabilitation outcomes. Attention to detail and appropriate pre- and postoperative care will help to avoid complications and improve rehabilitation potential following lower extremity amputation.

REFERENCES

1. Leonard JA Jr, Meier RH. Upper and lower extremity prosthetics. In: DeLisa JA, ed. Rehabilitation Medicine: Principles and Practice. 3rd ed. Philadelphia: Lippincott-Raven, 1998.
2. Mayfield JA, Reiber GE, Maynard C, et al. Trends in lower limb amputation in the Veterans Health Administration, 1989–1998. J Rehabil Res Devel 2000; 37.
3. Malone JM, Ballard JL. Complications of lower extremity amputation. In: Bernhard VM, Towne JB, eds. Complications in Vascular Surgery. St Louis: Quality Medical Publishing, 1991:313–329.
4. Most RS, Sinnock P. The epidemiology of lower extremity amputations in diabetic individuals. Diabetes Care 1983; 6:87.
5. Coletta EM. Care of the elderly patient with lower extremity amputation. J Am Board Fam Pract 2000;1323–34.
6. Berardi RS, Keonin Y. Amputations in peripheral vascular occlusive disease. Am J Surg 1978; 135:231–234.
7. Malone JM, Moore WS, Goldstone J, et al. Therapeutic and economic impact of a modern amputation program. Ann Surg 1979; 189:798–802.
8. Yekutiel M, Brooks ME, Ohry A, et al. The prevalence of hypertension, ischemic heart disease, and diabetes in traumatic spinal cord injured patients and amputees. Paraplegia 1989; 27:57.
9. Evans WE, Hayes JP, Vermilion BD. Rehabilitation of the bilateral amputee. J Vasc Surg 1987; 5:589.
10. Roon AJ, Moore WS, Goldstone J. Below-knee amputation. A modern approach. Am J Surg 1977; 134:153.
11. Steinberg FU, Sunwool I, Roettger RF. Prosthetic rehabilitation of geriatric amputee patients: A follow-up study. Arch Phys Med Rehabil 1985; 66:742.
12. Burgess EM, Matsen FA, Wyss CR, et al. Segmental transcutaneous measurements of P_{O_2} in patients requiring below the knee amputation for peripheral vascular insufficiency. J Bone Joint Surg 1982; 64:378.
13. Durham JR. Lower extremity amputation levels: Indications, methods of determining appropriate level, technique, and prognosis. In: Rutherford RB, ed. Vascular Surgery. 3rd ed. Philadelphia: Saunders, 1989.
14. Malone JM, Leal JM, Moore WS, et al. The "gold standard" for amputation level selection: Xenon-133 clearance. J Surg Res 1981; 30:449.
15. Lalka SG, Malone JM, Anderson GG, et al. Transcutaneous oxygen and carbon dioxide pressure monitoring to determine severity of limb ischemia and to predict surgical outcome. J Vasc Surg 1988; 7:507.
16. Eneroth M, Persson BM. Risk factors for failed healing in amputation for vascular disease: A prospective, consecutive study of 177 cases. Acta Orthop Scand 1993; 369.·
17. Dickhaut SC, DeLee JC, Pate CP. Nutritional status: Importance in predicting wound-healing after amputation. J Bone Joint Surg 1984; 66A:71.
18. Hansen ES, Wethelund JD, Skajaa K. Hemoglobin and hematocrit as risk factors in below-knee amputations for incipient gangrene. Arch Orthop Trauma 1988;10792.

19. Malone JM, Moore WS, Leal JM, et al. Rehabilitation for lower extremity amputation. Arch Surg 1981; 116:93.

20. McIntyre KE, Bailey SA, Malone JM, et al. Guillotine amputation in the treatment of non-salvageable lower extremity infections. Arch Surg 1984; 119:450–453.

21. Ruckley CV, Stonebridge PA, Prescott RJ. Skewflap versus long posterior flap in below-knee amputations: Multicenter trial. J Vasc Surg 1991; 13:423.

22. Gottschalk FA, Fisher DF Jr. Complications of amputation. In: Rutherford RB, ed. Vascular Surgery. 5th ed. Philadelphia: Saunders, 2000.

23. Fisher DF Jr, Clagett GP, Fry RE, et al. One-stage versus two-stage amputation for wet gangrene of the lower extremity: A randomized study. J Vasc Surg 1988; 8:428–433.

24. Desai Y, Robbs JV, Keenan JP. Staged transtibial amputations for septic peripheral lesions due to ischemia. Br J Surg 1986; 73:392.

25. Sonne-Holm S, Boeckstyns M, Menck H, et al. Prophylactic antibiotics in amputation of the lower extremity for ischemia. A placebo-controlled, randomized trial of cefoxitin. J Bone Joint Surg 1985; 67:800–803.

26. Norlin R, Fryden A, Nilsson L, et al. Short-term prophylaxis reduces the failure rate in lower limb amputations. Acta Orthop Scand 1991; 62:509.

27. Rubin JR, Yao JST, Thompson RG, et al. Management of infection of major amputation stump following failed femoro-distal grafts. Surgery 1985; 98:810.

28. Sherman RA, Sherman CJ, Parker L. Chronic phantom and stump pain among American veterans. Results of a survery. Pain 1984; 18:83.

29. Jensen TS, Brebs B, Nielsen J, et al. Immediate and long-term phantom limb pain in amputees: Incidence, clinical characteristics and relationships to preamputation limb pain. Pain 1985; 21: 267.

30. Esquenazi A, Meier RH III. Rehabilitation in limb deficiency. Arch Phys Med Rehabil 1996; 77(suppl):18.

31. Mooney V, Harvey JP Jr, McBride E, et al. Comparison of postoperative stump management: Plaster vs. soft dressings. J Bone Joint Surg 1971; 53A:241.

32. Cutson TM, Bongiorni DR. Rehabilitation of the older lower limb amputee: A brief review. J Am Geriatr Soc 1996; 44:1388.

33. Leung EC-C, Rush PJ, Devlin M. Predicting prosthetic rehabilitation outcome in lower limb amputee patients with the functional independence measure. Arch Phys Med Rehabil 1996; 77:605.

34. Taylor LM Jr, Chitwood RW, Dalman RL, et al. Antiphospholipid antibodies in vascular surgery patients: A cross-sectional study. Ann Surg 1994; 220:544.

35. Yeager RA, Moneta GL, Edwards JM, et al. Deep vein thrombosis associated with lower extremity amputation. J Vasc Surg 1995; 22:612.

36. Pernot HF, de Witte LP, Lindeman E, et al. Daily functioning of the lower extremity amputee: an overview of the literature. Clin Rehabil 1997; 11:93–106.

37. National Diabetes Data Group. Diabetes in America. 2d ed. Bethesda, MD: National Institutes of Health, 1995.

23

Complications of Vascular Access

Mark B. Adams, Christopher P. Johnson, and Allan M. Roza

Medical College of Wisconsin, Milwaukee, Wisconsin, U.S.A.

Currently more than 280,000 patients are maintained on chronic hemodialysis in the United States. Approximately 27,571 other patients undergo acute dialysis or hemofiltration in the treatment of a variety of conditions ranging from acute renal failure to drug overdose (1,2). Obtaining vascular access, temporary or permanent, in order to institute treatment in these patients requires the implementation of prosthetic devices, specific knowledge, and careful monitoring. Many of the complications related to vascular access are specific to the access technique, device, and site.

I. TEMPORARY ACCESS

Temporary access techniques use external prosthetic devices, such as Mahurkar catheters, that are not intended to be used on a permanent basis. With the advent of these temporary venous access devices, previous techniques, such as Scribner shunts and their variants, have fallen into disuse.

The most common form of temporary vascular access currently in use is the percutaneous subclavian or femoral dialysis catheter. Femoral catheters are not used as often as subclavian catheters because they are associated with a high rate of infection and thrombosis and are difficult to immobilize. Femoral catheters are often placed at the beginning of each dialysis treatment and removed at the end or after several treatments. Their use may lead to iliofemoral venous thrombosis, with its attendant risk of pulmonary embolism, and may also be the cause of significant retroperitoneal hemorrhage. The major advantage of using femoral catheters is avoidance of the risks associated with subclavian and jugular punctures. Iliofemoral thrombosis may become particularly problematic if and when the patient comes to renal transplantation.

Subclavian venous catheters remain a popular choice for temporary access. Subclavian catheters are introduced using standard subclavian technique over a guidewire. These are usually double-lumen catheters with the two lumens separated by 3–4 cm. The double-lumen catheter allows the patient to be dialyzed using the standard two-needle machine technique. Single-lumen catheters require a different technique, which generally gives a lower clearance rate and causes an increased recirculation effect. Because subclavian temporary (Mahurkar) catheters are associated with a high incidence of subclavian vein stenosis or occlusion, they should be avoided whenever possible. A better choice is an internal jugular catheter directed into the superior vena cava. One disadvantage of this placement is that the catheter protrudes near the patient's ear, making it annoying and difficult to dress.

Temporary dialysis catheters are available in a variety of models but have several characteristics in common. They must be of sufficient caliber to support the high flow rates required for adequate hemodialysis (greater than 200 mL/min) and rigid enough to prevent collapse when drawing pressures become high (3). The most commonly used temporary catheter is the Quinton-Mahurkar polyurethane double-lumen catheter (Quinton Instrument Co., Seattle, WA).

With careful nursing and patient management, these catheters may be left in place for 4–6 weeks, which is usually sufficient time to construct a permanent fistula.

There has been an increasing incidence of patients starting hemodialysis using a central venous catheter. In addition, a large percentage of patients are dependent on temporary catheters while obtaining permanent access at various times during their dialysis course (USRDS data).

Because Mahurkar catheters do not have a Dacron cuff, which functions as a barrier to bacterial colonization, they are associated with a high infection rate if left in place for more than a short time. Cuffed catheters (see below) provide longer and more reliable central venous access.

As the importance of reliable vascular access has become well accepted, a number of major efforts to promote a rational approach to the placement and maintenance of such access have been made. Notable have been the DOQI Guidelines of the National Kidney Foundation. This document stands as the best reference to vascular access in patients with end-stage renal disease (see clinical practice guidelines at www.kidney.org).

A. Complications

1. Infection

Infection represents the most common complication of temporary vascular access and requires the removal or replacement of the catheter. Infection will eventually occur in most percutaneously placed temporary access catheters. The clinical impact of infection related to the catheter can be minimized by early removal whenever signs of fever, pericatheter exudate, or erythema appear. In situations where the access site is of great clinical importance and another access site would be difficult to obtain, replacement of the catheter over a guidewire and careful observation with antibiotic coverage may allow continued use of the site for at least a short time.

As an additional barrier to infection, some dialysis catheters are manufactured with a proximal cuff (e.g., PermCath; Quinton Instrument Co., Seattle, WA). The cuff becomes incorporated into the subcutaneous tissue and retards the migration of bacteria along the catheter surface. The incidence of infection appears to be reduced with this modification, but these catheters remain prone to thrombosis and failure as a result of fibrin sheath formation at the tip. In general, their use is limited to patients in whom all other routes for permanent vascular access have been exhausted or in those patients in whom permanent access will not be usable for 6–8 weeks. The presence of a cuffed catheter lowers the risk of infection and usually provides reliable access at least until a permanent access site can be developed. These catheters have also been advocated for permanent use. In our hands, they have not worked well in this role. Other reports are more optimistic (4,5). However, they do not achieve flow rates or dialysis adequacy equal to that of peripheral access (6).

Cuffed subclavian dialysis catheters are often placed percutaneously using large dilators and peel-away sheaths. The size (20F) and rigidity of these sheaths are troublesome, however. Disruption of the subclavian veins and/or the superior vena cava have occasionally occurred. The safest way to place such catheters is using ultrasound imaging for initial placement with the additional use of fluoroscopy. Patients with a listing of multiple previous catheters are at significantly increased risk of complications and should have placement in a well-equipped interventional suite.

Internal jugular placement of both uncuffed and cuffed central catheters for dialysis has significantly lowered the incidence of central venous stenosis and/or occlusion. At present, most patients have a previous history of central venous catheters and up to 30% will have either central venous stenosis or occlusion (7). Because of this, further central catheter placement is best done with access to both ultrasound and angiography.

The way in which a subclavian dialysis catheter is cared for and flushed will, in many cases, determine its useful life span. Temporary subclavian catheters should be handled in an aseptic manner and flushed routinely with high-dose heparin solution (5000 U/mL). Care must be taken to aspirate the residual heparin before using the catheter for any purpose other than dialysis. Often the patient or a relative can handle flushing of the catheter, but in most cases qualified medical personnel should be responsible for the dressing change, since this requires knowledge and practice of sterile technique.

Recently, the LifeSite Hemodialysis Access System has been introduced as an alternative to cuffed catheters. The LifeSite is an implantable port (one or two valves), that can be accessed by subcutaneous puncture with a 14-gauge needle. In initial trials, this device was associated with lower infection rates than percutaneous catheters. The luminal diameter is slightly larger than that of conventional catheters, which also increases the effective flow rate on dialysis. However, this has raised concerns regarding central vein thrombosis (8,9).

2. Bleeding

The surgeon performing vascular access will undoubtedly become involved in situations where uremic patients experience excessive and prolonged bleeding. Most commonly, this occurs following percutaneous placement of access catheters.

Bleeding is more likely with temporary hemodialysis catheters of the uncuffed type than with other central venous catheters because of their size and rigidity and the manipulation that inevitably occurs. Bleeding can be minimized by careful handling of the catheter during dialysis. When bleeding occurs, it can usually be controlled by local pressure and correction of any coagulation abnormalities.

Uremic patients have a well-known tendency toward increased bleeding (10,11). The precise derangements are not entirely understood but predominantly relate to primary hemostasis (i.e., platelet-vessel interaction and platelet aggregation). The single best test that quantitatively measures this platelet dysfunction is the skin bleeding time. Other hemostatic defects that have been identified include abnormally increased production of prostaglandin I_2 by the uremic vessel wall, decreased production of platelet thromboxane A_2, changes in the von Willebrand factor (vWf) molecule, and decreased platelet factor III.

Presumably, the platelet dysfunction in uremia allows improved patency of vascular access. Observations that support this theory include the well-known propensity of fistulas to clot following successful renal transplantation and the generally accepted difficulty of maintaining vascular access in preuremic individuals.

Platelet transfusions will have little beneficial effect in these circumstances since, in the uremic milieu, normal platelets acquire the characteristics of uremic platelets. Cryoprecipitate is a plasma derivative and is a good source of factor VIII and vWf. Infusion of cryoprecipitate shortens the bleeding time of uremic patients, with the peak effect seen 4–6 h after infusion.

Desmopressin (DDAVP) is a synthetic derivative of an antidiuretic hormone and acts to increase plasma concentrations of vWf by releasing it from endothelial storage sites (12). Administration of DDAVP intravenously (0.3 /kg) temporarily corrects prolonged bleeding time and has a more rapid onset of action (peak effect, 1 h) than cryoprecipitate. DDAVP can also be given intranasally or subcutaneously at 10 times the intravenous dose.

Conjugated estrogens can normalize bleeding time for 3–10 days in patients with chronic renal failure. The mechanism of this effect is unknown but may relate again to an alteration of vWf. A single oral dose of estrogen (Premarin 25 mg) or intravenous doses (3 mg/kg) divided over 5 consecutive days may be effective and long-lasting (13).

Whenever bleeding occurs that is not easily controlled by pressure or is of high volume, the possibility of major vessel injury and/or coagulopathy should be considered. A bleeding time, prothrombin time, and partial thromboplastin time should be obtained and corrected with appropriate therapy. Most patients on dialysis have a significant qualitative platelet defect. Even if platelet counts are adequate, DDAVP or cryoprecipitate will often reduce bleeding that is otherwise difficult to control. Bleeding that occurs following dialysis or catheter flushing is often related to the effect of heparin and can be corrected by protamine. Heparinized patients usually respond to protamine. As in other surgical situations, however, it is unwise and unsafe to attribute ongoing bleeding to coagulopathy alone. If bleeding fails to come under control and the patient is in jeopardy, operation or interventional radiological approaches are indicated.

Major hemorrhage related to vessel injury is rare and most often occurs as a complication of venous perforation. Catheter removal, application of pressure, and correction of coagulation defects is the usual treatment. If the bleeding is vigorous and the catheter has been in place for some time, the possibility that injury or erosion into an artery has occurred should be considered. Several units of blood can easily be lost into the pleural space or retroperitoneum with few outward signs. Rarely, these patients require surgery to control arterial or venous lacerations. Operation should not be delayed if bleeding cannot be readily controlled.

3. Pneumothorax/Hemothorax

When the procedure is performed by experienced physicians hemothorax and pneumothorax are relatively uncommon complications of subclavian placement of temporary access (14). When it is performed by those with little experience or in patients with central venous problems from previous catheters, it is doubly dangerous because these complications are not only more likely to occur but also are often not immediately recognized. A postplacement chest x-ray should be obtained both to locate the catheter and to rule out hemorrhage or pneumothorax. These complications should be suspected whenever a patient complains of shortness of breath and/or when hypotension develops after catheter placement. The postplacement film should be carefully analyzed to make sure that the catheter has not transgressed the vessel wall into the pleural space.

The diagnosis can be difficult, since many of these catheters are placed just before the initiation of dialysis and patients may experience brief episodes of hypotension during hemodialysis as a result of reactions to materials in the dialysis system or to fluid shifts. The chance of a major hemorrhage is also increased in this setting because the patient is often systemically anticoagulated during dialysis. When hemothorax or pneumothorax is suspected, it should be treated by removal of the catheter and placement of a chest tube. X-ray film documentation should not delay appropriate treatment.

Catheter perforation of the superior vena cava is best treated by placing the patient in an upright position, inserting a chest tube, and removing the catheter. Hypotension should be rapidly corrected before placing the patient in an upright position, since this positional change can be dangerous in the hypovolemic patient.

4. Thrombosis

Catheter Thrombosis. Thrombosis of the catheter is a frequent problem encountered in patients with temporary central venous access. It can be treated by aggressive flushing with normal saline solution; enzymatic digestion with streptokinase, urokinase, or tissue plasminogen activator (TPA); or reestablishment of a lumen with a large guidewire. If these measures fail, the catheter can often be stripped angiographically via a femoral approach using a looped stripping device. If this is unsuccessful, the catheter will need replacement.

Subclavian Thrombosis. Acute subclavian thrombosis is not uncommon in patients with temporary access because of the size and mechanical properties of these catheters. If subclavian thrombosis/stenosis occurs, the catheter should be removed and another route of dialysis used. The administration of anticoagulation therapy (heparin) in this setting is controversial but should be considered. Pulmonary embolism in dialysis patients appears to be extremely rare. Patients with massively swollen arms may benefit symptomatically from a short course of heparin.

Replacement of the subclavian catheter on the opposite side may be unwise in such situations, since occlusion of both subclavian veins may lead to a superior vena cava syndrome. Also, bilateral subclavian thrombosis severely limits future choices for the site of permanent access but unfortunately may be unavoidable. When repeated thromboses occur, a primary hypercoagulable state should be suspected (e.g., antithrombin III deficiency, antiphospholipid syndrome, or protein C or S deficiency) (15). Such individuals frequently have associated heavy proteinuria (16). Antithrombin deficiencies can be effectively treated by administering fresh frozen plasma at the time of access placement and until conversion to long-term warfarin (Coumadin) therapy is complete.

With the increased use of subclavian dialysis catheters for initial vascular access in the patient presenting for dialysis, the incidence of subclavian thrombosis has increased, and may be as high as 30%. Creation of an arteriovenous fistula (AVF) distal to an occluded subclavian vein usually results in marked edema of the extremity and the eventual necessity of fistula takedown. Since subclavian dialysis catheters have been used previously in many patients currently referred for permanent access placement, the access surgeon must document that the subclavian vein is patent before proceeding with fistula formation. Verification of patency is most easily accomplished with duplex ultrasonography and can also be obtained with venography. The latter is more accurate than ultrasound, which has only an 80% sensitivity for proximal central vein obstruction (17). In the current milieu of ready placement of subclavian access, the importance of this step cannot be overemphasized.

5. Pulmonary Embolism

Pulmonary embolism appears to be rare in uremic patents because of their platelet dysfunction, but it should be suspected in any patient with a long-standing indwelling central venous or femoral catheter who experiences symptoms such as dyspnea or chest pain. Pulmonary embolism should also be suspected when thrombectomy of venous access catheters or a polytetrafluoroethylene (PTFE) graft is associated with dyspnea, hemoptysis, or deteriorating pulmonary function. The small size of these emboli makes death from a single embolus unlikely. However, repeated thrombectomy declotting could potentially produce a volume of embolus sufficient to produce chronic pulmonary hypertension.

II. PERIPHERAL ACCESS

Permanent vascular access is any type of access used frequently and repeatedly for an extended or indefinite period of time. Forms of permanent access include both autogenous AVFs and fistulas constructed with prosthetic material (PTFE, umbilical vein, Dacron) (18).

An autogenous AVF should be constructed even in patients undergoing peritoneal dialysis. Patients on peritoneal dialysis may have episodes of peritonitis or other complication, that temporarily interrupt their treatment. The average time patients who are started on peritoneal dialysis are able to be adequately managed via this modality is usually not more than a year or two. For most patients, peritoneal dialysis will not be their long-term means of renal replacement therapy. Because reliable autogenous access becomes increasingly difficult with time, all patients presenting for dialysis should be evaluated for autogenous access placement unless they can rapidly proceed to living donor transplantation. In addition, since patients with end-stage renal disease (ESRD) are experiencing increased longevity, cephalic veins are frequently used for intravenous therapy, usually resulting in thrombosis. The best time for fistula placement is when the patient initially presents with renal failure.

With more patients in renal failure presenting without adequate vessels available for autogenous fistula construction, the use of synthetic material has increased (19). The most common synthetic materials currently in use for access are PTFE (Gore-Tex, W. L. Gore and Associates, Inc., Elkton, MD; Impra, Impra, Inc., Tempe, AZ), tetrafluoroethylene (Medtronic, Minneapolis, MN; etc.), and tanned human umbilical vein (Biograft). PTFE is overwhelmingly the most commonly used material. Dacron has not proved useful because of the associated high rate of infection and pseudoaneurysm formation.

Theses materials are readily available and most vascular surgeons have experience with them in peripheral vascular reconstruction. Such fistulas have the advantage of being large and therefore easily palpated and cannulated. They can also be used soon after placement (20,21). This is particularly useful when a patient with advanced uremia is referred for urgent access, which has increasingly become the case. Synthetic grafts have their own significant and somewhat unique problems, however (22).

A. Choice of Access Location and Type—Autogenous

Permanent autogenous access is preferably placed at the wrist in the nondominant arm. This allows use of the dominant arm during dialysis and may lessen the chance of trauma to the fistula during daily activities. Unfortunately, in many patients, the cephalic vein at one or both wrists is unavailable for use, usually as the result of injudicious placement of intravenous lines by the time the patients are seen by a vascular surgeon. In these patients, obtaining autogenous vascular access becomes a challenge.

If neither wrist has a patent cephalic vein, the antecubital space is the next best site. An AVF at this site is constructed between the brachial artery and the cephalic vein or between the brachial artery and a connecting branch, such as the median antecubital vein. It is important to disconnect the new fistula from the deep venous system by ligation of deep veins going into the forearm to prevent the subsequent development of venous hypertension. This preferentially directs blood up the upper arm cephalic vein, which becomes the cannulation site.

Fistulas constructed between the brachial artery and the basilic vein or another deep vein are generally not successful, since dialysis personnel cannot consistently gain access to the deep venous system. In addition, because the vein is adjacent to the brachial artery, cannulation carries a risk of arterial injury.

Occasionally, the basilic vein in the upper arm can be transposed superficially by dissecting it out for a distance of 10–15 cm and then bringing it into a superficial position, where it is easy to cannulate. This procedure may lead to wound complications (seroma, hematoma, arm swelling) because of the extent of dissection required and the rich lymphatic network around the brachial and axillary arteries.

While upper arm cephalic vein fistulas have the advantages of high flow and earlier maturity, they may be difficult to cannulate reliably in obese patients.

When there are no usable veins in the arms for fistulas, a decision must be made whether to continue to pursue autogenous access or to construct access with prosthetic material. Although it is almost always easier to use prosthetic grafts, their useful life is not as good as that of autogenous access (23). Prosthetic AVFs generally last half as long and require twice as many interventions as autogenous AVFs.

Autogenous access occasionally can be constructed using the saphenous vein. It can be mobilized completely to the knee and then looped subcutaneously on the anterior surface of the thigh and anastomosed to the superficial femoral artery just distal to the bifurcation of the common femoral artery. Alternatively, in a thin patient, the saphenous vein can be left in situ and anastomosed end to side to the distal superficial femoral artery at the level of the adductor canal. It is unnecessary to ligate venous branches, since their presence only increases the venous outflow from the fistula. This particular procedure can easily be accomplished with the patient under local anesthesia and provides good length for easily accessible cannulation sites in a thin patient. The saphenous vein can also be harvested and transplanted to the arm for use as autogenous fistula graft material.

B. Prosthetic Arteriovenous Fistula

In the event that an autogenous fistula cannot be constructed, most surgeons prefer PTFE for prosthetic material. PTFE has generally outperformed most other prosthetic materials in terms of long-term patency. Many different sizes and shapes are currently available, including straight, tapered, stepped, and externally reinforced grafts as well as grafts with a hooded configuration at the venous end. No single form of PTFE has demonstrated clear superiority over others (24–26). Thicker-walled grafts are generally preferable because of their increased durability with repeated cannulations.

Forearm constructions include straight grafts (radial artery to antecubital vein) and loops (brachial artery looping back into antecubital vein). Loop grafts have the theoretical advantage of higher flow because of the larger artery on which they are based. However, this is a theoretical consideration, and loop grafts have not been proved to be superior over straight grafts.

Straight grafts have the advantage that, in the event of infection, graft removal is safer, since the radial artery can frequently be ligated without placing the hand in jeopardy. Ligation of the brachial artery will often result in tissue loss, especially in diabetic patients with extensive upper extremity peripheral vascular disease.

Upper arm loop prosthetic fistulas are based on the more proximal brachial artery and generally return into the basilic or deep venous system. Sites lower in the forearm should be selected first, since, with each successive access placement, the vein distal to the arteriovenous anastomosis is ligated to prevent venous hypertension. Therefore an upper arm loop generally precludes further attempts distally in the same arm.

When an upper arm loop PTFE fistula is being created, it is generally easier to perform both venous and arterial anastomoses at the same level (through the same incision medially on the upper arm). We usually do this with the venous anastomosis directed toward the heart and the arterial anastomosis situated deep to it. There may be some advantage in performing end-to-end venous anastomoses, although this has not been proved.

In general, it is unwise to cross joints with prosthetic graft material. Prolonged flexion at the joint, such as that which occurs during sleep, may lead to graft occlusion. However, use of spiral-wrapped reinforced PTFE can help to prevent kinking. Unfortunately, spiral-reinforced PTFE has an increased tendency to erode through the skin especially if placed too superficially or in thin elderly patients.

If access cannot be obtained in either upper extremity, more exotic maneuvers will need to be undertaken. It behooves the surgeon performing access to frequently remind his medical colleagues of the importance of preserving cephalic veins in those patients with renal disease, because once the cephalic vein is lost, obtaining good autogenous access becomes difficult.

C. Complications

1. Problems Associated with Cannulation

Because the technique for cannulation of synthetic grafts is different from that of autogenous AVFs, dialysis units with less experienced personnel have a high rate of perigraft hematomas, pseudoaneurysm formation, and graft infection.

Perigraft hematoma results from cannulation with the needle entering parallel to the graft and lacerating a portion of the graft wall. The result may be external bleeding or hematoma. Graft infection occurs when less than ideal aseptic technique is used during cannulation and dialysis. Proper technique involves puncturing the graft perpendicular to the long axis of the graft and then changing the angle of the needle once its tip has entered the graft lumen. It is important to avoid repeated punctures at the same site, since extensive damage to the graft wall will eventually result in pseudoaneurysm formation and/ or localized infection. The failure to rotate sites has increased during the last decade in the United States.

Perigraft hematomas should be treated conservatively unless signs of infection appear; if infection occurs, incision and drainage are required. Infected perigraft hematomas usually necessitate graft revision or removal. It is wise to avoid the use of a fistula with a large perigraft hematoma; temporary access should be obtained until the hematoma has resolved.

D. Maintenance/Surveillance

Once a fistula has been successfully constructed, the surgeon has an ongoing responsibility to the patient to ensure that the fistula lasts as long as possible. To maximize fistula longevity, the surgeon must consider three important points. First, the new fistula should not be used until it has had sufficient time to mature. Maturation of autogenous fistulas usually takes 2–3 months. In many cases the fistula can be easily palpated and cannulated before this time; however, the vein wall requires 2–3 months (DOQI) to sufficiently enlarge and arterialize. Early use frequently results in hematoma formation around the fistula, which may progress to scarring and stenosis and markedly shortens the useful life of the fistula. Fistulas constructed with prosthetic material usually require 10–14 days for sufficient incorporation of the foreign material. Premature puncture of the graft commonly leads to perigraft hematoma formation and a greater likelihood of infection.

Second, and whenever possible, the surgeon should ensure that dialysis personnel use proper aseptic technique at the time of cannulation and that they rotate puncture sites. Continual cannulation of a site leads to degeneration of the vessel or prosthetic graft wall, with pseudoaneurysm formation and/or infection. This is a matter of education and communication, which is the surgeon's as well as the nephrologist's responsibility. It is also important to avoid cannulation in the vicinity of the anastomotic sites to prevent cutting a suture and causing disruption.

Third, the dialysis nurses and technicians should be informed of the need to contact the surgeon whenever a problem with the fistula occurs. Early detection of changes in the hemodynamic characteristics of the fistula—such as high venous pressures, which frequently precede thrombosis—is vital. Correction of the abnormality before the fistula clots will markedly improve the useful life of the access site.

E. Thrombosis

Thrombosis is the most common problem with hemodialysis access. The majority of patients on hemodialysis will need revision or thrombectomy of their access at some time or other. Once thrombosis occurs, performance of a fistulogram is useless. Early surgical exploration or declotting by percutaneous intervention yields the highest salvage rates. At exploration, a careful search will usually determine the cause of thrombosis. Unless the cause is discovered and the problem corrected, thrombectomy will be unsuccessful in reestablishing a usable fistula. This cannot be overemphasized.

In most cases, the existing graft or fistula can be salvaged with thrombectomy and revision. AVFs that have been clotted longer than 24–48 h have a lower rate of salvage, probably because of the intimal damage that occurs when clot is present in the vessel lumen. Even in patients who present late following thrombosis of an AVF, unless overt phlebitis is evident, an attempt at thrombectomy or reconstruction should usually be made. Interventional approaches to declotting of autogenous AVFs (especially radiocephalic ones) are not often successful. Therefore, a long-standing autogenous AVF that occludes should generally be approached surgically.

Thrombosis of synthetic AVFs occurs frequently enough that many surgeons view it as a routine part of the management of fistulas made with synthetic material. In most cases, such grafts can be successfully thrombectomized if both arterial and venous connecting vessels are patent and thrombectomy is accomplished before clot has propagated and occluded the proximal venous runoff or before extensive intimal damage has occurred in the runoff vessel. Recently placed grafts are easy to thrombectomize. Older grafts may accumulate thick layers of pseudointima, which is difficult to remove. When this is the situation, it usually is better to excise and replace the graft or to place another fistula elsewhere.

It is important to remove all thrombus from the arterial and venous ends of the fistula. Visualization of the arterial end can be difficult once blood flow is restored. One way to obtain a good look at the arterial anastomosis is to temporarily occlude arterial flow with a proximal sterile tourniquet, which allows complete inspection and calibration of the arterial anastomosis with a minimal amount of blood loss. Calibration can be performed with a balloon catheter or coronary dilator. Both anastomoses should be directly visualized. When there is less than a clear, strong, palpable thrill proximally in the fistula, an operative fistulogram should be obtained.

The most common cause of graft thrombosis with synthetic material is stenosis at or proximal to the venous anastomosis. This probably represents a form of pseudointimal hyperplasia often seen in PTFE peripheral arterial reconstructions. Correction requires angioplasty, bypass, or movement of the anastomosis to another outflow vein.

Assessment of what constitutes adequate venous runoff is probably the single most difficult decision in creating a permanent venous access. Calibration of the outflow tract with coronary artery dilators is useful. A critical property of the outflow vein is elasticity. Free passage of anything smaller than a No. 3 coronary dilator is probably insufficient. If the graft or vein has a strong pulse but no thrill, venous outflow obstruction is present.

The interventional radiologist has gained a significant role in the management of access problems. This has had both positive and negative effects. On the positive side, the current ability to percutaneously perform thrombectomy, diagnostic angiography, and/or angioplasty with or without stenting has prolonged the life of many access sites. Negative effects include cost as compared to surgical thrombectomy/revision and lack of planning that incorporates important aspects of the patient's history and prognosis. We utilize a system in which the patient is first evaluated by a surgeon, who decides the best course of action for the patient based on past history, physical examination, performance in dialysis, etc. Repeated interventional thrombectomies are rarely justified.

III. USE OF DIALYSIS HISTORY AND PHYSICAL EXAMINATION

A. Arterial or Inflow Stenosis

Arterial or inflow stenosis may be diagnosed by noting that before occlusion the fistula was not providing adequate inflow into the dialysis machine (frequent "negative pressures"). On physical examination before occlusion, the fistula usually appears somewhat collapsed or has a weak pulse when occluded downstream. Such inflow stenoses are most common in radial artery–based fistulas. Treatment usually involves revision of the fistula with anastomosis to a more proximal area of the radial artery. If there is no associated venous stricturing, the cephalic vein can be thrombectomized and will provide excellent outflow. Because the vein is already arterialized, such a fistula can be used immediately following revision.

B. Venous or Outflow Stenosis

This situation is diagnosed by noting that before occlusion, high venous (or "return") pressures were present. In autogenous fistulas, venous stenoses are usually caused by premature cannulation of an inadequately arterialized vein or by repeated punctures at the same site. Occasionally it is possible to revise the anastomosis or bypass the area of stenosis. However, in many cases the stenoses are multiple and cannot be bypassed; therefore the fistula must be moved to another site. In PTFE fistulas, neointimal hyperplasia at the distal venous anastomosis is the common cause of stenosis; it is best treated by patch angioplasty or revision with bypass of the area of stenosis. Alternatively, balloon angioplasty and stenting can be used.

C. Hypotension

Patients undergoing hemodialysis frequently experience episodes of hypotension due to the removal of extracellular fluid during dialysis or occasionally from sepsis. AVFs may thrombose during these events. If the fistula was functioning well before thrombosis, thrombectomy is frequently successful. As noted earlier, it is wise to carefully evaluate both arterial and venous limbs at the time of thrombectomy to rule out mechanical obstruction as a predisposing factor. Hypotension on dialysis is usually due to aggressive fluid removal. This sometimes is the result of the patient having gained significant weight between dialysis treatments. It is more often a problem in small patients who are noncompliant with fluid restrictions and following the treatment occurring after a 2-day gap (e.g., Monday for a patient on M-W-F dialysis).

D. Hypercoagulable State

Hypercoagulable states are not uncommon in dialysis patients and should be considered in two situations: (a) when a well-functioning fistula suddenly thromboses and cannot be salvaged even though the thrombectomy or revision seems adequate intraoperatively and (b) when a patient on chronic hemodialysis presents with a history of repeated unsuccessful attempts at obtaining vascular access by experienced vascular surgeons.

Any patient in whom a technically adequate AVF has failed to remain patent should be suspected of having a hypercoagulable state. "Technically adequate" is defined as the operative documentation of a palpable thrill or postoperative presence of a clearly audible bruit in the AVF and/or intraoperative measurement of adequate blood flows. If an adequate thrill and bruit are present but are subsequently lost in the early postoperative period, the patient should be evaluated for a coagulation abnormality. An "adequate thrill or bruit" should be present throughout the entire cardiac cycle, indicating sufficient arterial inflow and low outflow resistance.

The two most common abnormalities resulting in hypercoagulability and access thrombosis are antithrombin III deficiency and heparin-induced platelet aggregation. Patients with antithrombin deficiency can usually be managed by perioperative infusion of fresh frozen plasma to supply the missing factors, followed by warfarin therapy. Patients with heparin-induced platelet aggregation often have a history of frequent blockage of dialysis coils by clots. If hemodialysis is the only means for maintenance dialysis, these patients can usually be dialyzed without the use of heparin; however, this situation presents difficulties for most dialysis units. Many of these patients will eventually require peritoneal dialysis. Most patients with a hypercoagulable state will need long-term warfarin anticoagulation. Additionally, patients with repeated episodes of graft thrombosis of unknown origin are best served by chronic anticoagulation.

E. Erythropoietin

Because erythropoietin is now administered to most hemodialysis patients, they are usually not as anemic as before its availability. Anemia contributes to impaired coagulation in uremic patients and thus promotes patency of AVFs (27). Vigorous correction of anemia using erythropoietin therapy may therefore serve to potentiate thrombosis. However, it has been our experience that patients on erythropoietin therapy in whom the fistula thromboses have a technical abnormality that explains the incident.

F. Pseudoaneurysm Formation

Pseudoaneurysms occur commonly in AVFs that have been used for vascular access over a prolonged period. They occur in both autogenous and prosthetic fistulas and can result from improper technique in graft cannulation, failure to rotate sites, and the nonhealing nature of prosthetic material. If pseudoaneurysms erode through overlying skin, the result may be life-threatening hemorrhage. The risk of erosion is best judged by whether the skin over the pseudoaneurysm is fixed or movable. Skin that is firmly fixed and thin should prompt corrective action. Once this condition is diagnosed, it can be corrected by by-passing or replacing the involved segment with new material or, when the pseudoaneurysm involves an anastomosis, by reconstructing that portion of the AVF.

Occasionally, a pseudoaneurysm is so large and complex that it requires sacrificing the fistula. The principal risks of pseudoaneurysm are continued enlargement with throm-bosis, rupture, or distal embolization. Dialysis personnel should be cautioned to avoid repeated cannulation of areas of pseudoaneurysm because of the risk of skin breakdown and rupture.

G. Infection

Infection can occur in any fistula but is more common with vascular access using synthetic graft material or in lower extremity AVFs, particularly in obese patients. It is usually related to lack of proper aseptic technique at the time of cannulation (28). Repeated cannulations at the same site and poor sterile technique (e.g., poor skin preparation, touching the prepared site with an ungloved finger) also place the fistula at higher risk for infection. Such infections can occasionally be managed by excision of the involved segment if the graft has been well incorporated before onset of the infection and the infected area does not involve an anastomosis to a host vessel.

More often, infection in prosthetic material involves one or both anastomoses and the whole graft must be removed. Before a wound with a suspected prosthetic graft infection is opened, a proximal tourniquet should be readily available. At the time of removal, a small rim (2–3 mm) of prosthetic material may be left attached to the artery to provide a secure closure. It is technically difficult to excise all the PTFE and close the arteriotomy without occluding it because of the arterial wall retention, which occurs after the PTFE-to-artery anastomosis. Infected wounds are best left open and allowed to heal secondarily. However, it is a good idea to cover the arterial closure with soft tissue.

Infection that occurs in an autogenous fistula is usually the result of a secondary infection of a hematoma surrounding the fistula caused by repeated cannulation of the same segment of vein. Because of the autogenous nature of the infection, these can often be treated with antibiotics and local care unless hemorrhage is threatened or has occurred.

When prosthetic materials are inserted, perioperative coverage with systemic anti-biotics is recommended. A single dose of an antibiotic with gram-positive coverage (first-generation cephalosporin, nafcillin, or vancomycin) is probably sufficient. The surgeon should try to anticipate when prosthetic material might be used so that antibiotics can be administered before the skin is incised.

Infection involving a major artery, such as the brachial artery at its bifurcation or the superficial femoral artery, may place a limb in jeopardy. With synthetic grafts placed in the groin, the arterial anastomosis should be made to the superficial femoral artery and not to the common femoral artery. In this way, if graft infection should occur and ligation of the donor vessel becomes necessary, it may be done with a lesser chance of limb compromise. In general, it is better to avoid placing any prosthetic material in the groin for vascular access if alternate sites are available in the upper body.

H. Venous Hypertension

Venous hypertension results from either high flow into a venous bed distal to the AVF and/ or proximal venous occlusion (29). Occasionally both conditions may be present. Patients usually present with redness and edema of a hand or arm, and stasis ulcers may actually develop. Other signs of venous stasis include rapid capillary filling time, cyanosis, brawny edema, and ecchymosis. If the AVF is placed at the wrist, there prominent pulsatile veins are usually palpable through the edema on the dorsum of the hand. When an antecubital fistula is the source of venous hypertension, patients more commonly present with edema of the hand and forearm and a vigorous thrill at the site of the fistula extending distally into the forearm.

Attention to detail at the time of initial access placement can usually avoid post-operative venous hypertension. Distal venous branches from the fistula should be ligated unless such branches allow for the filling of vessels that will be needed for access. The most common example of this situation is the lateral ulnar vein on the dorsum of the forearm, which in some cases will fill through a branch off the distal cephalic vein proximal to the fistula. In the case of an antecubital AVF, the distal cephalic vein extending to the forearm may provide excellent sites for cannulation and should be preserved. However, venous branches going deep in to the forearm and proximally along any major arteries should be ligated. Even though there is no apparent flow at the time of fistula construction, as veins dilate, venous valves may become incompetent, resulting in distal flow and venous hypertension.

If a patient with a previously functioning AVF suddenly presents with venous hypertension, deep venous occlusion should be suspected. This serious situation can be resolved only by takedown of the fistula on the affected side. If the fistula is patent at the time, it may be possible to secure new access elsewhere before taking down the fistula causing venous hypertension. Delay in takedown in this situation may put the patient at risk for subsequent skin necrosis.

I. Fistulogram

A fistulogram is a radiographic contrast study of the AVF to define arterial and venous anatomy. Although noninvasive techniques such as color duplex ultrasound scanning can provide similar information, a fistulogram provides the precise anatomical information that the surgeon requires. A fistulogram may play an important role in diagnosing and treating venous hypertension and the failing fistula. It aids in both locating venous branches supplying the distal venous bed and documenting the presence or absence of proximal deep venous occlusion.

The technique is simple and can be done without formal arteriography. A needle is placed into a vein connecting with the AVF or into the prosthetic graft itself and a blood pressure cuff is placed high on the upper arm and inflated above systolic pressure. Intra-vascular contrast (usually full-strength) is injected into the needle, thus filling both veins and arteries supplying the fistula. More than a single view may be necessary to demonstrate the relevant anatomy. The fistulogram is rarely of use in the evaluation of a thrombosed fistula and its use in this situation should be abandoned.

Immediately following thrombectomy and/or revision, the surgeon may wish to perform an intraoperative arteriogram. This often proves useful because unsuspected stenoses may be identified and corrected before the next episode of thrombosis occurs. It is rarely necessary to perform angiography. Venography is occasionally of use in the evaluation of veins preoperatively in obese patients in whom physical examination alone is inconclusive.

Many dialysis units now monitor blood flows ultrasonically and send patients with lower blood flows for study by fistulogram. Hopefully, this practice will identify problematic AVFs before occlusion occurs, allowing correction of abnormalities.

J. Steal Syndromes

Steal syndromes occur most often in elderly and/or diabetic patients with advanced peripheral atherosclerosis involving the arteries of the upper extremities. Patients at high risk usually have skin changes typical of diabetes and at operation have heavily calcified atherosclerosis of even 2- to 3- mm vessels. These patients can usually be identified preoperatively by careful palpation of the radial artery and/or by the examination of x-ray films of the forearms for vascular calcifications. Attempts to obtain vascular access for hemodialysis are often unsuccessful in these patients. However, some individuals with calcified vessels can still undergo successful fistula placement. A more precise approach is the use of vascular laboratory measurements of finger pressures on both sides. The side with the least severe disease can be chosen for placement of the fistula. In extremities with finger pressures below 90 mmHg, the results will predictably be poor. Any fistula placed in a patient with arterial insufficiency of the limb places distal tissue at risk; such placement should be avoided. Some patients may not have an acceptable site for vascular access and will need to have peritoneal dialysis or dialysis via a central catheter.

If the access has already been placed and ischemic changes of the hand or fingers develop, the fistula should be taken down urgently. Once ischemic neuropathy or gangrene develops, many of these patients will eventually require amputation of fingers and, on occasion, a hand. Attempts at downsizing a fistula in this situation are usually unsuccessful and prolong the period of ischemia.

IV. THE FAILING FISTULA

Many episodes of access failure can be prevented if the surgeon, nephrologist, and dialysis personnel work in concert to identify and correct access problems before thrombosis occurs. This same principle has been shown to apply in peripheral arterial bypass surgery (30). The role of noninvasive evaluation of access function has been unclear. Early studies suggested that routine Doppler evaluation of AVFs was useful in predicting which AVFs were at risk for problems. These efforts were short-lived because of lack of reimbursement for this surveillance. Venous pressure measurements during hemodialysis became the main surveillance technique used by dialysis personnel. Recently there has been increased use of ultrasonic measurements of access blood flow to predict thrombosis (31,32). This has the advantage of quantitating a change over time for a given patient. It requires relatively little time and effort and can serve to identify a patient's risk for access failure. Timely referral to a vascular surgeon should be made. Often the problem can be diagnosed by history and physical examination. If not, a fistulogram should be performed. If the fistulogram identifies a problem amenable to angioplasty/stenting, it can be performed at the same sitting. If not, plans can be made for surgical revision or new AVF placement. Access issues should be viewed as urgent and dealt with accordingly. Delay often complicates both the problem and the solution.

Vascular surgeons are frequently called to evaluate patients with "failing fistulas," that is, AVFs that previously provided adequate sites for cannulation and flow on dialysis for prolonged periods of time but have become difficult to cannulate or are not providing enough flow for adequate dialysis. In these situations it is important to speak directly with the dialysis nurse or technician to determine the exact nature of the problem, in addition to performing a careful physical examination, since a number of different situations may exist to cause this problem. With a dialysis history and physical examination, a fistulogram is not necessary to formulate a diagnosis. However, it may be useful for operative planning.

A. High Venous Pressure

The AVF may have developed high venous resistance to the reinfusion of blood. For this reason, extra pressure is required to reinfuse blood into the patient, resulting in ultrafiltration. A rising venous pressure over a period of weeks to months should be a clue that venous outflow obstruction is developing and revision should be undertaken before the access fails completely.

A fistulogram to delineate the site of stenosis is often useful in this setting. If the area of venous stenosis is single and located near a radiocephalic anastomosis, it will be possible, in most cases, to reconstruct the fistula proximal to the stenosis. This will usually provide a number of sites for cannulation. If the area causing the problem is some distance from the anastomosis and is too proximal to bypass readily, it may be possible to perform an angioplasty or resect the area of stenosis. Often there are several stenotic areas with surrounding scar, and a new AVF will need to be reconstructed at another site.

Venous stenosis occurring proximal to the venous anastomosis of a PTFE graft may occur at one site or multiple sites. The single-site stenosis can be corrected by bypassing it or performing patch angioplasty. Balloon angioplasty of venous stenoses is frequently performed but the long-term success rates are not good (25% patency at 1 year) (33,34). Problems on the venous side of a fistula are usually more serious than arterial problems in terms of maintaining adequate vascular access in the same general area.

B. Poor Arterial Inflow

The second type of problem occurs when there is insufficient or failing arterial inflow to the dialysis machine. Useful access requires arterial inflow of at least 200 mL/min. Problems with arterial inflow present with collapse of the arterial segment of the dialysis circuit because the inflow pressure becomes negative with respect to the dialysis pump. Here, as in the case when there is a high venous pressure, a fistulogram will usually provide useful information regarding the location of the problem.

The radiologist should be informed that special attention must to be paid to the arterial segment of the fistula. Occasionally additional films will be required to demonstrate the full arterial anatomy apart from overlying veins. Unless the patient is diabetic, the stenosis most often occurs in the vicinity of the anastomosis and can be corrected by reconstructing the fistula proximal to the original site.

If the problem is extensive atherosclerosis, it will usually be necessary to create a new fistula at another site. The hemodynamic effects of sequential stenoses are greater than the severity of any single stenosis would suggest (35).

C.   Difficulty in Cannulation

The final problem that occurs in the dialysis unit and causes a "failing fistula" is increased difficulty with cannulation. This is more common in units with less experienced personnel or with an uncooperative or obese patient. It is important to carefully examine the involved extremity. Not infrequently, the problem is progressive scarring around a site that has been used for an extended period of time. There are often additional viable sites proximal to the favored one.

If, in fact, the fistula is patent but cannot be reliably cannulated, a new one will have to be constructed, usually at a different site. A fistula that can be cannulated only with difficulty by the most experienced nurse or technician is inadequate, regardless of its hemodynamic characteristics once cannulated. Before another fistula is constructed, a concerted attempt should be made to use the existing access site. The performance of a fistulogram may be useful, followed by a cannulation demonstration of the access site by the surgeon or nephrologist and/or their marking of new sites for dialysis personnel.

D.   Congestive Heart Failure

Congestive heart failure is a rare complication of an AVF created for hemodialysis access (36). A well-developed AVF may obligate as much as 20% of the cardiac output. Rarely, flow through a large antecubital or femoral loop fistula can develop to greater than 2 L/min. If the patient is small or has significant organic heart disease, this can result in high-output cardiac failure. The diagnosis is missed only when it is not considered. It is suggested by a drop in heart rate with temporary occlusion of the fistula. The diagnosis can be more difficult in patients receiving beta blockers in whom the heart rate response to fistula occlusion is muted. Thermodilution cardiac output measurements may be useful in selected situations.

If vascular access is still required, two alternatives exist; either the fistula may be ligated after usable access (either temporary or permanent) is obtained or the flow through the existing access site may be decreased by downsizing the fistula. This can be done by direct reconstruction of the anastomosis or by banding the outflow vein to a smaller diameter. It is difficult to adequately judge the degree to which the fistula can be diminished without causing thrombosis; this is one situation in which Doppler flow probes may be of use. The best intraoperative information supporting adequate diminution of flow is a significant decrease in heart rate.

E.   Takedown of Arteriovenous Fistulas

If the AVF is no longer needed (resolution of renal failure, permanent peritoneal dialysis, successful renal transplant), takedown of the AVF may be indicated. This may be done either for cosmetic reasons or because of the possibility of hemorrhage from minor trauma. In addition, there is some evidence that closure of AVFs may be beneficial in reducing myocardial workload and left ventricular hypertrophy (37).

In general, fistula takedown following renal transplantation should not be considered until renal function has been stable for at least 1 year without significant complications relating to immunosuppression or recurrent renal disease. A patient's history of vascular access should be considered in deciding whether to remove a fistula. Patients in whom it has been difficult to obtain and maintain vascular access should usually not have the fistula removed.

AVF takedown can easily be done as an outpatient procedure with the patient under local anesthesia. A pneumatic tourniquet should be considered as a safety precaution, but it should be deflated unless needed. Ligation of outflow veins will accomplish takedown. Arterial flow to the hand should be preserved by reconstruction or preservation of the artery. Alternatively, venovenous reanastomosis and arterial reconstruction may preserve the vein and artery for future use and requires little extra time or effort.

Following fistula takedown or ligation, the large venous conduit becomes relatively stagnant and thrombosis with rather pronounced phlebitis frequently occurs. This can be lessened by elastic compression dressings placed at the time of fistula takedown. The treatment for this condition is symptomatic and the patient should be reassured that the problem will resolve.

F. Preservation of Cephalic Veins

In any patient with abnormal renal function or a disease process likely to lead to renal failure, all cephalic veins should be carefully preserved. This is often difficult to accomplish, since the cephalic veins are the most readily accessible intravenous sites. Often, by the time the surgeon has been consulted regarding vascular access, both cephalic veins are thrombosed because of ill-advised placement of intravenous sites. Obtaining an AVF in this situation becomes more difficult. It is important to constantly remind those taking care of patients with any renal abnormality or with the potential for it that the need for quality permanent vascular access requires preservation of all cephalic veins.

G. Neurological Sequelae

The patient should be informed that the position of the radial cutaneous nerve puts it at risk for injury during fistula formation or takedown. Injury results in a small area of decreased sensation on the back of the thumb. Careful preservation of the radial cutaneous nerve at operation will minimize the risk of this complication. This nerve is more often injured during takedown than during formation of AVF's, probably because of the scar tissue created by the original operation through which the takedown dissection must proceed.

Rarely, a patient with marked distal arterial insufficiency due to the AVF will present with palsy of the radial or median nerve. Nerve conduction studies will demonstrate abnormalities that cannot be related to the same level for both nerves. When nerve palsy occurs, the fistula must be taken down urgently and another form or site of dialysis undertaken.

H. Carpal Tunnel Syndrome

For unknown reasons, carpal tunnel syndrome occurs more commonly in hemodialysis patients than in the general population. Since the syndrome occurs as commonly on the side without the fistula, it is probably not related to its presence.

Treatment of carpal tunnel syndrome in a wrist with a functioning fistula requires planning. Since this syndrome is best treated surgically under tourniquet hemostasis, attention must be given to preservation of the fistula. We handle this problem by injecting the fistula with heparin before inflating the tourniquet. Using this technique, we have not lost a fistula even with up to 20 min of tourniquet occlusion.

V. CONCLUSION

Complications common to all areas of vascular surgery occur frequently in vascular access patients. Morbidity rarely involves limb loss, as it does in peripheral reconstructive surgery, but it represents significant problems nevertheless. Because these vessels or grafts are routinely cannulated, sometimes under less than ideal conditions, infection and pseudoaneurysm formation are not common.

The usable life of any vascular access depends to a large extent on how it is handled by personnel in the dialysis unit. The vascular surgeon's responsibility to the patient continues beyond the point at which usable vascular access is obtained. It is important to continually remind dialysis personnel of the rules in handling and cannulating AVFs and to remind physicians caring for these patients not to use any cephalic veins for intravenous sites. A well-constructed and cared for autogenous fistula can last for many years.

REFERENCES

1. www.usrds.org.
2. Shrier RW, Gottschalk CW. Diseases of the Kidney. 4th ed. Boston: Little, Brown, 1988:1526.
3. Bour ES, Weaver AS, Yang HC, Gifford RRM. Experience with the double lumen Silastic catheter for hemoaccess. Surg Gynecol Obstet 1990; 17(1):33–39.
4. Schwab ST, Buller GI, McCann RL, Bollinger RL, Stickel DL. Prospective evaluation of a Dacron cuffed hemodialysis catheter for prolonged use. Am J Kidney Dis 1988; 11:166–169.
5. Mendes RR, Farber MA, Marston WA, Dinwiddie LC, Keagy BA, Burnham SJ. Prediction of wrist arteriovenous fistula maturation with preoperative vein mapping with ultrasonography. Vasc Surg 2002; 36(3):460–463.
6. Atherikul K, Schwab SJ, Conlon PJ. Adequacy of hemodialysis with cuffed central-vein catheters. Nephrol Dial Transplant 1998; 13(3):745–749.
7. Hirsch DJ, Bergen P, Jindal KK. Polyurethane catheters for long-term hemodialysis access. Artif Organs 1997; 21(5):349–354.
8. Schwab SJ, Weiss MA, Rushton F, Ross JP, Kapoian T, Yegge J, Rosenblatt M, Reese WJ, Soundararajan R, Pedan A, Moran JA. Multicenter clinical trial results with the LifeSite hemodialysis access system. Kidney Int 2002; 62(3):1026–1033.
9. Beathard GA, Posen GA. Initial clinical results with the LifeSite Hemodialysis Access System. Kidney Int 2000; 58(5):2221–2227.
10. Castaldo PA. Homeostasis and kidney disease. In: Tatnoff DO, Forbes CD, eds. Disorders of Hemostasis. Orlando, FL: Grune and Stratton, 1984:473–483.
11. Livio M, Benigni A, Remuzzi G. Coagulation abnormalities in uremia. Semin Nephrol 1985; 5:82–90.
12. Mannucci PM, Remuzzi G, Pusiner F, Lombardi R, Valsecchi C, Mecca G, Zimmerman TS. Deamino-8-D-arginine vasopressin shortens the bleeding time in uremia. N Engl J Med 1983; 308:8.
13. Liu KY, Kosfeld RE, Marcum SG. Treatment of uremic bleeding with conjugated oestrogen. Lancet 1984; 2:887–890.
14. Kappes S, Towne JB, Adams MB, Kauffman HM, Maierhofer W. Perforation of the superior vena cava: a complication of subclavian dialysis. JAMA 1983; 249:2232–2233.
15. Joseph RE, Radhakrishnan J, Appel GB. Antiphospholipid antibody syndrome and renal disease. Curr Opin Nephrol Hypertens 2001; 10(2):175–181.
16. Kauffman HM, Elborn GA, Adams MB, Hussey CV. Hypercoagulability: A cause of vascular access failure. Proc Clin Dialysis Transplant Forum 1979; 9:28.
17. Passman MA, Criado E, Farber MA, Risley GL, Burnham CB, Marston WA, Burnham SJ, Keagy BA. J Vasc Surg 1998; 28(5):869–875.

18. Giacchino JL, Geis P, Buckingham JM, Vertumo VL, Bansal VK. Vascular access: Long-term results, new techniques. Arch Surg 1979; 114:403–409.
19. Konner K. Vascular access in the 21st century. J Nephrol 2002; 15(suppl 6):S28–S32.
20. Anderson CB, Etheredge EE, Sicard GA. One hundred polytetrafluoroethylene vascular access grafts. Dialysis Transplant 1980; 9.
21. Tellis VA, Kohlberg WI, Bhat DJ, Driscoll B, Veith FJ. Expanded polytetrafluoroethylene graft fistula for chronic hemodialysis. Ann Surg 1979; 189:101–105.
22. Morgan AP, Dammin GJ, Lazarus JM. Failure modes in secondary vascular access for hemodialysis. Am Soc Artif Int Organs 1978; 1:44–52.
23. Johnson CP, Zhu YR, Matt C, Pelz C, Roza AM, Adams MB. Prognostic value of intra-operative blood flow measurements in vascular access surgery. Surgery 1998; 124(4):729–737. Discussion 737–738.
24. Glickman MH, Stokes GK, Ross JR, Schuman ED, Sternbergh WC III, Lindberg JS, Money SM, Lorber MI. Multicenter evaluation of a polytetrafluoroethylene vascular access graft as compared with the expanded polytetrafluoroethylene vascular access graft in hemodialysis applications. J Vasc Surg 2001; 34(3):465–472. Discussion 472–473.
25. Almonacid PJ, Pallares EC, Rodriguez AQ, Valdes JS, Rueda Orgaz JA, Polo JR. Comparative study of use of Diastat versus standard wall PTFE grafts in upper arm hemodialysis access. Ann Vasc Surg 14(6):659–662.
26. Lemson MS, Tordoir JH, van Det RJ, Welten RJ, Burger H, Estourgie RJ, Stroecken HJ, Leunissen KM. Effects of a venous cuff at the anastomosis of polytetrafluoroethylene grafts for hemodialysis vascular access. J Vasc Surg 2000; 32(6):1155–1163.
27. Livio M, Gotti R, Marchesi D, Mecca de Gaetano G. Uremic bleeding: Not of anemia and beneficial effect of red cell transfusions. Lancet 1982; 2:1013–1015.
28. Appel GB. Vascular access infections with long-term hemodialysis. Arch Intern Med 1978; 138:1609–1610.
29. Wilson SE. Complications of vascular access procedures. In: Wilson SE, Owens MI, eds. Vascular Access Surgery. Chicago: Year Book, 1980:185–207.
30. Bandyk DF, Schmitt DD, Seabrook GR, Adams MB, Towne JB. Monitoring functional patency of in situ saphenous vein bypass: The impact of a surveillance protocol and elective revision. J Vasc Surg 1989; 9:286–296.
31. Krivitski NM, Gantela S. Access flow measurement as a predictor of hemodialysis graft thrombosis: making clinical decisions. Semin Dialysis 2001; 14(3):181–185.
32. Steuer RR, Miller DR, Zhang S, Bell DA, Leypoldt JK. Noninvasive transcutaneous determination of access blood flow rate. Kidney Int 2001; 60(1):284–291.
33. Lombardi JV, Dougherty MJ, Veitia N, Somal J, Calligaro KD. A comparison of patch angioplasty and stenting for axillary venous stenoses of thrombosed hemodialysis grafts. Vasc Endovasc Surg 2002; 36(3):223–229.
34. Clark TW, Hirsch DA, Jindal KJ, Veugelers PJ, LeBlanc J. Outcome and prognostic factors of restenosis after percutaneous treatment of native hemodialysis fistulas. J Vasc Intery Radiol 2002; 13(1):51–59.
35. Beckmann CF, Levin DC, Kubicka RA, Henschke CI. The effect of sequential arterial stenoses on flow and pressure. Radiology 1981; 140:655–658.
36. Fee HJ, Levisman JE, Doud RB, Golding AL. High output congestive failure from femoral arteriovenous shunts for vascular access. Ann Surg 1976; 183:321–323.
37. Unger P, Wissing KM, de Pauw L, Neubauer J, van de Borne P. Reduction of left ventricular diameter and mass after surgical arteriovenous fistula closure in renal transplant recipients. Transplantation 2002; 74(1):39–73.

24

Complications of Thoracic Outlet Surgery

David Rigberg

UCLA Medical Center, Los Angeles, California, U.S.A.

Julie Freischlag

Johns Hopkins School of Medicine, Baltimore, Maryland, U.S.A.

I. INTRODUCTION

Perhaps no disorder is as vexing to the vascular surgeon as the thoracic outlet syndrome (TOS). Although the venous (Paget-Schroetter) and arterial sequelae of thoracic outlet compression have clear objective signs, the more common neurogenic form requires a clinical diagnosis. There is considerable controversy regarding this diagnosis, and editorials by physicians experienced in treating these patients can be found warning clinicians of both over- and underdiagnosing of neurogenic TOS (1,2).

As discussed further on, TOS stems from the compression of several important structures traversing the thoracic outlet. Over the years, operative treatment has evolved from more radical therapies, such as bilateral claviculectomies, to the currently practiced approaches: transaxillary first rib resection and supraclavicular scalenectomy with or without first rib resection. The complications of these two procedures are the focus of this chapter, and these procedures are performed in a similar fashion for whichever form of TOS is being treated. In addition, recurrent TOS is considered an operative complication for the purposes of this review.

With regard to the operative treatment of other consequences of TOS, complications tend to mirror these procedures in other, non-TOS settings. Examples of these include resection of subclavian aneurysms, lysis and later venoplasty of axillo-subclavian thrombosis, or even the need for upper extremity sympathectomy. The one caveat is that the long-term success of most of these procedures depends on adequate decompression of the inciting TOS, without which recurrence or even primary treatment failure can be expected.

Most patients with neurogenic thoracic outlet syndrome never require operative intervention, as physical therapy tends to have good results in this setting. Physical therapy programs designed to open the anatomical confines of the thoracic outlet were originally described by Peet, who also coined the term *TOS* in 1956 (3). These programs are designed to relax muscle groups that tighten the thoracic outlet while conditioning those that open it. Aligne and Barral further described a program in which the trapezius, levator scapulae, and sternocleidomastoid muscles are strengthened and the middle scalene, subclavian, and pectoralis muscles are relaxed (4). These goals can be met by many different protocols, usually with a combination of supervised and at-home exercises. Complications from such treatment are minimal, although improperly performed physical therapy can lead to worsening of neurogenic TOS symptoms. The injection of botulinum toxin (Botox) provides another nonoperative intervention for TOS, although there is little experience with this modality's long-term results. Even with the considerable number of patients helped by conservative therapies, there are several tertiary referral centers with large series of TOS patients who have remained symptomatic.

II. ANATOMY

The limited space and large number of important structures that must traverse the neck and chest areas on their way to the arm make the thoracic outlet an area like no other in the body. Although there are any number of anatomical anomalies that predispose to or directly cause compression of the neural, venous, and arterial structures within its confines, the normal anatomy itself does not leave much room for stress positioning. Any of the structures within the thoracic outlet can be injured operatively, so a thorough appreciation of the region's anatomy is required before these procedures are performed.

Definitions may vary from author to author, but it is generally accepted that the thoracic outlet is the area from the edge of the first rib extending medially to the upper mediastinum and superiorly to the fifth cervical nerve. The clavicle and subclavian muscles can be pictured as forming a roof, while the superior surface of the first rib forms the floor (Fig. 1). Machleder's description of the thoracic outlet as a triangle with its apex pointed

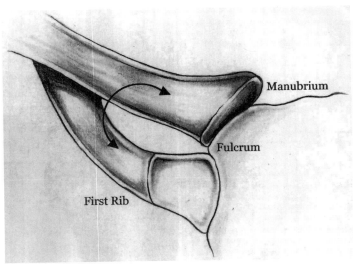

Figure 1 A schematic representation of the fulcrum and "scissoring" effect of the first rib and the clavicle is shown. As can be seen from the diagram, decompression can be accomplished via removal of either of these structures.

toward the manubrium is helpful in visualizing the three-dimensional orientation of the structures as well as the dynamic changes that can lead to injury (5). In this model, the clavicle and its underlying subclavian muscle and tendon form the superior limb, while the base is the first thoracic rib.

Although most cases of TOS are neurogenic, almost any structure that travels through the thoracic outlet can be involved with the disease or, as previously mentioned, injured when treating the disorder. Moving from medially to laterally, one first encounters the exiting of the subclavian vein, usually positioned adjacent to the region where the first rib and claivicular head fuse to form a fibrocartilagenous joint with the manubrium. Immediately lateral to the vein is the anterior scalene muscle, which inserts onto a prominence on the first rib. Lateral to this site is the subclavian artery, so that the anterior scalene muscle lies between the subclavian artery and vein, with the artery deep, lateral and somewhat cephalad. The brachial plexus is the next structure encountered (Fig. 2). The C4-C6 roots are superiorly oriented, and the C7-T1 roots inferiorly. Posterior and lateral to the plexus, there is a generally rather broad attachment of the middle scalene to the first rib. This is an area of particular importance during operative decompression of the thoracic outlet, for it is here that the long thoracic nerve can be inadvertently injured as it travels to the serratus anterior muscle (Fig. 3).

Other structures encountered in the thoracic outlet include the phrenic and dorsal scapular nerves, the stellate ganglion, the thoracic duct, and the cupola of the lung. The phrenic nerve lies between the prescalene fat pad and the anterior scalene muscle (Fig. 4).

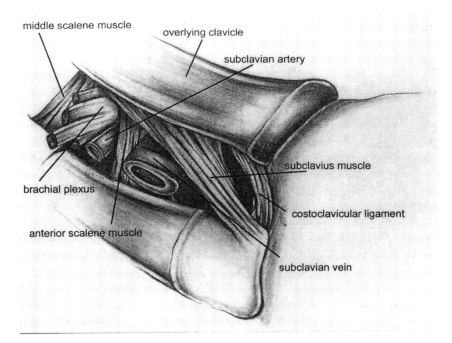

Figure 2 The anatomy of the thoracic outlet involves the passing of many important structures in close proximity on their way to the upper extremity and chest. Particular note should be made of the relationships between the major neurovascular structures and the scalene muscles.

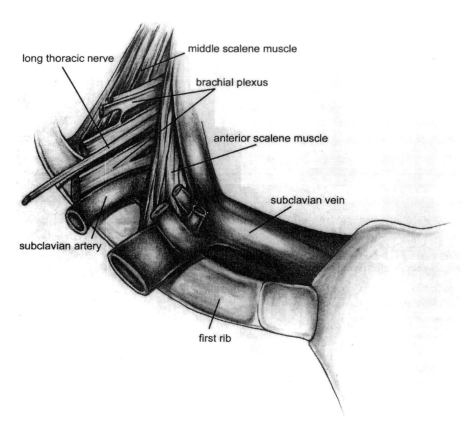

Figure 3 This diagram, an antero-posterior view of the thoracic outlet with the clavicle and subclavius muscle removed, also shows the proximity of the long thoracic nerve and suggests how injury to this structure can occur. Note should also be made of the broad insertions of the anterior and middle scalene muscles.

Compression of this structure does not generally occur, but it can be injured during supraclavicular approaches and must be left intact while the underlying scalene muscle is dissected. The dorsal scapular nerve comes off the brachial plexus on its way to innervate the medially inserting muscles of the scapula (rhomboids and levator scapulae). It is usually neither involved nor encountered. The stellate ganglion is found along the sympathetic chain. This structure can be involved in compression, and occasionally a cervicothoracic sympathectomy is part of the treatment plan for TOS. The thoracic duct may be encountered if a left supraclavicular approach is undertaken, and care must be taken not to injure it or to ligate it if injury occurs. Finally, one must watch for pleural injury in any approach to TOS and be prepared to evacuate pneumothoraces when indicated.

III. OPERATIONS

As previously described, there are two primary operations for decompressing the thoracic outlet, transaxillary first rib resection and supraclavicular scalenectomy with or without first

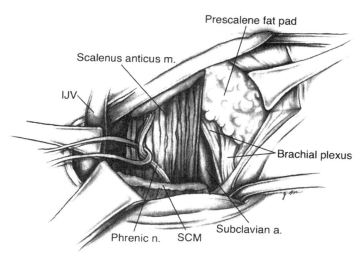

Figure 4 This surgical view represents the anatomy as seen via the supraclavicular route for scalenectomy with or without 1st rib resection. The prescalene fat pad must be divided with caution, as the phrenic nerve runs directly on top of the underlying anterior scalene muscle. The internal jugular vein typically serves as the median extent of the dissection. This exposure affords better access to the brachial plexus, particularly when neurolysis is to be included as part of the decompressive procedure.

rib resection. Various groups favor one operation over the other, but it appears they are similarly effective. Most surgeons treating recurrent TOS use the route not previously used, so that clinicians with a sizable TOS practice are versed in both approaches. Complications of thoracic outlet decompression do differ significantly based on the approach used, as would be expected based on the differences in the anatomy one encounters. These differences are pointed out below where appropriate.

IV.   COMPLICATIONS

A.   Operative Injuries

Any structure encountered in the dissection for first rib resection is a potential site of injury. The catastrophic complications of brachial plexus, subclavian artery, and subclavian vein injury occur infrequently. Concern about brachial plexus injury dates back to the early days of first rib resection. Particularly in the neurology literature, this has been a controversial topic. For a number of years there were only a few case reports of plexus injuries. However, Dale in 1982 published the results of a survey of thoracic surgeons performing first rib resections and discovered 273 injuries, 19% of which were permanent (6). While this study certainly suggested underreporting of this complication, reports of plexus injuries remained low, although not at the almost negligible rate that had been accepted.

What is most notable about the publications that followed is that no mention is made of the incidence of this injury. Wilbourn in 1988 reported on eight patients with plexus injuries form the Cleveland Clinic. They underwent first rib resection at some time between

1974 and 1983, but the total number of procedures performed is not given (7). Likewise, Horowitz reported on four cases of plexus injury, but no figures are given regarding the number of procedures performed from which these patients were taken (8). The same can be said of the four cases reported by Cherington in 1986 (9). In several large recent surgical series, most notably that of Roos, the incidence of such injuries is very low (0–2%). In the experience of the University of California–Los Angeles (UCLA), there have been no such injuries. It is fair to say that plexus injuries certainly do occur but that the risk of the injury must be weighed against the possible benefits of the procedure.

Another issue regarding plexus injuries is that of retraction. It is more than likely that most of the neurological injuries were related to stretching of the perineurium, with resultant ischemia. During the transaxillary approach, a considerable amount of stretch is applied to the arm; most surgeons relieve the traction intermittently to allow blood flow. This was not necessarily the case when an assistant was retracting. Specialized retraction systems, such as the Machleder retractor, allow for periods of extremity relaxation with easy repositioning to continue the procedure.

The incidence of major arterial or venous injury during first rib resection is also difficult to determine. It is clear that these injuries can and do occur and that they demand immediate attention. In a review of 2445 cases, Roos reported only 3 instances of major injuries of this nature (0.12%) (10). In all 3 cases, the patients had full recovery. Delayed bleeding, usually from a small subclavian branch or intercostal artery, is also seen. Roos reported 7 cases in the same series (0.2%). The patients also had complete recovery. In Green's review of 136 patients, there were no major vascular injuries (11). UCLA reported one such injury in their series over 10 years of operations. If the artery is injured during surgery via the transaxillary route, a supraclavicular incision must be made to allow for proximal control of the vessel. Major venous injuries can usually be addressed through the transaxillary incision and repaired. If better exposure is needed, the medial third of the clavicle can be removed to aid in visualization. Rarely if ever does the vein need to be ligated.

Injuries to other nerves occur, particularly the long thoracic. Roos reported a 0.12% incidence, with two of the patients having complete recoveries and one lost to follow-up. In Sharp's series of 36 patients, there was one such injury (12). Most of these tend to be temporary, but a permanently winged scapula can occur. Treatment of these injuries with nerve grafting can sometimes be successful. Injuries to the phrenic nerve are not common and are more associated with the anterior approach, particularly with reoperative cases. Most of these injuries result in temporary, subclinical diaphragmatic paralysis, although complete division with permanent injury is possible.

The most common nerve injury is not a true complication but a by-product of the operation; division of intercostal brachial cutaneous branches leading to cutaneous numbness. This occurs to some extent in most patients, not unlike that which occurs with axillary dissection for other disease states. It is usually well tolerated and resolves.

Reports of patients with postoperative causalgia or other pains are also difficult to place into clinical perspective. In most series, they are unusual. Significant causalgia is usually attributed to brachial plexus injury and thus should parallel the incidence of that injury. In the Washington State workers' compensation study of patients with neurogenic TOS, 6% of patients were reported to have causalgia and 13% had "other pains." It is not clear what these represented (13). Green's series of 136 cases had 3 patients with some form of postoperative vasospasm. Finally, postoperative Horner's syndrome occurs in from 0.5 to 2% of patients in most series. In almost all reported cases, it is self-limited.

Entry into the pleural space occurs in as many as 30% of cases. This is usually recognized and easily evacuated at the time of operation without the need for a chest tube. The highest reported incidence of postoperative pneumothorax is 5%.

As mentioned previously, there are reports of injuries to all of the structures encountered during first rib resection. Thus, supraclavicular approaches can lead to thoracic duct or even recurrent laryngeal nerve injury, although these injuries are rare. The risk of complications is increased with reoperative surgery. Many structures tend to be adherent in a particular pattern during these procedures, for example, the subclavian artery to the anterior scalene muscle. Care must be taken in these cases to identify all structures adequately.

B.   Treatment for Recurrent TOS

Recurrence of TOS following operative intervention is not uncommon. Published series have reported rates as low 2.2%, but most are on the range of 15–20% (14–17). Defining recurrence in this situation is frequently difficult, because it is not always clear that the patient's symptoms ever improved. Scalene block has utility as a predictor of surgical outcome for neurogenic TOS, with relaxation of the anterior scalene muscle approximating the decompression achieved with first rib resection/scalenectomy. Patients are given a series of injections of either lidocaine or saline and then pain with provocative maneuvers is assessed [generally the elevated arm stress test (EAST)]. Machleder and colleagues reported on 122 patients in whom this technique was used and found a 90% positive predictive value for correlation with the clinical diagnosis of TOS (18). In addition, for patients undergoing first rib resection for TOS, those with a positive scalene block had a much greater chance of a good outcome (94%) than those with a negative preoperative scalene block (50%). This test can be positive with other disorders, particularly radiculopathies, but is a useful adjunct to not only the diagnosis of TOS but also in gauging the likelihood of surgical benefit. This can reduce the number of recurrent or, more accurately, unimproved cases of TOS following surgery.

It is also of paramount importance that patients have realistic expectations before surgery. A discussion of the risks should include the possibility of no improvement, worsening of the symptoms, or later recurrence. Armed with this information, the patient is in a much better position to make an informed decision.

Recurrent symptoms tend to be similar to the original complaints, with paresthesias of the hand and pain of the neck and shoulder being the most common manifestations. The etiology of recurrence is usually not clear, although postoperative scarring is considered one of the main culprits. In this setting, there is generally a relatively long asymptomatic period (1–2 years) before the symptoms return. Several studies have looked at the implications of a long posterior stump to the first rib, but there is little correlation with return of symptoms. Other reported etiologies include middle scalene reattachment, calcified rib masses, and missed cervical ribs or cervical rib stumps. Some have drawn a distinction between a spontaneous recurrence, attributable to scar, and a recurrence secondary to a traumatic insult. In the latter situation, the patient again tends to have the original symptoms, despite the fact that the thoracic outlet has already been decompressed. A whiplash type injury frequently occurs in this scenario.

The workup for recurrence is essentially the same as for untreated disease. Special emphasis should be placed on ruling out other causes, as a percentage of patients failing treatment will have done so on the basis of a faulty diagnosis. Iatrogenic injury to the plexus, carpal tunnel syndrome, tendinitis, cervical arthritis or spine injury must be sought before treatment for the recurrence is started. A conservative plan is initially undertaken, although the overwhelmingly positive response seen with physical therapy in TOS patients who avoid the original operation is not reproduced here. It is worth noting that intense postoperative physical therapy, if properly prescribed and performed, is thought to decrease the incidence of recurrent symptoms after both initial and "redo" operations. If conservative methods fail in treating recurrent symptoms, reoperation is considered, although it should be noted that only a 50% improvement rate is quoted for these patients. In addition, at least a year should be allowed to pass before surgical intervention is again performed.

Although clinical practices vary, many surgeons have adopted an algorithm for reoperation (Fig. 5). If the original operation was via a transaxillary approach, a supraclavicular approach is taken. Care is taken to identify any remaining first rib and to resect it all the way to the transverse process. If the patient's original operation did not include first rib resection, it is removed now. Most surgeons also add some form of neurolysis to the reoperation, whereby the scar around the nerves is carefully removed. Some surgeons

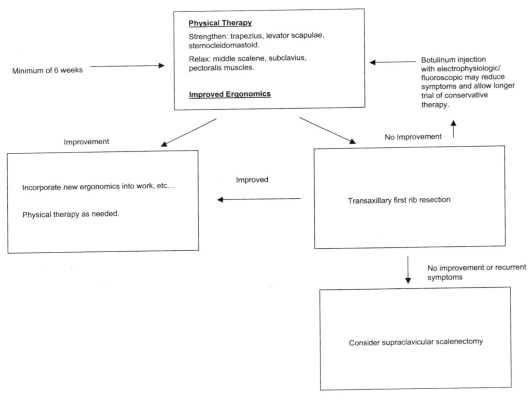

Figure 5   This algorithm incorporates the important modalities for treating TOS. This includes treating recurrence of symptoms following operative decompression. Note should be made that physical therapy should be utilized following operation and can decrease the incidence of recurrent symptoms. Physical therapy should also be considered for treating recurrent symptoms before further operation is undertaken.

remove the middle scalene during the course of reexploration. If the supraclavicular approach was already used, the transaxillary is utilized for the second operation. Again, care is taken to remove the entire first rib, any remaining attachments and scar. Neurolysis can be performed via this route, with some advocating that it be done over the supraclavicular route, particularly when ulnar symptoms predominate.

Several methods have been tried to prevent the formation of scar tissue and adhesions following thoracic outlet decompression, particularly in the face of reoperation. After the nerve roots are cleared, they are usually covered with the overlying adipose tissue, although the benefit of this technique has never been documented. Similarly, care is taken to replace the scalene fat pad, but this does not appear to influence the formation of scar. Attempts to control scarring with the administration of exogenous agents, including steroids, have also been disappointing. Sheets of polytetrafluoroethylene (PTFE) have been used to cover the nerves, but this technique has been abandoned by most and probably leads to additional scar formation. The use of hyaluronic acid gels showed some promise several years ago, but it is not clear whether these products are particularly helpful and they are not approved by the U.S. Food and Drug Administration for this use.

Brief mention should be made here of the treatment of bilateral TOS. For neurogenic disease, the initial procedure is performed on the most symptomatic side. Only 10% of patients require bilateral operations for this disorder, and the second side should be treated no sooner than 12 months following the first. Patients who have bilateral operations within less than 12 months will have difficulty regaining strength and stability of the neck and shoulders and take a longer time to recuperate from the second operation. Even more rarely do patients have venous compression on the opposite side. If this is demonstrated by provocative noninvasive testing, first rib decompression can be done prophylacticaly no sooner than 12 months later. Bilateral arterial TOS is practically never seen.

V. CONCLUSIONS

It has been demonstrated that decompression of the thoracic outlet can be safely accomplished in most patients with TOS. However, two factors dictate that surgeons performing these procedures be well trained in them and strive to minimize morbidity. The first is the abundance of critical structures in a confined space and the devastating consequences of harming them. The second is the subjective nature of neurogenic TOS and the importance of not replacing a patient's symptoms with a different problem, a situation that is fortunately not common. For a controversial clinical entity such as TOS, it is difficult to objectively demonstrate posttreatment improvement. However, it is not difficult to demonstrate many of the potential complications of therapy. Careful patient selection and meticulous technique are needed to ensure that the risk-benefit ratio of these procedures continues to justify operative intervention for neurogenic TOS in particular.

REFERENCES

1. Wilbourn AJ. Thoracic Outlet Syndrome is overdiagnosed. Muscle Nerve 1999; 22:130–136.
2. Roos DB. Thoracic Outlet Syndrome is underdiagnosed. Muscle Nerve 1999; 22:126–129.
3. Peet RM, Hendricksen JD, Anderson TP, et al. Thoracic outlet syndrome: Evaluation of the therapeutic exercise program. Mayo Clin Proc 1956; 31:281–287.
4. Aligne C, Barral X. Rehabilitation of patients with thoracic outlet syndrome. Ann Vasc Surg 1992; 6:381–389.

5. Machleder HI. Vascular Disorders of the Upper Extremity. 3d ed. Mt Kisco, NY: Futura Press, 1999.

6. Dale WA. Thoracic outlet compression syndrome. Arch Surg 1982; 164:149–153.

7. Wilbourn AJ. Thoracic outlet syndrome surgery causing severe brachial plexopathy. Muscle Nerve 1988; 11:66–74.

8. Horowitx SH. Brachial plexus injuries with causalgia resulting from transaxillary rib resection. Arch Surg 1985; 120:1189–1191.

9. Cherington M, Happer I, Machanic B, et al. Surgery for thoracic outlet syndrome may be hazardous to your health. Muscle and Nerve 1986; 9:632–634.

10. Roos DB. Thoracic outlet nerve compression. In: Rutherford RB, ed. Vascular Surgery. 3d ed. Philadelphia: Saunders, 1989:858–875.

11. Green RM, McNamara J, Ouriel K. Long-term follow-up after thoracic outlet decompression: An analysis of factors determining outcome. J Vasc Surg 1991; 14:739–746.

12. Sharp WJ, Nowak LR, Zamani T, et al. Long-term follow-up and patient satisfaction after surgery for thoracic outlet syndrome. Ann Vasc Surg 2001; 15:32–36.

13. Franklin GM, Fulton-Kehoe D, Bradley C, et al. Outcome of surgery for thoracic outlet syndrome in Washington State workers' compensation. Neurology 2000; 54:1252–1257.

14. Lindgren KA, Leino E, Lepantalo M, et al. Recurrent thoracic outlet syndrome after first rib resection. Arch Phy Med Rehabil 1991; 72:208–210.

15. Roos DB. Recurrent thoracic outlet syndrome after first rib resection. Acta Chir Belg 1980; 79:363–372.

16. Sessions RT. Recurrent thoracic outlet syndrome: Causes and treatment. South Med J 1982; 75:1453–1461.

17. Sanders RJ, Monsour JW, Gerber FG, et al. Scalenectomy versus first rib resection for treatment of the thoracic outlet syndrome. Surgery 1979; 85:109–121.

18. Jordan SE, Machleder HI. Diagnosis of thoracic outlet syndrome using electrophysiologically guided anterior scalene blocks. Ann Vasc Surg 1998; 12:260–264.

25

Stroke as a Complication of Noncerebrovascular Surgery

Sukru Dilege

Istanbul Medical Faculty, Istanbul, Turkey

Matthew I. Foley and Gregory L. Moneta

Oregon Health & Science University, Portland, Oregon, U.S.A.

Although improvements in perioperative care have resulted in the ability to perform complex operations in elderly, high-risk patients, serious complications can occur. One such complication is perioperative stroke. Most strokes occur 3–30 days following a surgical procedure. Perioperative stroke complicating noncerebrovascular surgery is uncommon, but it can be associated with devastating disability and high mortality (1). With the exception of death, long-term neurological disability following postoperative stroke is undoubtedly an elderly patient's most feared perioperative complication (2). Patients who have suffered a perioperative stroke can present a formidable social and financial burden to the family and community. All surgeons who operate on elderly, high-risk patients must be familiar with the risk factors for stroke, the incidence of perioperative stroke associated with various procedures, and variables that can be modified to reduce the risk of perioperative stroke.

I. STROKE DEMOGRAPHICS

Stroke is the third leading cause of death in the United States. In 1999, 167,366 people died of stroke-related causes (3). Each year, about 600,000 people suffer a stroke, and 82% of these strokes are initial events. Persons with hemorrhagic strokes have a higher 30-day mortality than those with ischemic strokes (4). Among patients with a first ischemic stroke, the stroke itself is the most common cause of early death (5).

A marked decrease in stroke mortality occurred in the United States, Canada, and western Europe during the 1970s and early 1980s. Stroke mortality, however, actually increased in eastern European countries (6–8). Japan and Finland, especially, have been very successful in reducing their stroke mortality rates (6). In the United States, the stroke-related death rate decreased 13.0%, but the actual number of stroke-related deaths increased

8.6% from 1989 to 1999 (3). Although the decline in stroke mortality rates in the United States is encouraging and the lowest in the industrialized world, recent evidence suggests that stroke rates have stabilized (3,4,6,9).

In addition to mortality, stroke remains a major source of disability. In 1999, more than 1,100,000 Americans who suffered strokes were affected with functional limitations, many with moderate to severe permanent neurological deficits (3).

II. ETIOLOGY OF STROKE

Vascular events were the cause of more than 90% of acute neurological deficits in the late 1970s (10) and continue to be so today. In the National Heart Lung and Blood Institute's Atherosclerosis Risk in Communities cohort, causes of stroke in middle-aged adults were reported as ischemic in 83%, intracerebral hemorrhage in 10%, and subarachnoid hemorrhage in 7% (4). In a study by Petty et al. (11), the underlying cause of ischemic stroke was cervical or intracranial large vessel atherosclerosis with stenosis in 16%, cardioembolic in 29%, lacunar in 16%, and other in 3%. The cause was uncertain in 36% of patients. Principal etiologies of stroke in young patients are extracranial arterial dissection, cardioembolism, premature atherosclerosis, hematological and immunological diseases, migraines, and drug abuse (12). Heavy consumption of alcohol predisposes to both hemorrhagic and nonhemorrhagic stroke (13). Less than half of thromboembolic events appear to originate from the extracranial cerebrovascular system and thus are potentially amenable to preoperative surgical correction (10,14).

III. RISK FACTORS FOR STROKE

Sacco et al. published a consensus in 1997 entitled "Risk Factors in Stroke"(15). This and other reports have concluded that risk factors for stroke have not changed for the last 20 years. Nonmodifiable and modifiable risk factors have been identified and are listed in Table 1.

A. Nonmodifiable Risk Factors

Age is the single most important nonmodifiable risk factor for stroke. Stroke risk increases with age. Stroke is more common in men than women except for in the very old. In the United States, approximately 1% of people between ages 65 and 75 die from a stroke annually. Some 22% of men and 25% of women die within the first year of having a stroke. In 1999, a total of 38.5 and 61.5% of deaths from stroke were in men and women, respectively (3). In the Framingham Study, a family history of stroke was associated with an increased stroke risk (16). Age-standardized mortality rates for all stroke subtypes are higher in blacks than in whites (17). Blacks have a 38% greater risk of first stroke than whites (4). Stroke incidence and mortality rates vary dramatically from one population or racial group to another. However, some of these risks for stroke may be related to environmental factors or inherited risk factors other than race.

B. Modifiable Risk Factors

One of the most important modifiable risk factors for stroke is hypertension, even at borderline levels. The risk of stroke seems to be directly related to the magnitude of blood pressure elevation (18,19). An analysis of seven studies has estimated the stroke risk from

Table 1   Risk Factors for Stroke

Non-modifiable	Age, male sex, race	
Modifiable (potentially)	Hypertension	
	Cardiac disease	
		Atrial fibrillation
		Cardiac valve abnormalities
		Coronary artery disease
		Left ventricular hypertrophy
		Congestive heart failure
	Aortic arch plaque	
	Diabetes	
	Low HDL[a]	
	Elevated homocysteine	
	Cigarette smoking	
	Alcohol abuse	
	Cocaine	
	Obesity	
	Physical inactivity	

[a] High-density lipoprotein.

the lowest to the highest blood pressure ranges to increase about 10-fold (15). Isolated systolic hypertension in the elderly may engender less risk of stroke than sustained diastolic hypertension (20). About half of those who have a first stroke have blood pressures higher than 160/95 mmHg (3). Women do not appear to tolerate hypertension any better than men. A higher percentage of men have high blood pressure until age 55, when the prevalence increases in women and surpasses that in men (3). In women taking oral contraceptives, hypertension is two to three times more common than in age-matched controls. In a metanalysis of 17 treatment trials of hypertension throughout the world involving nearly 50,000 patients, there was a 38% reduction in all strokes and a 40% reduction in fatal stroke in subjects treated for their hypertension (21). It appears that optimal prevention of late-life stroke will likely require control of midlife blood pressure (22).

Cardiac disease, especially atrial fibrillation (AF), has a definite effect on stroke rates. It is estimated that almost half of all cardioembolic strokes occur in the setting of AF. The incidence and prevalence of AF increase with age. A study from Denmark suggests that patients with an in-hospital diagnosis of AF have an increased risk of stroke that is greatest during the first year after discharge (23). In the Framingham Study, patients with nonvalvular AF had 3–5 times the risk of stroke (24). To prevent stroke in AF, it is advised to offer warfarin to patients and reserve aspirin for young subjects at low risk of stroke and those with contraindications to warfarin use (25). Cardiac valve abnormalities (especially mitral stenosis), coronary artery disease, left ventricular hypertrophy, and congestive heart failure are additional cardiac risk factors for stroke.

Proximal atherosclerotic plaque of the aorta is also associated with an increased risk of ischemic stroke in the elderly. One study suggests that aortic plaques are significantly more frequent in men than in women (26).

Diabetes mellitus is another risk factor for stroke. However, other risk factors for stroke such as hypertension, obesity, and hyperlipidemia are prevalent in patients with diabetes (15). Stroke risks from hypertension and diabetes mellitus are difficult to separate and probably have joint effects on the development of atherosclerosis in the cerebrovascular system.

Although there is a positive correlation between total cholesterol and the extent of extracranial carotid atherosclerosis, analysis of the EUROSTROKE project could not identify an association between total cholesterol with fatal or nonfatal, hemorrhagic, or ischemic strokes (27,28). HDL cholesterol was inversely related to stroke in men but not in women (28). Increased HDL levels are associated with a reduced risk of ischemic stroke in the elderly (29).

Elevated levels of homocysteine have been found to be associated with an increased risk of carotid artery disease and stroke. Recently, the British Regional Heart Study showed a strong, independent, graded relationship between homocysteine levels and stroke risk among middle-aged men (30). Randomized, controlled trials of homocysteine-lowering interventions are in progress to determine whether stroke incidence can be reduced (31).

Significant cigarette smoking increases the risk of stroke twofold. There is a dose-response relationship between cigarette smoking and the extent of extracranial cerebrovascular atherosclerosis (32). Moderate consumption of alcohol may be protective against cardiovascular disease, including stroke. Heavy alcohol consumption, however, increases the risk of intracranial hemorrhage (33). Cocaine abuse is also a major social and human health problem associated with stroke (34).

The independent effects of oral contraceptives are unclear. According to most studies, low-dose oral contraceptives (< 50 µg estrogen) do not increase risk of stroke (35,36). In the Heart and Estrogen-progestin Replacement Study (HERS), hormone therapy with conjugated equine estrogen and progestin had no significant effect on the risk of stroke among postmenopausal women with coronary artery disease (37).

Obesity and physical inactivity are associated with an increased stroke risk. The role of lifestyle modification in the primary prevention of stroke cannot be overemphasized (38).

C. Carotid Artery Disease

Asymptomatic carotid artery atherosclerosis is common; it is often discovered incidentally or found in a patient with a cervical bruit. The prevalence of carotid stenosis ranges from 0.5% in people under 60 years old up to 10% in those over age 80 (39). Although the prevalence is high, the degree of stenosis in most is not severe (40). Patients of advanced age, and those with histories of cigarette smoking, hypertension, and low HDL have a much higher incidence carotid artery stenosis (41,42).

The prevalence of a carotid bruit is 5% in persons more than 50 years old. However, less than a quarter of patients with a carotid bruit have greater than 50% internal carotid artery stenosis. A carotid bruit has a sensitivity of 63–76% and a specificity of 61–76% for predicting > 70% carotid artery stenosis (43).

Carotid ulceration has been implicated as a risk factor for stroke, especially when the ulcerations are large. This may be true even without concomitant severe stenosis (44,45). However, the added risk of ulceration, if any, is not firmly established. Certain plaque characteristics, such as echolucency, have also been implicated as a risk factor for stroke (46).

The risk of stroke among patients with asymptomatic carotid artery stenosis is relatively low. Some 45% of strokes in patients with stenosis of 60–99% are attributable to lacunar infarcts or cardioembolism (47). Several different randomized trials have compared aspirin therapy with endarterectomy in patients with asymptomatic carotid artery stenosis (48–51).

The Asymptomatic Carotid Atherosclerosis Study (ACAS) randomized 1662 patients with asymptomatic carotid stenosis of 60% or greater to medical management or medical management plus carotid endarterectomy (51). This study suggested a benefit of surgery, reducing the risk of ipsilateral stroke or death at 5 years from 11 to 5.1%. The absolute reduction in major stroke and death over 5 years in ACAS was insignificant. The benefit of endarterectomy for asymptomatic carotid stenosis remains controversial at present (52).

D. Transient Ischemic Attacks

A transient ischemic attack (TIA) is a temporary focal neurological deficit caused by a brief interruption of local cerebral blood flow. A significant percentage of TIAs occur in the absence of detectable significant extracranial carotid artery disease. Patients with TIAs have significantly more hypertension, cardiac disease, and diabetes than age-matched controls (53). One study demonstrated a 7% annual stroke risk for patients experiencing TIAs (54). Recent or multiple TIAs have a higher short-term risk for ischemic stroke than a remote TIA, and the same may be true for "crescendo" TIAs (15,55). The risk of stroke associated with TIAs is highest in the first year following TIA.

E. Previous Stroke

Patients with prior strokes are at much higher risk for a new cerebral infarction than patients without prior strokes (3). There is a 5–20% annual recurrence risk for patients experiencing stroke (3,53,56).

At least three prospective randomized clinical trials comparing carotid endarterectomy versus medical management for the treatment of symptomatic carotid artery stenosis have been completed (54,57,58). The North American Symptomatic Carotid Endarterectomy Trial (NASCET) demonstrated a major advantage of endarterectomy plus medical management over medical management alone in patients with greater than 70% stenosis and neurological symptoms referable to the stenosed artery (54). The cumulative risk of ipsilateral stroke at 2 years in patients with 70–99% stenosis was 26% in the medical group and 9% in the surgical group. Endarterectomy was also beneficial in symptomatic patients with 50–69% stenosis, but the absolute risk reduction (6.5%) was not as pronounced (59). The European Carotid Surgery Trial (ECST) and Veterans Affairs Cooperative Symptomatic Trial showed similar results (57,58).

IV. STROKE IN NONCEREBROVASCULAR SURGERY

The incidence and mechanism of stroke in patients undergoing noncerebrovascular surgery depends on the primary operative procedure.

A. Etiology of Perioperative Stroke

The pathogenesis of perioperative stroke is often not known with certainty. The currently recognized ischemic stroke mechanisms are decreased perfusion, embolism, and thrombosis. Lacunar infarction (infarct size ≤1.5 cm) may be associated with all three mechanisms.

The mechanism of perioperative stroke is predominantly embolic, although hypoperfusion may play a role (60). Acute hypotension in the setting of chronic hypertension has been implicated as a cause of stroke (61). A patient who undergoes a difficult procedure associated with significant intraoperative blood loss and hypotension followed by a post-operative neurological deficit will generally have the stroke ascribed to intraoperative hypotension. However, such patients are unusual. Severe alteration in blood pressure in direct proximity to stroke occurrence is an infrequent finding in perioperative cerebral infarction. Reviews of patients with perioperative cerebral infarction following aortoiliac procedures indicate that neurological events almost always occur after a variable lucid interval, not intraoperatively (1,62,63). Hart and Hindman (64) identified 12 perioperative strokes associated with 24,500 general surgical procedures. Although intraoperative hypotension was frequent, the onset of the neurological deficit was intraoperative in only 17% of the cases; the deficit clearly occurred postoperatively in 83%. Larsen et al. (65) found that 6 of 2463 patients suffered perioperative stroke after noncardiac, noncerebrovascular surgery; all 6 of these did so late in the postoperative period, between 5 and 26 days after surgery. Gerraty et al. (66) feel that cerebrovascular hemodynamics are important in that patients with severe symptomatic carotid disease may be at high risk for perioperative watershed infarction.

One explanation of the infrequent association of intraoperative hypotension with perioperative stroke is that agents used for general anesthesia may have cerebral protective effects. Furthermore, most cases of intraoperative hypotension are transient and may be of little overall hemodynamic significance. Hypotension in the postoperative recovery period can, however, be associated with stroke (67).

Embolism to the brain is often cardiac in origin. Commonly recognized cardiac sources of embolism include atrial fibrillation, sinoatrial disorder, recent acute myocardial infarction (AMI), subacute bacterial endocarditis, cardiac tumors, and valvular disorders affecting both native and artificial valves (68). Hart and Hindman (64) identified cardiac embolization as the underlying mechanism of stroke in 42% of their noncardiac, non-cerebrovascular perioperative stroke patients. Larsen et al. (65) and Parikh et al. (69) emphasized the role of atrial fibrillation in perioperative stroke. Platelet emboli from atheromatous arterial plaques have been suggested as a cause of perioperative stroke as well (64,67).

The role, if any, of a perioperative hypercoagulable state in the occurrence of perioperative cerebral infarction is unknown. Recent evidence suggests that perioperative alterations in blood rheology and transient postoperative hypercoagulable states may contribute to the risk of postoperative stroke. Such speculation is consistent with the observation that perioperative stroke is nearly always thrombotic or embolic in origin.

Blood rheology appears chronically altered in patients with previous stroke, TIAs, or significant risk factors for cerebrovascular disease (70–72). Whole blood and plasma viscosities are significantly elevated in such patients as compared with normal controls. The effect appears to be independent of the hematocrit and primarily associated with elevated plasma fibrinogen and a decreased albumin/globulin ratio (73).

The postoperative state is also associated with a number of alterations in the coagulation system. Gibbs et al. (74) compared postoperative changes in procoagulant, anticoagulant, and antifibrinolytic factors in patients undergoing peripheral vascular surgery. There was an increase in plasma fibrinogen and factor VIII levels, whereas antithrombin III and protein C levels decreased. The results suggest that peripheral vascular procedures are associated with an increased potential for thrombosis due to increases in procoagulant factors. Specific acquired hypercoagulable conditions such as antiphospholipid antibodies, which clearly predispose surgical patients to postoperative thrombotic complications, are being recognized with increasing frequency (75).

One can postulate that the increase in perioperative blood viscosity and coagulation factor abnormalities following vascular and general surgical procedures may predispose patients to thrombotic or embolic stroke.

B. Cardiac Surgery

Although stroke rates have declined with the improvements in surgical techniques and advances in myocardial protection, stroke remains a major complication of cardiac surgery. The majority of these strokes result in temporary, minor cognitive and psychiatric dysfunction. In a prospective study of perioperative stroke in cardiac surgery, less than 5% of neurological deficits consisted of a central focal deficit (76). In experienced centers, the contemporary stroke risk for patients undergoing coronary artery bypass grafting (CABG) is reported to be less than 2%. Estimates of the perioperative stroke risk of CABG in the presence of hemodynamically significant carotid stenosis generally vary from 6 to 16% (77). The risk of stroke associated with cardiac surgery clearly increases with patient age. Age > 75 is associated with an increased risk of nonembolic stroke after myocardial revascularization (76,78,79). The risk of stroke in this group reaches a disturbing incidence of 3.2–10% (80–83). In addition to previous stroke or transient ischemic attack, peripheral vascular disease, emergency operation, diabetes, and a left ventricular ejection fraction < 40% are independent predictors of stroke after cardiac surgery (84,85). Duration of cardiopulmonary bypass in excess of 2 h increases the probability of neurological damage (78,86). Engelman et al. found that perioperative TIA or stroke during the cardiac operation was associated with postoperative low cardiac output and atrial fibrillation (80). Finally, Hogue et al. (87) reported that female gender was associated with a 6.9-fold increased risk of early stroke and a 1.7-fold increased risk of delayed stroke.

The incidence of stroke during valvular surgery has decreased with time, despite the increased prevalence of risk factors. The overall risk of perioperative stroke with valve replacement is two to three times greater than the risk with coronary artery bypass. Patients with single valve replacement have a lower incidence than combined procedures with CABG (1.2 vs. 7.6%) (88). Causes of stroke in valve surgery are atherosclerotic emboli, septic emboli, and shock (79).

Early studies have mainly focused on intraoperative events, but symptoms may develop later in the postoperative period (88). Some 70% of strokes associated with cardiac surgery occur intraoperatively; the remaining 30% develop more than 24 h post-operatively (88–90). Intraoperative events are attributed most frequently to technical prob-lems with aortic clamping or cannulation, inadequate venting of the heart of air and debris at the completion of the reconstruction, and occasionally hypoperfusion associated with cardiac bypass. Borger et al. have suggested that macroemboli from the ascending aorta are the predominant cause of stroke during coronary bypass surgery (79).

The role of extracranial cerebrovascular disease in the etiology of stroke associated with cardiac surgery is not clear at present. Generally, detectable carotid artery stenosis coexists with significant coronary artery disease in 15% of coronary disease patients. Schwartz et al. found carotid atherosclerosis to be a risk factor for hemispheric stroke in patients under-going cardiopulmonary bypass (91). The risk of hemispheric stroke in patients with unilateral 80–99% stenosis, bilateral 50–99% stenosis, or unilateral occlusion with con-tralateral 50% or greater stenosis was 5.3%. Scotnicki et al. (92) reported that patients with as asymptomatic carotid bruit can safely undergo coronary artery surgery. In the group of patients without preoperative neurological symptoms, postoperative neurological deficits were rarely caused by carotid occlusive disease. Patients with asymptomatic bruits can be safely screened with ultrasonic carotid duplex scanning and do not require arteriography prior to cardiopulmonary bypass (93).

C. Noncerebrovascular Vascular Surgery

The increased mortality observed among claudicants is most often a consequence of atherosclerotic disease in other vascular beds. Myocardial infarction and cerebrovascular accidents are the cause of death in at least 50% of patients with peripheral vascular disease. About 20% of vascular surgery patients have a cervical bruit (94). Using continuous-wave Doppler examinations, Hennerici et al. (95) found a 32.8% incidence of vertebral or carotid artery disease (> 50% stenosis) in 325 patients undergoing peripheral vascular surgery. In 264 patients with severe coronary artery disease documented by angiography, these investigators found similar carotid disease in only 6.8%. Barnes and Marszalek (96) detected > 50% carotid stenosis in 17.2% of 116 patients undergoing peripheral vascular reconstruction and in 10.6% of 198 patients undergoing coronary bypass.

Plate and Hollier et al. (97) found 8.2% late mortality from stroke in 1112 patients operated upon for abdominal aortic aneurysms. The incidence of cerebrovascular accident (CVA) was 4.2 and 9.5% within 5 and 10 years, respectively. Advanced age, hypertension, and heart disease carried a greater risk for this complication.

Despite the prevalence of extracranial vascular disease and associated risk factors for stroke in peripheral vascular surgery patients, the overall incidence of perioperative stroke in noncerebrovascular vascular surgery patients is surprisingly low. Perioperative strokes occur in around 1% of peripheral vascular surgery patients, as shown in Table 2. Harris et al. (98) found only 13 perioperative neurological events associated with 1390 (0.9%) non-carotid vascular surgery procedures. There were 2 TIAs, 10 anterior circulation strokes, and 1 posterior circulation stroke. The neurological deficit developed in the immediate postoperative period in 31%, more than 4 h but less than 72 h postoperatively in 54%, and within 3–14 days postoperatively in 15%. Of these strokes, 27% were fatal. These investigators established that new anterior circulation strokes in vascular surgical patients tended to be associated with intra-abdominal procedures, perioperative hypotension, and the presence of

Table 2 Incidence of Perioperative Strokes Following Noncerebrovascular Surgery

Procedure	Patients	Stroke (%)
Cardiac valve replacement	1,343	4.1
CABG	41,769	1.5
Elective AAA	2,210	0.7
Ruptured AAA	437	1.3
Aortofemoral bypass	2,464	0.8
Infrainguinal bypass	2,246	0.5
Thoracoabdominal aneurysm	706	1.8
Other[a]	26,336	0.06

[a] Includes general surgical and subspecialty procedures (orthopedic, urologic).
Abbreviations: CABG, coronary artery bypass grafting; AAA, abdominal aortic aneurysm.

a greater than or equal to 50% ipsilateral internal carotid artery stenosis. Many vascular surgery patients are hypertensive, have suffered a previous stroke, or have significant cardiac dysfunction, all of which are risk factors for stroke independent of carotid artery disease. Preoperative knowledge and correction of modifiable risk factors can potentially reduce the incidence of perioperative stroke (99).

D. General Surgery

Perioperative stroke as a complication of general surgery is infrequent, with a reported incidence between 0.08 and 2.9% (69,100). Landercasper et al. (67) reported no perioperative strokes in 7517 consecutive patients without a prior history of stroke who underwent nonneurosurgical, noncardiac, and noncerebrovascular procedures while under general anesthesia. The incidence of perioperative stroke in 173 patients with a previous history of stroke was 2.9%. In another study, it was found that 2.1% of 279 patients with a history of cerebrovascular disease developed a new stroke in the perioperative period (65).

Ischemic strokes after general surgery most commonly occur after an asymptomatic interval (69,65). Parikh et al. (69), in a study involving 24,641 patients, found that majority of perioperative strokes occurred late in the postoperative period. The average time to the occurrence of perioperative stroke is 7 days (2). Patients with previous cerebrovascular disease, atrial fibrillation, hypertension, advanced age, or atherosclerosis were found to have an increased risk. Limburg et al. (100) described three major risk factors for perioperative stroke: prior CVA, chronic obstructive pulmonary disease, and peripheral arterial disease.

V. MINIMIZING PERIOPERATIVE STROKE

Despite the low incidence of perioperative stroke in noncerebrovascular surgery, certain steps may decrease the risk of perioperative stroke.

A. Patient Selection

An important factor in reducing the incidence of perioperative stroke is careful patient selection. A prior neurological event, carotid artery stenosis, diabetes mellitus, and advanced age have been found to increase susceptibility to perioperative stroke in many studies. By the avoidance of all but essential surgery in stroke-prone patients (patients of advanced age, especially greater than 75 years and those with a history of recent myocardial infarction, previous stroke, atrial fibrillation, or known thrombotic tendencies), the incidence of perioperative stroke can likely be reduced. Stroke is an important complication in patients with acute myocardial infarction, occurring in 1–3% of all infarctions. Most strokes occur in the first weeks after the infarction, but the risk for stroke remains for an indefinite time. Therefore all major surgical interventions should be postponed as long as possible in such patients.

Preoperative optimization of the patient by identifying and treating coexisting medical conditions such as coronary artery disease, hypertension, and atrial fibrillation is very important for reducing perioperative stroke (2). Preoperative patients with atrial fibrillation should be considered for conversion to sinus rhythm or for anticoagulation (69). Anesthesia and surgery are best delayed for 4–6 weeks after an acute CVA.

B. Intraoperative Management

Although most perioperative strokes do not occur intraoperatively, some obviously do. Certainly in cardiac surgery, extreme care must be exercised in manipulating the ascending and transverse aorta, and the heart must be well flushed of air and debris before circulation is restored. Careful attention should be given to maintaining proper mean arterial pressure during cardiac bypass, and pump times should be kept as short as possible (78,86).

Intraoperatively, the noncardiac surgery patient should be maintained as close to his or her resting physiological state as possible. Both mean arterial pressure and arterial carbon dioxide should be maintained within the patient's usual range. Blood pressure control and optimal cerebral oxygen delivery are crucial factors to prevent stroke. Wide variations may alter cerebral autoregulation and increase susceptibility to stroke. Blood glucose levels should be maintained at normoglycemic levels, because hyperglycemia exacerbates ischemic neurological damage.

Choice of anesthetic technique and agents may be of importance in high-risk patients. The major volatile anesthetic agents produce cerebral vasodilatation and decrease cerebral oxygen consumption. These agents can cause stealing of blood from peri-infarcted areas in patients with recent cerebral infarctions (2). Anesthetic agents or techniques may influence the incidence of perioperative stroke, but results from prospective controlled trials are not available. Hypocapnia and hypercapnia should be avoided (2).

C. Prophylactic Carotid Endarterectomy

Current data suggest that the >80% asymptomatic lesions have the highest potential to result in a neurological event during follow-up (Table 3). However, even if prophylactic carotid endarterectomy were to be offered to all patients with asymptomatic carotid artery stenosis, as many as one-third of strokes in this population would remain unavoidable because of their occurrence in a different vascular territory. Moreover, some additional strokes would result from surgery itself (106). The absolute reduction in major stroke and death due to surgery over 5 years in ACAS was small and surgery may result in other nonfatal complications (cranial nerve injury, myocardial infarction). In addition, the low complication rate of the ACAS-selected surgeons is not likely to reflect the typical risk of endarterectomy in the community. Therefore the optimal management of high-grade asymptomatic carotid disease prior to noncerebrovascular surgery still remains questionable.

In 1998, Benavante et al. (39) reported a metanalysis of six randomized clinical trials. The results of this metanalysis suggest that carotid endarterectomy should not be routinely recommended for unselected patients with asymptomatic carotid stenosis despite the substantial reduction in the risk of ipsilateral stroke by surgery. The incidence of ipsilateral stroke was relatively low in those patients who did not undergo the operation; hence the

Table 3 Annual Stroke Risks in Patients with >80% Asymptomatic Internal Carotid Artery Stenosis

Author	Stroke risk (%)
Cambers and Norris (101)	5.5
Bogousslavsky et al. (102)	4.2
Henneirci et al. (103)	8.1
Moneta et al. (104)	12; 4[a]
Caracci et al. (105)	9

[a] First year, 12%; second year; 4%.

benefit of carotid endarterectomy will remain small until high-risk subgroups are identified.

It seems reasonable to perform carotid endarterectomy before another operative procedure under certain circumstances. First, in patients with symptomatic carotid lesions, the performance of carotid endarterectomy can be justified on the basis of the carotid disease alone. Second, the patient should be a good operative risk and the operating surgeon should have a record of a low complication rate with carotid artery surgery. Third, the performance of carotid endarterectomy should not place the patient at significantly increased risk resulting from the inherent delay in performing the other indicated operative procedure.

D. Combined Carotid/Coronary Surgery

There is a close relationship between carotid and coronary artery disease. O'Donnell et al. (107) pointed out that 66% of patients undergoing carotid artery surgery had clinical evidence of coronary artery disease. Hertzer et al. (108) reported that coronary artery bypass grafting (CABG) might be indicated in as many as 37% of carotid endarterectomy patients. In the presence of significant carotid artery stenosis, the stroke rate of patients undergoing CABG varies from 6 to 16% (109). It is generally accepted that combined carotid endarterectomy and CABG procedures have higher stroke and death rates than isolated procedures. This is hardly surprising, since each operation carries an inherent risk of stroke. Brow et al. (110). found that risk factors are more prevalent in the combined endarterectomy and CABG group. Some investigators suggest that the difference between isolated and combined procedures is not significant if the carotid disease is asymptomatic (111). Patients with significant bilateral carotid artery disease have a worse stroke risk whether undergoing combined or isolated procedures (112,113). A metanalysis of 11 series determined that patients with unilateral carotid artery stenosis have a 6.9% stroke risk for combined procedures compared to 12.7% for patients with bilateral disease. The highest-risk group included patients with an occluded carotid and contralateral stenosis. These patients experienced a 29% stroke rate with combined procedures (114).

The authors of a retrospective German study of 313 simultaneous carotid endarterectomy and myocardial revascularization procedures concluded that combined procedures are justified. The risk of myocardial infarction, stroke, or mortality was not significantly different than reported with isolated procedures (115). Khaitan et al. (116) reported 121 consecutive combined operations with a perioperative neurological event rate of 5.8%. Two patients had transient ischemic attacks. The procedure-related mortality rate was 5.8%.

In summary, the available data suggest that for a majority of patients, combining CABG with carotid endarterectomy will not result in a substantial improvement in the incidence of stroke following CABG. No conclusions can be drawn for patients with severe bilateral carotid artery stenosis or those with symptomatic carotid disease who require urgent coronary revascularization. Combining CABG and carotid artery surgical procedures under these circumstances may be appropriate in centers with adequate expertise in both procedures.

VI. CONCLUSION

Perioperative stroke following noncerebrovascular surgery is an infrequent problem. Its incidence is about 4% for cardiac valvular surgery, 1–2% for CABG, and 0.2–0.5% for other surgical procedures. The risk of perioperative stroke is increased in older patients,

patients with prior stroke, and those with multiple risk factors for stroke. With the exception of cardiac procedures, perioperative strokes occur mainly in the postoperative period. There does not appear to be a consistent relationship between perioperative stroke and carotid bruit or asymptomatic carotid stenosis, although only a few patients with very high grade carotid stenosis have been studied. Prophylactic carotid endarterectomy in preparation for another procedure should be performed only when the extent of the carotid disease itself is adequate justification for carotid surgery and when delaying the primary procedure does not endanger the patient.

REFERENCES

1. Carney WI, Stewart WB, De Pinto DJ, Mucha SC, Roberts B. Carotid bruit as a risk factor in aortoiliac reconstruction. Surgery 1977; 81:567–570.
2. Kam PCA, Calcroft RM. Peri-operative stroke in general surgical patients. Anaesthesia 1997; 52:879–883.
3. American Heart Association. 2002 Heart and Stroke Statistical Update. Dallas: American Heart Association, 2001.
4. Rosamond WD, Folsom AR, Chambless LE, Wang CH, McGovern PG, Howard G, Copper LS, Shahar E. Stroke incidence and survival among middle-aged adults: 9-year follow-up of the Atherosclerosis Risk in Communities (ARIC) cohort. Stroke 1999; 30:736–743.
5. Hartmann A, Rundek T, Mast H, Paik MC, Boden-Albala B, Mohr JP, Sacco RL. Mortality and causes of death after first ischemic stroke: The Northern Manhattan Stroke Study. Neurology 2001; 57:2000–2005.
6. Sarti C, Rastenyte D, Cepaitis Z, Tuomilehto J. International trends in mortality from stroke, 1968 to 1994. Stroke 2000; 31:1588–1601.
7. Mihalka L, Smolanka V, Bulecza B, Mulesa S, Bereczki D. A population study of stroke in West Ukraine: Incidence, stroke services, and 30-day case fatality. Stroke 2001; 32:2227–2231.
8. Stegmayr B, Vinogradova T, Malyutin S, Peltonen M, Nikitin Y, Asplund K. Widening gap of stroke east and west. Eight years trends in occurrence and risk factors in Russia and Sweden. Stroke 2000; 31:2–8.
9. Howard G, Howard WJ, Katholi C, Oli MK, Huston S. Decline in US stroke mortality: An analysis of temporal patterns by sex, race, and geographic region. Stroke 2001; 32:2213–2220.
10. Mohr JP, Caplan LR, Melski JW, Goldstein RJ, Duncan GW, Kistler JP, Pessin MS, Bleich HL. The Harvard Cooperative Stroke Registry: A prospective registry. Neurology 1978; 28:754–762.
11. Petty GW, Brown RD Jr, Whisnant JP, Sicks JD, O'Fallon WM, Wiebers DO. Ischemic stroke subtypes: A population-based study of incidence and risk factors. Stroke 1999; 30:2513–2516.
12. Martin PJ, Enevoldson TP, Humphrey PR. Causes of ischemic stroke in the young. Postgrad Med J 1997; 73:8–16.
13. Gill JS, Shipley MJ, Tsementzis SA, Hornby RS, Gill SK, Hitchcock ER, Beevers DG. Alcohol consumption-a risk factor for hemorrhagic and non-hemorrhagic stroke. Am J Med 1991; 90:489–497.
14. Heyman A, Fields WS, Keating RD. Joint study of extracranial arterial occlusion. VI Rapid differences in hospitalized patients with ischemic stroke. JAMA 1972; 222:285–289.
15. Sacco RL, Benjamin EJ, Broderick JP, Dyken M, Easton JD, Feinberg WM, Goldstein LB, Gorelick PB, Howard G, Kittner SJ, Manolio TA, Whisnant JP, Wolf PA. Risk factors. Panel. Stroke 1997; 28:1507–1517.
16. Kiel DK, Wolf PA, Couples LA, Beiger AS, Myers RH. Familial aggregation of stroke: The Framingham Study. Stroke 1993; 24:1366–1371.
17. Ayala C, Greenlund KJ, Croft JB, Keenan NL, Donehoo RS, Giles WH, Kittner SJ, Marks

    JS. Racial/ethnic disparities in mortality by stroke subtype in the United States, 1995–1998. Am J Epidemiol 2001; 154:1057–1063.

18. Kannel WB, Wolf PA, Verter J, McNamara PM. Epidemiologic assessment of the role of blood pressure in stroke: The Framingham Study. JAMA 1970; 214:301–310.

19. Garraway WM, Whisnant JP. The changing pattern of hypertension and the declining incidence of stroke 1987; 258:214–217.

20. Perry HM, Smith WM, Mc Donald RH, Black D, Cutler JA, Furberg CD, Greenlick MR, Kuller LH, Schnaper HW, Schoenberger JA. Morbidity and mortality in the systolic hypertension in the elderly program (SHEP) pilot study. Stroke 1989; 20:4–13.

21. MacMahon S, Rodgers A. The epidemiological association between blood pressure and stroke: Implications for primary and secondary prevention. Hypertens Res 1994; 17(suppl 1):23–32.

22. Seshadri S, Wolf PA, Beiser A, Vasan RS, Wilson PW, Kase CS, Kelly-Hayes M, Kannel WB, D'Agostino RB. Elevated midlife blood pressure increases stroke risk in elderly persons: The Framingham Study. Arch Intern Med 2001; 161:2343–2350.

23. Frost L, Ingham G, Johnson S, Muller H, Hosted S. Incident stroke after discharge from the hospital with a diagnosis of atria fibrillation. Am J Med 2000; 108:36–40.

24. Wolf PA, Abbott RD, Kennel WB. Atria fibrillation as an independent risk factor for stroke: The Framingham Study. Stroke 1991; 22:983–988.

25. American College of Physicians. Guidelines for medical treatment for stroke prevention. Ann Intern Med 1994; 121:54–55.

26. Di Tullio MR, Sacco RL, Savoia MT, Sciacca RR, Homma S. Gender differences in the risk of ischemic stroke associated with aortic atheromas. Stroke 2000; 31:2623–2627.

27. Heiss G, Sharrett AR, Barnes R, Chambless LE, Szklo M, Alzola C. Carotid atherosclerosis measured by B-mode ultrasound in populations: Associations with cardiovascular risk factors in the ARIC study. Am J Epidemiol 1991; 134:250–256.

28. Bots ML, Elwood PC, Nikitin Y, Salonen JT, Freire de Concalves A, Inzitari D, Sivenius J, Benetou V, Tuomilehto J, Koudstaal PJ, Grobbee DE. Total and HDL cholesterol and risk of stroke. EUROSTROKE: A collaborative study among research centers in Europe. J Epidemiol Commun Health 2002; 56(suppl 1):19–24.

29. Sacco RL, Benson RT, Kargman DE, Boden-Albala B, Tuck C, Lin IF, Cheng JF, Paik MC, Shea S, Berglund L. High-density lipoprotein cholesterol and ischemic stroke in the elderly: The Northern Manhattan Stroke Study. JAMA 2000; 285:2729–2735.

30. Perry IJ, Refsum H, Morris RW, Ebrahim SB, Ueland PM, Shaper AG. Prospective study of serum total homocysteine concentration and risk of stroke in middle-aged British men. Lancet 1995; 346:1395–1398.

31. Perry IJ. Homocysteine and risk of stroke. J Cardiovasc Risk 1999; 6:235–240.

32. Wolf PA, D'Agostino RB, Kannel WB, Bonita R, Belanger AJ. Cigarette smoking as a risk factor for stroke: The Framingham Study. JAMA 1988; 259:1025–1029.

33. Gorelick PB. Does alcohol prevent or cause stroke? Cerebrovascular Diseases 1995; 5:379.

34. Kelly MA, Gorelick PB, Mirza D. The role of drugs in the etiology of stroke. Clin Neuropharmacol 1992; 15:249–275.

35. Petitti DB, Sidney S, Bernstein A, Wolf S, Quesenberry C, Ziel HK. Stroke in users of low-dose oral contraceptives. N Engl J Med 1996; 335:8–15.

36. Leblanc ES, Laws A. Benefits and risks of third-generation oral contraceptives. J Gen Intern Med 1999; 14:625–632.

37. Simon JA, Hsia J, Cauley JA, Richards C, Harris F, Fong J, Barrett-Connor E, Hulley SB. Postmenopausal hormone therapy and risk of stroke: The Heart and Estrogen-progestin Replacement Study (HERS). Circulation 2001; 103:620–622.

38. Paganini-Hill A, Perez Barreto M. Stroke risk in older men and women: Aspirin, estrogen, exercise, vitamins, and other factors. J Gend Specif Med 2001; 4:18–28.

39. Benavente O, Moher D, Pham B. Carotid endarterectomy for asymptomatic carotid artery stenosis: A meta-analysis. Br Med J 1998; 317:1477–1480.

40. Pujia A, Rubba P, Spencer MP. Prevalence of extracranial carotid artery disease detectable by echo-Doppler in an elderly population. Stroke 1996; 23:818–822.

41. Fine-Edelstein JS, Wolfe PA, O'Leary DH, Poehlman H, Belanger AJ, Kase CS, D'Agustino RB. Precursors of extracranial carotid atherosclerosis in the Framingham Study. Neurology 1994; 44:1046–1050.

42. Prati P, Vanuzzo D, Casaroli M, Di Chiara A, Di Basi F, Feruglio GA, Toubol PJ. Prevalence and determinants of carotid atherosclerosis in a general population. Stroke 1992; 23:1705–1711.

43. Sauve JS, Lauoacis A, Ostbye T, Feagan B, Sackett DL. Does this patient have a clinically important carotid bruit? JAMA 1993; 270:2843–2845.

44. Dixon S, Pais SO, Raviola C, Gomes A, Machleder HI, Baker JD, Busuttil RW, Barker WF, Moore WS. Natural history of nonstenotic asymptomatic ulcerative lesions of the carotid artery. Arch Surg 1982; 117:1493–1498.

45. Moore WS, Boren C, Malone JM, Roon AJ, Eisenberg R, Goldstone J, Mani R. Natural history of nonstenotic asymptomatic ulcerative lesions of the carotid artery. Arch Surg 1978; 113:1352–1359.

46. Liapis CD, Kakisis JD, Kostakis AG. Carotid stenosis: Factors affecting symptomatology. Stroke 2001; 32:2782–2786.

47. Inzitari D, Eliasziw M, Gates P, Sharpe BL, Chan RK, Meldrum HE, Barnett HJ. The causes and risk of stroke in patients with asymptomatic internal-carotid-artery stenosis. North American Symptomatic Carotid Endarterectomy Trial Collaborators. N Engl J Med 2000; 342:1693–1700.

48. Mayo Asymptomatic Carotid Artery Study Group. Results of a randomized controlled trial of carotid endarterectomy for asymptomatic carotid stenosis. Mayo Clin Proc 1992; 67:513–518.

49. The CASANOVA Study Group. Carotid surgery versus medical therapy in asymptomatic carotid stenosis. Stroke 1991; 22:1229–1235.

50. Hobson RW, Weiss DG, Fields WS, Goldstone J, Moore WS, Towne JB, Wright CB. Efficacy of carotid endarterectomy for asymptomatic carotid stenosis. The Veterans Affairs Cooperative Study Group. N Engl J Med 1993; 328:221–227.

51. Asymptomatic Carotid Atherosclerosis Study Group. Carotid endarterectomy for patients with asymptomatic internal carotid artery stenosis. JAMA 1995; 273:1421–1428.

52. The European Carotid Surgery Trialists Collaborative Group. Risk of stroke in the distribution of an asymptomatic carotid artery. Lancet 1995; 345:209–212.

53. Dyken ML, Wolf PA, Barnett HJ. Risk factors in stroke: A statement for physicians by the Subcommittee on Risk Factors and Stroke of the Stroke Council. Stroke 1984; 15:1105–1111.

54. North American Symptomatic Carotid Endarterectomy Trial Collaborators. Beneficial effect of carotid endarterectomy in symptomatic patients with high-grade carotid stenosis. N Engl J Med 1991; 325:445–453.

55. Estol CJ, Pessin MS. Anticoagulation: Is there still a role in atherothrombotic stroke. Stroke 1990; 21:820–824.

56. Sacco RL, Wolf PA, Kennel WB, McNamara PM. Survival and recurrence following stroke: The Framingham study. Stroke 1982; 13:290.

57. ECSTCG. MRC European Carotid Surgery Trial: Interim results for symptomatic patients with severe (70–99%) or with (0–29%) carotid stenosis. Lancet 1991; 337:1235–1243.

58. Mayberg MR, Wilson ES, Yatsu F, et al. Carotid endarterectomy and prevention of cerebral ischemia in symptomatic carotid stenosis. JAMA 1991; 266:3289–3294.

59. North American Symptomatic Carotid Endarterectomy Trial Collaborators: Benefit of carotid endarterectomy in patients with symptomatic moderate or severe stenosis. N Engl J Med 1998; 339:1415–1425.

60. Barbut D, Grassineau D, Lis E, Heier L, Hartman GS, Isom OW. Posterior distribution of infarcts in strokes related to cardiac operations. Ann Thorac Surg 1998; 65:1656–1659.

61. Kelly RE, Kovacks AG. Mechanism of in-hospital cerebral ischemia. Stroke 1986; 17:430–433.
62. Barnes RW, Liebman PR, Marszalek PB, Kirk CL, Goldman MH. The natural history of aymptomatic carotid disease in patients undergoing cardiovascular surgery. Surgery 1981; 90:1075–1081.
63. Bernhard VM. Discussion of Turnipseed WD, Berkoff HA, Belzer FO, Postoperative stroke cardiac and peripheral vascular disease. Ann Surg 1980; 192:367.
64. Hart R, Hindman B. Mechanisms of perioperative cerebral infarction. Stroke 1982; 13:766–773.
65. Larsen SF, Zaric D, Boysen G. Postoperative cerebrovascular accidents in general surgery. Acta Anaesthesiol Scand 1988; 32:698–701.
66. Gerraty RP, Gilford EJ, Gates PC. Watershed cerebral infarction associated with perioperative hypotension. Clin Exp Neurol 1993; 30:82–89.
67. Landercasper J, Merz BJ, Cogbill TH, Strutt PJ, Cochrane RH, Olson RA, Hutter RD. Perioperative stroke in 173 consecutive patients with a past history of stroke. Arch Surg 1990; 125:986–989.
68. Mohr JP, Albers GW, Amarenco P, Babikian VL, Biller J, Brey RL, Coull B, Easton JD, Gomez CD, Helgason CM, Kase CS, Pullicino PM, Turpie AGG. Etiology of stroke. Stroke 1997; 28:1501–1506.
69. Parikh S, Cohen JR. Perioperative stroke after general surgical procedures. N Y State J Med 1993; 93:162–165.
70. Coull BM, Beamer N, de Garmo P, Sexton G, Nordt F, Knox R, Seaman GV. Chronic blood hyperviscosity in subjects with acute stroke, transient ischemic attacks and risk factors for stroke. Stroke 1991; 22:162–168.
71. Tanahashi N, Gotoh F, Tomita M, Shinohara T, Terayama Y, Mihara B, Ohta K, Nara M. Enhanced erythrocyte aggregability in occlusive cerebrovascular disease. Stroke 1989; 20: 1202–1207.
72. Antonova N, Velcheva I. Hemorheological disturbances and characteristic parameters in patients with cerebrovascular disease. Clin Hemorheol Microcirc 1999; 21:405–408.
73. Beamer N, Coull BM, Sexton G, de Garmo P, Knox R, Seaman G. Fibrinogen and the albumin-globulin ratio in recurrent stroke. Stroke 1993; 24:1133–1139.
74. Gibbs NM, Crawford GP, Michalopoulos N. A comparison of postoperative thrombotic potential following abdominal aortic surgery, carotid endarterectomy, and femoro-popliteal bypass. Anaesth Intens Care 1996; 24:11–14.
75. Coull BM, Clark WM. Abnormalities of hemostasis in ischemic stroke. Med Clin North Am 1993; 77:77–94.
76. Roach GW, Kanchuger M, Mangano CM, Newman M, Nussmeier N, Wolman R, Aggarval A, Marschall K, Graham SH, Ley C. Adverse cerebral outcomes after coronary bypass surgery. Multicenter study of Perioperative Ischemia Research Group and the Ischemia Research and Education Foundation Investigators. N Engl J Med 1996; 335:1857–1863.
77. Faggioli GI, Curl GR, Ricotti JJ. The role of carotid screening before coronary artery bypass. J Vasc Surg 1990; 12:724.
78. Pompilio G, Lotto AA, Agrifoglio M, Antona C, Alamanni F, Spirito R, Biglioli P. Non-embolic predictors of stroke risk in coronary artery bypass patients. World J Surg 1999; 23: 657–663.
79. Borger MA, Ivanov J, Weisel RD, Rao V, Peniston CM. Stroke during coronary bypass surgery: Principal role of cerebral macroemboli. Eur J Cardiothorac Surg 2001; 19:627–632.
80. Engelman DT, Cohn LH, Rizzo RJ. Incidence and predictors of tias and strokes following coronary artery bypass grafting: Report and collective review. Heart Surg Forum 1999; 2:242–245.
81. Gardner TJ, Horneffer PF, Manolio TA, Hoff SJ, Pearson TA. Major stroke after coronary artery bypass surgery: Changing magnitude of the problem. J Vasc Surg 1986; 3:684–689.
82. Horneffer PF, Gardner TJ, Manolio TA. The effects of age on outcome after coronary bypass surgery. Circulation 1987; 76(suppl V):V6–V12.

83. Rao V, Christakis GT, Weisel RD, Ivanov J, Peniston CM, Ikonomidis JS, Shirai T. Risk factors for stroke following coronary artery bypass surgery. J Card Surg 1995; 10(suppl 4): 468–474.

84. Borger MA, Ivanon J, Weisel RD, Peniston CM, Mickleborough LL, Rambaldini G, Cohen G, Rao V, Findel CM, David TE. Decreasing incidence of stroke during valvular surgery. Circulation 1998; 98(suppl 19):II137–II143.

85. Salasidis GC, Latter DA, Steinmetz OK, Blair JF, Graham AM. Carotid artery duplex scanning in preoperative assessment for coronary artery revascularization: The association between peripheral vascular disease, carotid artery stenosis, and stroke. J Vasc Surg 1995; 21: 154–160.

86. Libman RB, Wirkowski E, Neystat M, Barr W, Gelb S, Graver M. Stroke associated with cardiac surgery. Determinants, timing, and stroke subtypes. Arch Neurol 1997; 54:83–87.

87. Hogue CW Jr, Murphy SF, Schechtman KB, Dávila-Román VG. Risk factors for early or delayed stroke after cardiac surgery. Circulation 1999; 100:642–647.

88. Ahlgren E, Aren C. Cerebral complications after coronary artery bypass and heart valve surgery: Risk factors and onset of symptoms. J Cardiothorac Vasc Anesth 1998; 12:270–273.

89. Reed GL, Singer DE, Pickard EH, DeSanctis RW. Stroke following coronary artery bypass surgery: A case control estimate of the risk from carotid bruits. N Engl J Med 1988; 319:1246–1250.

90. Gonzales-Scarano F, Hurtig HI. Neurologic complications of coronary artery bypass grafting: Case control study. Neurology 1981; 31:1032–1035.

91. Schwartz LB, Bridgman AH, Kieffer RW, Wilcox RA, McCann RL, Tawil MP, Scott SM. Asymptomatic carotid artery stenosis and stroke in patients undergoing cardiopulmonary bypass. J Vasc Surg 1995; 21:146–153.

92. Skotnicki SH, Schulte BP, Leyten QH, Tacke TJ, Arntz IE. Asymptomatic carotid bruit in patients who undergo coronary artery surgery. Eur J Cardiothorac Surg 1987; 1:11–15.

93. Ivey TD, Strandness E, Williams DB, Langlois Y, Misbach GA, Kruse AP. Management of patients with carotid bruit undergoing cardiopulmonary bypass. J Thorac Cardiovasc Surg 1984; 87:183–189.

94. Hart RG, Easton JD. Management of cervical bruits and carotid stenosis in preoperative patients. Stroke 1982; 14:290–297.

95. Hennerici M, Aulich A, Sandmann W, Freund HJ. Incidence of asymptomatic extracranial arterial disease. Stroke 1981; 12:750–758.

96. Barnes RW, Marszalek PB. Asymptomatic carotid disease in the cardiovascular surgical patients: Is prophylactic endarterectomy necessary? Stroke 1981; 12:497–500.

97. Plate G, Hollier LH, O'Brien PC, Pairolero PC, Cherry KJ. Late cerebrovascular accidents after repair of abdominal aortic aneurysms. Acta Chir Scand 1988; 154:25–29.

98. Harris EJ Jr, Moneta GL, Yeager RA, Taylor LM Jr, Porter JM. Neurologic deficits following noncarotid vascular surgery. Am J Surg 1992; 163:537–540.

99. Van den Brande P, Vanhandenhove I. The vascular surgical patient: problems in the management of coronary and cerebrovascular risk. Acta Chir Belg 1988; 88:359–362.

100. Limburg M, Wijdicks EF, Li H. Ischemic stroke after surgical procedures: Clinical features, neuroimaging, and risk factors. Neurology 1998; 50:895–901.

101. Chambers BR, Norris JW. Outcome in patients with asymptomatic neck bruits. N Engl J Med 1986; 315:860–865.

102. Bogousslavsky J, Despland PA, Regli F. Asymptomatic tight stenosis of the internal carotid artery: Long-term prognosis. Neurology 1986; 36:861–863.

103. Hennerici M, Hulshhomer H-B, Hefter H, et al. Natural history of asymptomatic extracranial arterial disease: Results of a long term prospective study. Brain 1987; 110:777–791.

104. Moneta GL, Taylor DC, Nicholls SC, et al. Operative versus nonoperative management of asymptomatic high-grade internal carotid artery stenosis: Improved results with endarterectomy. Stroke 1987; 18:1005–1010.

105. Caracci BF, Zukowski AJ, Hurley JJ, et al. Asymptomatic severe carotid stenosis. J Vasc Surg 1989; 9:361–366.
106. Warlow C. Endarterectomy for asymptomatic carotid stenosis? Lancet 1995; 345:1254–1256.
107. O'Donnell TF Jr, Callow AD, Willet C, Payne D, Cleveland RJ. The impact of coronary artery disease on carotid endarterectomy. Ann Surg 1983; 198:705–712.
108. Hertzer NR, Loop FD, Beven EG, et al. Coronary angiography in 506 patients with extracranial cerebrovascular disease. Arch Intern Med 1985; 145:849–852.
109. Faggioli GI, Curl GR, Ricotti JJ. The role of carotid screening before coronary artery bypass. J Vasc Surg 1990; 12:724.
110. Brow TD, Kakkar VV, Pepper JR, Das SK. Toward a rational management of concomitant carotid and coronary artery disease. J Cardiovasc Surg 1999; 40:837–844.
111. Terramani TT, Rowe VL, Hood DB, Eton D, Nuno IN, Yu H, Yellin AE, Starnes VA, Weaver FA. Combined carotid endarterectomy and coronary artery bypass grafting in asymptomatic carotid artery stenosis. Am Surg 1998; 64:993–997.
112. Hertzer NR, Loop FD, Beven EG, O'Hara PJ, Krajewski LP. Surgical staging for simultaneous coronary and carotid disease: A study including prospective randomization. J Vasc Surg 1989; 9:455–463.
113. Rizzo RJ, Whittemore AD, Couper GS, Donaldson MC, Aranki SF, Collins JJ Jr, Mannick JA, Cohn LH. Combined carotid and coronary revascularization: The preferred approach to the severe vasculopath. Ann Thorac Surg 1992; 54:1099–2108.
114. Brener BJ, Brief DK, Alpert J, Goldenkranz RJ, Parsonnet V. The risk of stroke in patients with asymptomatic carotid stenosis undergoing cardiac surgery: A follow-up study. J Vasc Surg 1987; 5:269–279.
115. Evagelopoulos N, Trenz MT, Beckmann A, Krian A. Simultaneous carotid endarterectomy and coronary artery bypass grafting in 313 patients. Cardiovasc Surg 2000; 8(1):31–40.
116. Khaitan L, Sutter FP, Goldman SM, Chamogeorgakis T, Wertan MA, Priest BP, Whitlark JD. Simultaneous carotid endarterectomy and coronary revascularization. Ann Thorac Surg 2000; 69:421–424.

26

Complications of Repair of the Supra-Aortic Trunks and the Vertebral Arteries

Jeffery B. Dattilo

Vanderbilt University Medical Center, Nashville, Tennessee, U.S.A.

Richard P. Cambria

Massachusetts General Hospital and Harvard Medical School, Boston, Massachusetts, U.S.A.

I. INTRODUCTION

The supra-aortic trunks (SATs) are defined as those arteries that originate from the aortic arch and course through the mediastinum, terminating just proximal to the carotid bifurcation or the origin of the vertebral arteries. Atherosclerotic occlusive disease of the SATs or vertebral arteries may lead to a variety of cerebral or peripheral symptoms. Patients may demonstrate symptoms of either carotid or posterior circulation ischemia or upper extremity vascular insufficiency. Hypoperfusion and microembolic phenomena are mechanisms by which symptoms are generated. Such symptoms occur across a spectrum of patient subsets, including the arteritities, among which Takayasu arterititis is more frequent in the younger population.

The anatomical locations of these lesions vary depending upon the vessel involved. The vast majority of SATs and vertebral lesions are diagnosed incidentally in conjunction with a workup for more distal circulatory pathology, specifically the internal carotid. Consequently, little is known about the natural history of morphology of these lesions. Stenosis of these arteries usually occurs at the origin of the vessel and often involves more than one artery. The Joint Study of Extracranial Arterial Occlusion reported the specific anatomical locations and incidence of lesions in patients with symptoms (1) (see Table 1).

The frequency of SAT lesions is relatively lower than that of carotid bifurcation lesions. Further, patients with supra-aortic trunk lesions are generally asymptomatic at the time of presentation. Even if the patient has symptoms of arm claudication or vertebrobasilar ischemia, nonoperative approaches are often chosen. Indications for open surgical repair of lesions of the SAT include flow-limiting stenosis greater than 70% with mor-

Table 1 Number of Lesions of SATs from 168 Patients
Studied

Location	Number of lesions
Left subclavian	129
Innominate or right subclavian	73
Right common carotid	27
Left common carotid	28
Right vertebral	34
Left vertebral	27

Source: Ref. 1.

phology of the plaque consisting of ulceration or surface irregularities and symptoms relating to the lesion such as distal embolization, preocclusive lesions of greater than 90%, or unique circumstances such as a subclavian artery that feeds an internal mammary graft. A relative indication for reconstruction of the vertebral artery is to treat vertebrobasilar ischemia. Of course, it is often difficult for the clinician to determine that the symptoms are secondary to a radiographically significant lesion of the vertebral artery. Further, radiographic subclavian steal is relatively common, but clinical sequelae are distinctly uncommon in these patients.

A major consideration in planning arterial reconstruction is whether to perform an anatomical reconstruction or extra-anatomical bypass. Generally, anatomical reconstructions are reserved for the younger, lower-risk patient who has an innominate artery lesion or multiple lesions. Further, the anatomical approach is prudent in a patient undergoing coronary artery bypass grafting where use of the mammary artery distal to the SAT lesion is planned. Extra-anatomical repairs are often reserved for the elderly patient in whom a thoracotomy or sternotomy would present too high a risk or for those who have had previous transsternal procedures. This chapter discusses the potential complications encountered perioperatively as well as issues of graft patency as they pertain to open surgical reconstruction.

II. EXTRA-ANATOMICAL REPAIRS OF THE SUPRA-AORTIC TRUNKS

Extra-anatomical repairs circumvent the normal human arterial anatomy. There are many described variations for bypassing these lesions (Table 2). The carotid-to-subclavian by-

Table 2 Extra-Anatomic
Reconstructions

Carotid to subclavian
Subclavian to carotid
Carotid to carotid
Axilloaxillary
Carotid subclavian transposition
Subclavian carotid transposition
Subclavian to subclavian
Femoral to subclavian

pass was originally described by Lyons in 1957 and popularized in the 1970s, and it became the standard of care for proximal subclavian lesions (2). The cervical approach causes less morbidity than an anatomical reconstruction. In modern surgical series, extra-anatomical reconstructions are generally reserved for high-risk patients with formidable cardiopulmonary risk factors that prevent transthoracic repair. Flow-dynamic advantages to these bypass grafts are short conduits in relatively large-bore, high-flow systems; historically, they perform well.

A. Technical Considerations

Technical complications of exposure of the supraclavicular carotid and subclavian arteries depend on a firm understanding of the anatomical relationships of the structures encountered during the dissection. Extrathoracic exposure of the subclavian artery starts with a supraclavicular incision centered over the clavicular head of the sternocleidomastoid muscle, which is then divided with impunity. Next, the prescalene fat pad is divided, with care taken to ligate all lymphatic channels. Dissection in the region of the thoracic duct on the left is to be avoided. The phrenic nerve, which typically lies on the anterior portion of the scalene fascia, must be identified and preserved, usually by medial retraction. Next, the anterior scalene muscle is divided, exposing the subclavian artery, which lies beneath. An understanding of the relationship of the brachial plexus as it exits laterally is also beneficial. The subclavian artery is then dissected proximally and distally, encountering the thyrocervical trunk, internal mammary artery, and vertebral artery medially and superiorly. The carotid artery can be mobilized from the carotid sheath using the same incision. Care must be taken in mobilizing the proximal carotid artery because the cervical sympathetic chain lies posterior to the verebral artery.

Most subclavian carotid or carotid subclavian bypasses are performed end to side, complemented by in-line ligation if there is a truly ulcerative lesions proximally, because of the risk of distal embolization. Further, early in the 1970s, the saphenous vein was used as the preferred conduit. However, because of problems such as mismatches in caliber, kinking, or compression of the vein, prosthetic materials were explored. Comparative studies have demonstrated impressive patency of prosthetics in this position, mainly because it is a relatively short and high-flow graft. It is currently used nearly exclusively in this position.

B. Perioperative Complications

1. Mortality

Mortality from extra-anatomic cervical repairs is low, ranging from 0–3% (3–6). The most common causes of perioperative death in these high-risk patients are myocardial infarction or stroke.

Since myocardial infarction is an important cause of death, consideration of cardiac risk stratification is appropriate, as in any vascular operation. Considerable controversy remains regarding what testing modalities are optimal for assessing coronary risk and whether such tests should be applied routinely. Perhaps the most prudent method is a selective approach to preoperative testing with dipyridamole-thallium imaging in patients undergoing vascular surgery, based on the presence of certain clinical markers of coronary artery disease such as overall functional status, age of 70 or greater, diabetes, Q wave on electrocardiography, history of angina, and ventricular ectopy—all of which have been shown to be independent predictors of perioperative ischemic events (7,8).

2. Stroke

The incidence of stroke has been reported to range from 0 to 3.3% (3,4). The mechanism of stroke is thromboembolism or ischemia. The role of intraoperative maneuvers to reduce the risk of stroke should be considered. Electroencephalographic monitoring, especially during carotid artery bypasses, should be considered to assist the clinician in determining candidates for intraoperative shunting. Basic vascular surgical tasks such as thorough antegrade and retrograde arterial flushing prior to completion of the anastomosis cannot be overemphasized.

3. Nerve Injury

Nerve injury is another complication related to extra-anatomical cervical repairs. The vagus nerve and its recurrent nerve branch are of particular risk of injury upon manipulation of the carotid sheath or the phrenic nerve during the anterior scalene maneuvers. Palsy of the recurrent and phrenic nerves ranges from 0 to 3% (4,5). Due to its relative clinical insignificance, it is probable that temporary palsy of the phrenic nerve is higher in incidence than has been reported. To avoid injury to the nerves involves avoidance of manual manipulation with instruments or vessel loops. Identification of these nerves without manipulation is often the best policy in carrying out the dissection or in the application of retractors for exposure.

Injury to the cords of the brachial plexus should also be considered in operating near the anterior scalene muscle for exposure of the subclavian artery. The reported risk of injury is typically quite low. It is only when the dissection is carried out too laterally or superiorly that the plexus is in danger of injury.

4. Lymphatic Injury

Lymphatic injury producing lymphocele or lymph leak ranges from 0 to 7% (3–11). This is the most common wound complication in operations conducted in the supraclavicular space. The mechanism is related unrecognized injury to the thoracic duct or the multitude of lymphatics associated with the scalene fad pad. Attention to detail with deliberate ligation of all lymphatic tissue during the original dissection is key to the prevention of these often troublesome injuries. We favor division under direct vision and ligation of the entirety of the scalene fat pad to minimize the risk of lymphatic injury. Reexploration with ligation of the source of the lymph leak may occasionally be required. Methylene blue can be used to detail the anatomy of the lymph leak for precise ligation.

5. Tunneling Complications

Certain extra-anatomical bypasses require tunneling of the graft in both subcutaneous and occasionally retropharyngeal tissue planes. Tunneling for an axillary-axillary bypass requires a subcutaneous tunnel. Routing of a carotid-carotid bypass requires a tunnel under the strap muscles. Crossing of the midline (i.e., trachea and sternum) can result in skin erosion and infectious complications (11). Additionally, these routes complicate subsequent surgical therapies such as tracheostomy, median sternotomy, and subsequent arch reconstructions.

6. Patency

Long-term patency varies with the extra-anatomical procedure undertaken as well as the chosen conduit (Table 3). Carotid subclavian bypass is well tolerated and has the best results of the extrathoracic approaches. Recently, AbuRahma from West Virginia reported a primary patency rate of 96 and 92% at 5 and 10 years in 51 patients (3). This

Table 3 Five-Year Patency of
Carotid Subclavian Bypass

Transposition	100%
PTFE	95%
Dacron	84%
Saphenous vein	65%

Source: Ref. 4.

study used only PTFE for conduit. Five-year patency rates for carotid subclavian bypass were 95% for bypass grafts using PTFE in the review by UCLA (4). Interestingly, Law and colleagues further reported that Dacron had a patency rate of 84% and saphenous vein graft of 65% in the carotid subclavian bypass position. Patency rates for 124 patients reviewed from the University of Arkansas was 95% at both 5 and 10 years, with 35% of grafts being constructed from PTFE and the remainder composed of Dacron (5). Finally, Perler reviewed the Johns Hopkins experience and found the 5-year patency of PTFE-constructed grafts to be 92 and the 8-year patency at 83% (6) (see Table 4).

Transposition appears to be superior in terms of patency even to bypass. The benefits seem to include both reduced morbidity and greater patency. Subclavian transposition in 178 procedures was reported by Edwards and coworkers (12). The mortality rate associated with the isolated subclavian-carotid transposition was 1.1%, and all but one artery

Table 4 Death, Stroke, and Patency Rates of Extra-anatomic Bypass

Series, year (Ref.)	Number of patients	Mortality (percent)	Stroke (percent)	5-year patency
Abu Rahma, 2000 (3) Carotid-subclavian bypass with PTFE	51	0	0	96
Law et al., 1995 (4) Carotid-subclavian and subclavian-carotid transposition and with differing conduits	60	1.7	3.3	87.5
Vitti et al., 1994 (5) Carotid-subclavian with Dacron or PTFE	124	0.8	0	95
Perler and Williams, 1990 (6) Carotid-subclavian with PTFE, Dacron vein, transpostion	31	3.2	3.2	92
Edwards et al., 1994 (12) Subclavian-carotid transposition	178	1.1	1	99[a]
Mingoli et al., 1999 (11) Axilloaxillary bypass	61	1.6	0	86.5

[a] 46 months.

remained patent after a mean follow-up of 46 months. Schardey and colleagues reviewed 108 patients who underwent subclavian artery transposition; they reported no strokes and patency of 100% at 70 months (13). Van der Vliet found patency differences in transposition compared to bypass to be 100% for transposition at 5 and 10 years compared to bypass patency of 62 and 52%, respectively (9). The risk of perioperative stroke maybe less with transposition than with bypass. Indeed, Kretschmer published a 5.3% stroke rate with bypass and a rate of zero with transposition (10). Disadvantages to transposition include preservation of the vertebral artery because of its medial location. Additionally, bypass grafting can preserve the internal mammary artery for future potential coronary artery bypass surgery.

Other extra-anatomical surgical strategies have less favorable patency rates. Indeed, axilloaxillary bypas has poor long-term results. Criado reported axilloaxillary bypass to have the worst patency of any extra-anatomical bypass (14). Mingoli and colleagues reported somewhat more favorable results, with 5-year patency rates nearing 86% (11). Probably the worst patency is related to the femoral-to-axillary bypass (15). Clearly, the retrograde flow and length of the bypass contribute to these poor results.

III. ASCENDING AORTIC OPERATIONS—INNOMINATE ARTERY ATHEROSCLEROSIS

Innominate artery atherosclerosis is uncommon. In a comprehensive review of nearly 2000 operations on the aortic arch branches, Wylie and associates found that lesions of the innominate artery occured in only 7.5% of the reported cases (16). Most patients undergoing innominate artery reconstruction, however, have multiple supra-aortic lesions. Indeed, it has been reported that 61–84% of patients have multiple arch lesions (1,17,18). Transthoracic reconstructions are the preferred treatment in Takayasu's arteritis, radiation arteritis, recurrent disease, and multiple-level disease. These axial reconstructions offer better inflow for multiple reconstruction if needed for multiple lesions.

A. Technical Considerations

Axial reconstruction may be accomplished by bypass grafting directly from the ascending aorta performing an endarterectomy. Endarterectomy is usually done at the aortic arch origin of the innominate artery and carried on to the right subclavian and/or the right common carotid artery. Endarterectomy is limited by the safe placement of the proximal clamp onto the often diseased aorta and the proximity to the left common carotid artery. Caution must be exercised in performing endarterectomy because of its technical hazards. Most vascular surgeons have abandoned endarterectomy in favor of bypass grafting.

Transthoracic bypass of the innominate artery or its branches begins with a median sternotomy and extension of the incision into the right subclavian fossa, depending on the extent of disease. After isolation of the proximal aorta and the distal target artery, a partial occlusion clamp is placed as proximal on the ascending aorta as possible. In our evaluation scheme of clamping strategies, we evaluate the ascending aorta for calcium and thrombus with either transesophageal echocardiography or spiral computed tomography. Dacron or externally supported PTFE is used if the bypass is a single one. Bifurcated Dacron grafts are used for multiple bypasses. The proximal anastomosis should be positioned on the right side of the very proximal intrapericardial ascending aorta to prevent compromise of the graft by closure of the sternum. Further, the graft should not be overstretched, as this may cause fibrosis and later kinking of the graft with movement of the head and neck. Distal anastomoses are created in one of two ways. If the disease proximally is thought to create atheroemboli, the surgeon may consider transecting the diseased artery at it origin and creating an end-to-end anastomosis with the graft. If thromboembolism is not a threat proximally, an end-to-side anastomosis can be created. Additionally, care and attention must be given to protecting the right vagus nerve during these manipulations.

Care must be exercised in tunneling the graft. The graft should not obstruct the innominate artery or internal jugular vein. In most circumstances, the graft should not be tunneled underneath the veins. Placing the graft ventral to the veins will avoid venous compression or obstruction. Another described technique is to ligate and divide the brachiocephalic vein. Although permanent arm swelling has been described, this is usually a transient problem that subsides over time.

Concomitant coronary artery disease occurs frequently in this patient population (18,19). It is often prudent to evaluate the patient for coronary artery disease angiographically prior to performing a median sternotomy. Recently, Takach and colleagues from the Texas Heart Institute reported a perioperative mortality of only 3.2% when direct revascularization of the SATs was performed along with coronary artery bypass grafting (20). Our practice is to routinely do at least a dipyridamole-thalliwm study if we do a sternotomy and then, if positive, to consider coronary angiography.

B. Mortality

Interest in ascending axial reconstructions of the innominate artery decreased in the 1970s because of the high mortality rate following those procedures (21). However, since the inception of the modern era of critical care and refined surgical techniques, the mortality rate for transthoracic procedures has diminished substantially. Mortality rate in a sampling of large contemporary series ranges from 0 to 14.7% (17–19,22–25) (see Table 5).

C. Stroke

Perioperative stroke ranges from 0 to 8% in the latest series (see Table 5). Frequently, these patients will have multiple other lesions, including carotid bifurcation lesions. We commonly use electroencephalographic control to detect global ischemia. It is often technically possible to shunt through the graft. In our experience with routine electroencephalographic monitoring, ischemic changes with clamping are seldom noted. This can be best explained by the external-to-internal carotid artery pathway above the clamps.

Table 5 Perioperative Stroke and Mortality Rates of Transthoracic Repair of Supra-aortic Trunks

Author, year (Ref.)	Number of patients	Stroke (percent)	Mortality (percent)
Berguer, 1998 (18)	100	8	8
Kieffer, 1995 (19)	148	5.4	5.4
Cherry, 1989 (17)	26	0	3.8
Brewster, 1985 (25)	29	6.9	3.4
Zelenock, 1985 (22)	17	5.9	0
Crawford, 1983 (24)	43	5.5	4.7
Vogt, 1982 (23)	34	0	14.7

D. Venous Problems

As mentioned previously, careful placement of the graft in relation to the brachiocephalic vein is critical in avoiding compression of the vein. Our stance is to place the graft over the vein. We have had no venous compression or thrombosis related to this technique.

E. Nerve Injury

The surgeon should have an understanding of the location of the vagus and recurrent laryngeal nerves as they course through the mediastinum. Additionally, if more distal exposure of the subclavian artery is necessary, the phrenic nerve must be identified and preserved.

F. Sternotomy Complications

Sternotomy issues that should be considered include graft kinking after the bypass, kinking of venous structures after the closure, and the periodically encountered sternal wound infections. The surgeon should be keenly aware of the right of domain of the mediastinum in constructing the bypass and prior to sternotomy closure. As discussed previously, reducing the amount of tissue in the mediastinum is crucial in preventing overcrowding in the mediastinum. Perhaps resecting the proximal diseased segment of the innominate artery would be helpful to get the graft to lie properly. Again, we routinely do end-to-end anastomosis as opposed to end-to-side, partially to help avoid these and other problems.

G. Patency

Direct transthoracic reconstruction of the supra-aortic trucks results in excellent patency rates (see Table 5). The best assessment of the modern surgical experience and long-term results of transthoracic anatomical reconstruction have been reported by the groups in Detroit and Paris (18,19). Primary patency in the series by Kieffer and collegues was 98.4 at 5 years and 96.3% at 10 years. Berguer and coworkers reported 94% and 88% patency rates at 5 and 10 years, respectively. In comparing endarterectomy to direct reconstruction, no difference in patency was found (17,25,26). This operation, however, is performed less often than anatomical reconstruction.

IV.   DIRECT VERTEBRAL ARTERY RECONSTRUCTION

Surgical treatment of vertebrobasilar insufficiency continues to generate a great deal of debate in the literature. Most agree, however, that if clinical manifestations and definitive objective imaging studies both confirm the diagnosis, surgical options should be considered. Depending on the level of disease, three open surgical options have been described: transposition of the vertebral to the common carotid artery, vertebral artery endarterectomy, or—for cervical segment disease—bony decompression. While large surgical series such those of Berguer et al. are noted, primary vertebral artery reconstruction is seldom required (27,28). Furthermore, while most respect Ramon Berguer's work, the fact is that direct surgical reconstruction is (in the hands of most) confined to the vertebral artery origin.

A.   Technical Considerations

The vertebral artery is approached through a standard supraclavicular incision. The sternocleidomastoid muscle laterally is divided. The anterior scalene muscle is likewise divided. Care is taken to avoid injury to the phrenic nerve, which is retracted laterally. If the thoracic duct is identified it is also ligated. The common carotid artery is mobilized from the carotid sheath. The origin of the vertebral artery is identified and ligated. The vertebral artery is then carefully mobilized and reimplanted into either the CCA or sometimes described a nondiseased external carotid artery. Other options include an interposition vein graft from the subclavian artery to the vertebral artery. Of note is the rather fragile nature to the vertebral artery. The wall of the vertebral artery is on the order of one-third the thickness of the saphenous vein; therefore clamping must be done carefully and untoward stretching avoided. Technical considerations of bypass or reconstruction of the distal vertebral artery are beyond the scope of this chapter.

B. Mortality/Stroke

The perioperative mortality rate of vertebral artery reconstruction is low, at around 0.6–3.2% (27). More recent reports claim lower mortality rates, near 0.6%, and state that this is due to modern anesthetic regimens and improved patient selection (28). The perioperative stroke rate of vertebral artery reconstruction ranges from 1.9 to 4.1% (27,28).

C. Other Complications

The left vertebral artery origin lies in close proximity to the thoracic duct. Often, if identified, the duct can be ligated to prevent the occurrence of a lymphocele. Local complications such as Horner's syndrome are due to manipulation or injury of the lower cervical sympathetics and are usually transient.

D. Patency

Patency rates of vertebral artery transposition are usually quite satisfactory, ranging from 90 to 97% at 5 years (27,28). Occlusion of these reconstructions is usually exclusively in patients in whom vertebral-to-carotid transposition is not possible and interposition vein graft is necessary.

REFERENCES

1. Fields WS, Lemak NA. Joint study of extracranial arterial occlusion. JAMA 1972; 222:1139.
2. Lyons C, Galbraith G. Surgical treatment of atherosclerotic occlusion of the internal carotid artery. Ann Surg 1957; 146:484–487.
3. AbuRahma AF, Robinson PA, Jennings TG. Carotid subclavian bypass grafting with PTFE grafts for symptomatic subclavian artery stenosis or occlusion: A 20 year experience. J Vasc Surg 2000; 32:411–419.
4. Law MM, Colburn MD, Moore WS, Quinones-Baldrich WJ, Machleder HI, Gelabert HA. Carotid subclavian bypass for brachiocephalic occlusive disease: Choice of conduit and long term follow-up. Stroke 1995; 26:1565–1571.
5. Vitti MJ, Thompson BW, Read RC, et al. Carotid-subclavian bypass: A twenty-two year experience. J Vasc Surg 1994; 20:411–418.
6. Perler BA, Williams GM. Carotid-subclavian bypass–A decade of experience. J Vasc Surg 1990; 12:716.
7. Eagle KA, Coley CM, Newell JB, et al. Combining clinical and thallium data optimizes preoperative assessment of cardiac risk before major vascular surgery. Ann Intern Med 1989; 110:859–866.
8. Cambria RP, Brewster DC, Abbott WM, L'Italien GJ, Megerman JJ, LaMuraglia GM,

Moncure AC, Zelt DT, Eagle K. The impact of selective use of dipyridamole-thallium scans and surgical factors on the current morbidity of aortic surgery. J Vasc Surg 1992; 15(1):43–50.

9. Van der Vliet JA, Palamba HW, Scharn DM, et al. Arterial reconstruction for subclavian obstructive disease: A comparison of extrathoracic procedures. Eur J Vasc Endovasc Surg 1995; 9:454–458.

10. Kretschmer G, Teleky B, Marosi L, et al. Obliterations of the proximal subclavian artery: To bypass or to anastomose? J Cardiol Surg 1991; 32:334–339.

11. Mingoli A, Sapienza P, Feldhaus RJ, Bartoli S, Palombi M, de Marzo L, Cavallaro A. Long-term results and outcomes of crossover axillo-axillary bypass grafting: A 24 year experience. J Vasc Surg 1999; 29:894–901.

12. Edwards WH, Tapper SS, Edwards WH Sr, Mulherin JL, Martin RS, Jenkins JM. Subclavian revascularization: A quarter-century experience. Ann Surg 1994; 219:673.

13. Schardey HM, Meyer G, Rau HG, et al. Subclavian caroted transposition: An analysis of a clinical series and a review of the literature. Eur J Vasc Endovasc Surg 1996; 12:431–436.

14. Criado FJ. Extrathoracic management of aortic arch syndrome. Br J Surg 1982; 69(suppl):45–51.

15. Sproul G. Femoral-axillary bypass for cerebral vascular insufficiency. Arch Surg 1971; 103:746–747.

16. Wylie EJ, Effeney DJ. Surgery of the aortic arch branches and vertebral arteries. Surg Clin North Am 1979; 59:669–680.

17. Cherry KJ Jr, McCullough JL, Hallet JW Jr, Pairolero P. Technical principles of direct innominate artery revascularization: A comparison of endarterectomy and bypass grafts. J Vasc Surg 1989; 9:718–724.

18. Berguer R, Flynn LM, Kline RA, Caplan L. Transthoracic repair of innominate and common carotid artery disease: immediate and long-term outcome for 100 consecutive surgical reconstructions. J Vasc Surg 1998; 27(1):34–41.

19. Kieffer E, Sabatier J, Koskas F, Bahnini A. Atherosclerotic innominate artery occlusive disease: Early and long term results of surgical reconstruction. J Vasc Surg 1995; 21:326–337.

20. Takach TJ, Reul GJ Jr, Cooley DA, et al. Concomitant occlusive disease of the coronary arteries and great vessels. Ann Thorac Surg 1998; 65:79–84.

21. Crawford ES, DeBakey ME, Morris GC, Howell JF. Surgical treatment of occlusion of the innominate, common carotid, and subclavian arteries: A 10-year experience. Surgery 1969; 65: 17–31.

22. Zelenock GB, Cronenwett JL, Graham LM, et al. Brachiocephalic arterial occlusions and stenosis. Arch Surg 1985; 120:370–376.

23. Vogt DP, Hertzer NR, O'Hara PJ, Beven EG. Brachiocephalic arterial reconstruction. Ann Surg 1982; 196:541–552.

24. Crawford ES, Stowe CL, Powers RW Jr. Occlusion of the innominate, common carotid and subclavian arteries: Long-term results of surgical treatment. Surgery 1983; 94:781.

25. Brewster DC, Moncure AC, Darling RC, et al. Innominate artery lesions: Problems encountered and lessons learned. J Vasc Surg 1985; 2:99–112.

26. Reul GJ, Jacobs MJHM, Gregoric ID, et al. Innominate artery occlusive disease: Surgical approach and long-term results. J Vasc Surg 1991; 14:405–412.

27. Berguer R, Morasch MD, Kline RA. A review of 100 consecutive reconstructions of the distal vertebral artery for embolic and haemodynamic disease. J Vasc Surg 1998; 27(5):852–859.

28. Berguer R, Flynn LM, Kline RA, Carplan L. Surgical reconstruction of the extracranial vertebral artery: Management and outcome. J Vasc Surg 2000; 31(1 Pt 1):9–18.

27

Prevention of Transient Ischemic Attacks and Acute Strokes After Carotid Endarterectomy: A Critique of Techniques for Cerebrovascular Protection During Carotid Endarterectomy

William H. Baker and Maureen Sheehan

Loyola University Medical Center, Maywood, Illinois, U.S.A.

The purpose of carotid endarterectomy is the prevention of stroke. The role of the operation has been well established by prospective, randomized studies in both symptomatic and asymptomatic patients (1–3). Newer antiplatelet agents, while effective, have not supplanted operation. Carotid dilatation and stenting is currently undergoing scrutiny in a prospective study sponsored by the National Institutes of Health.

If carotid endarterectomy is to remain the "gold standard" of treatment, stroke and death rates associated with operation must be kept to a minimum. Many Centers of Excellence report stroke and mortality rates of 1–3% following carotid endarterectomy. Older statistics of Medicare patients gathered by the Rand Corporation suggest an almost 10% combined stroke and mortality rate (4). The American Heart Association suggests that an operation-related stroke and death rate of 2–5% is acceptable in symptomatic patients (5). It is this author's opinion that the stroke and death rate ought to be below 3% in all circumstances. Thus it behooves all vascular surgeons to use the safest methods for cerebrovascular protection during operation. Although perioperative stroke rates may also be related to such factors as patient selection, anesthesia, and avoidance of cardiac complications, this chapter concentrates on those operative techniques that may correlate with intraoperative stroke.

I. TEMPORARY INDWELLING SHUNT

During the performance of a carotid endarterectomy, vascular clamps by necessity are applied to the common, external, and internal carotid arteries, resulting in cessation of flow in the ipsilateral internal carotid artery and a reduction of flow in the ipsilateral cerebral hemisphere. If the collateral cerebral circulation is adequate, no neurological sequelae result from this temporary reduction of flow. If the cerebral collateral circulation is inadequate, the patient is at risk for intraoperative stroke. In an effort to avoid stroke in patients in whom the cerebral collateral flow is inadequate, surgeons have used a temporary indwelling shunt (6). A variety of plastic tubes can be used to shunt blood from the common carotid artery to the distal internal carotid artery during the performance of endarterectomy. Whereas this technique does increase ipsilateral hemispheric flow during operation, the shunt itself may "snowplow" debris from the atheromatous intima into the ipsilateral cerebral circulation, causing hemispheric emboli. If air is inadvertently introduced during insertion of a shunt, air emboli may result. Finally, the shunt itself is an encumbrance during the performance of the endarterectomy. It can be easier to perform the operation without the presence of a plastic tube in the middle of the artery. Although the shunt does not preclude the performance of an adequate operation and, in fact, in some operations is easy to work around, it is simpler not to have it in the way. Furthermore, in some patients with a long tail of atheroma in whom the carotid bifurcation is situated quite high in the neck underneath the angle of the mandible, the operation is challenging even without the shunt in place. Use of a temporary indwelling shunt in this situation is almost impossible. To protect the brain during the performance of carotid endarterectomy, some surgeons usually use a temporary indwelling shunt (6), most surgeons use a shunt selectively for all the reasons enumerated above (7), and relatively few surgeons entirely avoid using a shunt (8).

Surgeons who always use a shunt find it is the easiest way to perform the operation, arguing that the labyrinth of data concerning selective shunt usage is inconsistent. Thus, rather than sift through this maze of statistics to determine indications for shunt usage, they use the shunt in every case. These surgeons suggest that with consistent shunt usage, they become more proficient and accustomed to the shunt's presence in the operating field, and they do not find it an impediment to the performance of the endarterectomy. They have developed techniques for its use even in the presence of a long atheroma located unusually high up in the neck. In these patients, carotid endarterectomy is performed expeditiously in the internal carotid artery, the distal endpoint is seen directly and tacked if necessary, and finally the distal end of the shunt is inserted under direct vision, taking care not to disturb the distal endpoint. Insertion time may be somewhat prolonged in this group; the total time of the decreased ipsilateral hemispheric blood flow is reduced markedly compared with that in patients in whom a shunt is not used. With a shunt in place, closure of the arteriotomy is said to be facilitated. However, most vascular surgeons currently use a patch angioplasty technique; thus compromise of the internal carotid artery is a rare occurrence. Closure after an eversion carotid endarterectomy is not facilitated by a shunt.

A. Criteria for Use

Most surgeons find that it is technically more pleasing to perform the operation without a shunt. Thus surgeons who recognize the occasional need for a shunt base their decisions for selective use on a variety of criteria.

One of the earliest criteria surgeons used was the observation of the back-bleeding from the internal carotid artery. Pulsatile blood flow that shot across the operative field clearly was adequate, whereas flow that seeped from the distal end of the internal carotid artery was inadequate. The exact distinction between adequate and inadequate is difficult to quantify using this method.

In an effort to quantify this back-bleeding, stump or distal internal carotid artery back pressures were measured. This method was first used by Moore and Hall (9) at the San Francisco Veterans Administration Hospital and reported in 1969. Their initial and subsequent experiences with the measurement of stump pressure in patients undergoing operation using local anesthesia indicated that if the stump pressure was greater than 25 mmHg, the operation could be performed without risk of intraoperative neurological deficit. Those patients with a reduced stump pressure were at an increased risk of intraoperative stroke. In the same city, the University of California at San Francisco group suggested, on the basis of their experience, that the safe level of stump pressure was 50 mmHg, not 25 mmHg (7). This latter pressure has become the accepted norm in this country. Most surgeons who practice this technique use mean pressure rather than systolic pressure.

This technique has its detractors also. Hobson et al. (10) reported that test occlusion will result in neurological symptoms even with a back pressure greater than 50 mmHg. Connelly and coworkers (11) have reported similar experiences. It would be interesting to know whether these authors tested the adequacy of carotid occlusion as reported by Archie (12). During measurement of stump pressure, Archie occludes the internal carotid artery with the pickups. If indeed the stump pressure does not become a straight line at zero, he repositions the clamp on either the external or common carotid artery to ensure that each is occluded.

Electroencephalography has also been used successfully to determine which patients require a temporary indwelling shunt. One champion of this technique is Callow (13) and his group at Tufts University Medical Center. The electroencephalogram is unquestionably accurate in detecting subtle abnormalities as they relate to cerebral circulation. Surgeons who use this technique to select patients for shunt usage find that up to one-third require a shunt. This number is quite high considering the number of patients in whom a shunt is used while under local anesthesia and the observance of neurological deficits (14). Thus it must be concluded that the electroencephalogram is hypersensitive to subtle changes resulting from decreased perfusion. Surgeons using this technique undoubtedly will use the shunt more often, but they should feel secure that their patients are carefully selected.

There are newer electroencephalograms in use that are easier for surgeons to interpret. They compress the tracings and interpret wave heights in numbers. Excellent results with this technique in carotid endarterectomy have been reported (15).

Many surgeons use local anesthesia in an awake patient to determine whether a shunt is indicated. A field block is used to anesthetize the neck, a routine exposure is performed, and the carotid artery is clamped. If indeed the patient exhibits a neurological deficit during the 3–5 min of test clamping, the clamps are removed and preparation is made for the use of a temporary indwelling shunt. Surgeons practicing this technique report that shunt usage is between 5 and 10%. Excellent results have been reported with the technique, but detractors point out that it is not suitable for all patients and that general anesthetic agents, although they are myocardial depressants, also depress the cerebral metabolic rate and may in themselves confer safety to the operation.

There are relatively few surgeons who never use a shunt. Initially our group opposed the use of shunts. We reasoned that the data were not precise in selecting who should and should not have a temporary indwelling shunt, and we elected not to use them. During that time we measured stump pressures in all patients. Interestingly, we came to the conclusion that in patients with contralateral carotid occlusion and a stump pressure below

50 mmHg, the stroke rate was sufficiently high (11%) to strongly consider the use of a temporary indwelling shunt (16). In a subsequent publication, our group reported an increased stroke risk in patients with a stump pressure below 25 mmHg regardless of the status of the contralateral carotid artery (17). These studies form the basis of our current pattern of selective shunt usage.

In the discussion of our initial results, we reasoned that if we had used a shunt in those patients with a low stump pressure and a contralateral carotid occlusion, the stroke rate in this subset would have been reduced from 11 to 2%. With the use of a shunt, seven patients who indeed had a stroke might have been spared this neurological deficit. Overall, this would have reduced the incidence of permanent neurological deficit from 2 to 1.1%. This small reduction in stroke, although significant, especially for those seven patients, underscores that there is a preeminent role for other factors in the production of operation-related stroke.

II. AVOIDANCE OF INTRAOPERATIVE EMBOLIZATION

What are these other factors? Most surgeons agree that they are the avoidance of intraoperative embolization and the performance of a technically perfect operation. The incidence of intraoperative embolization is increased if the surgeon is rough in handling the carotid bifurcation before the application of appropriate vascular clamps. Evans, of Columbus, Ohio, suggests that those surgeons who obtain superior results with local anesthesia may do so because local anesthesia forces them to be gentle during the performance of the operation (personal communication, 1981). We make a special effort not to dissect the carotid bulb until after the appropriate clamps have been placed to avoid the possibility of emboli. The incidence of embolization of air and atherosclerotic debris can be increased by the use of a temporary indwelling shunt unless the shunt is inserted perfectly.

III. THE TECHNICALLY PERFECT OPERATION

A technically superior operation can be performed with or without shunt usage. To assess our technical results in the operating room, we have increasingly used B-mode imaging. We find this technique to be superior to contrast radiology because of its ease of use and avoidance of the theatrics that sometimes accompany intraoperative arteriography. Initially we found several defects that required correction. Because of the use of this technique, we have routinely carried the proximal extent of endarterectomy more caudad in the common carotid artery. This has resulted in a proximal shelf of atheroma that is less prominent. This monitoring technique, like operative arteriography and imaging of distal bypass grafts, forces the surgeon to be extremely meticulous, knowing that his or her operative result will be scrutinized immediately. This protects against the possibility of early postoperative occlusion.

IV. CORRECTION OF NEUROLOGICAL DEFICITS

What if the patient has neurological deficit in the immediate postoperative period? Is there a "golden period" during which the surgeon can boldly act before such a neurological deficit becomes permanent? If the stroke is caused by intraoperative ischemia, clearly nothing can be done. If the stroke is the result of intraoperative embolization, any surgical actions taken postoperatively are akin to "closing the barn door after the horse has gone."

Thus the surgeon can positively affect a postoperative stroke only if indeed there is a mechanical blockage in the internal carotid artery at the operative site.

In prior years, all patients who awoke in the operating room with a neurological deficit were reexplored. We assumed that the patient with an internal carotid artery occlusion would benefit from this algorithm. Kwaan and colleagues have established that a prompt restoration of flow results in total reversal of a neurological deficit in selected patients (18). In all likelihood the duration of this golden period is 1–2 h. In some patients it is clearly much shorter. This policy is still used in many institutions and cannot either be faulted or proven to be efficacious (19).

At Loyola we have used intraoperative duplex to assess our technical result since 1988. During that time we have evolved a different therapeutic algorithm for the patient who has a stroke after carotid endarterectomy (20). Those patients who awaken in the operating room, sometimes within 15 min of a normal intraoperative duplex, are rarely reexplored. Of the 15 patients in our series who awoke from surgery with a related deficit, 5 were reexplored and all had patent internal carotid arteries. Nine of the remaining 10 had a duplex-proven patent internal carotid artery. One patient without lateralizing signs was found to have extensive thrombosis at postmortem.

However, those patients who awaken neurologically intact and then later, after a lucid period, exhibit a related neurological deficit are assumed to have an internal carotid artery occlusion and thus are returned to the operating room. We had 10 patients in this category; 6 were reexplored, and all had thrombosed internal carotid arteries. Of these 6 patients, 5 improved after thrombectomy. One of the patients who was not reexplored had an observed embolus during the original intraoperative duplex; a post operative duplex at the time of a neurological deficit revealed a perfectly normal internal carotid artery. The second patient had a transient ischemic attack and a duplex-proven normal internal carotid artery. Two additional patients had delayed recognition of their deficit (greater than 2 h) as well as a normal postoperative duplex and were not reexplored. The only patient of these 10 who did not improve neurologically was a man who was reexplored and had flow restored within 1 h of onset of his neurological deficit.

At reexploration, the surgeon often feels a pulse in the operating area. Our bias is that these arteries ought to be opened or at the very least be interrogated with intraoperative duplex. The pulse at the operative site may be associated with a distal thrombus. If a technical cause for the thrombosis cannot be found, it is our habit to reclose the arteries with a vein patch. Occasionally the artery is replaced with either vein or polytetrefluoroethylene.

Patients who exhibit a postoperative transient ischemic attack with rapid normalization of their neurological function pose a special problem. Most patients do not have a preoperative arteriogram; their surgery is based solely on duplex ultrasonography. Many patients do not have preoperative computed tomography or magnetic resonance imaging. Thus, such patients need a complete workup to ensure that the operative site is pristine and that other unrecognized pathology is not present.

A. Neurological Rescue

Many patients who undergo exploration for stroke after carotid endarterectomy will have a relatively clean endarterectomy site. Many may have had intracranial embolization. In prior years, emboli were treated with heparin, and sometimes these patients were switched to warfarin. At the present time invasive neuroradiologists are able to traverse the endarterectomy site and identify thrombi in the anterior and/or middle cerebral arteries.

Either by mechanically passing a catheter through the clot or direct administration of thrombolytic therapy, these clots can often be dissolved or broken up to restore flow to the affected brain. Thus it is our current practice to call neuroradiology when we begin an exploration for a stroke after carotid endarterectomy. If, at the end of the procedure, we suspect that the patient has had an embolism and this same patient awakens with a significant neurological deficit, the patient is transported directly to the neuroradiology suite from the operating room. A repeat arteriogram is then performed; if a distal embolus is identified, the embolus is treated as outlined above.

Direct intervention for an intracerebral embolus is debatable in neurological circles and is clearly not the standard of care for a post–carotid endarterectomy embolus in 2002. However, neurorescue as described above may be the most promising therapy on the horizon. Fortunately this situation is rare. We have only embarked on this therapy in one patient to date and cannot comment on its efficacy.

V. CONCLUSION

The main methods used to avoid stroke during carotid endarterectomy are the use of an indwelling shunt during the performance of the operation to prevent intraoperative ischemia, avoidance of intraoperative embolization by gentle operative techniques, and performance of a technically perfect operation that prevents early postoperative occlusion. A variety of methods may safely predict who should and should not require a temporary indwelling shunt. Surgical technique that avoids trauma to the carotid bifurcation must be learned but cannot be monitored. Intraoperative arteriography, B-mode imaging, and other imaging techniques are of great assistance in detecting defects that could lead to postoperative stroke and are recommended especially for those centers whose existing morbidity and mortality rates are judged to be excessive. If indeed postoperative stroke occurs, especially after a period during which the patient was neurologically intact, immediate reexploration of a totally thrombosed carotid and reestablishment of cerebral blood flow may result in total or partial restoration of function.

REFERENCES

1. North American Symptomatic Carotid Endarterectomy Trial Collaborators. Beneficial effect of carotid endarterectomy in symptomatic patients with high-grade carotid stenosis. N Engl J Med 325(7):445–451.
2. North American Symptomatic Carotid Endarterectomy Trial Collaborators. Benefit of carotid endarterectomy in patients with symptomatic moderate or severe stenosis. N Engl J Med 339(20):1415–1425.
3. Executive Committee for Asymptomatic Carotid Artery Stenosis. Endarterectomy for asymptomatic carotid artery stenosis. JAMA 1995; 273(18):1421–1428.
4. Winslow CM, Solomon DH, Chassin MR, et al. The appropriateness of carotid endarterectomy. N Engl J Med 1988; 318:721–727.
5. Beebe HG, Clagett P, DeWeese JA, Moore W, et al. Assessing risk associated with carotid endarterectomy. Stroke 1989; 20:314–315.
6. Thompson JE, Talkington CM. Carotid endarterectomy. Ann Surg 1976; 184:1–15.
7. Hays RJ, Levinson SA, Wylie EJ. Intraoperative measurement of carotid back pressure as a guide to operative management for carotid endarterectomy. Surgery 1972; 72:593.
8. Ott DA, Cooley DA, Chapa L, et al. Carotid endarterectomy without temporary intraluminal shunt: Study of 309 consecutive operations. Ann Surg 1980; 191:708–714.

9. Moore WS, Hall AD. Carotid artery back pressure: A test of cerebral tolerance to temporary carotid occlusion. Arch Surg 1969; 99:702–710.

10. Hobson RW, Wright CB, Jublett JW, et al. Carotid artery back pressure and endarterectomy under regional anesthesia. Arch Surg 1974; 109:682.

11. Connelly JE, Kwaan JH, Stemmer EA. Improved results with carotid endarterectomy. Ann Surg 1977; 186:334.

12. Archie JP. Technique and clinical results of carotid back pressure to determine selective shunting during carotid endarterectomy. J Vasc Surg 1991; 13:319–327.

13. Callow AD. The Leriche Memorial Lecture. J Cardiovasc Surg 1980; 21:641–658.

14. Imparato AM, Ramirez A, Riles T, et al. Cerebral protection in carotid surgery. Arch Surg 1982; 117:1073–1078.

15. Tempelhoff R, Modica PA, Grubb RL, et al. Selective shunting during carotid endarterectomy based on two-channel computerized electroencephalographic compressed spectral array analysis. Neurosurgery 1989; 24:339–344.

16. Baker WH, Littooy FN, Hayes AC, et al. Carotid endarterectomy without a shunt: The control series. J Vasc Surg 1984; 1:50–56.

17. Littooy FN, Halstuk KS, Mamdani M, et al. Factors influencing morbidity of carotid endarterectomy without a shunt. Am Surg 1984; 50:350–353.

18. Kwaan JH, Connolly JE, Sharefkin JB. Successful management of early stroke after carotid endarterectomy. Ann Surg 1979; 190:676–678.

19. Edwards WH, Jenkins JM, Edwards WH Sr, et al. Prevention of stroke during carotid endarterectomy. Am Surg 1988; 54:125–128.

20. Sheehan MK, Littooy FN, Greisler HP, et al. The effect of intraoperative duplex upon the treatment of post carotid endarterectomy stroke. Presented at the 59th annual meeting of the Central Surgical Association, March 9, 2002.

28

Nonstroke Complications of Carotid Endarterectomy

Caron Rockman and Thomas S. Riles

New York University School of Medicine, New York, New York, U.S.A.

The benefits of carotid endarterectomy (CEA) over the medical treatment of patients with both symptomatic and asymptomatic carotid stenosis have been confirmed by randomized, prospective clinical trials (1,2). However, the advantage of surgical therapy is achieved only if the complications of carotid surgery are maintained at an extremely low level. Particularly in asymptomatic patients, in whom the margin of benefit in stroke prevention is less remarkable, reducing the incidence of post-CEA complications is critical. The most commonly discussed and analyzed complication of CEA is, of course, stroke. However, a variety of other complications can occur and can cause considerable morbidity in both the short and long term. This chapter reviews the nonstroke complications that can compromise the outcome of CEA.

The general complications of CEA can be divided into neurological and nonneurological complications. Neurological complications include cranial nerve injury, the cerebral hyperperfusion syndrome, and ischemic stroke. Nonneurological complications of CEA include perioperative myocardial infarction and other cardiac complications; cardiopulmonary events as a complication of vascular surgical procedures in general are covered in another chapter of this book. However, perioperative hemodynamic instability consisting of either postoperative hyper- or hypotension is specific to CEA as opposed to other vascular surgical procedures and is discussed below. Other nonneurological complications of CEA include wound complications as well as complications related to patch material, hematoma, and postoperative infection. Finally, the development of recurrent carotid stenosis can be considered a late complication of CEA; this topic is addressed elsewhere in this book.

I. NEUROLOGICAL COMPLICATIONS

A. Cranial Nerve Injury

Although not a frank cerebral infarction, the rare permanent, severe cranial nerve injury following CEA can have equally devastating consequences to a patient's quality of life. Cranial nerve injury following CEA is well documented in the literature. However, it is usually a transient neuropraxia: the mechanism of injury is thought to be most often related to stretch, retraction, or clamping of the involved nerve rather than outright transection of the structure (3). Given the familiarity of most carotid surgeons with the anatomy of the neck, severe cranial nerve injuries most often occur in unusual circumstances such as reoperative carotid surgery or surgery involving unusually high lesions (4). The reported incidence of cranial nerve dysfunction following CEA varies widely from approximately 3–23% in representative series (5–16); the discrepancy in the reported incidence of this complication most likely depends on the exact methodology by which cranial nerve dysfunction is defined and diagnosed. The true incidence of clinically significant cranial nerve injuries is more difficult to ascertain and is likely much lower.

The cranial and cervical nerves at risk during CEA include the following: the hypoglossal, vagus, recurrent laryngeal, marginal mandibular, superior laryngeal, glossopharyngeal, spinal accessory, transverse cervical, and greater auricular nerves. Severe injuries to the hypoglossal, vagus, recurrent laryngeal, or glossopharyngeal nerves have the potential to result in distressing clinical consequences. Severe injury to the hypoglossal nerve can result in tongue clumsiness and biting, dysarthria, and impaired mastication and deglutition (3). Vagal and/or recurrent laryngeal nerve injury can result in vocal cord paralysis, hoarseness, or airway obstruction when bilateral. Glossopharyngeal injury most often results from unusually high dissection during CEA, especially if the posterior belly of the digastric muscle is divided (3). Symptoms of glossopharyngeal injury can range from dysphagia to recurrent aspiration, respiratory failure, and malnutrition. Tracheostomy and feeding jejunostomy may rarely be required.

Injury to the spinal accessory nerve is rare, given its typical location away from the field of the routine CEA. Injury to the superior laryngeal branch of the vagus can result in subtle voice changes that may be troublesome to singers or public speakers (3). Injuries to the transverse cervical and greater auricular nerves produce generally benign sensory losses. Injury to the marginal mandibular branch of the facial nerve is usually transient and of mainly cosmetic concern.

Several recent prospective studies have specifically examined the incidence and etiology of cranial nerve injuries following CEA. Maroulis, et al. (14) prospectively evaluated 269 operations. They found a 5.6% incidence of documented injury, including unilateral vocal cord paralysis (2.6%), hypoglossal palsy (3.3%), glossopharyngeal injury (0.7%), and marginal mandibular palsy (0.4%). All patients showed improvement within a few weeks, and none had residual disability at times ranging from 2 weeks to 14 months. Ballotta, et al. (15) prospectively reviewed 200 consecutive CEAs. They report a 12.5% incidence of injuries, with 5.5% hypoglossal, 4% recurrent laryngeal, 1% superior laryngeal, 1% marginal mandibular, and 1% greater auricular nerve injuries. All nerve dysfunctions were transient; two patients with recurrent laryngeal nerve dysfunction had prolonged but full recoveries within 37 months. Forssell et al. (16) prospectively studied 689 operations. Injuries were found in 11.4% of cases, including hypoglossal (10.7%), recurrent laryngeal (1.2%), glossopharyngeal (0.3%), and superior laryngeal (0.3%) injuries. One hypoglossal and one recurrent nerve injury were permanent. Nerve injury was more frequent in operations performed with a shunt ($p = 0.05$), with patch closure ($p = 0.01$), and by a junior surgeon ($p = 0.05$). Finally, AbuRahma et al. (4), in a prospective study of 89 carotid reoperations, reported a 21% rate of cranial nerve injury, with 3 permanent injuries.

In summary, cranial nerve dysfunction following CEA is relatively common, but most injuries are transient and do not have great clinical significance. Treatment when required, is expectant and supportive. In the case of planned bilateral CEAs, care must be taken to document vocal cord recovery prior to proceeding with contralateral surgery. Severe cranial nerve injuries can best be avoided by excellent knowledge of the variations in cranial and cervical nerve anatomy, attention to detail in dissection and retractor placement, and meticulous placement of vascular clamps.

B. Cerebral Hyperperfusion Syndrome

The cerebral hyperperfusion syndrome with resulting intracerebral hemorrhage (ICH) is one of the most feared complications by surgeons who perform CEAs. Although relatively infrequent, this complication can have tremendous and often fatal sequelae, and it remains a significant cause of neurological morbidity following CEA. ICH following cerebral revascularization was recognized as early as 1964 by Wylie et al. (17) and was found to be a common and catastrophic complication in patients who underwent CEA or carotid thrombectomy for an acute stroke (18). In 1984, Bernstein, et al. (19) reported the first CEA patient with the classic symptoms of postoperative unilateral head, face, and eye pain; the patient subsequently developed seizures and delayed ICH and then died. Cerebral hyperperfusion from lack of vascular autoregulation was proposed as the mechanism of this hemorrhage, which occurred in the absence of other, previously identified risk factors (18,19). The common denominator in the pathophysiology of the syndrome appears to be reactive hyperemia. In its less severe forms, hyperperfusion can result in mild cerebral edema, headache, and seizures. When an abnormal, hyperperfused vessel ruptures, ICH results (18).

The true incidence of the cerebral hyperperfusion syndrome following CEA is unknown. In its mild form, it is probably more common than clinically recognized. The reported incidence from several large series ranges from 0.4 to 2% (18). In the authors' institution, an evaluation of 1500 CEAs performed between 1975 and 1984 identified 11 patients with ICH, for an incidence of 0.7% (20). However, the mortality rate among these patients was 36%. A more recent review of 2024 CEAs performed between 1985 and 1997 identified only 5 patients with intracranial hemorrhage (0.3%). However, ICH still accounted for 5 of 38 perioperative neurological deficits that occurred after CEA during this period (13.2%) (18). An additional report by Ouriel et al. (21) revealed an incidence of 0.75% in 1471 patients during a 6-year period, with massive hemorrhage and death occurring in 4 cases. Considering the severe morbidity of this particular complication, it is critically important to understand which patients are at increased risk.

The most commonly identified factors that predispose a patient to the development of the cerebral hyperperfusion syndrome include a history of stroke, especially when recent; relief of a severely stenotic lesion (>90%); severe intraoperative and postoperative hypertension; anticoagulant use; severe chronic cerebral ischemia; and perhaps occlusion of the contralateral carotid artery (18,20). In the report by Ouriel et al. (21), five factors were associated with a statistically increased risk of intracranial bleeding: increased age, a history of hypertension, a high degree of ipsilateral stenosis, a high degree of contralateral stenosis, and contralateral carotid occlusion. Of course, one or more of these recognized risk factors are often present in many patients undergoing CEA. Clinically evident hyperperfusion does not occur in the majority of patients in whom one or even more of these risks exist. However, awareness of the early symptoms of the syndrome is important in these cases.

In the authors' series (18), most postoperative neurological deficits related to thrombosis or embolization occurred within the first 4 h after operation. In marked contrast, three of five intracranial hemorrhage occurred on postoperative day 4 or later.

These patients presented with headaches, seizures, progressive obtundation, or hemiparesis. It appears that the symptoms of cerebral hyperperfusion are more likely to occur somewhat later in the postoperative course than deficits associated with thromboembolization and are also more likely to present with either headache or seizures than with hemiparesis alone. The diagnosis of the syndrome is often clinical and rests heavily on the surgeon's suspicion in a patient with appropriate risk factors. Computed tomograpy (CT) scanning to evaluate for hemorrhage or edema is the test of choice in any patient who presents with severe frontoparietal or orbital pain or seizure activity. Electroencephalography may reveal lateralizing epileptiform discharges or frank seizure activity.

Prophylaxis is difficult because it would require predicting which patients will sustain such an event. However, in patients thought to be at increased risk, certain measures are reasonable: strict blood pressure control, judicious use of anticoagulants and antiplatelet agents, and close monitoring of the neurological status are indicated. In patients with headaches only, simple analgesia may suffice. In patients with more severe symptoms, antihypertensives and anticonvulsant medications may be warranted. If cerebral edema is significant, diuretics and anti-inflammatory medications may be utilized. If petechial or small cerebral hemorrhages occur, the above measures will often suffice (21). However, if massive hemorrhage occurs, neurosurgical intervention may become necessary. However, in all reported series, the prognosis of massive ICH after CEA is exceedingly poor (18).

II. NONNEUROLOGICAL COMPLICATIONS

A. Vein Patch Rupture

Patch angioplasty reconstruction of the carotid artery following CEA is an accepted technique and may reduce the incidence of postoperative thrombosis, embolization, and recurrent carotid artery stenosis. However, the ideal material for patch reconstruction remains to be defined. Certainly the greater saphenous vein has the advantages of being autologous, readily available, and easy to use. However, a rare but potentially life-threatening complication of its use is rupture of the vein patch following CEA. Its reported incidence in the literature ranges from 0 to 4.0% (22–27). Manifestations of vein patch rupture in the early postoperative period obviously include massive hemorrhage into the neck with airway compromise, respiratory arrest, and possible death.

Yamamoto et al. (25) reported 5 postoperative vein ruptures among 2888 CEAs (0.17%). All ruptures occurred within 4 days of surgery, including 2 during the first 24 h. All patients were found to have intact suture lines and tears in the middle of the grafts. Two patients died. Tawes et al. (26) reported a combined experience of 1760 operations, in which vein patch rupture occurred in 13 patients (0.7%). In 12 of these, the saphenous vein was harvested from the ankle. All ruptures occurred from a split in the center of the vein patch. Four patients died (30.7%), and three had strokes but survived. Riles et al. (27) reported a series of 2275 CEAs; in 3 patients out of 75 in whom the vein patch had been harvested from the ankle, rupture of the patch occurred. In all cases, reoperations revealed necrosis of the central portion of the vein with no evidence of infection. O'Hara et al. (23) reported 8 postoperative ruptures after 1691 CEAs in which saphenous vein patch angioplasty was used (0.5%). In each case, the vein had been harvested distal to the knee. Of the patients in whom rupture occurred, 29% either died or sustained strokes.

Based on the above studies as well as his own experience, Archie prospectively established diameter criteria for the use of the saphenous vein as a patch material (22). In a 7-year prospective study of 614 CEAs, using only greater saphenous veins with a distended diameter of greater than 3.5 mm, no ruptures occurred. This compared favorably with our own prior experience with 3 patch ruptures in 239 cases when no vein diameter criteria were utilized ($p = 0.03$).

In summary, although saphenous vein is an excellent patch material, its results may be compromised by the devastating complication of early patch rupture. This complication often results in death or severe morbidity. The incidence of vein patch rupture can probably be reduced or nearly eliminated by using greater saphenous vein harvested from the thigh or using only vessels greater than 3.5 mm in diameter when vein must be harvested from below the knee. Late aneurysmal degeneration of vein patching for CEA, with the potential for thrombus formation and thromboembolization, has been reported in the literature as well (28).

B. Postoperative Hematoma

Wound hematoma following CEA has not been extensively studied specifically. However, because of the risk of airway compromise with hemorrhage into the neck, this complication can be life-threatening. The incidence of wound hematoma reported in the literature varies from 1 to 4.5% (29–32). Risk factors reported include perioperative hypertension, lack of reversal of intraoperative heparinization with protamine sulfate, and postoperative resumption of anticoagulation with heparin and/or warfarin for treatment or prophylaxis of arterial or venous thromboembolization.

Treiman et al. (29) reported a study on the influence of protamine use following CEA on postoperative stroke and wound hematoma. A review of 697 operations was performed, in which 328 patients received protamine and 369 did not based on the practices and judgment of the individual operating surgeons. The incidence of stroke was similar between the groups. Thirty patients (4.3%) experienced a postoperative wound hematoma requiring reoperation. The incidence of wound hematoma was 1.8% in patients given protamine and 6.5% in patients not given protamine, and this difference was statistically significant ($p = 0.004$). In this series, all patients were intubated without difficulty. However, if intubation is difficult or impossible, the authors recommend opening the wound using local anesthesia prior to intubation and reoperation. No complications occurred in this series from evacuation of a wound hematoma.

The successful management of wound hematoma following CEA centers on immediate recognition of the complication and return to the operating room for hematoma evacuation. Even a hematoma that initially appears benign can rapidly progress to stridor and respiratory compromise. Although these hematomas are most often related to seemingly minor venous bleeding or diffuse bleeding from residual heparin effect, their consequences can be severe if not treated expeditiously.

C. Infectious Complications

While vein has long been considered the optimal standard for arteriovascular bypasses elsewhere in the arterial tree, concerns have arisen regarding the use of saphenous vein for carotid reconstruction. Specifically, reports of late aneurysmal dilatation and patch rupture, as described previously, have led to investigations for alternative acceptable patch materials. Harvest site morbidity and the need for venous conduits for subsequent coronary or lower extremity revascularizations have also been cited as reasons to consider prosthetic patch options.

Prosthetic patches such as polytetrafluoroethylene (PTFE) and polyester are attractive alternatives to vein in that they are readily available, technically easy to use, and may reduce the risk of patch rupture or aneurysmal dilatation. While several studies have shown that knitted polyester has been comparable to vein in rates of restenosis, potential drawbacks to prosthetic materials include possible increases in recurrent stenosis, increased thrombogenicity, and infection.

While potential infectious complications remain a significant concern, there have been very few reported series of infected prosthetic patch infections, and their true incidence is unknown. Several recent case series of carotid prosthetic patch infections have addressed this issue (33–35). Naylor et al. (34) report that 8 of 936 CEAs performed with prosthetic patch material developed a patch infection (0.85%). Responsible organisms included primarily *Staphylococcus* and *Streptococcus* species. Surgical repair consisted of carotid ligation in 3 cases and reconstruction with autologous material in 5; 1 patient suffered a disabling postoperative stroke following reoperations, and 2 had transient cranial nerve injuries. Rizzo et al. (35) reported an additional 8 patients with infected Dacron patches. Of these cases from their own institution, 6 represented 1.8% of 340 synthetic patches utilized. As in the prior series, gram-positive organisms predominated; in this series, all carotid arteries were reconstructed with autologous material. Again, two temporary cranial nerve injuries occurred.

The authors' institution is in the process of completing a report of 10 patients who required reoperations and management of postoperative Dacron patch infections following CEA (33). Half of these patients presented early with cellulitis and abscess formation within several weeks following the original operation. However, the remaining half presented with draining sinus tracts 1–2 years following surgery. All patients had their carotid arteries reconstructed with autologous material, with no significant morbidity. In all three of these reports (33–35), all patients remain free of infection following surgical management and removal of the patch.

Infection of a prosthetic patch is a rare but serious complication following CEA. However, it can be successfully managed with an acceptably low complication rate. Although infection of prosthetic patches is probably more common that infection of autologous patch material, the latter has in fact been reported (36).

D. Perioperative Blood Pressure Instability

Blood pressure instability following CEA may contribute to morbidity, increase length of hospital stay, increase costs, and occasionally result in mortality (37). Carotid baroreceptor dysfunction and impaired cerebral autoregulation following manipulation of the carotid bulb and carotid sinus nerve have been implicated in the etiology of both hyper- and hypotension post-CEA.

Reported risk factors for postoperative hypertension include having undergone an eversion endarterectomy (38) and having undergone surgery under general as opposed to regional anesthesia (39). Postoperative hypertension in particular has been shown to be associated with increased postoperative stroke and death and also with postoperative cardiac complications (40). In a report by Wong et al. (40), independent risk factors for postoperative hypertension included angiographic intracranial carotid stenosis greater than 50%, cardiac dysrhythmia, preoperative systolic blood pressure greater than 160 mmHg, neurological instability, and renal insufficiency. Postoperative hypotension and bradycardia did not correlate with perioperative outcome.

Management of post-CEA patients must include aggressive treatment of hemodynamic instability in order to prevent secondary complications. In addition to potential cardiac complications, severe hypotension may theoretically predispose toward thrombosis of the arterial reconstruction, and severe hypertension can increase the chance of cerebral hyperperfusion and intracranial hemorrhage.

III. CONCLUSIONS

In addition to stroke, CEA has the potential to result in a wide variety of neurological and nonneurological complications that have the potential to cause significant morbidity or mortality. In order for CEA to achieve success in stroke prevention, potential perioperative complications other than stroke must also be appropriately appreciated, recognized, and managed in order to minimize their occurrence and the resulting morbidity.

REFERENCES

1. The Executive Committee for the Asymptomatic Carotid Atherosclerosis Study. Endarterectomy for asymptomatic carotid artery stenosis. JAMA 1995; 273:1421–1428.
2. North American Symptomatic Carotid Endarterectomy Trial Collaborators. Beneficial effect of carotid endarterectomy in symptomatic patients with high-grade carotid stenosis. N Engl J Med 1991; 325:445–453.
3. Schauger MD, Fontenelle LJ, Solomon JW, Hanson TL. Cranial/cervical nerve dysfunction after carotid endarterectomy. J Vasc Surg 1997; 25:481–487.
4. AbuRahma AF, Chouerie MA. Cranial and cervical nerve injuries after repeat carotid endarterectomy. J Vasc Surg 2000; 32:649–654.
5. Maniglia AJ, Han AP. Cranial nerve injuries following carotid endarterectomy: An analysis of 336 procedures. Head Neck 1991; 13:121–124.
6. Hertzer NR, Feldman BJ, Beven EG, Tucker HM. A prospective study of the incidence of injury to the cranial nerves during carotid endarterectomy. Surg Gynecol Obstet 1980; 151:781–784.
7. Knight FW, Yeager RM, Morris DM. Cranial nerve injuries during carotid endarterectomy. Am J Surg 1987; 154:529–532.
8. Verta MJ Jr, Applebaum EL, McClusky DA, Yao JST, Bergan JJ. Cranial nerve injury during carotid endarterectomy. Ann Surg 1977; 185:192–195.
9. Dehn TCB, Taylor GW. Cranial and cervical nerve damage associated with carotid endarterectomy. Br J Surg 1983; 70:365–368.
10. Massey EW, Heyman A, Utley C, Haynes C, Fuchs J. Cranial nerve paralysis following carotid endarterectomy. Stroke 1984; 15:157–159.
11. Lusby RJ, Wylie EJ. Complications of carotid endarterectomy. Surg Clin North Am 1983; 63:1293–1301.
12. Rodgers W, Root HD. Cranial nerve injuries after carotid endarterectomy. South Med J 1988; 81:1006–1009.
13. Evans WE, Mendelowit DS, Liapis DS, Wolf V, Florence CL. Motor speech deficit following carotid endarterectomy. Ann Surg 1982; 196:461–463.
14. Maroulis J, Karkanevatos A, Papakostas K, Giling-Smith GL, McCormick MS, Harris PL. Cranial nerve dysfunction following carotid endarterectomy. Int Angiol 2000; 19:237–241.
15. Ballotta E, Da Giau G, Renon L, Narne S, et al. Cranial and cervical nerve injuries after carotid endarterectomy: A prospective study. Surgery 1999; 125:85–91.
16. Forssell C, Kitzing P, Bergqvist D. Cranial nerve injuries after carotid artery surgery. A prospective study of 663 operations. Eur J Vasc Endovasc Surg 1995; 10:445–449.
17. Wylie EJ, Hein MF, Adame JE. Intracranial hemorrhage following surgical revascularization for treatment of acute strokes. J Neurosurg 1964; 21:212–215.
18. Rockman CB, Riles TS. Cerebral hyperperfusion syndrome after carotid endarterectomy. In:

Ernst CB, Stanley JC, eds. Current Therapy in Vascular Surgery. 4th ed. St. Louis: Mosby, 2001:69–71.

19. Bernstein M, Fleming JFR, Deck JHN. Cerebral hyperperfusion after CEA: A cause of cerebral hemorrhage. Neurosurgery 1984; 15:50–56.

20. Pomposelli FB, Lamparello PJ, Riles TS, et al. Intracranial hemorrhage after CEA. J Vasc Surg 1988; 7:248–255.

21. Ouriel K, Shortell CK, Illig KA, et al. Intracerebral hemorrhage after carotid endarterectomy: Incidence, contribution to neurologic morbidity, and predictive factors. J Vasc Surg 1999; 29:82–89.

22. Archie JP. Carotid endarterectomy saphenous vein patch rupture revisited: Selective use on the basis of vein diameter. J Vasc Surg 1996; 24:346–352.

23. O'Hara PJ, Hertzer NR, Krajewski LP, Beven EG. Saphenous vein patch rupture after carotid endarterectomy. J Vasc Surg 1992; 15:504–509.

24. Lawhorne TW Jr, Brooks HB, Cunningham JM. Five hundred consecutive carotid endarterectomies: emphasis on vein patch closure. Cardiovasc Surg 1997; 5:141–144.

25. Yamamoto Y, Piepgras DG, Marsh WR, Meyer FB. Complications resulting from saphenous vein patch graft after carotid endarterectomy. Neurosurgery 1996; 39:670–676.

26. Tawes RL Jr, Treiman RL. Vein patch rupture after carotid endarterectomy: A survey of the Western Vascular Society members. Ann Vasc Surg 1991; 5:71–73.

27. Riles TS, Lamparello PJ, Giangola G, Imparato AM. Rupture of the vein patch a rare complication of carotid endarterectomy. Surgery 1991; 107:10–12.

28. Rockman CB, Riles TS, Landis R, Lamparello PJ, Giangola G, Adelman MA, Jacobowitz GR. Redo carotid surgery: An analysis of materials and configurations used in reoperative carotid surgery and their effects on perioperative stroke and subsequent recurrent stenosis. J Vasc Surg 1999; 29:72–81.

29. Treiman RL, Cossman DV, Foran RF, Levin PM, Cohen JL, Wagner WH. The influence of neutralizing heparin after carotid endarterectomy on postoperative stroke and wound hematoma. J Vasc Surg 1990; 12:440–446.

30. Kunkel JM, Gomez ER, Spebar MJ, et al. Wound hematomas after carotid endarterectomy. Am J Surg 1984; 148:844–847.

31. Welling RE, Ramadas HS, Gansmuller KJ. Cervical wound hematoma after carotid endarterectomy. Ann Vasc Surg 1989; 3:229–231.

32. Oller DW, Welch H. Complications of carotid endarterectomy. A military hospital experience. Am Surg 1986; 52:479–484.

33. Rockman CB, Wu WT, Domenig C, et al. Postoperative infection associated with polyester patch angioplasty following carotid endarterectomy. J Vasc Surg 2003; 38:251–256.

34. Naylor AR, Payne D, London NJM, et al. Prosthetic patch infection after carotid endarterectomy. Eur J Vasc Endovasc Surg 2002; 23:11–16.

35. Rizzo A, Hertzer NR, O'Hara PJ, Krajewski LP, Beven EG. Dacron carotid patch infection: A report of eight cases. Dacron carotid patch infection: a report of eight cases. J Vasc Surg 2000; 32:602–606.

36. Motte S, Wautrecht JC, Bellens B, Vincent G, Dereume JP, Delcour C. Infected false aneurysm following carotid endarterectomy with vein patch angioplasty. J Cardiovasc Surg 1987; 28:734–736.

37. Nowak LR, Corson JD. Blood pressure instability after carotid endarterectomy. In: Ernst CB, Stanley JC, eds. Current Therapy in Vascular Surgery. 4th ed. St. Louis: Mosby, 2001:71–73.

38. Mehta M, Rahmani O, Dietzek AM, et al. Eversion technique increases the risk for post–carotid endarterectomy hypertension. J Vasc Surg 2001; 34:839–845.

39. Sternbach Y, Illig KA, Zhang R, et al. Hemodynamic benefits of regional anesthesia for carotid endarterectomy. J Vasc Surg 2002; 35:333–339.

40. Wong JH, Findlay JM, Suarez-Almazor ME. Hemodynamic instability after carotid endarterectomy: Risk factors and association with operative complications. Neurosurgery 1997; 41:35–43.

29

Radiation Exposure and Contrast Toxicity

Evan C. Lipsitz, Frank J. Veith, and Takao Ohki

Montefiore Medical Center and the Albert Einstein College of Medicine, Bronx, New York, U.S.A.

I. RADIATION EXPOSURE

A. Introduction

Endovascular repair of aortoiliac aneurysms has gained widespread acceptance and the number of investigational devices as well as devices approved by the U.S. Food and Drug Administration for this procedure is growing. Other endovascular procedures for the treatment of such entities as aortoiliac occlusive disease and renal artery stenosis are also being employed more frequently. It has been estimated that the vast majority of abdominal aortic aneurysms are amenable to treatment with an endovascular graft and that, in the near future, 40–70% of all vascular interventions will be performed by an endovascular method, including an increasing number of peripheral and cerebrovascular interventions (1). These procedures require the use of digital cine-fluoroscopy, which exposes both the patient and staff to ionizing radiation.

B. Units of Measurement

Several different measures are used in the evaluation of radiation exposure. Absorbed dose is the energy delivered to an organ divided by the mass of the organ, expressed in grays (Gy). Equivalent dose is the average absorbed dose in an organ or tissue multiplied by a radiation weighting factor, expressed in sieverts (Sv). Since radiation used in medicine generally has a weighting factor of 1, the absorbed dose and the equivalent dose are considered equal. Total effective dose (TED) is the sum of the equivalent doses in all tissues and organs multiplied by a tissue weighting factor for each organ or tissue. It is this value that is used to evaluate total body exposure (2).

C. Biological Effects

The biological effects of radiation can be divided into two types, deterministic and stochastic (2). Deterministic effects are observed only when many cells in an organ or tissue are killed by virtue of a dose that is above a given threshold. Stochastic effects are due to radiation-induced injury to the DNA of a single cell. In this setting there is no threshold below which the risk is eliminated. However, the probability of an effect occurring is small. Stochastic effects may be somatic, affecting somatic cells, or hereditary, affecting germ cells. It is these stochastic effects that are of special concern, because there is no threshold below which their occurrence can be prevented.

There are many sources of radiation present within the environment, both naturally occurring and man-made. These are collectively referred to as *background radiation*. Radon gas constitutes the single most important source of naturally occurring external background radiation, followed closely by solar, cosmic, and galactic radiation (3). Natural atmospheric radiation and radionuclides also contribute to background radiation, as do terrestrial nuclides. Nuclear reactors and nuclear weapons testing also add to background radiation.

Radiation exposure is cumulative and its effects are permanent. The total exposure for an individual performing fluoroscopic procedures is the sum of his or her exposure during these procedures plus the background exposure as well as any incidental medical exposure—e.g., diagnostic chest x-rays—incurred by the individual. In the United States, the average person receives approximately 3.5 millisieverts (mSv) per year in background exposure. This dose increases with altitude, doubling at every 2000 m. Other local effects, such as radionuclides in the soil, can affect the background radiation significantly. Table 1 highlights the currently recommended dose limits for both the occupational and civilian settings.

D. Specific Recommendations

1. General Principles

Fluoroscopy Time. Radiation exposure is proportional to total fluoroscopy time. Therefore the most effective way to reduce exposure to both the patient and staff during endovascular procedures is to reduce the total fluoroscopy time. Several steps can be taken toward this end. Catheter-guidewire exchanges with a stable wire position do not need to be visualized in their entirety. When repositioning the field of interest either by moving the table or the C-arm, the desired position should be estimated and then fine-tuned under fluoroscopy rather than imaged along the entire course. This is also true when obtaining oblique or angled projections. In performing cine-acquisition, each screening should be carefully planned and have a specific objective. Poorly planned runs add no information to

Table 1 Yearly Recommended Dose Limits

Application	Dose limit (mSv/year)	
	Occupational	Public
Effective dose	20	1
Equivalent dose		
lens of eye	150	15
skin	500	50
hands and feet	500	—

Source: From Ref. 2.

the procedure and increase exposure, contrast load, and operative time. For example, a subtraction run over the upper abdomen without holding the respirations—either by anesthesia in the intubated patient or voluntarily in the awake patient—is likely to produce a useless image. All individuals involved in the procedure must be constantly aware of when the fluoroscope is on. When the fluoroscope is on, they must evaluate whether or not essential information is being obtained or if it is necessary for the technical performance of the procedure. Simply measuring the fluoroscopy time on a routine basis may increase awareness enough to reduce overall fluoroscopy time. Because radiation is not detectable by any of the five senses, coupling the fluoroscopy "on" setting to a detectable signal facilitates control of exposure. Hough et al. found that the use of audible dose-sensitive radiation monitors led to a significant reduction in exposure to the staff wearing them (4).

Distance from Source. The next most effective way to reduce exposure is to increase the distance from the source. The exposure to the operator resulting from scatter decreases with the square of the distance from the source. This is known as the inverse square law. There is a substantial drop in scattered radiation to an operator when he or she moves to between 30 and 50 cm from the scatter source (5,6). For most endovascular interventions, the working distance from the source is largely fixed by the distance between the area of interest and the arterial access site (Fig. 1). The radiation dose to the operator during cardiac interventions has been shown to increase by 1.5–2.6 times when the operator moves from the femoral to the subclavian position (7). Kuwayama found that radiation to the operator was increased by approximately two to three times when a transcarotid versus

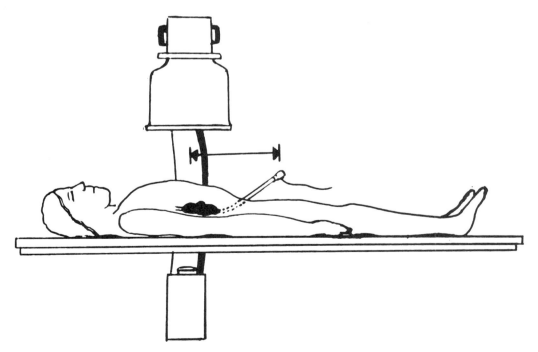

Figure 1   Showing fixed working distance from the sheath to the area of interest, in this case the abdominal aorta.

a transfemoral route was used for neuroradiological procedures (8). In this same study, the transcarotid approach led to a tenfold increase in exposure to the hands due to proximity to the beam.

Endovascular aortoiliac aneurysm repair requires prolonged imaging over the abdomen and pelvis. Penetration of these tissues requires more energy and results in a significantly higher exposure than imaging the periphery (9).

2. Use of the Fluoroscope and Patient Positioning

The radiation exposure of the operator is proportional to that of the patient. Therefore reducing the patient exposure will also reduce the operator exposure. Several methods can be used to achieve these ends. The beam should be positioned under the patient—i.e., posteroanterior imaging (Fig. 2A). This will decrease scatter as well as exposure of the operator's hand. Placing the beam in the anteroposterior position (source anterior to patient, image intensifier posterior to patient, patient supine) results in approximately four times greater exposure to the operator's head, neck, and upper extremities (Fig. 2B) (5). Not only is the exposure higher but these areas are far more difficult to shield than the area below the waist. Obtaining oblique views will also impact on the scattered radiation dose. The right anterior oblique view will result in significantly more scatter to an operator standing on the patient's left than the left anterior oblique view. The reverse is true when the operator stands on the patient's right (10).

The image intensifier should be positioned as close as possible to the patient. This reduces the amount of scatter by allowing for a lower entrance exposure. This positioning also results in a sharper image (Fig. 3A and B). Pulse-mode fluoroscopy at rates of 15–30 frames per second or lower greatly reduces exposure as compared to continuous mode.

A larger image intensifier mode requires less radiation than a smaller one. The radiation dose approximately doubles with each successively smaller image intensifier setting—i.e., increasing the magnification (11). Large image intensifier sizes should be used whenever possible. Avoid excessive use of high-level or cine-fluoroscopy mode. This mode should be used only for essential acquisitions.

The amount of radiation produced by the fluoroscope is dependent on the energy used to generate the beam. The factors determining this are the milliamperes (mA) and kilovolts (kV). The mA setting controls the number of photons produced (11). Low mA produces a mottled image, which can be eliminated by increasing the mA at the cost of higher radiation. The kV control determines the penetration of the beam and image contrast. For most fluoroscopic units, the mA and kV settings are determined by an automatic brightness control, which sets the values using feedback from the image obtained. However, where these are not set, the use higher kV and lower mA techniques will reduce exposure while not greatly affecting image quality. One study found that increasing the fluoroscopy voltage from 75 to 96 kV decreased the entrance dose by 50% (12).

There are factors intrinsic to the fluoroscopic unit itself that affect the radiation dose. These include the design and manufacture of the unit. Mehlmen et al. found that deep and shallow unprotected collar exposure as well as eye exposure were increased by at least 1.5 times when using an OEC 9600 as compared to a Philips BV 29 (6). There was also a substantial increase in deep and shallow unprotected waist exposure. These differences are likely accounted for by the increased mA generated by the OEC 9600 (3.3 mA/69 kV) as compared to the Philips (2.7 mA/72 kV). Newer models include a "low-dose" button, which allows the operator to reduce the exposure without significantly compromising image quality. In another study, Watson et al. found a statistically significant difference

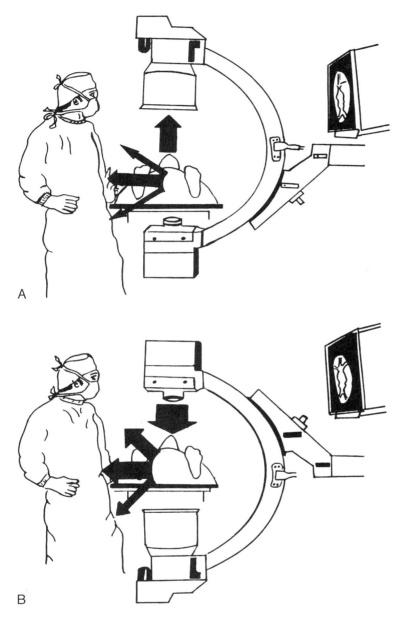

A

B

Figure 2   A. Posteroanterior imaging showing the majority of scatter directed at the level of the patient and below. B. Anteroposterior imaging showing the majority of scatter directed at the level of the patient and above.

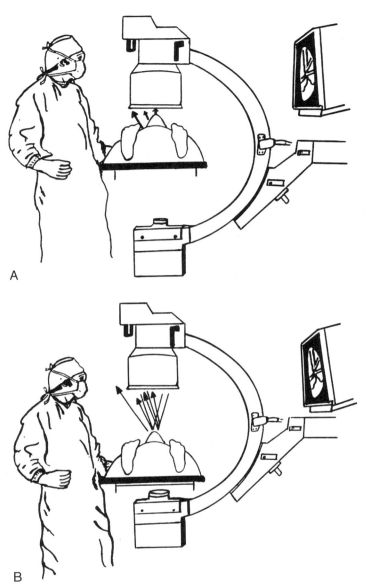

A

B

Figure 3 A. Image intensifier located close to the patient. Less energy is required for tissue penetration because scatter is reduced, resulting in a clearer image with decreased dose. B. Image intensifier located far away from the patient. More energy is required for tissue penetration because of increased scatter, resulting in increased exposure to obtain adequate image quality.

between two wall-mounted units that used different imaging technologies (13). A General Electric LU-C MPX/L500 PULSCAN 17178 Video Processor using pulsed progressive fluoroscopy showed a 45% higher dose per case than a Philips DCI-S Poly-Diagnostic using digital imaging technology. This difference was largely due to differences in the techniques used for image acquisition, since progressive pulsed fluoroscopy generally reduces radiation exposure. Finally, a heavier patient will require greater radiation energy to penetrate the tissues, with a consequent increase in radiation exposure to the patient and staff. We have found increased doses in heavier patients, although the amount is difficult to quantify because of the variability in the amount of high-level fluoroscopy used in each case.

Although the collimation of all fluoroscopic units is regulated by federal law, the ratio of the field of view to the total exposed area is not 1:1. Granger et al. found that the percent difference between the total exposed area and the field of view may be quite significant even though the fluoroscopic unit is in compliance with federal regulations (14). They evaluated 18 fluoroscopic units from different manufacturers and of different ages and found that only 67% of the units met federal compliance standards. For units not in compliance, the measured difference between the total exposed area and the field of view ranged from 22 to 48%. For units in compliance, the difference ranged from 5 to 32%. This excess exposed area provides no additional clinical information, increases the radiation doses to the patient and staff, and reduces image contrast and quality. After the units were serviced, a 40% average reduction in beam area was achieved and 100% of the units met compliance standards.

Although automatic collimation is part of all current systems, reducing the field size by using manual collimation will greatly decrease exposure and has the added benefit of enhancing image quality by reducing stray radiation. Lindsay et al. found that by collimating the field of image during radiofrequency catheter ablation procedures, the radiation dose to the patient and staff was reduced by 40% (7).

Antiscatter grids mounted in front of the input screen decrease the amount of scatter reaching the image intensifier and improve image quality by doing so. They also greatly increase both the required radiation to obtain a satisfactory image and the backscatter to the patient and staff (15). Removal of these grids can reduce the radiation dose by factor of 2–4, but with some loss of resolution. This is not the case during pediatric procedures, where grids can and should be removed without loss of image quality (15).

The fluoroscope should undergo at least biannual inspection and calibration, as required by law. More frequent quality-control checks are probably in order. If the unit requires service and any components are replaced, the fluoroscope should be recalibrated.

3. Radiological Protection

Protective barriers must be readily available and used consistently. The most important of these is the lead apron. These are generally available in 0.5- and 0.25-mm thicknesses. In optimal circumstances, the 0.5-mm thickness has the ability to attenuate 98–99.5% of the radiation dose, while the 0.25-mm thickness attenuates approximately 96% of the dose (11,16). Deterioration of the apron's lead lining occurs with use and is increased by rough handling or improper storage. Aprons should undergo periodic screening and replacement if inadequate protection is found. Many aprons are not of the wraparound type and as such do not provide circumferential protection. Scattered radiation from the sides may produce unprotected exposure. A thyroid collar and "protective" glasses are essential. These glasses are highly variable in the amount of protection afforded and allow for anywhere from 3–98% transmission of the radioactive beam (17). The greatest protective effect is obtained with glasses containing lead. Glasses at the lower end of this spectrum may provide protection against ultraviolet (UV) but not against ionizing radiation. Also of note is that a significant amount of the ocular exposure, up to 21%, is the result of scatter from the operator's head (17). Depending on the head position of the operator during the procedure, side shields or wraparound configurations are necessary to provide adequate protection. A lead acrylic shield, which can either be ceiling-mounted or on a mobile floor stand, should be placed between the operator and patient to further reduce exposure. Eye radiation can be reduced by a factor of 20–35 with the use of a ceiling-suspended lead glass shield (7,10). Lead-lined gloves also help to reduce exposure but can be cumbersome. Because back-scattered radiation is more intense than forward-scattered radiation, and because with the C-arm in the posteroanterior orientation the greatest exposure due to scatter occurs from under the table, we use a lead drape suspended from the operating table on the operator's side to reduce this exposure (18). Use of this additional shield eliminates a significant amount of this scatter (5).

4. Role of Experience

Certain endovascular procedures may be quite complex and require lengthy fluoroscopy times. This may be the case especially at tertiary referral centers, which generally have affiliated training programs. In a study of radiation exposure during cardiology fellowship training, Watson et al. found a statistically significant increase in exposure for cases done in the first versus the second year of fellowship (13). This difference was largely accounted for by an increase in fluoroscopy time but not cine time, reflecting an increased time for the less experienced operators to position the catheters. These results have implications for fellowship training programs, where the teaching of less experienced operators will result in increased radiation exposure for the patients and staff alike. The needs of training must be balanced against the increased fluoroscopy times and resulting exposure.

5. Patient and Staff Monitoring

The use of radiation badges by all persons working with fluoroscopy is mandatory and required by law. The position of the badges is important. A badge must be worn at waist level under the lead apron. Additional badges should also be worn on the collar to monitor the head dose and to aid in calculating the total effective dose, since there is a large and variable difference between the over- and under-lead doses (19). Ring badges are also advisable. Waist and collar badges should be worn toward the operator's left side in working on the patient's right side and toward the operator's right side in working on the patient's left side—i.e., the badge should face the source directly. Ring badges should be worn on the hand most likely to be exposed. A self-retaining device to stabilize the sheaths may also reduce exposure. Monitoring of all at-risk body positions is essential, since doses to the fingers of the dominant hand have been shown not to correlate with doses estimated by shoulder badges in interventionalists performing percutaneous drainage procedures (20). Although the use of badges is mandated, it is the responsibility of the individual to wear them and of the institution to have a monitoring program with feedback to the exposed individuals in place.

In general, the patient is exposed only once. Many patients undergoing these procedures are in an older age range and are less likely to suffer from potential malignancies. However, because of the long screening times, patients should be warned about transient skin erythema, which may present up to several weeks following the procedure, and other skin conditions.

In one large prospective study of interventional radiologists, Marx et al. found that the only variable correlating with the over-lead collar dose was number of procedures performed per year and the only variable correlating with the under-lead waist dose was the thickness of the lead apron (0.5 vs. 1 mm) (19). This study also included a questionnaire that inquired about the practice habits of the interventional radiologists involved. Nearly half of the respondents reported rarely or never wearing their radiation badges. Half of the respondents either had exceeded or did not know whether they had exceeded monthly or quarterly occupational dose limits at some time within the past year. With regard to protection habits, 30% rarely or never wore a thyroid shield, 73% rarely or never wore lead glasses, 70% rarely or never used a ceiling-mounted lead shield, and 83% rarely or never wore leaded gloves. These results indicate that there can be significant complacency even among the most at-risk population of physicians who have had substantial background and education in radiation safety and physics.

We reviewed our own radiation exposure incurred during 47 endovascular aortic and/ or iliac aneurysm repairs performed over a 1-year period (21). We did not include other fluoroscopic procedures we routinely perform, such as diagnostic or completion angiography, iliac or renal artery angioplasty and stenting, fluoroscopically assisted thromboembolectomy, and inferior vena cave filter placement.

Each of three surgeons wore three radiation dosimeters (Landauer, Inc., Glenwood, IL), as follows: (a) on the waist under the lead apron, (b) on the waist outside the lead apron, and (c) on the collar outside the thyroid shield. A ring dosimeter was worn on the ring finger of the left hand by each surgeon. Additional badges were placed around the operating room to estimate the exposure to the scrub and circulating nurses. Patient entrance doses were calculated using the fluoroscopic energies and positions recorded during each case. Total effective doses (TEDs) were calculated and compared to standards established by the International Commission on Radiological Protection (ICRP) (2).

Yearly TEDs for the surgeons (under lead) ranged from 5 to 8% of the ICRP occupational exposure limit. Outside lead doses for all surgeons approximated the recommended occupational limit. Ring and calculated eye doses ranged from 1 to 5% ICRP occupational exposure limits. Lead aprons attenuated 85–91% of the dose. Patient entrance doses averaged 360 mSv per case (range 120–860). Outside lead exposure to the scrub and circulating nurses were 4 and 2% of ICRP occupational limits respectively.

Our results suggested that a team of surgeons could perform 386 h of fluoroscopy per year, or 587 endovascular aortoiliac aneurysm repairs per year, and remain within occupational exposure limits. This does not take into account other endovascular procedures performed by the surgeons, which would reduce these figures accordingly.

6. Additional Equipment to Help Reduce Exposure

Several available devices not directly related to the fluoroscopic unit are helpful in reducing the total exposure. A floating table simplifies positional changes and reduces the need to constantly adjust the fluoroscope. A power injector (Contrast injection system, Acist Medical Systems, Minneapolis, MN) ensures that an adequate volume of contrast is delivered, which maximizes image quality and reduces the need for multiple screening runs. This is especially important in imaging the thoracic or abdominal aorta and it branches. A power injector may actually reduce the overall contrast required to perform the procedure by eliminating the need for multiple image acquisitions. An equally important benefit is that a power injector allows the operator to increase his or her distance from the source. The same effect can be achieved by adding extension tubing to the catheter injection port during manual injection technique. The tabletop should be maximally radiolucent. The equipment used (stent grafts, guidewires, catheters) should be well marked with radio-opaque indicators that are easily visualized, such that one does not have to strain or increase the image intensifier size to see them.

Noninvasive vascular imaging techniques such as duplex Doppler and intravascular ultrasound contribute information that can aid in the performance of endovascular procedures and lessen the fluoroscopic time. Often these modalities are complementary; the information gained from duplex, for example, can be used to limit the contrast load as well as both fluoroscopy and procedural time. These modalities, however, may not always provide the same anatomical detail as angiography. Finally, marking appropriate landmarks on the screen with an erasable pen allows one to work under regular fluoroscopy rather than road mapping, which may lead to increased exposure.

7. Summary

It is critical to remember that radiation exposure is cumulative and the effects permanent. The major factors increasing exposure include increased fluoroscopy time and the proximity of the surgeon to the operative field. The maximum allowable occupational and civilian radiation exposure doses as defined by the various regulatory agencies have been lowered with time. It is likely that with increasing knowledge concerning the effects of radiation, this trend will continue. We recommend keeping exposure to less than 10–20% of established occupational limits. All centers performing endovascular procedures should actively monitor their effective doses and educate personnel in methods for reducing exposure.

II. CONTRAST TOXICITY

A. Introduction

The recent increasing number and complexity of endovascular interventions being performed means that patients are being exposed to radiological contrast agents in greater numbers and with larger doses. There has been much improvement in the production of contrast agents since the first use of an iodinated contrast agent 70 years ago. This has led to a reduction in the overall toxicity of these agents (22). Adverse reactions to contrast agents vary widely in their severity and clinical presentation, from minimal, transient elevations in serum creatinine to major anaphylactic reactions.

B. Types of Reaction

1. Systemic

Many systemic reactions begin with isolated endothelial, hematological, or cardiac toxicity and may progress to a systemic response. Although immunological responses occur, they are not felt to be traditional allergic reactions for two major reasons (23): (a) antibodies to contrast agents and additives have been identified in only a few cases and (b) repeat contrast administration leads to a response in less than 50% of cases. Systemic reactions to contrast agents may be mild, moderate, or severe. Mild reactions include pain, heat, itching, and pallor. Moderate reactions include hypotension and wheezing. Severe reactions include unresponsiveness, arrhythmias, and cardiac arrest. Many minor reactions to contrast agents are related to the osmolality of the agent. Specifically, pain is greatly reduced with the use of low-osmolality agents.

The occurrence of severe reactions is more difficult to predict. Several risk factors are associated with the development of systemic reactions, including severe allergies, active asthma, and cardiac disease. Shellfish allergies have traditionally been thought to be closely associated with contrast sensitivity, but this has not been shown to be a stronger risk factor than the presence of any other severe allergy (24). Additionally, although a prior contrast reaction does increase the likelihood of a subsequent reaction, it does not help to predict the severity of such a reaction (23).

The treatment of systemic contrast reactions is dictated by the nature and severity of the episode. Vasovagal reactions can be treated with Trendelenburg positioning and fluids. Respiratory reactions may resolve spontaneously but should be treated to prevent progression to a more severe reaction. Adrenergic inhalers are the first line of treatment, which can be followed by intramuscular or intravenous epinephrine if these local measures fail. Cardiopulmonary reactions may require full cardiopulmonary resuscitation.

2. Hematological

There are a myriad of effects on the vessel wall and hematological system, all of which appear to be insignificant when contrast agents are administered at the doses generally required for routine imaging studies (23). For example, while early studies using high doses of contrast with stagnant flow showed endothelial damage, these results were not borne out in studies using more clinically relevant doses in the presence of blood flow (25–28). Additionally, the incidence of venous thrombosis in the setting of high-volume, high-concentration, slow infusions with high-osmolality nonionic agents has been reported to be as high as 30%; however, with a reduction in contrast osmolality and alteration of technique, this figure can be reduced sixfold (29–32). For arterial injections, these concerns are not as relevant, since these agents are cleared rapidly by high flow and hence reduced exposure time to the contrast. In fact, with ionic agents there seems to be a mild, transient anticoagulant effect, which once again is not clinically significant (33). Any significant thrombotic or anticoagulation effects of these agents are far outweighed by the technique used, the state of the vessels being evaluated, and the presence of the catheters and guidewires used in the procedure.

3. Cardiac

As is the case for hematological effects, cardiac toxicity is generally not significant at clinically relevant doses; the osmolality of the contrast agent employed is the most important factor determining toxicity. These effects are a more pronounced during the performance of cardiac catheterization that during peripheral angiography. For example, injection of contrast into the left ventricle leads to a fall in heart rate and blood pressure with a slight increase in diastolic pressure, all of which return to baseline within 30 s to 3 min. Similar but far less notable effects are noted with the injection of contrast into the periphery. Although the results vary depending on the model used, studies with isolated heart perfusion show that almost all contrast agents suppress both myocardial and coronary artery contractility and that the effects increase with the osmolality of the contrast agent (23). Another possible cardiac effect is the development of electromechanical dissociation—which can mimic an anaphylactic response—due to a rapid drop in the serum calcium concentration. This can occur during angiography, because many contrast agents contain calcium chelating agents that are used to stabilize the solution (34). Newer agents have a reduced amount of such compounds and therefore pose a reduced risk of this complication.

While perhaps not strictly considered a contrast reaction, fluid overload, especially in patients with congestive heart failure, must be guarded against. Contrast agents can be a significant volume load both in terms of pure volume as well as the osmotic activity of the agents. This is yet another reason to minimize contrast load whenever possible. Thus respiratory difficulty during an angiographic examination may represent a reaction to contrast or simply fluid overload (35).

4. Nephrotoxicity

Contrast nephrotoxicity is the third leading cause of acute renal failure in hospitalized patients and has been reported to occur in up to 6% of unselected patient populations and up to 50% of high-risk populations receiving radiological contrast agents (36–39). Because many of the patients undergoing these interventions fall into the high-risk category due to the underlying nature of their disorder, the incidence of contrast nephrotoxicity is significant (40).

Clinical Course, Pathogenesis, and Risk Factors. Although nearly all patients receiving radiographic contrast experience a small, transient decreases in glomerular filtration, the exact definition of contrast nephropathy varies. It is generally defined as a rise in the serum creatinine to >25% or >0.5 mg/dL above baseline in the absence of other inciting events (41). The elevation in creatinine typically occurs within 24–48 h of contrast administration. The peak increase occurs between 3 and 5 days, with a return to baseline by 7–10 days. In the majority of cases the renal failure is nonoliguric and entirely reversible. The urinalysis may be unremarkable but is usually consistent with acute tubular necrosis, showing coarse granular casts and renal tubular epithelial cells. A small percentage of patients may present with more severe renal failure, with symptoms manifesting within 24 h of contrast administration. Less than 1% of patients with contrast nephropathy will require dialysis, but in this setting the mortality is approximately 30% (42). Lactic acidosis resulting from contrast nephropathy in diabetic patients who take the oral hypoglycemic medication metformin is a rare complication (43). It has been recommended by some that patients discontinue this medication 24 h prior to any contrast study, while others have suggested that patients not restart the medication until 48 h following the procedure, and then only if there is no evidence of nephrotoxicity (41).

Contrast agents are excreted by glomerular filtration alone without undergoing tubular resorption or secretion. Contrast nephrotoxicity occurs due a combination of alterations in renal hemodynamics and direct tubular epithelial cell toxicity. There is a biphasic response to the administration of contrast in the renal vasculature, with an initial brief period of vasodilatation followed by a more prolonged but variable period of vasoconstriction. These changes are most likely mediated by alterations in nitric oxide, endothelin, adenosine, or prostaglandin metabolism (41). Direct cellular toxicity is inferred from in vitro and in vivo studies showing increased excretion of enzymes and low-molecular-weight proteins in the urine in addition to pathological changes seen on histology (44).

The most important risk factor for the development of contrast nephrotoxicity is the presence of preexisting renal insufficiency (45,46). Patients with a creatinine level of >1.5 mg/dL have up to a 21-fold increase risk of contrast nephropathy compared to patients with a normal creatinine level. There are several other important factors that may increase the risk for the development of contrast nephropathy including dehydration, diabetes mellitus, contrast volume, congestive heart failure, and concurrent exposure to other nephrotoxic agents (Table 2). Many of these factors act synergistically. For example, diabetic patients without preexisting renal insufficiency do not seem to be at increased risk of

Table 2 Risk Factors for Contrast Nephropathy

Preexisting renal insufficiency
Volume of contrast
Intravascular volume depletion
Diabetes mellitus
Concurrent administration of other nephrotoxic agents
Repeat contrast procedures
Congestive heart failure
Abnormal liver function
Multiple myeloma
Nephrosis
Nonsteroidal anti-inflammatory drugs
Angiotensin-converting enzyme inhibitors

contrast nephropathy, while those with renal insufficiency are at higher risk than in the presence of renal insufficiency alone (45,46). One study of patients undergoing cardiac catheterization found that the risk of renal failure ranged from 1 to 100% as the number of risk factors increased (47).

Prevention. The principles in the prevention of contrast nephrotoxicity include selection of the appropriate diagnostic and/or therapeutic modality, preprocedural correction of risk factors, ensuring adequate hydration, eliminating or reducing any additional nephrotoxic agents, limiting the amount of contrast administered, and close follow-up of serum creatinine postprocedurally.

All patients undergoing contrast procedures should receive adequate hydration either orally or intravenously at the time of the procedure, such that positive fluid balance and high urine output are achieved. Patients with preexisting renal insufficiency should be hydrated well before and after these procedures. Patients with cardiopulmonary dysfunction must be monitored closely while receiving hydration. There are many different protocols for hydration, but in general the use of 0.45% saline at 1–1.5 mL/Kg/h beginning 1–2 h prior to the procedure and continuing for up to 6 h (outpatients) or 24 h (inpatients) are acceptable. The urine volumes should be approximately 0.75–1.25 mL/h (40,41,48–50).

The use of low-osmolality nonionic contrast media has also been advocated for the prevention of contrast nephropathy. The impetus for the development of these agents was the high incidence of side effects associated with the earlier agents. However, their high cost raised concern for their routine use. Additionally, large studies have shown a significant risk reduction only in patients with preexisting renal dysfunction (51,52). Because of these factors, low-osmolality nonionic contrast agents may best be reserved for use in patients with underlying renal dysfunction, especially diabetics and patients with potential hemodynamic instability.

Diuretics have been proposed as a method to reduce contrast nephropathy based on the theoretical advantage that loop diuretics (e.g., furosemide) might decrease medullary oxygen consumption and hence the potential for ischemic injury during contrast studies (53,54). Mannitol, alone or in conjunction with loop diuretics, has also been proposed to reduce contrast nephropathy. In one large study, patients with creatinine >1.6 mg/dL undergoing cardiac catheterization were randomized to three groups. One group received hydration alone, one received hydration plus mannitol, and one received hydration plus furosemide. A significant increase in creatinine was noted in 11% of the patients who received hydration alone, 28% of the patients receiving hydration plus mannitol, and 40% of the patients who received hydration plus furosemide (50). In another study, a similar cohort of patients was treated with hydration alone versus a regimen of hydration, mannitol, furosemide, and renal-dose dopamine. In this study, urine output was replaced with saline to control for dehydration effects. There was no significant difference between the groups in terms of increase in creatinine; however, there was a higher incidence of contrast nephropathy in patients with a lower (<150 mL/h) as opposed to a higher urine output, suggesting some protective effect of maintaining a good urine output (55). One additional study did find that the risk of contrast nephropathy was reduced by mannitol in nondiabetic azotemic patients (56). Presently there is no evidence to suggest that the use of either mannitol or diuretics reduces the risks of contrast nephropathy; they may, in fact, increase the risk by their tendency to produce negative fluid balance and dehydration.

Based on studies suggesting that reactive oxygen species may play a major role in the pathogenesis of contrast nephropathy, the antioxidant N-acetylcysteine has been evaluated for a potential protective effect. Two recent studies, one in patients undergoing contrast computed tomography scanning and one in patients undergoing cardiac catheterization, both showed some reduction of contrast nephropathy (57,58).

Another approach to the prevention of contrast nephropathy involves the use of agents that selectively increase renal blood flow. Low-dose dopamine is one such agent. Despite its theoretical advantages, studies using low-dose dopamine have failed to show a clear-cut benefit in terms of preventing contrast nephropathy or in providing a protective effect once contrast nephropathy has occurred (56,59). In one of these studies, diabetic patients actually had a higher rate of contrast nephropathy with dopamine, while nondiabetic patients had a lower rate (56). These results plus other studies suggest that dopamine may be of some benefit in preventing contrast nephropathy in nondiabetic patients, although its routine use has not been advocated (60,61). It is not recommended for prevention of contrast nephropathy in diabetic patients (40,41).

Fenoldopam is a selective dopamine-1 (DA-1) receptor agonist approved for the treatment of systemic hypertension. It is given parenterally but has no stimulatory effect on dopamine-2 (DA-2) or adrenergic receptors (both cause vasoconstriction), as does dopamine at higher doses (40). Fenoldopam has been found to increase renal blood flow and improve glomerular filtration rate while reducing both systolic and diastolic blood pressure in hypertensive patients (62–66). Blood pressure reductions are only mild in normotensive patients. Fenoldopam also prevents shunting of blood flow from the medulla to the cortex, permitting maintenance of medullary oxygenation. Several recent studies have shown significant reductions in the incidence of contrast nephropathy with the use of fenoldopam (67–69).

Various other agents have been used in an attempt to reduce the incidence of contrast nephropathy. Atrial natriuretic peptide is another agent that increases renal blood flow and was found to reduce contrast nephropathy in animal studies. However, in a recent randomized, double-blind, placebo-controlled study, atrial natriuretic peptide was not shown to decrease the incidence of contrast nephropathy, even across subgroup analysis for diabetic patients (70). Theophylline was hypothesized to have a role in the reduction of contrast nephropathy, since it is an adenosine antagonist. Adenosine is thought to contribute to the renal vasoconstriction seen in contrast nephropathy. Some studies have shown benefit with the use of theophylline, while others have not. In the absence of prospective trails, theophylline has not been recommended. The use of calcium channel blockers, which have been demonstrated to attenuate the reductions in renal blood flow associated with contrast administration in laboratory studies, have similarly not been shown to have a significant effect in clinical studies. Endothelin antagonists have also not shown benefit in clinical studies.

C. Summary

As is the case with any medication and/or imaging modality, the best way to reduce toxicity is to use the lowest possible volume and concentration of the agent while still obtaining an adequate diagnostic or therapeutic result. Many different agents are undergoing evaluation for their role in reducing contrast nephropathy, but more long-term studies are needed to clarify their efficacy. At the present time, maintenance of adequate hydration is the most important factor in preventing contrast nephropathy.

REFERENCES

1. Veith FJ. Presidential address: Charles Darwin and vascular surgery. J Vasc Surg 1997; 25(1):8–18.
2. The International Committee on Radiological Protection. Radiological protection and safety in medicine. A report of the International Commission on Radiological Protection. Ann ICRP 1996; 26(2):1–47.
3. National Council on Radiation Protection and Measurements. Ionizing Radiation Exposure of the Population of the United States. NCRP Report No. 93, 1987. Bethesda, MD: NCRP, 1987.
4. Hough DM, Brady A, Stevenson GW. Audible radiation monitors: The value in reducing radiation exposure to fluoroscopy personnel. AJR 1993; 160:407–408.
5. Boone JM, Levin DC. Radiation exposure to angiographers under different fluroscopic imaging conditions. Radiology 1991; 180:861–865.
6. Mehlman CT, DiPasquale TG. Radiation exposure to the orthopaedic surgical team during fluoroscopy: "How far away is far enough?" J Orthop Trauma 1997; 11(6):392–398.
7. Lindsay BD, Eichling JO, Ambos HD, Cain ME. Radiation exposure to patients and medical personnel during radio frequency catheter ablation for supraventricular tachycardia. Am J Cardiol 1992; 70:218–223.
8. Kuwayama N, Takaku A, Endo S, Nishljima M, Kamei T. Radiation exposure in endovascular surgery of the head and neck. Am J Neuroradiol 1994; 15:1801–1808.
9. Ramalanjaona GR, Pearce WH, Ritenour ER. Radiation exposure risk to the surgeon during operative angiography. J Vasc Surg 1986; 4(3):224–228.
10. Pratt TA, Shaw AJ. Factors affecting the radiation dose to the lens of the eye during cardiac catheterization procedures. Br J Radiol 1993; 66:346–350.
11. Aldridge HE, Chisholm RJ, Dragatakis L, Roy L. Radiation safety in the cardiac catheterization laboratory. Can J Cardiol 1997; 13(5):459–467.
12. Heyd RL, Kopecky KK, Sherman S, Lehman GA, Stockberger SM. Radiation exposure to patients and personnel during interventional ERCP at a teaching institution. Gastrointest Endosc 1996; 44:287–292.
13. Watson LE, Riggs MW, Bourland PD. Radiation exposure during cardiology fellowship training. Health Phys 1997; 73(4):690–693.
14. Granger WE, Bednarek DR, Rudin S. Primary beam exposure outside the fluoroscopic field of view. Med Phys 1997; 24(5):703–707.

15. Coakley KS, Ratcliffe J, Masel J. Measurement of radiation dose received by the hands and thyroid of staff performing gridless fluoroscopic procedures in children. Br J Radiol 1997; 70: 933–936.

16. Kicken PJ, Bos AJJ. Effectiveness of lead aprons in vascular radiology: Results of clinical measurements. Radiology 1995; 197:473–478.

17. Cousin AJ, Lawdahl RB, Chakraborty DP, Koehler RE. The case for radioprotective eyewear/facewear: Practical implications and suggestions. Invest Radiol 1987; 22:688–692.

18. Lo NN, Goh SS, Khong KS. Radiation dosage from use of the image intensifier in orthopaedic surgery. Singapore Med J 1996; 37:69–71.

19. Marx MV, Niklason L, Mauger EA. Occupational radiation exposure to interventional radiologists: A prospective study. J Vasc Intervent Radiol 1992; 3:597–606.

20. Vehmas T, Tikkanen H. Measuring radiation exposure during percutaneous drainages: Can shoulder dosimeters be used to estimate finger doses? Br J Radiol 1992; 65(779):1007–1010.

21. Lipsitz EC, Veith FJ, Ohki T, et al. Does the endovascular repair of aortoiliac aneurysms pose a radiation safety hazard to vascular surgeons? J Vasc Surg 2000; 32:704–710.

22. Osborne ED, Sutherland CG, Scholl AJ, Rowntree LD. Roentgenography of the urinary tract during excretion of sodium iodine. JAMA 1923; 80:368–373.

23. Bettmann MA. Physiologic effects and systemic reactions. In: Baum S, ed. Abrams' Angiography. 4th ed. Philadelphia: Lippincott Williams & Wilkins, 1996:22–33.

24. Lasser EC, Berry CC, Talner LB, et al. Pre-treatment with corticosteroids to alleviate reactions to intravenous contrast material. New Engl J Med 1987; 317:845–849.

25. Merseredu WA, Robertson HR. Observations on venous endothelial injury following the injection of various radiographic contrast media in the rat. J Neurosurg 1961; 18:289–294.

26. Laerum F. Cytotoxic effects of six angiographic contrast media on human endothelium in culture. Acta Radiol 1987; 28:99–105.

27. Morgan DML, Bettmann MA. Effects of x-ray contrast media and radiation on human vascular endothelial cells in vitro. Cardiovasc Intervent Radiol 1989; 12:154–160.

28. Thiesea B, Muetzer W. Effects of angiographic contrast media on venous endothelium of rabbits. Invest Radiol 1990; 25:121–126.

29. Albrechtsson U, Olsson C-G. Thrombotic side effects of lower limb phlebography. Lancet 1976; 1:723–724.

30. Laeram F, Holm HA. Postphlebographic thrombosis: A double blind study with methylglucamine metrizoate and metrizamide. Radiology 1981; 140:651–654.

31. Bettmann MA, Salzman EW, Rosenthal D, et al. Reduction of venous thrombosis complicating phlebography. AJR 1980; 134:1169–1172.

32. Bettmann MA, Robbins A, Braun SD, Wetzner S, Dunnick NR, Finkelstein J. Comparison of the diagnostic efficacy, tolerance and complication rates of a nonionic and an ionic contrast agent for leg phlebography. Radiology 1987; 165:113–116.

33. Mamoa JF, Hoppensteadt MS, Fareed J, Moncada R. Biochemical evidence for a relative lack of inhibition of thrombin formation by nonionic contrast media. Radiology 1991; 179:399–402.

34. Bourdillon PD, Bettmann MA, McCracken S, Poole-Wilson PA, Grossman W. Effects of a new ionic and a conventional ionic contrast agent on coronary sinus ionized calcium and left ventricular hemodynamics in dogs. J Am Coll Cardiol 1985; 6:845–853.

35. Rosen RJ. Angiography: General techniques, complications, and risk management. In: Taveras JM, et al., eds. Radiology. Vol. 2. Philadelphia: Lippincott Williams & Wilkins, 2002: 2–4.

36. Hou SH, Bushinsky DA, Wish JB, Cohen JJ, Harrington JT. Hospital-acquired renal insufficiency: A prospective study. Am J Med 1983; 74:243–248.

37. Davidson CJ, Hlatky M, Morris KG, et al. Cardiovascular and renal toxicity of a nonionic radiographic contrast agent after cardiac catheterization: A prospective trial. Ann Intern Med 1989; 110:119–124.

38. Lautin EM, Freeman NJ, Schoenfeld AH, et al. Radiocontrast-associated renal dysfunction: Incidence and risk factors. AJR 1991; 157:49–58.

39. Weisberg LS, Kurnik PB, Kurnik BRC. Risk of radiocontrast nephropathy in patients with and without diabetes mellitus. Kidney Int 1994; 45:259–265.

40. Waybill MM, Waybill PN. Contrast media-induced nephrotoxicity: Identification of patients at risk and algorithms for prevention. J Vasc Intervent Radiol 2001; 12(1):3–9.

41. Murphy SW, Barrett BJ, Parfrey PS. Contrast nephropathy. J Am Soc Nephrol 2000; 11(1): 177–182.

42. McCullough PA, Wolyn R, Rocher LL, Levin RN, O'Neill WW. Acute renal failure after coronary intervention: Incidence, risk factors, and relationship to mortality. Am J Med 1997; 103:368–375.

43. Thomsen HS, Morcos SK. Contrast media and metformin: Guidelines to diminish the risk of lactic acidosis in non-insulin-dependent diabetics after administration of contrast media. ESUR Contrast Media Safety Committee. Eur Radiol 1999; 9:738–740.

44. Humes HD, Hunt DA, White MD. Direct toxic effect of the radiocontrast agent diatrizoate on renal proximal tubule cells. Am J Physiol 1987; 252:F246–F255.

45. Parfrey PS, Griffiths SM, Barrett BJ, Paul MD, Genge M, Withers J, Farid N, McManamon PJ. Contrast-material induced renal failure in patients with diabetes mellitus, renal insufficiency, or both: A prospective controlled study. N Engl J Med 1989; 320:143–149.

46. Rudnick MR, Berns JS, Cohen RM, Goldfarb S. Contrast-media associated nephrotoxicity. Semin Nephrol 1997; 17:15–26.

47. Rich MW, Crecelius CA. Incidence, risk factors, and clinical course of acute renal insufficiency after cardiac catheterization in patients 70 years of age or older. Arch Intern Med 1995; 150: 1237–1242.

48. Eisenberg RL, Bank WO, Hedgock MW. Renal failure after major angiography can be avoided with hydration. AJR 1981; 136:859–861.

49. Taylor AJ, Hotchkiss D, Morse RW, McCabe J. PREPARED: Preparation for Angiography in Renal Dysfunction. A randomized trial of inpatient vs outpatient hydration protocols for cardiac catheterization in mild-to-moderate renal dysfunction. Chest 1998; 114:1570–4574.

50. Solomon RC, Werner C, Mann D, D'Elia J, Silva P. Effects of saline, mannitol, and furosemide on acute decreases in renal function induced by radiocontrast agents. N Engl J Med 1994; 331:1416–1420.

51. Barrett BJ, Carlisle EJ. Meta-analysis of the relative nephrotoxicity of high- and low-osmolality iodinated contrast media. Radiology 1993; 188:171–178.

52. Rudnick MR, Goldfarb S, Wexler L, Ludbrook PA, Murphy MJ, Halpern EF, Hill JA, Winniford M, Cohen MB, VanFossen DB. Nephrotoxicity of ionic and nonionic contrast in 1196 patients: A randomized trial. Kidney Int 1995; 47:254–261.

53. Heyman SN, Brezis M, Epstein FH, Spokes K, Silva P, Rosen S. Early renal medullary hypoxic injury from radiocontrast and indomethacin. Kidney Int 1991; 40:632–642.

54. Barrett BJ. Contrast nephrotoxicity. J Am Soc Nephrol 1994; 5:125–137.

55. Stevens MA, McCullough PA, Tobin KJ, Speck JP, Westveer DC, Guido-Allen DA, Timmis GC, O'Neill WW. A prospective randomised trial of prevention measures in patients at high risk for contrast nephropathy. J Am Coll Cardiol 1999; 33:403–411.

56. Weisberg LS, Kurnik PB, Kurnik BRC. Dopamine and renal blood flow in radiocontrast–induced nephropathy in humans. Renal Failure 1993; 15:61–68.

57. Tepel M, Van Der Giet M, Schwarzfeld C, Laufer U, Liermann D, Zidek W. Prevention of radiographic-contrast-agent–induced reductions in renal function by acetylcysteine. New Engl J Med 2000; 343:180–184.

58. Diaz-Sandoval LJ, Kosowsky BD, Losordo DW. Acetylcysteine to prevent angiography-related renal tissue injury (the APART trial). Am J Cardiol 2002; 89:356–358; 2000; 343:180–184.

59. Abizaid AS, Clark CE, Mintz GS, Dosa S, Popma JJ, Pichard AD, Satler LF, Harvey M, Kent KM, Leon MB. Effects of dopamine and aminophylline on contrast-induced acute renal failure after coronary angioplasty in patients with preexisting renal insufficiency. Am J Cardiol 1999; 83:260–263.

60. Hans SS, Hans BA, Dhillon R, Dmuchowski C, Glover J. Effect of dopamine on renal function after arteriography in patients with pre-existing renal insufficiency. Am Surg 1998; 64:432–436.

61. Hall KA, Wong RW, Hunter GC, Camazine BM, Rappaport WA, Smyth SH, Bull DA, McIntyre KE, Bernhard VM, Misiorowski RL. Contrast–induced nephrotoxicity: The effects of vasodilator therapy. J Surg Res 1992; 53:317–320.

62. Barkis GL, Lass NA, Glock D. Renal hemodynamics in radiocontrast medium–induced renal dysfunction: A role for dopamine-1 receptors. Kidney Int 1999; 56:206–210.

63. Panacek EA, Bednarczyk EM, Dunbar LM, Foulke GE, Holsclaw TL. Randomized, prospective trial of fenoldopam vs. sodium nitroprusside in the treatment of acute severe hypertension. Acad Emerg Med 1995; 2:959–965.

64. Post JB, Frishman WH. Fenoldopam: A new dopamine agonist for the treatment of hypertensive urgencies and emergencies. J Clin Pharmacol 1998; 38:2–13.

65. Singer I, Epstein M. Potential of dopamine A-1 agonists in the management of acute renal failure. Am J Kidney Dis 1998; 31:743–755.

66. Mathur VS, Ellis D, Fellmann J, Luther RR. Therapeutics for hypertensive urgencies and emergencies-fenoldopam: A novel systemic and renal vasodilator. Cardiovasc Intervent Radiol 1998; 1:43–53.

67. Madyoon H. Clinical experience with the use of fenoldopam for prevention of radiocontrast nephropathy in high-risk patients. Rev Cardiovasc Med 2001; 2(suppl 1):S26–S30.

68. Tumlin JA, Wang A, Murray PT, Mathur VS. Fenoldopam mesylate blocks reductions in renal plasma flow after radiocontrast dye infusion: A pilot trial in the prevention of contrast nephropathy. Am Heart J 2002; 143:894–903.

69. Kini AS, Mitre CA, Kim M, Kamran M, Reich D, Sharma SK. A protocol for prevention of radiologic contrast nephropathy during percutaneous coronary intervention: Effect of selective dopamine receptor agonist fenoldopam. Cathet Cardiovasc Intervent 2002; 55:169–173.

70. Kurnik BRC, Allgren RL, Genter FC, Solomon RJ, Bates ER, Weisberg LS. Prospective study of atrial natriuretic peptide for the prevention of radiocontrast-induced nephropathy. Am J Kidney Dis 1998; 31:674–680.

30

Complications in Peripheral Thrombolysis

Kenneth Ouriel

The Cleveland Clinic Foundation, Cleveland, Ohio, U.S.A.

The principal goal of thrombolytic therapy is to dissolve intravascular thrombus. Thrombolytic agents are remarkably effective in accomplishing this goal, and they can do so in a minimally invasive fashion. Through percutaneous means alone, recanalization of an occluded bypass graft or artery can be achieved within a few hours and the thrombus can be completely dissolved over the course of 12–48 h (1). Culprit stenotic lesions become readily apparent after successful thrombolytic therapy; these lesions must be addressed to diminish the risk of reocclusion (2). The unmasked lesions can frequently be repaired percutaneously. Even when open surgical revascularization is necessary, it can often be performed on an elective basis, allowing ample time for patient preparation. Thrombolytic therapy can be employed to clear thrombus from small vessels that are inaccessible to standard balloon catheter thrombectomy, sometimes identifying target vessels for an operative bypass procedure (Fig. 1) (3). Clinical trials have proven thrombolytic therapy to be effective for the treatment of acute arterial occlusion, resulting in a reduction in mortality (4), limb loss (5), length of hospital stay (6), and the need for open surgical intervention (7).

But successful thrombolytic therapy cannot be separated from its major complication, the inextricable risk of life-threatening hemorrhage. In fact, other complications pale in comparison to bleeding, and the association between thrombolytic therapy and hemorrhage is the sole factor that has precluded the use of thrombolysis to an even broader number of patients (8). To understand the association between thrombolytic therapy and hemorrhage, it is beneficial to first consider the biochemistry underlying the mechanism of action of thrombolytic agents. The fundamental physiology of dissolving (a) pathological intravascular thrombi and (b) desirable plugs sealing remote sites where vascular integrity has been lost is virtually identical. Herein lies the failure of thrombolytic therapy: how does one effect dissolution of "bad" thrombus without causing distant hemorrhage due to the dissolution of "good" thrombus sealing small vascular defects in the gastrointestinal tract, at the catheter insertion site, or, most importantly, within the calvarium?

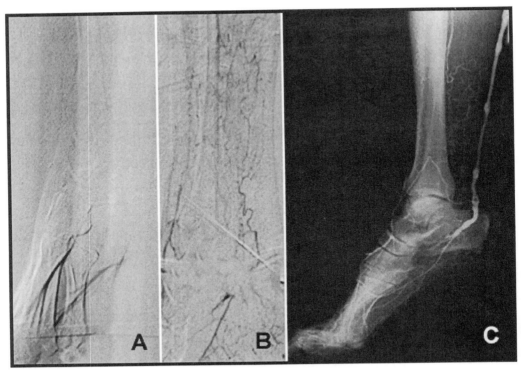

Figure 1 Thrombolytic therapy can clear thrombus from small vessels inaccessible to balloon catheter thrombectomy. A. This patient had no identifiable vessels below the popliteal, even on delayed views. B. Following thrombolysis, a lateral plantar artery was identified in this patient. C. A saphenous vein popliteal–plantar artery bypass was now possible.

I. BIOCHEMISTRY OF THROMBOLYTIC AGENTS

The sum and substance of intravascular thrombus is fibrin, a polymerized meshwork of cross-linked protein interspersed with abundant platelets and occasional red and white blood cells. The pharmacologic goal of thrombolytic therapy is to digest this meshwork, breaking the bonds on which the integrity of the thrombus depends. In this manner, the thrombolytic agents convert the highly insoluble fibrin-platelet mass into microscopic fragments of degenerated thrombus and, preferably, soluble breakdown products that wash into the circulation and are cleared by the kidney and liver.

It is important to emphasize that all clinically available thrombolytic agents do not degrade thrombus directly. Rather, each is a "plasminogen activator." As such, they do not directly degrade fibrinogen, and without plasminogen they are inert. The thrombolytic agents comprise trypsin-like serine proteases that have high specific activity directed at the cleavage of a single peptide bond in the plasminogen zymogen, converting it to plasmin (9). Importantly, plasmin is the active molecule that cleaves fibrin polymer to cause the dissolution of thrombus. Milstone first recognized the importance of plasminogen in 1941, when it was noted that clots formed with highly purified fibrinogen and thrombin were not lysed by streptococcal fibrinolysin unless a small amount of human serum (plasminogen) was added (10). Recognizing this direct role of plasminogen, early investigators attempted to dissolve occluding thrombi with the administration of exogenous plasmin (11). Free plasmin administered intravenously is ineffective as a thrombolytic agent, accounting for the failure of these attempts. Effective thrombolysis was achieved only when *fibrin-bound* plasminogen was converted to active plasmin at the site of the thrombus (9).

The dependence of fibrinolysis on adequate circulating levels of plasminogen is best illustrated by studies of the fibrinolytic potential of blood drawn from patients receiving intravenous of thrombolytic agents after acute myocardial infarction (12). Blood obtained soon after the start of the administration of these agents displayed a great degree of in vitro fibrinolytic potential. Aliquots of plasma drawn from the patients and then added to radiolabeled clots in test tubes produced rapid dissolution of the clots. By contrast, similar aliquots drawn from patients after 20 min of thrombolysis had considerably less thrombolytic potential. The explanation for this observation relates to the amount of plasminogen present in the blood. Prolonged thrombolysis consumed all of the endogenous plasminogen and, despite continued administration of the thrombolytic agent, no further clot lysis was possible.

II. SAFETY OF THROMBOLYTIC AGENTS IN CLINICAL TRIALS

There are few well-designed clinical comparisons of different thrombolytic agents for the treatment of peripheral arterial occlusion. By contrast, the literature is replete with a broad spectrum of in vitro studies and retrospective clinical trials, most pointing to improved efficacy and safety of urokinase and alteplase over streptokinase (13–16). In an analysis of data collected in a prospective, single-institution registry at the Cleveland Clinic Foundation, urokinase demonstrated a diminished rate of bleeding complications compared with alteplase (Table 1) (17).

There have been two prospective, randomized comparisons of urokinase and alteplase. Neither was blinded. Meyerovitz and associates from the Brigham and Women's Hospital randomized 32 patients with peripheral arterial or bypass graft occlusions of less than 90 days duration to alteplase (10 mg bolus, 5 mg/h to a maximum of 24 h) or urokinase (60,000 IU bolus, 4,000 IU/min for 2 h, 2000 IU/min for 2 h, then 1000 IU/min to a maximum of 24 h total administration) (18). There was significantly greater systemic fibrinogen degradation in the alteplase group ($p = 0.01$), indicating that the fibrin specificity of

Table 1   Relative Rate of Complications in 627 Patients Treated with Urokinase or Alteplase Between 1990 and 1998 at the Cleveland Clinic Foundation

Event	Urokinase $N = 483$	Alteplase $N = 144$	p Value
Bleeding requiring transfusion	12%	23%	0.004
Hematoma at catheter insertion site	22%	44%	<0.001
False aneurysm	1.7%	2.8%	Not significant
Intracranial bleeding	0.6%	2.8%	0.03
Death	2.7%	4.2%	Not significant

Source: Ref. 17.

Table 2 Complications Associated with Three Escalating Doses of Prourokinase (Initiated at 2, 4, or 8 mg/h) Versus Urokinase (Initiated at 240,000 IU/h) in the PURPOSE Trial

Site	2.0 mg	4.0 mg	8.0 mg	Urokinase
Epistaxis	0.0%	0.0%	3.8%	0.0%
Gastrointestinal	0.0%	0.0%	1.9%	0.0%
Gums	0.0%	0.0%	9.6%	0.0%
Intracranial	0.0%	0.0%	0.0%	0.0%
Hematuria	6.6%	7.3%	9.6%	8.3%
Retroperitoneum	1.6%	0.0%	3.8%	1.7%

Source: Ref. 22.

alteplase was lost at this dosing regimen. Alteplase patients achieved more rapid initial thrombolysis, but efficacy was identical in the two groups by 24 h. The trade-off to more rapid thrombolysis was a trend toward a higher rate of bleeding complications in the alteplase-treated patients.

The second randomized comparison of urokinase and alteplase was the STILE trial, a three-armed multicenter comparison of urokinase (250,000 IU bolus, 4000 IU/min for 4 h, then 2000 IU/min for up to 36 h), alteplase (0.05 to 0.1 mg/kg/h for up to 12 h) and primary operation (19). There was one intracranial hemorrhage in the urokinase group (0.9%) and two in the alteplase group (1.5%, no significant difference). Although actual rates of overall bleeding complications and efficacy were not reported for the two thrombolysis groups, the authors remarked that there were no significant differences detected in any of the outcome variables. In a subsequent "reanalysis" of the STILE data, reported in 1999, the frequency of complete clot lysis was similar with urokinase and alteplase at the time of the early arteriographic study (A.J. Comerota, personal communication). These recent data suggests that the rate of thrombolysis may be quite similar, in direct opposition to the popularly held view that alteplase is a much more rapidly acting agent.

A multicenter, blinded trial compared the results of thrombolysis with urokinase versus recombinant urokinase in 300 patients with peripheral arterial occlusion (20). These data were never published. No significant differences were noted between the two agents. A North American multicenter trial compared three different doses of prourokinase to urokinase in 241 patients with lower extremity arterial occlusions of less than 14 days duration (21). While the higher prourokinase dose was associated with slightly greater percentage of patients with complete (>95%) clot lysis at 8 h, there was a mild increase in the rate of bleeding complications compared with either the urokinase or the lower-dose prourokinase groups. The fibrinogen levels fell in the higher prourokinase group, suggesting that fibrin specificity was lost at the higher dose regimens for this compound (Table 2).

III. PREVENTING HEMORRHAGE DURING THROMBOLYSIS: POTENTIAL FOR THE FUTURE

There are several methods to consider in the quest to diminish the rate of distant hemorrhagic complications with thrombolytic therapy. First, one might strive to limit the "leak" of active thrombolytic agent into the systemic circulation. In fact this was the primary reason for considering the local, catheter-directed route for low-dose thrombolysis in the

1970s and 1980s (22,23). Clearly, the intrathrombus administration of thrombolytic agents is associated with improved efficacy (24). Whether increased safety has been achieved with this now ubiquitous method, however, remains to be established (Fig. 2).

The use of "fibrin-specific" agents was investigated to decrease the risk of distant bleeding (25). Fibrin specificity is quantified by the ratio of fibrin breakdown to fibrinogen breakdown. A fibrin-specific agent degrades fibrin but not fibrinogen. This property is accomplished through a variety of mechanisms. Alteplase was the first "designer" thrombolytic agent with fibrin-specific properties (26). Alteplase binds to fibrin but not to fibrinogen and attains plasminogenolytic activity only after binding. Tenectaplase, a modified form of alteplase, has even greater fibrin specificity, with very little reduction in fibrinogen concentration during therapy (27). Nevertheless, fibrin specificity has not resulted in a reduction in the risk of bleeding. The agents, in fact, may be associated with a greater

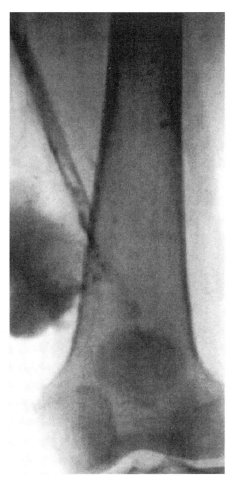

Figure 2   Thrombolysis-induced bleeding from the suture holes in a recently constructed polytetrafluoroethylene femoropopliteal bypass graft.

risk of distant hemorrhage, possibly related to the production of an intermediary fibrin breakdown product, fragment X (28). Fragment X is readily incorporated into existing distant thrombi, rendering the thrombi fragile and more susceptible to subsequent thrombolytic dissolution and hemorrhage. Interestingly, urokinase and streptokinase do not appear to generate significant quantities of fragment X during thrombolysis due to rapid conversion to smaller breakdown products. This mechanism might explain the putative lower incidence of distant bleeding with streptokinase and urokinase versus alteplase (29).

The use of concomitant systemic heparinization has been considered to reduce the rate of bleeding complications during thrombolytic therapy (30). The TOPAS trial was initially begun using full-dose systemic heparinization (7). The rate of intracranial bleeding decreased substantially when therapeutic heparinization was deleted from the protocol. Similar results were observed when heparin was decreased in the prourokinase trials for stroke (31). Recently, during peripheral arterial thrombolysis, a trend has emerged restricting heparin administration to an infusion rate of several hundred units per hour or less (32). Further, experience from the cardiology literature suggests that bleeding complications bear a greater relationship to heparin anticoagulation than to pharmacological thrombolysis (29).

The use of mechanical thrombectomy devices as adjuvants to pharmacological thrombolysis holds the potential to lower the rate of bleeding complications (33–35). Recognizing the link between duration of administration and hemorrhage, bleeding complications might be lower if mechanical adjuvants diminish thrombolytic exposure (36). As well, a new mechanical thrombectomy device utilizes proximal and distal balloon occlusion to limit the distribution of thrombolytic agent to the thrombosed vascular segment. Whether these mechanical adjuvants will result in a significant reduction in the risk of bleeding remains unproved; a critical analysis is not possible without a prospective trial.

Novel agents may diminish the risk of distant bleeding. For example, the agent alfimeprase, an analogue of fibrolase, is a direct fibrinolytic with activity that is independent of plasminogen (37). Circulating alpha2 macroglobulin inactivates alfimeprase. Systemic fibrinolysis will not occur as long as the dose of alfimeprase is kept below a threshold determined by available alpha2 macroglobulin. Like alfimeprase, plasmin analogues hold promise as alternative thrombolytic agents with a decreased risk of systemic bleeding. Plasmin, while ineffective when administered systemically, retains its activity when administered directly into the thrombus (38). As well, plasmin analogues may diminish the rate of distant bleeding as a result of systemic inactivation by circulating alpha2 antiplasmin (Fig. 3).

IV. NONHEMORRHAGIC COMPLICATIONS OF THROMBOLYTIC AGENTS

There are a wide variety of nonhemorrhagic complications associated with thrombolysis (39). Streptokinase is associated with allergic reactions in a significant percentage of patients, especially in those who have recently experienced a streptococcal infection and in those who undergo retreatment with the agent. Urokinase may be accompanied with rigors, especially in patients for whom the agent is administered in a large bolus dose. The target vessel or bypass graft may rethrombosis during thrombolytic infusion, a complication that occurs in approximately 8% of patients and seems to be reduced with heparin anticoagulation (21,30). The patient may sustain distal embolization of partially dissolved

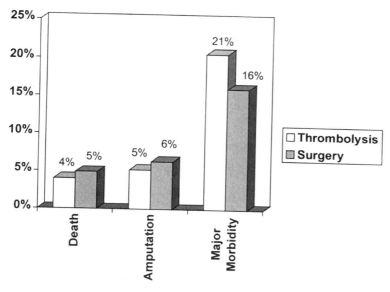

Figure 3 Complications in the STILE trial (19). Major morbidity was diminished in the surgery group, a finding that was related to a greater frequency of "ongoing ischemia" in the thrombolysis group. This did not translate into differences in the more important endpoints of death and major amputation.

thrombus, a problem that is noted in 10–20% of patients and one that appears to be diminished in frequency when a glycoprotein IIb/IIIa inhibitor is added to the thrombolytic regimen (21,40). Of importance, the amputation rate is higher when either rethrombosis or distal embolization develop during thrombolytic infusion (41). Last, technical complications may occur during percutaneous thrombolytic therapy, including catheter or wire perforation of the arterial wall (1%), arterial dissection (2%), pericatheter thrombosis (3%), and false aneurysm formation (1–3%) (17,21).

V. SUMMARY AND CONCLUSIONS

Thrombolytic therapy is associated with significant benefits to the patient, including (a) the ability to achieve restoration of blood flow in a minimally invasive fashion, (b) the identification of the culprit lesion responsible for the occlusive event, and (c) clearance of thrombus from small vessels inaccessible to balloon catheters. These benefits have culminated in a reduction in the rate of amputation (19) and death (1) for patients with acute limb ischemia. Complications, however, continue to occur at a relatively high frequency. Hemorrhage is the most frequent and clinically significant complication of thrombolytic therapy. The rate of hemorrhage can be diminished by avoiding therapeutic heparinization, decreasing the dose of thrombolytic agent, limiting the period of exposure, and prudent patient selection. Even with attention to these and other measures, bleeding, distal embolization, and rethrombosis will continue to occur with some frequency. These issues should be considered in presenting the therapeutic options to a patient, carefully weighing the risks versus the potential benefits prior to embarking on a particular treatment regimen.

REFERENCES

1. Ouriel K, Shortell CK, DeWeese JA, Green RM, Francis CW, Azodo MV, et al. A comparison of thrombolytic therapy with operative revascularization in the initial treatment of acute peripheral arterial ischemia. J Vasc Surg 1994; 19(6):1021–1030.
2. Sullivan KL, Gardiner GAJ, Kandarpa K, Bonn J, Shapiro MJ, Carabasi RA, et al. Efficacy of thrombolysis in infrainguinal bypass grafts. Circulation 1991; 83(suppl 2):99–105.
3. Garcia R, Saroyan RM, Senkowsky J, Smith F, Kerstein M. Intraoperative intra-arterial urokinase infusion as an adjunct to Fogarty catheter embolectomy in acute arterial occlusion. Surg Gynecol Obstet 1990; 171(3):201–205.
4. Ouriel K, Shortell CK, Azodo MV, Guiterrez OH, Marder VJ. Acute peripheral arterial occlusion: predictors of success in catheter-directed thrombolytic therapy. Radiology 1994; 193 (2):561–566.
5. Comerota AJ, Weaver FA, Hosking JD, Froehlich J, Folander H, Sussman B, et al. Results of a prospective, randomized trial of surgery versus thrombolysis for occluded lower extremity bypass grafts. Am J Surg 1996; 172(2):105–112.
6. Weaver FA, Comerota AJ, Youngblood M, Froehlich J, Hosking JD, Papanicolaou G. Surgical revascularization versus thrombolysis for nonembolic lower extremity native artery occlusions: results of a prospective randomized trial. The STILE Investigators. Surgery versus Thrombolysis for Ischemia of the Lower Extremity. J Vasc Surg 1996; 24(4):513–521.
7. Ouriel K, Veith FJ, Sasahara AA. A comparison of recombinant urokinase with vascular surgery as initial treatment for acute arterial occlusion of the legs. N Engl J Med 1998; 338:1105–1111.
8. Ricotta JJ, Green RM, DeWeese JA. Use and limitations of thrombolytic therapy in the treatment of peripheral arterial ischemia: results of a multi-institutional questionnaire. J Vasc Surg 1987; 6(1):45–50.
9. Alkjaersig N, Fletcher AP, Sherry S. The mechanism of clot dissolution by plasmin. J Clin Invest 1959; 38:1086.
10. Milstone H. A factor in normal human blood which participates in streptococcal fibrinolysis. J Immunol 1941; 42:116.
11. Cliffton EE. The use of plasmin in humans. Ann NY Acad Sci 1957; 68:209–229.
12. Onundarson PT, Haraldsson HM, Bergmann L, Francis CW, Marder VJ. Plasminogen depletion during streptokinase treatment or two-chain urokinase incubation correlates with decreased clot lysability ex vivo and in vitro. Thromb Haemost 1993; 70(6):998–1004.
13. van Breda A, Robison JC, Feldman L, Waltman AC, Brewster DC, Abbott WM, et al. Local thrombolysis in the treatment of arterial graft occlusions. J Vasc Surg 1984; 1(1):103–112.
14. Ouriel K, Welch EL, Shortell CK, Geary K, Fiore WM, Cimino C. Comparison of streptokinase, urokinase, and recombinant tissue plasminogen activator in an in vitro model of venous thrombolysis. J Vasc Surg 1995; 22(5):593–597.
15. Fox D, Ouriel K, Green RM, Stoughton J, Riggs P, Cimino C. Thrombolysis with prourokinase versus urokinase: an in vitro comparison. J Vasc Surg 1996; 23(4):657–666.
16. McNamara TO, Fischer JR. Thrombolysis of peripheral arterial and graft occlusions: Improved results using high-dose urokinase. AJR 1985; 144:769–775.
17. Ouriel K, Gray BH, Clair DG, Olin JW. Complications associated with the use of urokinase and recombinant tissue plasminogen activator for catheter-directed peripheral arterial and venous thrombolysis. Vasc Intervent Radiol 2000; 11:295–298.
18. Meyerovitz M, Goldhaber SZ, Reagan K, Polak JF, Kandarpa K, Grassi CJ, et al. Recombinant tissue-type plasminogen activator versus urokinase in peripheral arterial and graft occlusions: a randomized trial. Radiology 1990; 175:75–78.

19. Results of a prospective randomized trial evaluating surgery versus thrombolysis for ischemia of the lower extremity. The STILE trial. Ann Surg 1994; 220(3):251–266.

20. Abbott Laboratories Venture Group. A comparison of urokinase and recombinant urokinase in the treatment of peripheral arterial occlusion. Data on file. Abbott Park, IL: Abbott Laboratories, 1994.

21. Ouriel K, Kandarpa K, Schuerr DM, Hultquist M, Hodkinson G, Wallin B. Prourokinase versus urokinase for recanalization of peripheral occlusions, safety and efficacy: the PURPOSE trial. J Vasc Intervent Radiol 1999; 10(8):1083–1094.

22. Dotter CT, Rösch J, Seaman AJ. Selective clot lysis with low-dose streptokinase. Radiology 1974; 111:31–37.

23. Katzen BT, Edwards KC, Albert AS, van Breda A. Low-dose direct fibrinolysis in peripheral vascular disease. J Vasc Surg 1984; 1(5):718–722.

24. Graor RA, Risius B, Denny KM, Young JR, Beven EG, Hertzer NR, et al. Local thrombolysis in the treatment of thrombosed arteries, bypass grafts, and arteriovenous fistulas. J Vasc Surg 1985; 2(3):406–414.

25. Hoylaerts M, Rijken DC, Lijnen HR, Collen D. Kinetics of the activation of plasminogen by human tissue plasminogen activator: role of fibrin. J Biol Chem 1982; 257:2912.

26. Lijnen HR, Van Hoef B, De Cock F, Collen D. Effect of fibrin-like stimulators on the activation of plasminogen by tissue-type plasminogen activator (t-PA): Studies with active site mutagenized plasminogen and plasmin resistant t-PA. Thromb Haemost 1990; 64:61.

27. Cannon CP, Gibson CM, McCabe CH, Adgey AA, Schweiger MJ, Sequeira RF, et al. TNK-tissue plasminogen activator compared with front-loaded alteplase in acute myocardial infarction: Results of the TIMI 10B trial. Thrombolysis in Myocardial Infarction (TIMI) 10B Investigators. Circulation 1998; 98(25):2805–2814.

28. Owen J, Friedman KD, Grossman BA, Wilkins C, Berke AD, Powers ER. Quantitation of fragment X formation during thrombolytic therapy with streptokinase and tissue plasminogen activator. J Clin Invest 1987; 79(6):1642–1647.

29. The GUSTO Investigators. An international randomized trial comparing four thrombolytic therapies for acute myocardial infarction. N Engl J Med 1993; 329:673–682.

30. Ouriel K, Katzen B, Mewissen MW, Flick P, Clair DG, Benenati J, McNamara TO, Gibbens D. Initial experience with reteplase in the treatment of peripheral arterial and venous occlusion. J Vasc Intervent Radiol 2000; 11:849–854.

31. del Zoppo GJ, Higashida RT, Furlan AJ, Pessin MS, Rowley HA, Gent M. PROACT: a phase II randomized trial of recombinant prourokinase by direct arterial delivery in acute middle cerebral artery stroke. Stroke 1999; 29:4–11.

32. McNamara TO, Dong P, Chen J, Quinn B, Gomes A, Goodwin S, et al. Bleeding complications associated with the use of rt-PA versus r-PA for peripheral arterial and venous thromboembolic occlusions. Tech Vasc Intervent Radiol 2001; 4(2):92–98.

33. Kasirajan K, Haskal ZJ, Ouriel K. The use of mechanical thrombectomy devices in the management of acute peripheral arterial occlusive disease. J Vasc Intervent Radiol 2001; 12(4): 405–411.

34. Greenberg R, Ouriel K, Srivastava S, Shortell C, Ivancev K, Waldman D, Illig KA, Green RM. Mechanical versus chemical thrombolysis: an in vitro differentiation of thrombolytic mechanisms. J Vasc Intervent Radiol 2000; 11:199–205.

35. Silva JA, Ramee SR, Collins TJ, Jenkins JS, Lansky AJ, Ansel GM, et al. Rheolytic thrombectomy in the treatment of acute limb-threatening ischemia: immediate results and six-month follow-up of the multicenter AngioJet registry. Possis Peripheral AngioJet Study AngioJet Investigators. Cathet Cardiovasc Diagn 1998; 45(4):386–393.

36. Ansel GM, George BS, Botti CF, McNamara TO, Jenkins JS, Ramee SR, et al. Rheolytic thrombectomy in the management of limb ischemia: 30-day results from a multicenter registry. J Endovasc Ther 2002; 9(4):395–402.

37. Ahmed NK, Tennant KD, Markland FS, Lacz JP. Biochemical characteristics of fibrolase, a fibrinolytic protease from snake venom. Haemostasis 1990; 20(3):147–154.

38. Marder VJ, Stewart D. Towards safer thrombolytic therapy. Semin Hematol 2002; 39(3):206–216.
39. Sharma GVRK, Cella G, Parisi AF, Sasahara AA. Thrombolytic therapy. N Engl J Med 1982; 306:1268–1272.
40. Ouriel K. The RELAX Trial. Presented at the TCT Conference, Washington DC, Sept. 2002.
41. Galland RB, Earnshaw JJ, Baird RN, Lonsdale RJ, Hopkinson BR, Giddings AE, et al. Acute limb deterioration during intra-arterial thrombolysis. Br J Surg 1993; 80(9):1118–1120.

31

Complications of Sclerotherapy

John J. Bergan

*University of California, San Diego, School of Medicine,
San Diego, California, and Uniformed Services University of the Health Sciences,
Bethesda, Maryland, U.S.A.*

Mitchel P. Goldman

*University of California, San Diego, School of Medicine,
San Diego, California, U.S.A.*

I. INTRODUCTION

Venous insufficiency manifests itself in different ways. Its appearance varies from simple telangiectatic blemishes to severe chronic leg ulcer in an edematous, pigmented leg. Symptoms also vary from the essentially asymptomatic limb to that with disabling postexercise pain. Manifestations of venous insufficiency also vary and include those conditions—such as telangiectasias, varicose veins, and axial incompetence—that are usually well treated. In contrast, severe chronic venous insufficiency may be refractory to treatment. For example, the severely damaged postthrombotic limb manifests segmental occlusion in combination with universal reflux.

It is clear that treatment of varicose veins, primary venous insufficiency, and severe chronic venous insufficiency will involve sclerotherapy to a greater extent in the near future than in the recent past. Seventy years ago, sclerotherapy dominated treatment of venous insufficiency; however, through the 1950s, controlled trials comparing sclerotherapy with surgery revealed comparable short-term results but a much higher rate of recurrence after sclerotherapy than after surgery (1). Therefore interest in primary sclerotherapy declined and surgery became dominant.

Various disciplines including internal medicine, family practice, dermatology, general surgery, and vascular surgery have treated venous insufficiency to a greater or lesser extent. However, there is widely accepted and reasonable agreement among the various disciplines that treatment of large varicose veins and saphenous venous insufficiency should be treated surgically. It is small veins that might benefit from sclerotherapy. Dermatologists, for example, have taken up ambulatory phlebectomy for larger veins because of the influence of European dermatologists who invented specialized hook techniques for removing varicosities (2).

However, new stimuli are reviving sclerotherapy. One of these is the wide availability of ultrasound technology, which is used to guide sclerotherapeutic injections. Although some adverse sequelae have been seen with ultrasound-guided sclerotherapy, this has not deterred investigators (3). Large-vein sclerotherapy is liable to be associated with adverse reactions such as superficial thrombophlebitis, and hyperpigmentation of the skin; therefore surgery has remained the mainstay of treatment.

Recently a number of techniques have been developed to create sclerosant foam, which totally displaces the blood column and allows undiluted sclerosant agents to act on the endothelium and vein wall to produce both endothelial damage and venoconstriction (4). It is anticipated that sclerotherapy using foam will be increasingly popular and will largely replace surgery in the near future. This is truly minimally invasive and is perceived by patients and physicians alike as being very effective treatment.

The fundamental principle of sclerotherapy is obliteration of the lumen of the vein so that no blood can flow through it (5). Injection sclerotherapy has been used in the past for all sizes of varicose veins, ranging from protuberant saccular varicosities to minute telangiectasias. Gradually, principles have been developed that allow the successful performance of sclerotherapy.

II. PRINCIPLES OF SCLEROTHERAPY

In general, the first principle is the smaller the vessel to be destroyed, the greater the success of sclerotherapy. A second principle is that varicose veins treated by sclerotherapy will recur if axial reflux through the long and short saphenous veins is not controlled first. Following these principles relegates the sclerotherapy of varicose veins to a distant second place. It is most applicable in varicose veins that are persistent or recurrent following ambulatory surgery and varicose veins in the aged or infirm when these veins are symptomatic.

The fundamental mechanism of action of sclerotherapy is fibrotic obliteration of the vein lumen. The detergent sclerosants in use today denude the endothelium. If blood is present in the vein lumen, thrombus may form, and this thrombus may defeat the objectives of complete fibrosis. Such postinjection thrombosis is best referred to in the presence of the patient as "trapped blood." It is the most common side effect of sclerotherapy and is a causative factor in the development of postinjection pigmentation, which is discussed below. Veins larger than 1 mm and those raised above the skin surface are particularly prone to thrombosis. When this occurs, the vein becomes black, raised, and tender. In veins larger than 1 mm, a #18 needle can be introduced to allow external expression of the trapped blood.

One of the most common complications of sclerotherapy is postinjection hyperpigmentation (6). This is a product of the inflammatory process that obliterates the injected veins. There is no treatment for postinjection hyperpigmentation, but 90% of this will disappear within a year. Other side effects, including skin ulceration and postinflammatory telangiectatic matting, are less commonly seen.

For most injections, a 3- to 5- mL plastic syringe can be used, and this should be coupled to a 30-gauge hypodermic needle. The syringes are filled from vials of 3–5% solutions and diluted to appropriate strength. For sodium tetradecyl sulfate, this is 0.25% for telangiectasias and 0.5% for varices 1–3 mm in diameter. Equivalent strengths of other available sclerosants can be calculated.

There is much dogma surrounding the practice of sclerotherapy, most of it untrue. For example, there is no truth in the statement that crossing the legs brings on telangiectasias.

Similarly, the instruction for patients to walk around the clinic for 15–30 min and then come back for an evaluation is unnecessary. Most practitioners of the art of sclerotherapy believe that external compression is essential to the process, and a small but growing number of physicians believe that compression after the injection of telangiectasias is totally unnecessary.

Injection sclerotherapy does hold a rightful place in the treatment of venous insufficiency, but the rule still holds that the smaller the vessel, the more adaptable it is to sclerotherapy.

III. SCLEROTHERAPY COMPLICATIONS

As with any therapeutic technique, sclerotherapy carries with it a number of potential adverse sequelae and complications (Table 1). In addition to the previously mentioned cutaneous pigmentation, there can be edema of the injected extremity, pain with injection of certain sclerosing solutions, localized urticaria over injected sites, blisters or folliculitis caused by postsclerosis compression, recurrence of previously treated vessels, stress-related problems, and localized hirsutism. Relatively rare complications include localized cutaneous necrosis, systemic allergic reactions, clinically significant thrombophlebitis of the injected vessel, arterial injection with resultant necrosis, deep venous thrombosis, nerve damage, compartment syndrome, and air emboli. This chapter addresses the pathophysiology of some of these reactions, methods for reducing their incidence, and treatment of their occurrence.

A. Hyperpigmentation

This is a common occurrence after sclerotherapy of veins of all sizes; it occurs in approximately 10–80% of patients and can follow the use of any of the sclerosant agents. Its incidence appears to depend on technique and on the concentration of the sclerosant. The

Table 1 Complications of Sclerotherapy

Thrombosis, trapping
Post injection hyperpigmentation
Skin ulceration
Telangiectatic matting
Edema
Pain during injection
Localized urticaria
Blisters
Vein recurrence
Localized hirsutism
Localized skin necrosis
Systemic allergy
Superficial thrombophlebitis
Arterial injection
Deep venous thrombosis
Compartment syndrome
Air emboli

brown color, due entirely to hemosiderin deposition, may be linear or punctate and is reported to persist longer than 1 year in only 6% of patients (Fig. 1).

Reduction of pigmentation may be achieved by the use of lower concentrations of the sclerosant, by treating the source of proximal reflux first in order to reduce intravascular pressure, and by minimizing injection pressure. This last change can be accomplished by exerting less pressure on the plunger of the syringe and by using a larger syringe (2- to 3- mL syringes are recommended). The use of postsclerotherapy compression with a 30- to 40- mm graduated medical compression stocking has been associated with the development of less pigmentation.

Some patients are predisposed to the development of pigmentation, although the reasons for this are poorly understood (7). Certain medications (such as minocycline) may lead to the formation of a blue-gray discoloration in the skin following sclerotherapy. Certain stages of the menstrual cycle are associated with increased vessel fragility, which may lead to increased pigmentation.

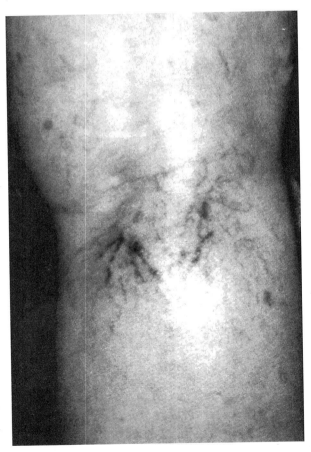

Figure 1 Linear brown streaks shown in this photograph are the product of intravascular thrombosis in large telangiectasias. (From Ref. 16.)

Removal of postsclerotherapy thrombi may decrease the incidence and intensity of pigmentation. The size of the thrombus may initially be minimized through the application of strong compression over treated veins, especially if the veins are >4 mm in diameter. Removal of thrombi may be easily accomplished by first locating the tender, often erythematous "lumpy" areas, infiltrating the tissue with lidocaine, and then using an 18-gauge needle or #11 blade or lancet to make a small puncture. The thrombus is then expressed with manual pressure. Thereafter compression may be reapplied for up to 3 days to decrease further thrombus accumulation.

Pigmentation usually lasts from 6 to 12 months. If it persists, one should search for a vessel with persistent reflux into the area. Bleaching agents are usually ineffective. Exfoliants (trichloroacetic acid) may hasten the resolution of pigmentation by decreasing the overlying cutaneous pigmentation, but they carry a risk of scarring or permanent hypo- or hyperpigmentation. Laser treatment has been shown to be effective in many cases.

B. Swelling

Multiple factors are responsible for swelling (edema) after sclerotherapy. Edema is most common when varicose veins or telangiectatic veins below the ankle are treated, especially when volumes greater than 1 mL are injected into the ankle or foot or when higher concentrations of sclerosing agents are utilized. It may be caused directly by the application of nongradient compression following sclerotherapy. Edema may be significantly reduced by the use of graduated compression stockings following sclerotherapy. Edema is self-limiting and generally resolves within several days to several months.

C. Telangiectatic Matting

The new appearance of previously unnoticed fine red telangiectatic veins occurs in many patients after sclerotherapy or surgery for varicose veins or telangiectatic veins (Fig. 2). These are sometimes referred to as *flares*, *telangiectatic matting*, *blushing*, or *postsclerotherapy neovascularization*. The reported incidence varies from 5 to 75%. Probable risk factors include obesity, use of estrogen-containing hormones, pregnancy, and a family history of telangiectatic veins. Excessive postsclerotherapy inflammation may also predispose to the development of matting.

New vessels can occur in 2–3 days or may not be visible for several weeks following treatment, and they can develop on any part of the leg. Generally, telangiectatic matting resolves in 3–12 months without any specific treatment. For persistent matting, one should first attempt to locate a source of reflux into the area, usually a feeding reticular vein, although matting may be a sign of underlying saphenous insufficiency. If matting persists, sclerotherapy treatment with a different sclerosant or pulsed-dye laser treatment may be effective.

D. Pain

Several variables may be altered to minimize the pain felt by the patient during sclerotherapy. The smallest needle possible should be used. If one inserts a needle multiple times, the needle should be changed frequently. Needles with an acute angle on the bevel and those coated with silicone generally cause in less pain. The preprocedure application of a topical anesthetic cream (EMLA) may be helpful in diminishing the pain with needle insertion. The cream must be applied in a thick layer 2 h before the procedure in order to be effective.

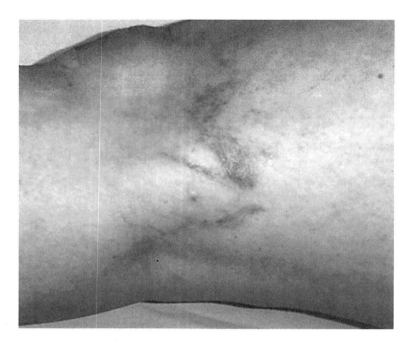

Figure 2 Telangiectatic matting is a common and disturbing complication of sclerotherapy. It consists of fine red intracutaneous vessels that are difficult to eradicate.

Choose the least painful sclerosing agent and dilute it with normal saline to the lowest effective concentration. Hypertonic agents frequently cause severe burning and muscle cramping, although this may be lessened with slower injection (8). Dilute sotradecyl or polidocanol in any concentration usually result in the least pain after injection. Burning or stinging pain resulting from any sclerosant may be diminished by firm pressure over the affected area or by rubbing the area with alcohol.

Aching in the legs is common for several hours to several days following sclerotherapy. This may be relieved by having the patient walk briskly and by the application of a 30- to 40- mmHg graduated medical compression stocking immediately following treatment. Aching that does not respond to these measures may indicate the presence of deep venous thrombosis.

E. Localized Urticaria

Localized urticaria occurs after injection of all sclerosing agents. It usually lasts less than 30 min and is probably the result of endothelial irritation. As it can occur with undiluted hypertonic saline, it should not be confused with a systemic allergic response to the sclerosant. Bothersome itching can be diminished by applying topical steroids immediately after injection and limiting the volume of additional injections.

F. Folliculitis

Occlusion of any hairy area by bandaging can promote the development of folliculitis, especially if the area becomes moist with perspiration. Treatment consists of removal of the dressing or compression and application of an antibacterial soap or topical antibiotic gel. The folliculitis usually disappears within a few days. If the itching is bothersome, a topical steroid preparation may be used. Systemic antibiotics will rarely be necessary.

G.   Localized Hirsutism

Hypertrichosis overlying a vein treated with sclerotherapy may occur, possibly due to improved cutaneous oxygenation or increased vascularity in the area. It may develop one or more months after treatment and is generally self-limiting.

H.   Cutaneous Necrosis

Ulceration of the skin may occur with the injection of any sclerosing agent even under ideal circumstances and does not necessarily imply physician error (Fig. 3). It is thought to be the result of extravasation of a sclerosing solution into the perivascular tissues. Injection into a dermal arteriole is more likely (Fig. 4). Otherwise it may be due to an arteriovenous anastomosis, severe vasospasm of the vessel, or excessive cutaneous pressure created by compression techniques.

Direct extravasation may be due to poor technique, leakage of the sclerosant through holes made in the vein from multiple prior injections or through-and-through perforation of the vein, tracking the solution into the tissues as the needle is withdrawn, or a "blowout" of a vessel due to the endothelial necrosis that may occur when strong sclerosants are used.

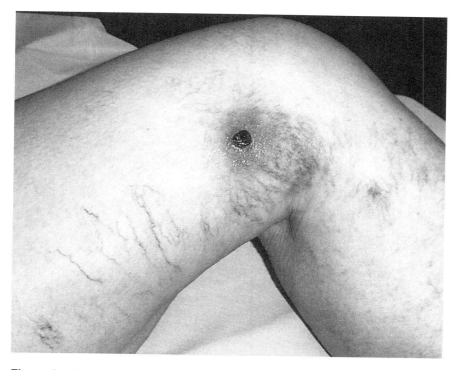

Figure 3   Cutaneous necrosis as shown here is a significant complication of sclerotherapy. It is a misunderstood and difficult-to-treat complication.

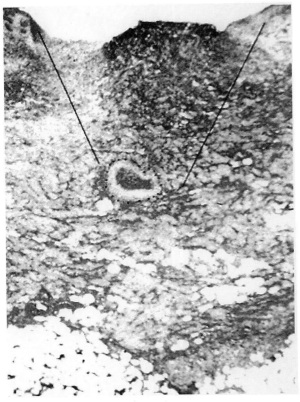

Figure 4 In this biopsy of an area of cutaneous necrosis, Goldman has shown a thrombosed arteriole in the base of the ulceration. (From Ref. 17.)

Some sclerosing agents are more caustic to the tissues—such as hypertonic saline, dextrose, or polyiodinated iodine—although cutaneous necrosis has been reported with all sclerosing solutions. If significant extravasation is suspected, the area should be infiltrated with normal saline in an attempt to dilute the sclerosant. Ten times the volume of extravasated solution must be used in order to dilute the sclerosant effectively. Infiltration of the area with 250 U of hydraluronidase may also be helpful due to the accelerated dilution, cellular stabilization, and wound repair properties of this agent (9).

Approximately 4% of telangiectatic veins are associated with a dermal arteriole. Thus, injection into an arteriovenous anastomosis is probably the most common cause of cutaneous ulcerations following sclerotherapy (Fig. 5). Reduction of the volume injected in each site along with a reduction of the pressure exerted on the plunger during injection may help to reduce this complication.

Rarely after injection, an immediate porcelain-white appearance to the skin is noted at the site of injection. A hemorrhagic bulla may form over this area within 2–48 h and later progress to an ulcer (Fig. 6). It is thought that this represents arterial spasm. In an attempt to reverse the spasm, vigorous massage may be directed to the area. To further reduce the likelihood of ulceration, one can rub a small amount of 2% nitroglycerin ointment into the area of blanching. This is usually successful in preventing an ulcer.

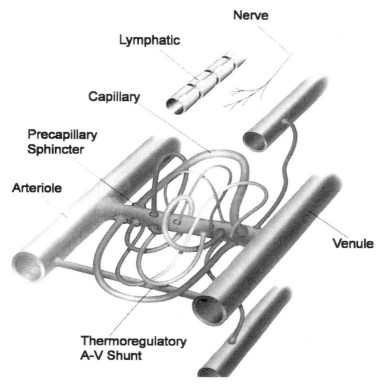

Figure 5 This diagram of a cutaneous thermoregulatory shunt explains why a true intravenous injection of sclerosant can be distributed by long-standing venous hypertension.

Excessive compression of the skin overlying the treated vein may produce tissue anoxia with the development of cutaneous ulceration. This is primarily found in patients with underlying arterial occlusive disease and most often occurs on the foot. Using inelastic compression, which does not exert any pressure on the foot or leg when the patient is supine, or using two 20- to 30- mmHg stockings during the day when the patient is upright and removing one of them at nighttime may prevent this complication.

Since most of these ulcerations are less than 4 mm in diameter, primary healing usually results in an acceptable scar. Larger ulcerations may be excised and closed for faster healing and a smaller scar. Application of hydrocolloid or hydrophilic dressings may reduce the pain associated with the ulcer and speed the rate of healing. Most ulcers will heal within 4 weeks to 4 months.

I. Systemic Allergic Reactions

Allergic reactions may occur following sclerotherapy with any of the sclerosants, even hypertonic saline. Minor reactions such as urticaria are easily treated with an oral antihistamine such as diphenhydramine (Benadryl) 25 to 50 mg PO or hydroxyzine (Atarax) 10 to 25 mg PO. If the reaction does not subside readily, a short course of prednisone 40–60 mg PO q.d. for one week in conjunction with the antihistamine is helpful.

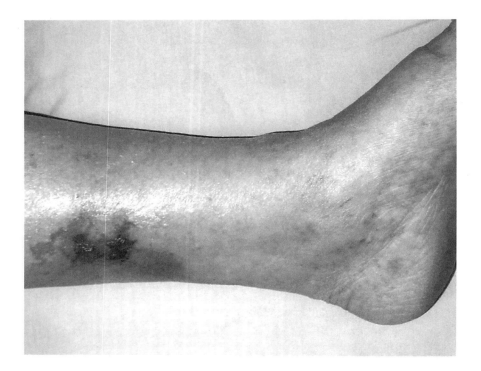

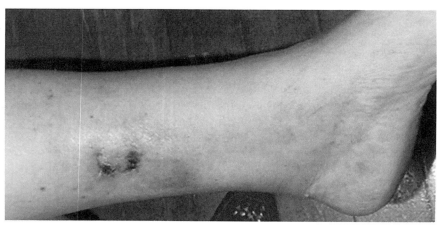

Figure 6 This area of tissue necrosis developed following ultrasound-guided injection of 2 mL of sclerosant foam equivalent to 0.5% STD.

Because of the possibility of angioedema or bronchospasm, each patient with an allergic reaction should be examined for stridor and wheezing by auscultation. Supine and seated pulse and blood pressure should be measured to rule out orthostatic changes, hypotension, or tachycardia that might result from the vasodilation that precedes ana-phylactic shock. If any of these more serious allergic reactions occur, an intravenous line should be started immediately. For angioedema with stridor, the patient should be given

Benadryl IV or IM and corticosteroids IV. A laryngoscope and endotracheal tube should be available. For bronchospasm, antihistamines and corticosteroids should be administered intravenously. A bronchodilator should be given either as an inhaler or nebulizer. If anaphylaxis is present, large volumes of intravenous fluids should be administered, along with 0.3–0.5 mL of epinephrine 1:1000 subcutaneously every 20–30 min as needed, up to three doses. If the reaction is feared to be life-threatening, 5 mL of epinephrine 1:10,000 should be administered intravenously every 5–10 min as needed. Obviously, patients with serious allergic reactions should be transferred to a hospital and observed for at least 6–12 h due to the biphasic nature of allergic reactions.

In addition to these general allergic reactions, there are point tenderness toxic reactions that may occur with all of the popular sclerosing agents. The physician should be familiar with these reactions and treat them if they occur.

J. Superficial Thrombophlebitis

Superficial thrombophlebitis may appear 1–3 weeks after injection as a tender, erythematous induration over the injected vein. This complication is observed less often if compression is maintained for an adequate period of time following sclerotherapy. The compression should be applied over the treated veins and even more proximally, as the sclerosing action may spread proximal to the injection site. When thrombophlebitis occurs, the thrombus should be evacuated and adequate compression and frequent ambulation should be maintained until the pain and inflammation subside. Aspirin or other nonsteroidal anti-inflammatory medication may be helpful in limiting both the inflammation and the pain. The concomitant presence of a deep venous thrombosis must be considered.

K. Arterial Injection

The most feared complication in sclerotherapy is inadvertent injection into an artery. Fortunately, this complication is very rare. Arterial injection of a sclerosing agent produces a sludge embolus that obstructs small arteries and the microcirculation. Experiments demonstrate little effect on the artery itself (10). The most common location for arterial injection is the posterior or medial malleolar region. Less common areas include the proximal thigh and popliteal fossa (the regions of the saphenofemoral junction and the saphenopopliteal junction). After intra-arterial injection, the patient will usually though not always note immediate pain. A dusky cyanotic hue may be noted at first, followed by pallor. Sloughing of the superficial tissues may result in significant scarring or even amputation of a limb. Occlusion of small arteries may lead to the development of a compartment syndrome with nerve damage and even paralysis.

Arterial injection is a true sclerotherapy emergency (11). The extent of cutaneous necrosis is usually related to the amount of solution injected (12). Efforts to treat this complications are usually unsatisfactory but should be made. Practical treatments include periarterial infiltration with 1 mL of procaine 3%, which will form a complex with sotradecyl and render it inactive. The affected area should be cooled with ice packs to minimize tissue anoxia. Immediate heparinization (continued for 6 days) and the administration of intravenous 10% dextran, 500 mL for 3 days, is recommended. Thrombolysis should be considered if no contraindication exists. Finally, use of prazosin, hydralazine, or nifedipine PO for 30 days should be considered.

L. Deep Venous Thrombosis

Pulmonary embolism and deep venous thrombosis are diagnosed very rarely after sclerotherapy (13). However, most cases of thrombosis and embolization go unnoticed, so the incidence is greater than statistics demonstrate (14). Sclerotherapy may affect all three components of the Virchow triad: Endothelial damage, vascular stasis, and changes in coagulability (15). Thus efforts to reduce the introduction of the sclerosant agent or a thrombus into the deep venous system should be a high priority. The volume of sclerosing agent per injection site should be limited in order to reduce the chance of its entering the deep venous system at a concentration sufficient to cause damage. Blood flow in the deep venous system must be rapidly stimulated with compression and muscle movement in an attempt to dilute any sclerosing agent that might be present. For this reason, some physicians ask patients to flex their ankles periodically during treatment. Patients should be asked to ambulate immediately and frequently after treatment. Postsclerotherapy compression may also reduce the incidence of thrombosis if applied in a graduated fashion. Sclerotherapy should be undertaken cautiously in patients with previous deep venous thrombosis or in those with a hypercoagulable state.

M. Nerve Damage

Because of their close proximity to the long and short saphenous veins, the saphenous and sural nerves may be damaged inadvertently during sclerotherapy. Injection into a nerve is very painful and may cause anesthesia and sometimes permanent interruption of nerve function. An area of paresthesia following sclerotherapy may result from perivascular inflammation extending from the treated vein to nearby superficial nerves. Nonsteroidal anti-inflammatory medications or high-potency topical corticosteroids may hasten resolution of this problem, which may take 3–6 months.

REFERENCES

1. Hobbs JT. The treatment of varicose veins: A random trial of injection compression therapy versus surgery. Br J Surg 1968; 55:777–780.
2. Neumann HAM, De Roos KP, Veraart JCJM. Muller's ambulatory phlebectomy and compression. Dermatol Surg 1998; 24:471–474.
3. Bergan JJ, Weiss RA, Goldman MP. Extensive tissue necrosis following high-concentration sclerotherapy for varicose veins. Dermatol Surg 2000; 26:535–542.
4. Tessari L, Cavezzi A, Frullini A. Preliminary experience with a new sclerosing foam in the treatment of varicose veins. Dermatol Surg 2001; 27:58–60.
5. Bergan JJ. Varicose veins: Treatment by surgery and sclerotherapy. In: Rutherford RB, ed. Vascular Surgery. 5th ed. Saunders, 2000:2007–2021.
6. Georgiev M. Post sclerotherapy hyperpigmentations: A one-year followup. J Dermatol Surg Oncol 1990; 16:608–610.
7. Lupo ML. Sclerotherapy: Review of results and complications in 200 patients. J Dermatol Surg Oncol 1989; 15:214–219.
8. Thibault P, Wlodarczky J. Post sclerotherapy hyperpigmentation: The role of ferritin levels and effectiveness of treatment with the copper vapor laser. J Dermatol Surg Oncol 1992; 18:47–52.
9. McCoy S, Evans A, Spurrier N. Sclerotherapy for leg telangiectasias: A blinded comparative trial of polidocanol and hypertonic saline. Dermatol Surg 1999; 25:371–386.
10. Zimmet SE. The prevention of cutaneous necrosis following extravasation of hypertonic saline and sodium tetradecyl sulfate. J Dermatol Surg Oncol 1993; 19:641–646.
11. MacGowan WAL, Holland PDJ, Browne HI, Byrnes DP. The local effects of intraarterial

injections of sodium tetradecyl sulphate (STD) 3%: An experimental study. Br J Surg 1972; 59:101–104.

12. Natali J, Farman T. Implications médico-légales au cours du traitement sclérosant des varices. J Malad Vasc 1996; 21:227–232.

13. Bergan JJ, Weiss RA, Goldman MP. Extensive tissue necrosis following high-concentration sclerotherapy for varicose veins. Dermatol Surg 2000; 26:535–542.

14. Yamaki T, Nozaki M, Sasaki K. Acute massive pulmonary embolism following high ligation combined with compression sclerotherapy for varicose veins: Report of a case. Dermatol Surg 1999; 25:321–325.

15. Feied CF. Deep venous thrombosis: The risks of sclerotherapy in hypercoagulable states. Sem Dermatol 1993; 12:135–149.

16. Weiss RA, Feied CF, Weiss MA. Vein Diagnosis and Treatment: A Comprehensive Approach. New York: McGraw Hill Medical Publishing Division, 2001.

17. Goldman MP, Bergan JJ, eds. Sclerotherapy Treatment of Varicose and Telangiectatic Leg Veins. 3rd ed. Mosby: St Louis, 2001.

32

Complications of Subfascial Endoscopic Perforator Vein Surgery and Minimally Invasive Vein Harvests

Peter Gloviczki and Manju Kalra

Mayo Clinic, Rochester, Minnesota, U.S.A.

Minimally invasive endoscopic procedures have been used for almost two decades for surgical treatment of both venous and arterial pathology. The primary aim of minimally invasive techniques is to reduce complications related to open surgical techniques. Endoscopic procedures are used to accelerate functional recovery, achieve a better cosmetic result, and enhance patient satisfaction.

Subfascial endoscopic perforator vein surgery (SEPS) was introduced in the mid-1980s by Hauer to treat incompetent perforating veins in patients with varicosity, advanced chronic venous insufficiency, and venous ulcers (1). Endoscopic techniques permitted interruption of incompetent perforating veins in the calf under direct vision with the help of an endoscope introduced through a small incision made proximal to the area of lipodermatosclerosis and venous ulcer. This technique was rapidly adopted and refined by several groups; in the past decade, SEPS has emerged as an effective minimally invasive technique to interrupt incompetent perforating veins (2–21).

Endoscopic vein harvesting (EVH) techniques to remove the great saphenous vein (GSV) were developed to decrease wound complications and improve patient satisfaction in those who undergo coronary artery bypass grafting (CABG) or lower extremity revascularization for critical limb ischemia. Experience using different endoscopic instrumentations to harvest the GSV has rapidly increased in the past decade (22–37).

In this chapter first we discuss current techniques and the associated complications of SEPS. We also describe the most frequently used techniques of EVH, discuss complications, and compare those with complications observed after traditional open vein harvesting techniques.

I. SUBFASCIAL ENDOSCOPIC PERFORATOR VEIN SURGERY

A. Surgical Techniques

Two main techniques for SEPS have been developed. The first is a single-scope technique, a refinement of the original work of Hauer (1), Fischer (2), and Jugenheimer (3) with further development by Bergan and his team (8,14,17) and by Wittens and Pierik (6,10,11). It uses a single scope with channels for the camera and working instruments, which sometimes makes visualization and dissection in the same plane difficult (Fig 1). Improvement in instrumentation for this technique now allows for carbon dioxide insufflation into the subfascial plane.

The second technique, using standard laparoscopic instrumentation, was introduced in the United States by O'Donnell (4) and developed simultaneously by Conrad in Australia (5) and by our team at the Mayo Clinic (7,16,20,21). This two-port technique employs one port for the camera and a separate port for instruments, thereby making it easier to work in the subfascial space. First the limb is exsanguinated with an Esmarque bandage and a thigh tourniquet is inflated to 300 mmHg to provide a bloodless field (Fig. 2A). A 10-mm endoscopic port is placed in the medial aspect of the calf 10 cm distal to the tibial tuberosity, 2 cm medial to the anterior edge of the tibia. Balloon dissection is used to widen the subfascial space and facilitate access after port placement (Fig 2B). The distal 5-mm port is now placed halfway between the first port and the ankle (about 10–12 cm apart), about 5–7 cm posterior to the anterior edge of the tibia, under direct visualization with the camera (Fig. 2C). Carbon dioxide is insufflated into the subfascial space and pressure is maintained at 30 mmHg to improve visualization and access to the perforators. Using laparoscopic scissors inserted through the 5-mm port, loose connective tissue between the calf muscles and the superficial fascia is sharply divided.

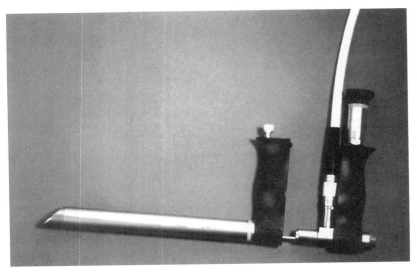

Figure 1   Olympus endoscope for the subfascial perforating vein interruption. The scope can be used with or without CO_2 insufflation. It has an 85-degree field of view and the outer sheath is either 16 or 22 mm in diameter. The working channel is 6 by 8.5 mm, with a working length of 20 cm. (From Ref. 43.)

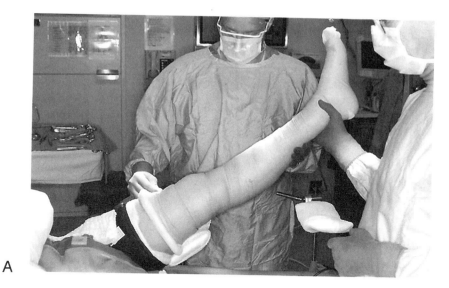

A

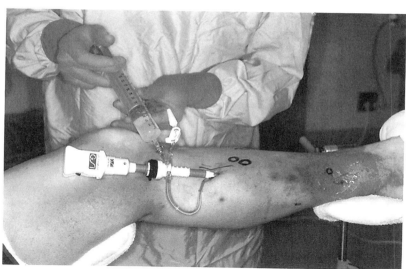

B

Figure 2 Two port technique of SEPS. A. A thigh tourniquet inflated to 300 mmHg is used to create a bloodless field. B. Balloon dissection is used to widen the subfascial space. C. SEPS is performed using two ports: a 10-mm camera port and a 5- or 10-mm distal port inserted under video control. Carbon dioxide is insufflated through the camera port into the subfascial space to a pressure of 30 mmHg to improve visualization and access to perforators. D. The subfascial space is widely explored from the medial border of the tibia to the posterior midline and down to the level of the ankle, and all perforators are interrupted using clips or harmonic scalpel. E. A paratibial fasciotomy is routinely performed to identify perforators in the deep posterior compartment. (From Ref. 44.)

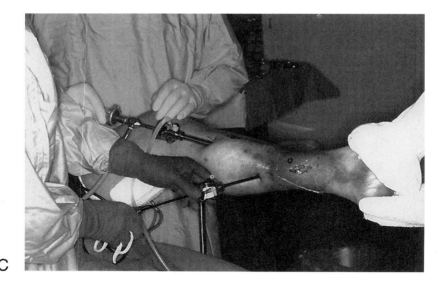

C

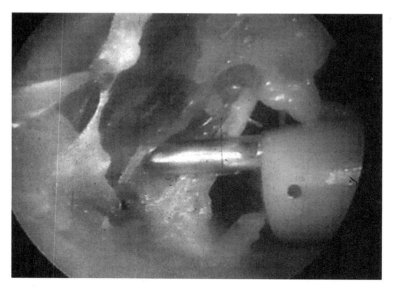

D

Figure 2 Continued.

The subfascial space is explored from the medial border of the tibia to the posterior midline and down to the level of the ankle. All perforators encountered are divided either with the harmonic scalpel or sharply between clips (Fig. 2D). A paratibial fasciotomy is next made by incising the fascia of the posterior deep compartment (Fig. 2E). The Cockett II and Cockett III perforators are located frequently within an intermuscular septum, and this has to be incised before identification and division of the perforators can be accomplished. The medial insertion of the soleus muscle on the tibia is also exposed proximally as high as possible to visualize proximal paratibial perforators. By rotating the ports cephalad and continuing the dissection up to the level of the knee, the more proximal perforators can also

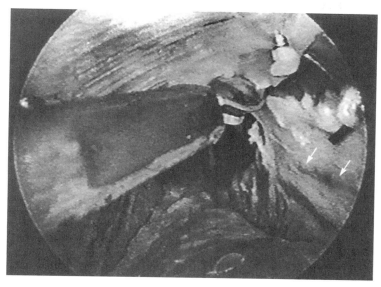

E

Figure 2   Continued.

be divided, although in our practice we seldom perform this part of the procedure. While the paratibial fasciotomy can aid in distal exposure, reaching the retromalleolar Cockett I perforator endoscopically safely is seldom possible.

After completion of SEPS, the instruments and ports are removed, the CO_2 is manually expressed from the limb and the tourniquet is deflated. For postoperative pain control, 20 mL of 0.5% bupivacaine (Marcain) solution is instilled into the subfascial space. Stab avulsion of varicosities in addition to high ligation and stripping of the great and/or small saphenous vein or radiofrequency closure of the saphenous vein is performed as needed. The wounds are closed and the limb is wrapped with an elastic bandage. Elevation is maintained at 30 degrees postoperatively for 3 hr, after which ambulation is permitted. The patients are usually discharged on the same day or occasionally next morning following overnight observation.

B.   Complications

SEPS may lead to systemic or local, nonvascular and vascular complications.

1.   Systemic Complications

Patient selection is important to prevent systemic complications and this procedure should not be done in those at high risk for general or epidural anesthesia or if unfit for surgical treatment. Using these criteria, mortality following SEPS is exceedingly rare. No deaths was reported in the North American SEPS registry and no pulmonary embolism was noted within 30 days in 148 patients who underwent 155 SEPS procedures (18,19). In our experience with over 150 SEPS procedures performed at our institution using general or epidural anesthesia, no death or pulmonary embolism was noted. One patient with known protein C deficiency with a history of multiple episodes of deep venous thrombosis developed recurrent popliteal vein thrombosis 2 months after the operation (20). Iafrati and O'Donnell reported on 51 SEPS procedures, with no deaths or cardiac, thromboembolic, or other systemic complications (15). To prevent deep vein thrombosis and pulmonary embolism, we give 3000 U of heparin before placement of the tourniquet for those patients who have underlying coagulation abnormality and postthrombotic syndrome. These patients also receive low-molecular-weight heparin postoperatively until full ambulation is resumed. In all others, leg elevation, early ambulation and elastic compression alone are used for thrombosis prophylaxis.

2. Local Complications

Local complications develop in 5–8% of the patients. Nonvascular local complications include cellulitis, wound dehiscence or infection, seroma or lymphocele, postoperative pain usually related to subfascial hematoma, saphenous nerve neuralgia, and injury to the tibial nerve. Vascular complications include thrombophlebitis, injury to the posterior tibial vessels, and deep venous thrombosis.

In the 148 registry patients, cellulitis occurred in 4 (3%) and wound infections in 8 (5%); five at port entry sites and three at other incisions (18). Wound infections after 30 days developed in 2 patients, one of whom also had early infection. Therefore the overall incidence of wound infection was at least 6% (9 of 148) (18). Of the 9 patients with wound infections, 7 had active ulcers at the time of the SEPS procedure. However, we failed to identify any clinical factors that predicted the development of wound infection in these patients (Table 1). Of the 10 patients with saphenous neuralgia, 9 underwent stripping of the GSV (8 from groin to knee, 1 from groin to ankle). Only avulsion of varicose veins was identified as a clinical variable significantly associated with saphenous neuralgia (Table 1). It is important, however, to avoid nerve injury at the time the proximal port is placed through the fascia.

A roll-on tourniquet caused skin necrosis in one patient (18), and this tourniquet is not used at our institution. A thigh tourniquet should be released after 90 min, and it should always be padded with gauze to protect the skin from pressure necrosis. No complication has been reported with pneumatic tourniquets, where constant pressure (200–300 mmHg) can be maintained and monitored during the procedure.

The registry reported superficial thrombophlebitis in 5 patients, of which 3 occurred within 30 days. Because all direct medial perforator veins join the paired posterior tibial veins (38), the potential for injury of the neurovascular bundle at that level exists. Geselschap et al. reported tibial nerve injury in one patient and injury to the posterior tibial artery in another (39). Dissection of the low medial perforators (Cockett II) should be done cautiously, since many times these perforators are located in the deep posterior compartment and the fascia overlying this compartment has to be incised to gain control of these important perforators (38). Interruption of all perforators must be done as close to the superficial fascia as possible to avoid injury to deep structures. As emphasized by Wittens and his team, one must be absolutely sure at this level that the divided structure penetrates the superficial fascia before clipping or division is done (39). Otherwise one can inadvertently injure the posterior tibial vessels or the tibial nerve.

A prospective randomized study between SEPS and open perforator ligation was performed in Holland and found less complications and shorter hospitalization following SEPS (11). The incidence of wound infections after open exploration was 53%, compared to 0% in the endoscopic group ($p < 0.001$). Patients in the open group needed longer hospital stays (mean, 7 days; range, 3–39 days) than patients in the endoscopic group (mean, 4 days; range, 2–6 days; $p = 0.001$).

With appropriate patient selection, adherence to the guidelines of endoscopic surgical techniques and thrombosis prophylaxis SEPS has a low complication rate and similar

Table 1 Association of Clinical Variables and Early Surgical Complications in the NASEPS
Registry

Clinical variables	Wound infection ($n = 8$)	p Value[a]	Saphenous neuralgia ($n = 6$)	p Value[a]
Ulcer				
Present	6/79 (7.6%)		3/79 (3.8%)	
Absent	2/29 (6.9%)	1.0	3/29 (10.3%)	0.340
Saphenous vein stripping				
Done	4/66 (6.1%)		6/66 (9.1%)	
Not done	4/42 (9.5%)	0.709	0/42 (0%)	0.080
High ligation				
Yes	1/10 (10.0%)		0/10 (0%)	
No	7/98 (7.1%)	0.553	6/98 (6.1%)	1.0
Tourniquet time				
> 60 min	1/22 (4.6%)		0/22 (0%)	
< 60 min	3/59 (5.1%)	1.0	6/59 (10.2%)	0.182
Endoscopes used				
One	4/55 (7.3%)		4/55 (7.3%)	
Multiple	4/53 (7.6%)	1.0	2/53 (3.9%)	0.679
CO_2 insufflation				
Yes	3/52 (5.8%)		2/52 (3.9%)	
No	5/56 (8.9%)	0.718	4/56 (7.1%)	0.680
Varicose vein avulsion				
Yes	4/53 (7.6%)		6/53 (11.3%)	
No	4/55 (7.3%)	1.0	0/55 (0%)	0.012
Diabetes				
Yes	0/4 (0%)		0/4 (0%)	
No	8/100 (8.0%)	1.0	6/100 (6.0%)	1.0
Gender				
Female	5/49 (10.2%)		5/49 (10.2%)	
Male	3/59 (5.1%)	0.464	1/59 (1.7%)	0.09

[a] Fisher's exact test.

long-term clinical outcome as open interruption of incompetent perforators (11). Although
foam sclerotherapy is emerging as potentially acceptable minimally invasive alternative
therapy, that procedure is not without complications and the recurrence rate is not yet
known. The minimally invasive SEPS remains the treatment of choice for perforator
interruption in 2003.

II. ENDOSCOPIC SAPHENOUS VEIN HARVESTING

A. Surgical Techniques

Several instruments are available for endoscopic saphenous vein harvesting (EVH), including instrumentation of Ethicon Endo-Surgery Inc. (Cincinnati, OH) and the Vaso View
System (Guidant Cardiac and Vascular Surgery, Menlo Park, CA), among others. Our
technique using the Ethicon instrumentation for EVH has been previously described (27).
The principal instrument is a disposable subcutaneous retractor, which incorporates a 5-mm

straight or a 30-degree angled endoscopic camera for viewing. This retractor is available in two different sizes. The endoscopic instruments include a pigtail dissector (a modified Mayo vein stripper) (Fig. 3), an endoscopic clip applier (5-mm Allport Clip applier) and endoscopic scissors (Ethicon Endo-Surgery, Inc., Cincinnati, OH). A 2.5 cm long incision is first made in the groin crease, the saphenofemoral junction is identified and all tributaries of the GSV are ligated proximally and distally. A subcutaneous tunnel is developed caudally over the anterior surface of the GSV with the aid of the endoscopic retractor containing the 5-mm videoscope (Fig. 3). The retractor is advanced distally to dissect and retract the tissues along the anterior surface of the vein. A gentle upward pressure has to be applied on the retractor to avoid injury to the saphenous vein by stripping its adventitia. All tributaries are clipped distally and divided. Only few very large tributaries need to be double clipped before division. The GSV must not be held under great tension during dissection to avoid adventitial and endothelial damage.

Once the limits of the retractor are reached (about 30 cm), the pigtail dissector is inserted to free up the vein circumferentially (Fig. 4). Additional lateral and any posterior tributaries are dissected, clipped, and divided (Fig. 5). Since clips are placed only laterally on the tributaries, the pigtail dissector can be advanced over the GSV without danger of vein injury. Nevertheless, smaller tributaries are frequently avulsed during dissection, and this renders in situ bypass rather difficult to perform because of bleeding in the tunnel through these sites.

When the entire length of the exposed vein is mobilized, additional distal incisions are made to insert the scope for further dissections. A longer incision at the knee level is frequently needed because of multiple genicular tributaries at this level. The adjacent saphenous nerve should be protected at the knee and the calf during vein dissection.

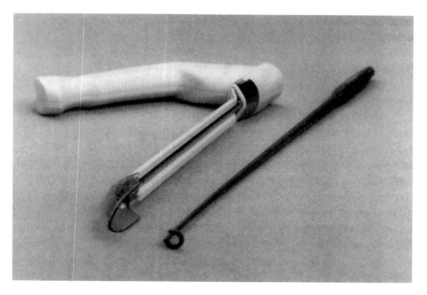

Figure 3 Instruments for endoscopic vein harvest (Ethicon Endosurgery, Inc., Cincinnati, OH). Left. Endoscopic dissector/retractor with a port for a 5- by 300-mm videoscopic lens. Right. A pigtail dissector (a modified Mayo vein stripper). (From Ref. 45.)

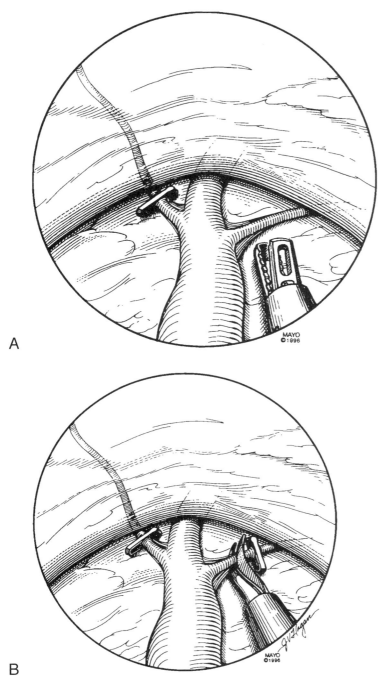

A

B

Figure 4 A and B. After the side branches are clipped with an endoscopic clip applier on the side of the body, they are divided with endoscopic scissors on the side of the vein. Venospasm and competent valves minimize blood loss. (From Ref. 45.)

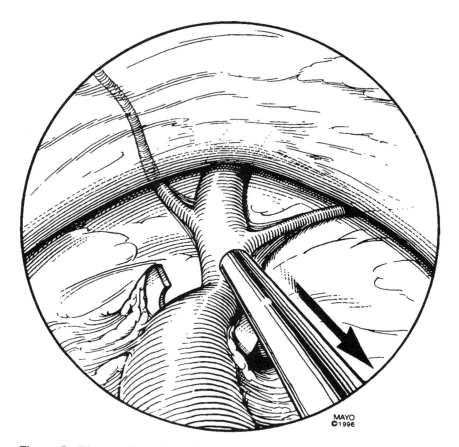

Figure 5 The anterior surface of the saphenous vein has been dissected using an endoscopic dissector. The vein is encircled with the open circle of the pigtail dissector, gently dissected from surrounding soft tissue, and the branches identified. (From Ref. 45.)

Upon completion of the vein dissection, high ligation and division of the proximal tributaries is performed, the vein is divided and clipped distally, and is removed. The vein is distended with heparinized saline/papaverine solution (our vein solution contains 1000 U of heparin sodium and 30 mg of papaverine in 400 mL of normal saline). Inflation over arterial pressure (120 mmHg) is avoided by using a syringe with a pressure gauge. Previously transected tributaries are ligated with 3-0 or 4-0 silk ties. Any tear in the vessel is repaired with 7-0 monofilament polypropylene sutures.

The technique of the Vaso View (Guidant Cardiac and Vascular Surgery, Menlo Park, CA) was described by several authors, including Bitondo et al. (37). This group uses a 2- to 2.5-cm transverse incision made just above the knee, where the vein is identified first. With the aid of carbon dioxide insufflation, a dissection cannula is used to isolate the vein and its surrounding branches. Once isolation of the vein is achieved, a second endoscopic instrument is used through which scissors connected to a bipolar cautery is inserted to cauterize and cut the tributary branches. A 1- to 1.5-cm incision is made in the groin to perform high ligation and division of the proximal saphenous vein and an additional 1-cm incision is made in the lower leg to expose the end of the vein for ligation and division. Metal clips can also be used to clip distal tributaries of the vein. After hemostasis is confirmed, the tunnel is irrigated with antibiotic solution and the incision closed with one or two interrupted, absorbable subcutaneous stitches and a running, 4-0 absorbable suture for the subcuticular layer. A drain is used only occasionally in obese patients or those with bleeding tendency. If the EVH was performed for CABG, the leg is wrapped immediately after skin closure with an elastic bandage that is used for at least 2 days.

B. Complications

Since EVH is done in patients who undergo lower limb revascularization or CABG, systemic complications are usually the results of the primary operation. Local complications of EVH are listed in Table 2 and range from wound dehiscence, infection, lymphocele, and lymphorrhea to wound necrosis, graft failure and even limb loss.

There is increasing evidence that EVH is associated with a reduced rate of wound complications. Most reports emphasize improved patient comfort, early mobility, decreased length of hospital stay, and superior cosmetic results (22–37). In early reports, Lumsden et al. observed only 3 wound complications following endoscopic removal of the GSV in 30 limbs. Two of these patients had cautery burns and one patient had injury to the saphenous vein (23). In a prospective series of 68 consecutive GSV harvests for lower extremity revascularization, Jordan et al. reported a wound complication rate of 8.8% (22). No graft failure or, more importantly, no graft harvest–related wound complications were noted, saphenous neuralgia appeared to decrease and hospitalization was also reduced (22). In a recent study, Alcocer and Jordan reported results in 185 operations using EVH (40). Only 16 patients (8.6%) had minor wound complications, including drainage, erythema, hematoma, and mild inflammation. Eleven patients had prolonged hospitalization or readmission because of wound complications. All complications were managed easily without further complications or wound dehiscence. The authors concluded that pain and perioperative complications were reduced after EVH compared to their own experience with open harvesting of the saphenous vein.

Table 2 Complications of Great Saphenous Vein Harvest

Wound infection
Cellulitis
Lymphangitis
Skin necrosis
Wound dehiscence
Lymphorrhea
Lymphocele
Seroma
Hematoma
Abscess
Saphenous neuralgia
Paresthesia
Graft failure
Limb amputation

In a prospective nonrandomized study Bitondo et al. studied wound complications and compared results of EVH in 92 patients to those with open vein harvesting (OVH) in 133 (37). Wound complications (dehiscence, drainage for greater than 2 weeks post-operatively, cellulitis, hematoma, and seroma/lymphocele) were significantly less in the endoscopic vein harvest group (9 of 133, 6.8%) versus the open vein harvest group (26 of 92, 28.3%). The 9 complications in the EVH group included seroma in 6 and dehiscence, lymph drainage and cellulites in one patient each. By multivariable analysis with logistic regression, the open vein harvest technique was the only risk factor for postoperative leg wound complication (relative risk 4.0). These results were confirmed in prospective randomized trials by Allen et al. (28) and in another by Puskas et al. (31), who observed more drainage from leg incisions at hospital discharge in the open harvest group (34%) versus EVH group (8%; $p = 0.001$), but more ecchymosis in the EVH group. This study did not find reduced leg incision pain in the EVH group, and there was no statistically significant difference in pain or in the quality of life measured at any point in time. In addition, there was no difference between groups in readmission to hospital, administration of antibiotics, or incidence of leg infection. Mean hospital charges for the EVH group were approximately $1500 greater than for OVH; this difference however, did not reach statistical significance. These authors concluded that EVH is a safe, reliable, and cost-neutral method for saphenous vein harvest, but commented that the best indication for EVH may be in patients who are at increased risk for wound infection and in those for whom cosmesis is a major concern.

In another prospective randomized trial, Schurr et al. recently compared EVH to traditional open harvesting technique for patients who underwent CABG. In this trial, 140 CABG patients were randomized into two groups, 80 EVH and 60 open vein harvest (OVH). There was a 7% conversion of EVH patients to OVH. EVH time was significantly longer than OVH time (45 +/− 6.2 min vs. 31.1 +/− 6.5 min). However, morbidity was significantly lower, with reduced pain and better cosmetic results following EVH. Bleeding complications were less frequent and no local infections or wound complications were observed in the EVH group versus 11 (18%) cases in the OVH group. Two OVH cases (3.6%) were readmitted for wound debridement. These authors concluded EVH is a safe and efficient technique for patients who require CABG. While these studies performed in patients who underwent EVH for CABG are convincing, EVH continues to be avoided by many vascular surgeons. Increased cost, increased OR time, and the possibility of injury of a long conduit for infrainguinal bypass are continuing concerns that have prevented widespread acceptance of this technique by vascular surgeons who perform limb salvage procedures.

The pivotal issue that must be considered is the risk of endothelial injury and subsequent intimal hyperplasia in these patients, leading to failure of the grafts. There are obvious concerns that traction during adventitial dissection and manipulation of the vein will result in intimal trauma and secondary changes affecting long-term patency. Several studies have investigated the effects of minimally invasive GSV harvest on morphology and function of the veins and failed to show a deleterious effect. Meldrum-Hanna demonstrated preservation of intima by scanning electron microscopy (SEM) and observed a 93% graft patency rate at 10 days after surgery (25). In another histological study of vein samples performed using light microscopy and SEM, preservation of endothelial architecture, cell cohesion, and intercellular junctional gaps was observed (41). Functional studies from the Mayo Clinic of porcine venous endothelium confirmed, that endothelial release of vasoactive substances after endoscopic harvesting is similar to that after the traditional extended incision technique, and microscopy confirmed similar histology and integrity (27).

Vein injuries requiring vein patch angioplasty occurred in two patients in the series of Jordan et al. (22) One of the veins thrombosed at 5 months after operation. In that series, primary patency rate of femoropopliteal bypasses was 63% and secondary patency rate was 83% at a mean follow-up of 7.9 months. Long-term follow-up with 5 year results by the same group was recently reported (40,42). The 1-, 3-, and 5-year secondary patency rates of the infrainguinal vein grafts were 85, 74, and 68%. Of the 30 failed grafts, 7 (4%) failed in the first month related to inadequate runoff (4), cardiac instability (2), and an additional surgical procedure (1). Twenty-three late graft failures were salvaged in all but one patient. Five-year limb salvage was 89%.

With improvement in technology and decrease in cost, EVH may regain popularity among vascular surgeons and will be used even more frequently by our cardiac colleagues. Available evidence supports decreased wound complications with EVH compared to open harvesting techniques in patients who undergo CABG, and long-term graft patency and limb salvage in those who underwent EVH for lower extremity bypass does not appear to be adversely affected. Long-term randomized study of infrainguinal reconstructions with EVH and open techniques will still be required to provide the final answer.

Prevention of systemic and local complications of SEPS and EVH requires careful patient selection, adherence to open and minimally invasive surgical techniques, and appropriate postoperative care. Early recognition and correct management of complications will result in improved outcome and will avert potentially severe secondary complications, disability, limb loss, or even death. These minimally invasive procedures are here to stay, and with progress in technology, they have an excellent chance to be used more frequently in the future in cardiovascular surgery.

REFERENCES

1. Hauer G. Endoscopic subfascial discussion of perforating veins—Preliminary report. [German]. Vasa 1985; 14:59–61.
2. Fischer R. Surgical treatment of varicose veins: Endoscopic treatment of incompetent Cockett veins. Phlebologie 1989; 1040–1041.
3. Jugenheimer M, Junginger T. Endoscopic subfascial sectioning of incompetent perforating veins in treatment of primary varicosis. World J Surg 1992; 16:971–975.
4. O'Donnell TF. Surgical treatment of incompetent communicating veins. In: Atlas of Venous Surgery. Philadelphia: Saunders, 1992:111–124.
5. Conrad P. Endoscopic exploration of the subfascial space of the lower leg with perforator interruption using laparoscopic equipment: A preliminary report. Phlebology 1994; 9:154–157.
6. Wittens CH, Pierik RG, van Urk H. The surgical treatment of incompetent perforating veins. Eur J Vasc Endovasc Surg 1995; 9:19–23.
7. Gloviczki P, Cambria RA, Rhee RY, Canton LG, McKusick MA. Surgical technique and preliminary results of endoscopic subfascial division of perforating veins. J Vasc Surg 1996; 23:517–523.
8. Bergan JJ, Murray J, Greason K. Subfascial endoscopic perforator vein surgery: A preliminary report. Ann Vasc Surg 1996; 10:211–219.
9. Gloviczki P, Bergan JJ, Menawat SS, Hobson RW, Kistner RL, Lawrence PF, et al. Safety, feasibility, and early efficacy of subfascial endoscopic perforator surgery: A preliminary report from the North American registry. J Vasc Surg 1997; 25:94–105.

10. Pierik EG, Toonder IM, van Urk H, Wittens CH. Validation of duplex ultrasonography in detecting competent and incompetent perforating veins in patients with venous ulceration of the lower leg. J Vasc Surg 1997; 26:49–52.

11. Pierik EG, van Urk H, Hop WC, Wittens CH. Endoscopic versus open subfascial division of incompetent perforating veins in the treatment of venous leg ulceration: A randomized trial. J Vasc Surg 1997; 26:1049–1054.

12. Gloviczki P, Bergan JJ, Menawat SS, Hobson RW, Kistner RL, Lawrence PF, et al. Safety, feasibility, and early efficacy of subfascial endoscopic perforator surgery: A preliminary report from the North American registry. J Vasc Surg 1997; 25:94–105.

13. Stuart WP, Adam DJ, Bradbury AW, Ruckley CV. Subfascial endoscopic perforator surgery is associated with significantly less morbidity and shorter hospital stay than open operation (Linton's procedure). Br J Surg 1997; 84:1364–1365.

14. Sparks SR, Ballard JL, Bergan JJ, Killeen JD. Early benefits of subfascial endoscopic perforator surgery (SEPS) in healing venous ulcers. Ann Vasc Surg 1997; 11:367–373.

15. Iafrati MD, Welch HJ, O'Donnell TF Jr. Subfascial endoscopic perforator ligation: An analysis of early clinical outcomes and cost. J Vasc Surg 1997; 25:995–1000.

16. Rhodes JM, Gloviczki P, Canton LG, Rooke T, Lewis BD, Lindsey JR. Factors affecting clinical outcome following endoscopic perforator vein ablation. J Vasc Surg 1998; 176:162–167.

17. Murray JD, Bergan JJ, Riffenburgh RH. Development of open-scope subfascial perforating vein surgery: Lessons learned from the first 67 patients. Ann Vasc Surg 1999; 199:372–377.

18. Gloviczki P, Bergan JJ, Rhodes JM, Canton LG, Harmsen S, Ilstrup DM. Mid-term results of endoscopic perforator vein interruption for chronic venous insufficiency: Lessons learned from the North American subfascial endoscopic perforator surgery registry. The North American Study Group. J Vasc Surg 1999; 29:489–502.

19. Gloviczki P, Bergan JJ, Rhodes JM, Canton LG, Harmsen S, Ilstrup DM. Mid-term results of endoscopic perforator vein interruption for chronic venous insufficiency: Lessons learned from the North American subfascial endoscopic perforator surgery registry. The North American Study Group. J Vasc Surg 1999; 29:489–502.

20. Kalra M, Gloviczki PM, Noel AA, et al. Subfascial endoscopic perforator vein surgery (SEPS) in patients with post-thrombotic venous insufficiency—Is it justified? Vasc Endovasc Surg 2002; 36:41–50.

21. Kalra M, Gloviczki P. Subfascial endoscopic perforator vein surgery: Who benefits? Semin Vasc Surg 2002; 15:39–49.

22. Jordan WD, Voellinger DC, Schroeder PT, McDowell HA. Video-assisted saphenous vein harvest: The evolution of a new technique. J Vasc Surg 1997; 26:405–414.

23. Lumsden AB, Eaves FF, Ofenloch JC, Jordan WD. Subcutaneous, video-assisted saphenous vein harvest: Report of the first 30 cases. Cardiovasc Surg 1996; 4:771–776.

24. Cable DG, Dearani JA. Endoscopic saphenous vein harvesting: minimally invasive video-assisted saphenectomy. Ann Thorac Surg 1997; 64:1183–1185.

25. Meldrum-Hanna W, Ross D, Johnson D, Deal C. An improved technique for long saphenous vein harvesting for coronary revascularizaiton. Ann Thorac Surg 1986; 42:90–92.

26. Cable DG, Dearani JA, Pfeifer EA, Daly RC, Schaff HV. Minimally invasive saphenous vein harvesting: endothelial integrity and early clinical results. Ann Thorac Surg 1998; 66:139–140.

27. Cho JS, Gloviczki P. Techniques for harvesting the GSV. In: Whittemore AD, ed. Advances in Vascular Surgery. St. Louis: Mosby, 1998:171–140.

28. Allen KB, Griffith GL, Heimansohn DA, et al. Endoscopic versus traditional saphenous vein harvesting: A prospective randomized trial. Ann Thorac Surg 1998; 66:26–32.

29. Crouch JD, O'Hair DP, Keuler JP, et al. Open versus endoscopic saphenous vein harvesting: Wound complications and vein quality. Ann Thorac Surg 1999; 68:1513–1516.

30. Kan CD, Luo CY, Yang YJ, et al. Endoscopic saphenous vein harvest decreases leg wound complication in coronary artery bypass grafting patients. J Card Surg 1999; 14:157–162.

31. Puskas JD, Wright CE, Miller PK, et al. A randomized trial of endoscopic versus open saphenous vein harvest in coronary bypass surgery. Ann Thorac Surg 1999; 68:1509–1512.

32. Vitali RM, Reddy RC, Molinaro PJ, et al. Hemodynamic effects of carbon dioxide insufflation during endoscopic vein harvesting. Ann Thorac Surg 2000; 70:1098–1099.

33. Meyer DM, Rogers TE, Jessen ME, et al. Histologic evidence of the safety of endoscopic saphenous vein graft preparation. Ann Thorac Surg 2000; 70:487–491.

34. Alwari SJ, Samee M, Raju R, et al. Intercellular and vascular cell adhesion molecule levels in endoscopic and open saphenous vein harvesting for coronary artery bypass surgery. Heart Surg Forum 2000; 3:241–245.

35. Fabricius AM, Diegeler A, Doll N, et al. Minimally invasive saphenous vein harvesting techniques: Morphology and postoperative outcome. Ann Thorac Surg 2000; 70:473–478.

36. Patel AN, Hebeler RF, Hamman BL, Hunnicutt C, Williams M, Liu L, Wood RE. Prospective analysis of endoscopic vein harvesting. Am J Surg 2001; 182(6):716–719.

37. Bitondo JM, Daggett WM, Torchiana DF, Akins CW, Hilgenberg AD, Vlahakes GJ, Madsen JC, MacGillivray TE, Agnihotri AK. Endoscopic versus open saphenous vein harvest: a comparison of postoperative wound complications. Ann Thorac Surg 2002; 73(2):523–528.

38. Mozes G, Gloviczki P, Menawat SS, Fisher DR, Carmichael SW, Kadar A. Surgical anatomy for endoscopic subfasical division of perforating veins. J Vasc Surg 1996; 24:800–808.

39. Geselschap JH, van Gent WB, Wittens CH. Complications in subfascial endoscopic perforating vein surgery: A report of two cases. J Vasc Surg 2001; 33:1108–1110.

40. Alcocer F, Jordan WD. Long-term follow-up of endoscopically harvested vein graft. In: Pearce WE, Matsumura JS, Yao STJ, eds. Trends in Vascular Surgery. Chicago: Precept Press, 2002: 293–300.

41. Dimitri WR, West IE, Williams BT. A quick and atraumatic method of autologous vein harvesting using the subcutaneous extraluminal dissector. J Cardiovasc Surg 1987; 28:103–111.

42. Jordan WD Jr, Alcocer F, Voellinger DC, Wirthlin DJ. The durability of endoscopic saphenous vein grafts: A 5-year observational study. J Vasc Surg 2001; 34:434–439.

43. Bergan JJ, Ballard JL, Sparks S. In: Gloviczki P, Bergan JJ, eds. Atlas of Endoscopic Perforator Vein Surgery. London: Springer-Verlag, 1998:141–149.

44. Gloviczki P, Canton LG, Cambria RA, Rhee RY. Subfascial endoscopic perforator vein surgery with gas insufflation. In: Gloviczki P, Bergan JJ, eds. Atlas of Endoscopic Perforator Vein Surgery. London: Springer-Verlag, 1998:125–138.

45. Cho JS, Gloviczki P. Techniques for harvesting the greater saphenous vein. In: Whittemore AD, ed. Advanced in Vascular Surgery. St. Louis: Mosby, 1998:171–180.

33

Complications of Venous Endovascular Lysis and Stenting (Iliac, Subclavian)

Peter Neglén

River Oaks Hospital, Jackson, Mississippi, U.S.A.

Indications for percutaneous venous endovascular procedures are expanding and techniques for venous interventions are developing rapidly. This chapter will deal mainly with complications of procedures performed for acute or chronic obstruction of the venous outflow of the upper and lower extremities. Complications related to endovascular procedures for malfunctioning dialysis accesses and interruption of the inferior vena cava are discussed in Chapters 34 and 35, respectively.

The most frequent complications of endovascular venous procedures are related to cannulation of the vessel, as with arterial percutaneous interventions. In addition, administration of lytic agents through inserted catheters may lead to local or systemic bleeding complications, which mitigate potential benefits. Inadvertent events related to the venous balloon angioplasty are infrequent. Contrary to angioplasty of the arteries, clinical rupture of veins has to our knowledge not been reported. Dissection does not occur in veins, but embolization secondary to balloon dilation in chronic venous disease or after outflow thrombolysis, although extremely rare, may be of clinical importance in individual patients. Complications may also be related to the stent. Unlike arterial obstruction, a stent is always required in treating venous obstruction because the fibrous and elastic venous lesion often recoils after dilation alone. After the insertion, there is a potential risk for migration of the stent proximally or distally, fracture of the stent material, in-stent restenosis, and early or late occlusion. Patency rates of stents placed in the venous system may vary depending upon the anatomic location, etiology of the obstruction, development rate of neointimal hyperplasia, magnitude of venous inflow, and presence of concomitant diseases. The significance of many of these factors for the patency of stents placed in the venous system is not fully known and warrants further investigation.

I.   COMPLICATIONS RELATED TO VENOUS CANNULATION

Complications related to cannulation of the vein are inherent in all percutaneous procedures. Although the formation of hematomas or pseudoaneurysms and development of
traumatic arteriovenous fistulas are rare (<0.5%) (1), the frequency is higher with increasing
use of larger percutaneous instruments and more intensive anticoagulation. The rate of
hematoma formation appears to be less frequent in venous than in arterial interventions,
probably owing to the lower venous pressure and the ease with which compression can
control venous cannulation-site bleeding. We have found that the insertion of collagen plugs
(VasoSeal, Datascope Corp., Montvale, NJ) at the end of the procedure effectively controls
the bleeding at the venous cannulation site within a minute in the majority of limbs without
later rebleeding and obviates prolonged manual compression.

Formation of traumatic arteriovenous fistulas or pseudoaneurysms occurs when the
artery beside the vein is inadvertently injured during cannulation. Ultrasound-guided cannulation, either by ultrasound-tipped cannulas or special ultrasound probes, makes multiple
blind attempts unnecessary, puncture of the posterior wall is avoided, and the risk of arterial
injury is substantially decreased. Trauma to the artery is rare when ultrasound-guided
cannulation of the proximal femoral or popliteal veins is performed, but it may still occur
despite ultrasound guidance when it is necessary to access the distal femoral vein, which is
often hidden behind the artery at this location.

Both pseudoaneurysms and traumatic arteriovenous fistulas can be diagnosed by duplex Doppler ultrasound scan with high accuracy. Spontaneous thrombosis may occur in as
many as one-third of pseudoaneurysms. If the pseudoaneurysm persists, the next step is to
attempt ultrasound-guided manual compression or compression by the ultrasound probe
(2,3). Closure of the pseudoaneurysm is successful in the majority of cases since the inflow
channel of the pseudoaneurysm is very narrow and easily compressed. Compression time is
relatively long, averaging 40 min; the pressure is painful for the patient; and larger aneurysms (> 4 cm in diameter) are more difficult to close. A more expeditious and efficient
method is injection of thrombin under guidance of duplex scanning (4,5). The pseudoaneurysm closes within minutes. The rate of inadvertent arterial injection in one study was 4%
(4). Intra-arterial injection must be avoided, since it results in limb-threatening ischemia. If
these interventions are unsuccessful, the patients must undergo surgery, usually with simple
closure of the arterial defect.

The majority of traumatic arteriovenous fistulas are closed by open surgery. Short stent
grafts may be inserted intra-arterially to close the connecting tract. Closure is easily
achieved, but the long term patency has not been assessed.

II.   COMPLICATIONS RELATED TO LYSIS OF DEEP
   VEIN THROMBOSIS

The current standard of treatment for deep venous thrombosis remains anticoagulation
therapy with intravenous unfractionated or subcutaneous low-molecular-weight heparin,
followed by oral warfarin. It is clear, however, that anticoagulation therapy does not
actively promote fibrinolysis. Consequently, this method leaves clot behind, which undergoes retraction and organization and results in remaining obstruction and valve damage.
Only 20–30% of iliac veins completely recanalize spontaneously following thrombosis,
while the remaining veins recanalize partially and develop varying degrees of collateralization (6,7). When an early complete lysis of the clot can be achieved, improved patency of the

thrombosed vein and better preservation of the valve function are observed (8–10). This is the rationale behind actively attempting to dissolve a deep venous thrombus. Although no randomized prospective studies have been performed, thrombolysis of acute deep venous thrombosis (DVT) involving the iliofemoral and axillary–subclavian outflows is an attractive form of therapy. Results are similar to those achieved with surgical thrombectomy, a procedure that is scorned in the United States but still practiced in parts of Europe (11). With the introduction of the catheter-directed thrombolytic (CDT) techniques reported by Semba and Dake in 1994 (12), a better degree of lysis has been obtained than with the previously used systemic administration. By application of high concentrations of thrombolytic agent to the clot itself, the lysis rates have been improved and the duration of treatment reduced. The complication rate appears to be lower in CDT than that in systemic administration.

At present, the most common approach to the iliofemoral vein segment is ultrasound-guided cannulation of the ipsilateral popliteal vein with the patient in the prone position. When the popliteal vein is occluded, the ipsilateral posterior tibial vein is cannulated. The internal jugular access or contralateral femoral approach has now been abandoned because of the difficulty of pushing guidewires and catheters safely through a femoral thrombosis in a retrograde direction against the direction of the venous valves. A sheath is inserted and venography is performed, visualizing the distal extent of the clot. The thrombus is then crossed by a guidewire and catheter, through which the proximal extent is shown by repeat contrast dye injection. A multiside-hole catheter is then inserted into the thrombus, covering its entire extent if possible. A thrombolytic agent is then infused continuously or in a pulse-spray fashion. Concomitantly, heparin is infused intravenously. The extent of thrombolysis is assessed every 12 h with venography performed through the sheath. It may be necessary to reposition the infusion catheter into remaining thrombus or sometimes to gently macerate the thrombus with a balloon catheter. Typically, the thrombolysis is continued to complete lysis or terminated when no discernible progress is shown on consecutive venograms unless the lysis is interrupted because of complications. The duration of infusion is often 24–48 h. Heparin infusion is continued until therapeutic anticoagulation is achieved by oral warfarin administration.

General complications of lytic therapy are outlined in Chapter 30. Two major reports regarding specific complications of CDT of iliofemoral vein thrombosis have been published. A review by Grossman and McPherson of 15 studies, including 263 patients who had CDT using urokinase (234 patients) and rt-PA (29 patients) for iliofemoral thrombosis (13). This study was compiled before publication of the multicenter National Registry study by Mewissen et al., detailing the results of 473 patients treated by CDT with urokinase (8). Metanalysis in the Grossman-McPherson study (13) found an overall major bleeding rate (requiring transfusion) in 4.9% (13 of 263 patients). This rate is comparable to that reported for conservative treatment with unfractionated heparin, approximately 5% (14). Almost half the bleeding patients, however, were given rt-PA, resulting in bleeding rates for those treated by urokinase and rt-PA of 2.9% (7 of 234) and 21% (7 of 29), respectively. The mortality was 0.4 % (1 of 263, owing to cardiac ischemia). Symptomatic pulmonary embolism (PE) was observed in 0.8% (2 of 263), but none was fatal.

The prospective National Registry study (8) revealed a higher rate (11%) of major bleeding complications (4% at cannulation site, 1% spontaneous retroperitoneal bleeding, 3% gastrointestinal, genitourinary or musculoskeletal sites, 3% unknown sites) and a 16% rate of minor bleeding events (the majority at the cannulation site). Intracranial bleeding occurred in two patients (<1%, one fatal) and 1% had symptomatic pulmonary embolism (one fatal). Thus the mortality rate was the same in the two studies, i.e., 0.4%. The complication rate may appear high but should be compared to anticoagulation treatment alone, which also carries risk. Major bleeding risk requiring blood transfusion appears higher with urokinase CDT and even higher with rt-PA than with unfractionated heparin and certainly than with low-molecular-weight heparin (0.8–2.4%) (15). The rates of symptomatic and fatal pulmonary embolism are, however, higher with anticoagulation therapy alone (7.9 and 1.3%, respectively) (13).

Spontaneous intracranial hemorrhage is the most devastating and dreaded complication of thrombolytic therapy. Although it was not reported in the compiled study, it was observed in the national registry in <1%. Since urokinase was abruptly removed from the market in the United States in 1999, alteplase and reteplase replaced it and are now the preferred drugs for noncoronary thrombolysis. Initially, no intracranial bleedings or strokes were reported in the pilot studies. Rates of 0.8 and 1.4%, respectively, have been reported with reteplase treatment for acute myocardial infarction (14). The optimal dose and the effects of concomitant use of heparin in lysis of iliofemoral DVT were not fully defined initially, which probably led to an increased rate of bleeding complications, including intracerebral hemorrhage. It appears that the rate of bleeding complications is related to the dosage (16). The continuous evaluation of adequate dosage has led to a substantial reduction in the dosage of both rt-PA and concomitant heparin. The initial recommendation, for example, was to administer reteplase at 1 U/h to treat venous occlusion (16). With increased experience, most centers using this agent have successively decreased the dosage. In our service we now use ≤0.4 U/h of reteplase for CDT of deep vein thrombosis with apparently the same efficacy but fewer bleeding events. A similar development has occurred with alteplase. Just as we are learning how to use rt-PA, urokinase is apparently making a comeback in the United States. Its future role is not known at this time.

Bleeding complications related to the catheter insertion site can be minimized by careful needle access of the vein under ultrasound guidance to avoid inadvertent puncture of the adjacent vessels, multiple attempts, and puncture through the posterior wall. The systemic effect of the thrombolytic agents, which results in distant bleeding, is more difficult to avoid. It is important that an optimal dose with maximal efficacy and minimal bleeding rate be found for each thrombolytic agent and concomitant heparin. The patient must be meticulously supervised and frequently assessed for bleeding, including measurements of regular hemoglobin levels, hematocrit, platelet count, prothrombin time and partial prothrombin time. PTT is used to monitor intravenous unfractionated heparin infusion, but there is no reliable marker for the thrombolytic agent. The current recommendation is that the blood fibrinogen level be measured to assess the lytic state. When the level falls to 100–150 mg/dL, the dose may be reduced; below the level of 100 mg/dL, it may be prudent to stop the infusion altogether. Unfortunately, major bleeding complications do not appear to be directly related to the fibrinogen level (16–18). A low level does not necessarily lead to increased bleeding, and a major bleeding event may occur despite normal or near-normal fibrinogen levels. Therefore clinical surveillance is crucial. In addition, careful selection of patients for CDT treatment is important. It appears that elderly patients, especially those with arterial hypertension, are more prone to develop cerebral hemorrhage. The patient must also have a reasonable life expectancy, since the main impetus to perform CDT for deep venous thrombosis is the avoidance of future postthrombotic disease.

CDT for iliofemoral venous thrombosis appears to be a safe procedure with good short-term results when applied in patients with relatively acute clot formation (< 10 days). If the benefits are to surpass the risks, careful assessment of the thrombotic disease per se, appropriate dosage of the lytic agent administered, and evaluation of the patient's concomitant diseases are essential.

III. COMPLICATIONS RELATED TO STENTING OF ILIOFEMORAL VENOUS OUTFLOW CHANNEL

Experience from stenting of the venous system is collected mainly from treatment of large vein obstruction. As compared to more proximal veins, results of balloon angioplasty and stenting of femoropopliteal or brachioaxillary veins have not been encouraging. Both location and etiology of the obstruction appear to be important. The most commonly seen acute obstruction of the iliofemoral outflow channel is acute deep veinous thrombosis. Even after open venous thrombectomy or catheter-directed thrombolysis (CDT), a chronic venous stenosis is often "uncovered." The rate of rethrombosis is apparently less if this stenosis is controlled (8). The most commonly seen chronic obstruction is that due to postthrombotic disease. Following thrombosis that has been conservatively treated with anticoagulation alone, as many as 70–80% of iliac veins remain only partly recanalized or occluded, with varying degrees of collateral formation (6,7). Less frequently, benign or malignant masses, retroperitoneal fibrosis, iatrogenic injury, irradiation, cysts, and aneurysms may also cause blockage of the iliac vein. A "primary" nonthrombotic iliac vein obstruction [May-Thurner syndrome (19) or iliac compression syndrome (20)] has also been described and is probably more common than is recognized.

Balloon angioplasty alone of the iliofemoral vein was found to be insufficient early in the development of this technique. This procedure leads to immediate complete recoil in the majority of limbs and results in early restenosis. Stenting is therefore advised in all cases (21–24). Depending on the location of the obstruction, ultrasound-guided access to the vein below the obstruction is obtained. A guidewire is inserted, followed by a sheath, through which catheters, balloons, and stents are inserted. The guidewire must cross the obstruction in order for stenting to proceed, which may be difficult when complete obstruction is present. The details of the technique are described elsewhere (24–26). At least in the medium term, there appears to be good symptom relief following the intervention (27).

The nonthrombotic complication rate related to the endovascular intervention is presently minimal and comprises mostly cannulation site hematoma, although a few cases of retroperitoneal hematoma requiring blood transfusions have been described (24,28). As previously described, the utilization of ultrasound-guided cannulation and closure with collagen plugs have largely abolished these problems, reducing the nonthrombotic complication rate from 3 to <1%. The mortality has been zero. Iliac vein balloon dilation and stenting of an iliofemoral and caval vein obstruction is a safe, minimally invasive method with a low complication rate and no mortality.

Data regarding early rethrombosis (<30 days) after iliofemoral stenting are sparse. The rate was found to be 11% in the Creighton University experience following stenting after thrombolysis of an acute DVT (29) and 15% in the National Registry study (8). The early thrombosis rate was found to be lower (4%) when stenting was performed for chronic, nonmalignant iliac vein obstruction without preceding thrombolysis (25). All of the latter postoperative obstructions occurred in patients with chronic postthrombotic disease (8% thrombosis rate), while none occurred in nonposthrombotic limbs (0% thrombosis rate) with primary disease. Early failures appear more common with stents placed across complete occlusions than across stenoses (30). The occlusions appeared to be related to limbs with severe nonyielding stenoses or complete obstructions that could not be fully dilated. Thrombolysis of the newly formed clot may be attempted in initially technically successful limbs to reveal and treat unknown additional obstructions. Midterm patency apparently depends on the etiology of the obstruction, but results are generally encouraging. One-year primary patency after CDT of an acute DVT and iliofemoral stenting is 74–80% (8,29). Primary, assisted-primary, and secondary patency rates at 3 years after stenting for chronic nonmalignant obstructions were 75, 92, and 93%, respectively. Similarly, the rates at 32 months for limbs with nonthrombotic (primary) etiology of the obstruction was significantly better than for postthrombotic limbs (84 and 73%, 100 and 86%, and 100 and 86%, respectively) (25,31). Typically, the stented limbs that occluded were characterized by postthrombotic etiology, stent lengths >13 cm, and stent placement below the inguinal ligament. At the time of initial balloon angioplasty and stenting, the majority of the iliac veins were either completely occluded or had tight, nonyielding stenoses. The reason for late occlusions is probably multifactorial but appears to result mainly from a combination of development of in-stent restenosis and recurrent attacks of thrombosis in a patient with chronic postthrombotic disease. Iliofemoral occlusion caused by malignant pelvic tumors has poorer patency rates, with a 1–3 year secondary patency rate of 64–68% (32,33). Thrombolysis may be attempted to disobliterate the occluded stent vein and, if possible, treat underlying restenosis.

In-stent restenosis is a serious long-term complication, which may result in recurrence of symptoms and potential occlusion of the stent; further interventions may be required (Figs. 1 and 2). The nature of in-stent restenosis, rate of development, prevention, and treatment for stents placed in the venous vasculature are poorly understood. Symptomatic restenosis was observed in 9% of limbs 6–12 months after initial treatment in the Creighton University experience (29) and responded well after angioplasty. Based on venographic follow-up and survival analysis by the Kaplan-Meier method, only 23 % of limbs remained hyperplasia-free at 3 years follow-up (31). However, most stents with hyperplasia had only minimal development. At the same time interval, 61 and 15% of limbs had >20 and >50% diameter reduction, respectively. Probably a stenosis does not become symptomatic until it exceeds 50% narrowing. Increased hyperplasia formation has been observed in stents crossing thrombotic obstructions, in long stents extending below the inguinal ligament, and in the presence of hypercoagulable states. The observed in-stent restenosis may be due to true neointimal hyperplasia or a thrombotic lining of the stent. In the majority of narrowed stents, balloon angioplasty reveals a very tough stenosis, which is often nonyielding and largely recoiling, suggesting true neointimal hyperplasia formation. Despite this observation, balloon angioplasty alone will often improve outflow sufficiently to result in improvement of the patients' symptoms. The efficacy of covering the in-stent restenosis with an additional stent inside the previously inserted stent has not been adequately assessed. The role of drug therapy—e.g., with clopidogrel, placement of drug-eluting stents (now under development), or primary vascular brachytherapy of stents inserted in the venous system—is unknown. Experience from treatment of in-stent restenosis of coronary and noncoronary arterial stents cannot necessarily be extrapolated to the venous system.

Short migration of Wallstent endoprostheses placed over short and tight venous stenosis of the left common iliac vein at the vessel crossing close to the junction of the IVC (iliac vein compression syndrome) has been described (24,34). When the end of the stent was placed just at the confluence or slightly into the IVC, antegrade migration toward the

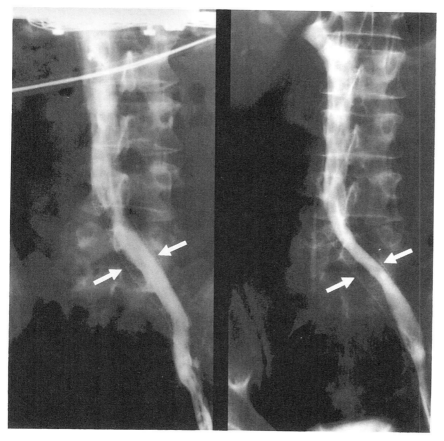

Figure 1 In-stent restenosis revealed by a transfemoral venogram in two patients with stents placed in the iliac veins because of postthrombotic obstruction. The arrows outline the outer limits of the Wallstent.

IVC was observed in 3 of 18 limbs (17%) and retrograde migration with recurrence of stenosis was found in 9 of 25 limbs (36%). The stent appears to be "squeezed" proximally or more commonly distally by the external compression (Fig. 3). This may be a result of the spiral configuration and the inherent, somewhat weaker radial force of the self-expanding Wallstent. The "recurrence" of the previously treated stenosis was easily corrected by placement of an additional stent. To avoid this migration, we have suggested that the stent should be placed well into the IVC in this type of stenosis when Wallstent endoprostheses are used. This IVC placement raises concern for risk of occlusion of the contralateral iliac vein in the long-term, although the stent does not appear to significantly impair the flow from the contralateral limb. The few cases of contralateral limb DVT observed appear to be caused by recurrent attacks of thrombosis. Longer follow-up is necessary, however, to fully assess outcome.

The Stanford group found that, over a 5-year period, major misplacement or migration occurred in 2.5% of 801 noncoronary vascular stent placements, the majority in the venous

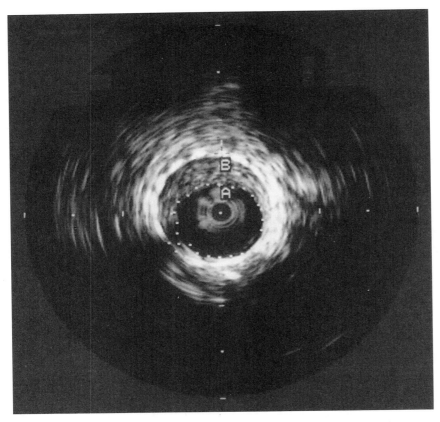

Figure 2 An image obtained by intravascular ultrasound (IVUS), distinctly showing the in-stent restenosis. Seen is the remaining cross area lumen (A) and the stent area (B); the center dark circle is the IVUS catheter. Commonly, the in-stent stenosis shown on IVUS is more severe than the venogram suggests.

system (35). "Lost" Palmaz stents could be managed by using a balloon catheter to reposition the stent, either in the intended vessel (not considered as misplaced) or in a stable alternate location (13 of 16). If the stent could be withdrawn into the sheath, it was removed percutaneously (2 of 16). One stent was surgically removed from the right ventricle. Eleven Wallstents were managed primarily with use of different snare techniques, well described in detail in the report. Nine stents were removed percutaneously and two were removed surgically after being repositioned percutaneously in the femoral vein and artery, respectively. Care was taken to avoid injury to the vessel wall during the procedure and the patients were fully anticoagulated. Investigations were performed in 13 patients, 2–65 months later indicating full patency after retrieval. To avoid gross misplacement/migration during insertion of venous stents and to facilitate retrieval, it is vital to maintain wire access across the stent throughout the entire procedure and to place the wire through the IVC and SVC to prevent stent migration into the heart and pulmonary arteries. The stent and balloon size should be carefully chosen to avoid undersizing the stent. A large stent (14–16 mm diameter) is recommended for the iliofemoral venous segment. The vein seems to accept

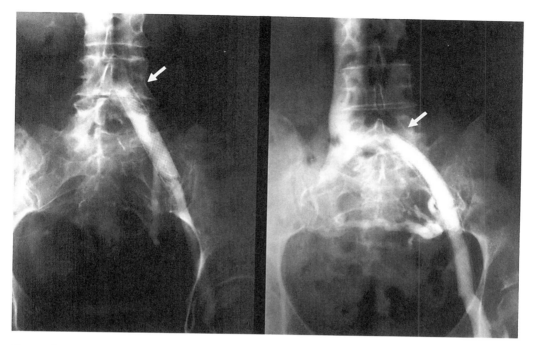

Figure 3 Two examples of recurrent stenosis (arrows) proximal to the stents previously inserted in the iliac vein. These stents were inserted flush with the IVC and appear to have been squeezed distally by a severe iliocaval junction stenosis (From Ref. 24).

extensive dilation without clinical rupture in contrast to the artery. No clinical rupture, of the vein has been reported to date, even when a total occlusion is recanalized and dilated up to 14–16 mm width.

Fracture of the inserted stent may occur owing to external pressure or metal fatigue of the stent. To our knowledge, fracture has not been described for stents placed below the inguinal ligament in the lower extremity venous outflow tract. There is concern that movement of the hip may compress a stent placed under the inguinal ligament. We have sometimes found it difficult to fully expand a stent under the inguinal ligament, but we have not observed any "crushed" stent in that position so far. A higher in-stent restenosis rate has been observed when the stent reaches below the inguinal ligament. It is, however, rare to have a stent placed for a localized stenosis under the ligament. When placed in this position, the stent is usually a distal extension of a proximal iliac stent. The problems with these long stents may be related less to external compression and more to the significant over-representation of postthrombotic etiology of the obstruction in these limbs (31).

There is concern that the enlarged uterus during pregnancy may compress an IVC filter placed in the infrarenal position (36). Similarly, a stent in the iliocaval vein could be compressed. In one report, a Palmaz stent placed in the iliocaval junction was crushed during pregnancy and resulted in thrombosis (34). The extent of this problem is not known. Placement of stent in women of childbearing age to treat iliac compression syndrome is increasingly performed. Some caution may be justified until further data have been collected.

Complications may occur due to the perioperative anticoagulation. Currently, we do not routinely anticoagulate the patient during diagnostic procedures, including intravascular ultrasound. All patients receive 2500 U of dalteparin, subcutaneously before surgery. When it is decided to continue with balloon angioplasty and stenting during the procedure, 5000 U of heparin and 30 mg of ketorolac are administered intravenously. Postoperatively, a foot compression device is applied, and dalteparin (2500 U) is given subcutaneously. During postoperative hospitalization, an additional dose of dalteparin (5000 U SQ) and a ketorolac injection are given the morning before discharge. Low-dose aspirin (81 mg PO) daily is started immediately after surgery and continued. Most patients have no additional anticoagulation. Only patients already on warfarin preoperatively are given warfarin postoperatively. These are a minority of patients with prior recurrent DVT and/or thrombophilia, which makes lifelong anticoagulation necessary. When warfarin is discontinued prior to surgery, dalteparin 5000 U is injected subcutaneously during the days warfarin is discontinued. This regimen appears to result in minimal bleeding problems and still prevent early thrombosis.

Venous balloon angioplasty and stenting of the IVC and iliac veins appears to be a safe, relatively simple, and efficient method to treat iliocaval vein obstruction in the midterm. An immediate or late failure of the procedure does not preclude later open surgery to correct the obstruction. Further studies are necessary to elucidate long-term clinical results and potential risks.

IV. COMPLICATIONS RELATED TO STENTING OF THE SUBCLAVIAN VEIN

Management of venous stenosis of the upper extremity owing to complications of placement of central venous access catheters or related to arteriovenous fistulas for dialysis access are described in Chapter 34. Acute obstruction of the venous outflow by a DVT results in sudden symptoms with swelling, stasis, and pain. Patients may also complain of intermittent swelling, bluish discoloration and pain on exertion owing to a slowly developing stenosis. The unique anatomical situation in the thoracic outlet makes treatment of venous obstruction of the upper extremity radically different from that of the lower extremity. Venous outflow obstruction in the arm is usually associated with subclavian vein compression in the thoracic outlet. Infrequently, it is caused by external compression or direct ingrowth by malignant and benign tumors. The entire neurovascular bundle may be compressed to varying degrees between the first rib and the clavicle. Abnormal soft tissue, muscles, and bands of fascia may also contribute. When a venous stenosis in this area is only balloon-dilated or stented, the vein will still be subjected to extrinsic compression between the clavicle and the first rib, and to flexion forces when the arm is abducted. This may lead to structural failure, restenosis, and occlusion.

With acute nonaccess related subclavian DVT, a catheter-directed thrombolysis is recommended in a fashion similar to that for acute DVT in the lower extremity. Complications due to thrombolysis are the same as described above. A successful lysis will often reveal an underlying stenosis due to thoracic outlet compression of the vein. It appears logical to alleviate the compression by removing the first rib (37,38). However, there is often a residual significant venous stenosis observed after release, even after early venous balloon angioplasty has been performed. This residual stenosis can then be corrected by insertion of a stent to ensure patency and prevent early rethrombosis. Although there is an increasing consensus that upper limbs with subclavian vein stenosis should be treated by first-rib resection, the issues of timing of balloon dilation of any remaining stenosis and whether a stent should be routinely inserted are still controversial (39,40). There is strong evidence, however, that venous balloon angioplasty alone does not always suffice in the thoracic outflow channel and that stent insertion is necessary (41). A stent should never be inserted into the thoracic outlet without decompressive surgery. The stent will inevitably fracture or be compressed by the strong extrinsic forces and ultimately fail (Fig. 4) (41–44). The decompression appears to prevent deleterious external stent compression but may not decrease the possibility of stent fracture due to metal fatigue following repeated stent flexion. Therefore the use of a rigid stent in the thoracic outlet is not advised. We favor the flexible, self-expanding type of stent. These stents do not appear to fracture because of repeated arm and neck movement so long as decompressive surgery has been performed.

Providing thoracic outlet decompression has been performed, a remaining subclavian venous stenosis of less than 50% is apparently acceptable. Kreienberg et al. (39) have reported that in all patients with less than 50% residual stenosis after percutaneous trans-luminal angioplasty (PTA), the subclavian vein was patent and the patient asymptomatic at a mean follow-up of 4 years. Conversely, almost one-third of stented patients (5 of 14) had occluded the stent during a similar follow-up. The stents were inserted in the subclavian vein because of a residual stenosis of more than 50% after PTA. This result could be blamed in part on the presence of thrombophilia in three patients and extensive brachio-axillary-subclavian venous involvement in all patients. The long-term in-stent restenosis rate has not been established and consequences of intimal reaction to the stents are unknown. On the other hand, patients with >50% stenosis remaining after release and balloon angioplasty appear to be at increased risk for rethrombosis. This finding, coupled with the fact that prognosis of a stent thrombosis appears not to be no worse than thrombosis of the vein itself, causes us to favor the use of stents in residual stenosis of >50% of the subclavian vein as measured by intravascular ultrasound providing that a first-rib resection has been performed.

V. COMPLICATIONS RELATED TO STENTING OF THE SUPERIOR VENA CAVA

By far the most common cause of SVC syndrome is malignancy (85–97% of cases) (45). The combination of thrombolysis, angioplasty, and stent insertion is the current "method of choice" for malignant obstruction, with a good technical success rate, primary patency rates of 50–100%, and improvement in secondary patency by subsequent procedures. The important observation is that all patients were symptom-free within 48 h of treatment and 90% remained symptom-free until death (usually within 1 year) (46). When treatment is performed for a benign lesion (mainly catheter—related obstructions), a secondary patency rate is 85% with relatively short follow-up (mean 17 months) in these patients with longer life expectancy (47). Although stents placed inside the thorax should be free from external forces, "crushing" of stents placed in the left brachiocephalic vein between the manubrium and the aortic arch has been described (48). Surgical bypass may be a better alternative for patients with benign obstruction.

Complications are similar to those described with previous venous procedures (a rate of 3.2% minor and 7.8% major complications) (49). Most complications are related to restenosis, early or late occlusion, stent displacement, and problems inherent in anti-

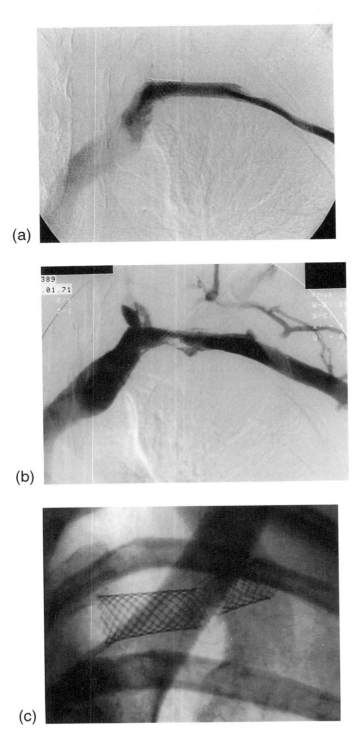

Figure 4 A 28-year-old woman with a subclavian vein thrombosis undergoing thrombolysis revealing a stenosis, which was successfully balloon-dilated and stented (a). No surgical decompression was performed. Control venogram 1 year later demonstrated a 50% stenosis (b). No additional treatment was performed. Follow-up with venogram another year later showed stent fracture and recurrent total occlusion by thrombosis (c)(From Ref. 44).

coagulation and thrombolysis. Complications specific to the SVC procedure include the infrequently seen mediastinal hematoma, hemopericardium with cardiac tamponade, and pulmonary edema following the increased venous return after disobliteration. If the patient collapses after the procedure, immediate ultrasound or thoracic CT/CT pulmonary angiography is recommended to detect these complications.

Undoubtedly, venous stenting appears to be a promising treatment, but some caveats are prudent. In comparison to coronary and arterial angioplasty and stenting, there is little information regarding the development of neointimal hyperplasia, long-term patency, and potential long-term risks with stent placement in the venous system. The technology is relatively recent; thus the follow-up period is limited. Monitoring for several more years is necessary to assess the efficacy and safety of this therapeutic modality in venous disease.

REFERENCES

1. Fellmeth BD, Roberts AC, Bookstein JJ, Freischlag JA, Forsythe JR, Buckner NK, Hye RJ. Postangiographic femoral artery injuries: Nonsurgical repair with US-guided compression. Radiology 1991; 178:671–675.
2. Dean SM, Olin JW, Piedmonte M, Grubb M, Young JR. Ultrasound-guided compression closure of postcatherization pseudoaneurysm during concurrent anticoagulation: A review of seventy-seven patients. J Vasc Surg 1996; 23:28–35.
3. Sorrell KA, Feinberg RL, Wheeler JR, Gregory RT, Snyder SO, Gayle RG, Parent NF III. Color-flow duplex-directed manual occlusion of femoral false aneurysms. J Vasc Surg 1993; 17:571–577.
4. Khoury M, Alanna R, Greene K, Rama K, Colaiuta E, Flynn L, Berg R. Duplex scanning-guided thrombin injection for the treatment of iatrogenic pseudoaneurysms. J Vasc Surg 2002; 35:517–521.
5. Liau C-S, Ho F-M, Chen M-F, Lee Y-T. Treatment of iatrogenic femoral artery pseudoaneurysm with percutaneous thrombin injection. J Vasc Surg 1997; 26:18–23.
6. Mavor GE, Galloway JMD. Iliofemoral venous thrombosis: Pathological considerations and surgical management. Br J Surg 1969;56:45–59.
7. Plate G, Åkesson H, Einarsson E, Ohlin P, Eklof B. Long-term results of venous thrombectomy combined with a temporary arterio-venous fistula. Eur J Vasc Surg 1990; 4: 483–489.
8. Mewissen MW, Seabrook GR, Meissner MH, Cynamon J, Labrapoulos N, Haughton SH. Catheter-directed thrombolysis for lower extremity deep venous thrombosis: Report of a national multicenter registry. Radiology 1999; 211:39–49.
9. Comerota AJ, Aldridge SC. Thrombolytic therapy for acute deep vein thrombosis. Semin Vasc Surg 1992; 5:76–81.
10. Meissner MH, Manzo RA, Bergelin RO, Markel A, Strandness DE Jr. Deep venous insufficiency: The relationship between lysis and subsequent reflux. J Vasc Surg 1993; 18:596–608.
11. Eklof B, Kistner RL. Is there a role for thrombectomy in iliofemoral venous thrombosis? Semin Vasc Surg 1996; 9:34–45.
12. Semba CP, Dake MD. Iliofemoral deep venous thrombosis: Aggressive therapy with catheter-directed thrombolysis. Radiology 1994; 191:487–494.
13. McPherson S, Grossman C. Safety and efficacy of catheter-directed thrombolysis for iliofemoral venous thrombosis. AJR 1999; 172:667–672.
14. INJECT Study Group. Randomised, double-blind comparison of reteplase double-bolus administration with streptokinase in acute myocardial infarction (INJECT): Trial to investigate equivalence. Lancet 1995; 346:329–336.
15. Siragusa S, Cosmi B, Piovella F, Hirsh J, Ginsberg JS. Low-molecular-weight heparins and

unfractionated heparin in the treatment of patients with acute venous thromboembolism: Results of a meta-analysis. Am J Med 1996; 100:269–277.

16. Ouriel K, Katzen B, Mewissen M, Flick P, Clair DG, Benenati J, McNamara TO, Gibbens D. Reteplase in the treatment of peripheral arterial and venous occlusions: A pilot study. J Vasc Intervent Radiol 2000; 11:849–854.

17. Ouriel K, Veith FJ, Sasahara AA. A comparison of recombinant urokinase with vascular surgery as initial treatment for acute arterial occlusion of the legs. N Engl J Med 1998; 338: 1105–1111.

18. Ouriel K, Kandarpa K, Schuerr DM, Hultquist M, Hodkinson G, Wallin B. Prourokinase vs. urokinase for revanalization of peripheral occlusions, safety and efficacy: The PURPOSE Trial. J Vasc Intervent Radiol 1999; 10:1083–1091.

19. May R, Thurner J. The cause of the predominantly sinistral occurrence of thrombosis of the pelvic veins. Angiology 1957; 8:419–428.

20. Cockett FB, Thomas ML. The iliac compression syndrome. Br J Surg 1965; 52:816–821.

21. Neglén P, Al-Hassan HKh, Endrys J, Nazzal MMS, Christenson JT, Eklof B. Iliofemoral venous thrombectomy followed by percutaneous closure of the temporary arteriovenous fistula. Surgery 1991; 110:493–499.

22. Wisselink W, Money SR, Becker MO, Rice KL, Ramee SR, White CJ, Kazmier FJ, Hollier LH. Comparison of operative reconstruction and percutaneous balloon dilatation for central venous obstruction. Am J Surg 1993; 166:200–205.

23. Marzo KP, Schwartz R, Glanz S. Early restenosis following percutaneous transluminal balloon angioplasty for the treatment of the superior vena caval syndrome due to pacemaker-induced stenosis. Cathet Cardiovasc Diagn 1995; 36:128–131.

24. Neglén P, Raju S. Balloon dilation and stenting of chronic iliac vein obstruction: Technical aspects and early clinical outcome. J Endovasc Ther 2000; 7:79–91.

25. Neglén P, Berry MA, Raju S. Endovascular surgery in the treatment of chronic primary and post-thrombotic iliac vein obstruction. Eur J Vasc Endovasc Surg 2000; 20:560–571.

26. O'Sullivan GJ, Semba CP, Bittner CA, Kee ST, Razavi MK, Sze DY, Dake MD. Endovascular management of iliac vein compression (May-Thurner) syndrome. J Vasc Intervent Radiol 2000; 11:823–836.

27. Raju S, Owen S Jr, Neglén P. The clinical impact of iliac venous stents in the management of chronic venous insufficiency. J Vasc Surg 2002; 35:8–15.

28. Hurst DR, Forauer AR, Bloom JR, Greenfield LJ, Wakefield TW. Diagnosis and endovascular treatment of iliocaval compression syndrome. J Vasc Surg 2001; 34:106–113.

29. Thorpe PE. Endovascular therapy for chronic venous obstruction. In: Ballard JL, Bergan JJ, eds. Chronic Venous Insufficiency. New York: Springer, 1999: 179–219.

30. Nazarian GK, Austin WR, Wegryn SA, Bjarnason H, Stackhouse DJ, Castaneda-Zuniga WR, Hunter DW. Venous recanalization by metallic stents after failure of balloon angioplasty or surgery: Four-year experience. Cardiovasc Intervent Radiol 1996; 19:227–233.

31. Neglén P, Raju S. In-stent restenosis in stents placed in the lower extremity venous outflow tract. J Vasc Surg 2003. In print.

32. Nazarian GK, Bjarnason H, Dietz CA Jr, Bernades CA, Hunter DW. Iliofemoral venous stenosis: Effectiveness of treatment with metallic endovascular stents. Radiology 1996; 200:193–199.

33. Carlson JW, Nazarian GK, Hartenbach E, Carter JR, Dusenbery KE, Fowler JM, Hunter DW, Adcock LL, Twiggs LB, Carson LF. Management of pelvic venous stenosis with intravascular steel stents. Gynecol Oncol 1995; 56:362–369.

34. Juhan C, Hartung O, Alimi Y, Barthelmy P, Valerio N, Portier F. Treatment of nonmalignant obstructive iliocaval lesions by stent placement: Mid-term results. Ann Vasc Surg 2001; 15:227–232.

35. Slonim SM, Dake MD, Razavi MK, Kee ST, Samuels SL, Rhee JS, Semba CP. Management of misplaced or migrated endovascular stents. J Vasc Intervent Radiol 1999; 10:851–859.

36. Greenfield LJ, Proctor MC. Suprarenal filter placement. J Vasc Surg 1998; 28:432–438.

37. Molina JE. Surgery for effort thrombosis of the subclavian vein. J Cardiovasc Surg 1992; 103:341–346.
38. Molina JE. Letter to the editor. J Vasc Surg 2001; 33:662–663.
39. Kreienberg PB, Chang BB, Darling RC III, Roddy SP, Paty PS, Lloyd WE, Cohen D, Stainken B, Shah DM. Long-term results in patients treated with thrombolysis, thoracic inlet decompression, and subclavian vein stenting for Paget-Schroetter syndrome. J Vasc Surg 2001; 33(suppl 2):S100–S105.
40. Rutherford RB. Primary subclavian-axillary vein thrombosis: The relative roles of thrombolysis, percutaneous angioplasty, stents, and surgery. Sem Vasc Surg 1998; 11:91–95.
41. Meier GH, Pollak JS, Rosenblatt M, Dickey KW, Gusberg RJ. Initial experience with venous stents in exertional axillary-subclavian vein thrombosis. J Vasc Surg 1996; 24:974–983.
42. Phipp LH, Scott DJA, Kessel D, Robertson I. Subclavian stents and stent-grafts: Cause for concern? J Endovasc Surg 1999; 6:223–226.
43. Dowling R, Mitchell P, Cox GS, Thomson KR. Complication of a venous Wallstent. Australas Radiol 1999; 43:246–248.
44. Maintz D, Landwehr P, Gawenda M, Lackner K. Failure of Wallstents in the subclavian vein due to stent damage. Clin Imaging 2001; 25:133–137.
45. Schindler N, Vogelzang RL. Superior vena cava syndrome: Experience with endovascular stents and surgical therapy. Surg Clin North Am 1999; 79:683–694.
46. Nicholson AA, Ettles DF, Arnold A, Greenstone M, Dyet JF. Treatment of malignant superior vena cava obstruction. Metal stents or radiation therapy. J Vasc Intervent Radiol 1997; 8:781–788.
47. Kee ST, Kinoshita L, Razavi MK, Nyman UR, Semba CP, Dake MD. Superior vena cava syndrome: Treatment with catheter-directed thrombolysis and endovascular stent placement. Radiology 1998; 187–193.
48. Hammer F, Becker D, Gofette, Mathurin P. Crushed stents in benign left brachiocephalic vein stenosis. J Vasc Surg 2000; 32:392–396.
49. Brant J, Peebles C, Kalra P, Odurny A. Hemopericardium after superior vena cava stenting for malignant SVC obstruction: The importance of contrast-enhanced CT in the assessment of postprocedural collapse. Cardiovasc Intervent Radiol 2001; 24:353–355.

34

Complications of Endovascular Intervention for AV Access Grafts

Abigail Falk

Mount Sinai Medical Center, New York, New York, U.S.A.

I. INTRODUCTION

The incidence of treated end-stage renal disease (ESRD) in the United States is 180 per million and it continues to rise at a rate of 7.8% per year (1). A majority of patents with ESRD require hemodialysis for survival. In such patients, the creation and maintenance of an arteriovenous (AV) access are two of the most difficult issues associated with their hemodialysis treatment. Hemodialysis vascular access dysfunction is a major clinical problem. Although current options for vascular access include an arteriovenous fistula (AVF), an arteriovenous graft (AVG), a venous catheter, or a totally subcutaneous catheter-based access system, approximately 70% of permanent dialysis vascular access in the United States is a polytetrafluoroethylene (PTFE) AVG. In general, such AVGs have dismal unassisted primary patency rates—50% at 1 year and 25% at 2 years—and require interventions for maintenance of adequate flow (2). Endovascular interventions, including balloon or percutaneous angioplasty (PTA) (intraluminal balloon dilatation), stent deployment (placement of a self-expanding or balloon expandable stent), pharmacological thrombolysis (catheter-directed infusion of thrombolytic agents), mechanical thrombolysis and thrombectomy (fragmentation, maceration, or mobilization of thrombus by mechanical means or devices), and pharmacomechanical thrombolysis (mechanical disruption of thrombus by fragmentation, maceration, or mobilization accompanied by catheter-directed administration of an agent that results in pharmacological thrombolysis) are the current standards of practice for AV access maintenance.

The natural history of all AVG is the gradual development of intimal hyperplastic stenoses, which will ultimately lead to AVG failure. Some 80% of all vascular access dysfunction in PTFE grafts is due to venous stenosis and thrombosis formation at the graft-vein anastomosis. The stenosis occurs as a result of venous neointimal hyperplasia, which is composed of smooth muscle cells and characterized by significant angiogenesis. While many local therapeutic approaches—including radiation therapy, gene therapy, and use of coated stents and polymeric drug delivery systems—are being investigated to combat this problem, balloon angioplasty (with or without lysis/thrombectomy when needed) and stent placement remain the current standard of care. The National Kidney Foundation's Diseases Outcomes Quality Initiative (K-DOQI) recommends surgery for correction of graft degeneration, infection, and pseudoaneurysms and endovascular intervention for correction of stenoses (3). Each of these interventions is itself associated with varying complications that require specific active management. This chapter focuses on endovascular interventions and their associated complications.

II. ENDOVASCULAR INTERVENTIONS

Intervention is mandated whenever stenosis becomes hemodynamically significant—i.e., when there is a $\geq$50% reduction of vessel or graft diameter along with abnormal changes in hemodynamic or clinical parameters (3). The K-DOQI guidelines recommend that a patient's AVG be routinely monitored for stenosis. Increased static or dynamic blood pressure, decreased blood flow, increased access recirculation, or swollen extremity are all abnormal changes indicative of possible underlying stenosis. If left untreated, the decreasing pressures within stenotic vessels become conducive to thrombus formation, progressive graft occlusion, and compromised dialysis. Balloon angioplasty is a well-recognized intervention for the maintenance of graft patency (4). When angioplasty remains unsuccessful or is required more than two times within a 3-month period, surgical revision should be attempted provided that the patient is a candidate for surgery (3). In cases where surgery is contraindicated or not possible, intragraft stent placement may be an option for improving patency. In patients with underlying thrombus, additional treatment directed toward the mechanical, pharmacological, or pharmacomechanical lysis of the thrombus is necessary to increase the duration of graft patency. Guideline 10 of the K-DOQI states that prospective surveillance of AVG for hemodynamically significant stenosis, when combined with correction, improves patency and decreases the incidence of thrombosis (3). Thus, maintenance of hemodialysis access requires both prospective surveillance and need-based intervention.

III. COMPLICATIONS OF ENDOVASCULAR INTERVENTIONS

A team approach is best for the successful management of complications associated with endovascular interventions. The concerted input of nephrologists, interventional radiologists, vascular and transplant surgeons, fellows, nurses, and physicians' assistants is important in achieving the overall goal of vascular access preservation.

A. General Complications

General allergic reactions to radiographic contrast media and fluid overload, with possible progression to congestive heart failure (CHF), are two overall complications to be cognizant of in this patient population regardless of the type of endovascular intervention. A history of moderate or severe reactions to contrast media or of asthma is considered an important risk factor for generalized contrast media reactions (5). Patients with such risk factors may be prophylactically treated with corticosteroids at least 11 h prior to the procedure and should preferably receive nonionic contrast media. Some physicians additionally use oral antihistamine treatment. In patients at high risk for reaction, a resuscitation team should be available at the time of the procedure. In those cases where an immediate need for intervention precludes steroid premedication, gadolinium may be used as a contrast agent, albeit with some compromise in resolution. Because of the risk of carbon dioxide reflux and arterial CO_2 embolism in the cerebral circulation, CO_2 is contraindicated for arterial use above the diaphragm and should not be used in upper extremity grafts. There is a potential for serious consequences with the use of CO_2. In one case, the use of CO_2 contrast during the declotting procedure of an upper arm AVG led to a CO_2 embolism of the vertebral artery and subsequent major stroke (A. Novick, personal communication, 1999).

Patients with ESRD requiring hemodialysis typically have poor cardiopulmonary function, and fluid overload during the interventional procedure may lead to increased cardiac burden and CHF. Monitoring of fluid delivery during endovascular interventions is thus critical in reducing cardiac complications.

B. The Nature of the Stenotic Lesion and Its Influence on Interventional Complications

Stenotic lesions in AVGs are typically concentric, intimal thickenings of the vein wall consisting of smooth muscle and extracellular matrix components. Although they can occur anywhere along the outflow circuit, stenotic lesions are more common at venous anastomoses (6). They are generally more difficult to treat than atherosclerotic lesions because of their aggressive development and greater resistance to balloon dilatation.

For treatment to be successful, it should be instituted early—i.e., before progression to thrombosis (7). When they are instituted later, interventions should restore patency as well address any underlying problem of thrombosis, since the risk for rethrombosis is generally 90% or greater. Anatomical success is defined as a less than 30% residual diameter stenosis (8). For stenosis with AVG thrombosis, restoration of flow combined with a less than 30% maximal residual stenosis should be considered successful. In all cases, restoration of hemodynamic and flow parameters is a measure of treatment or clinical success and helps prolong the duration of patency of AVGs. Prospective monitoring of graft function is recommended to facilitate early detection and intervention of stenosis in AVGs, since grafts treated with percutaneous transluminal angioplasty (PTA) alone have been shown to have a longer duration of patency than those treated with a combination of thrombolysis plus PTA.

C. Percutaneous Transluminal Angioplasty

The PTA of venous stenoses related to AVGs is well accepted, with technical success rates of 85–97%. While recurrent stenosis requiring repeat PTAs may be an issue, the rates of restenosis do not appear to be greater than with surgical intervention. The 6-month unassisted patency rate following PTA is between 40 and 50%. The intervention is relatively safe, with complications occurring in 2–4% of cases (9).

1. Complications

In general, percutaneous procedures are outpatient procedures, with reduced morbidity, reduced postprocedural pain, and little or no wound edema. However, since graft stenoses are intimal hyperplastic lesions of muscle and matrix material that form a concentric, focal thickening of the vein wall, high pressures are often needed to inflate the angioplasty balloon completely. These high inflation pressures are causative of a majority of complications associated with PTA intervention. First, the tremendous forces required to dilate stenotic lesions may directly cause a tear or perforation in the vascular wall. Second, vascular ruptures may also result from bursting of the angioplasty balloon during the dilatation procedure. As the balloon bursts, a fluid jet is released almost instantaneously with the burst. Since the balloon is tightly apposed to the endovascular wall at the time of balloon rupture, the pressurized fluid is directed at the adjacent vascular wall, causing a rupture of that wall. Fortunately, such complications are uncommon. Reported rates of incidence range from 0.7 to 4.5% (9).

In some cases, PTA-associated complications may become serious and lead to emergent crises. The Standards of Practice Committee of the Society of Cardiovascular and Interventional Radiology (SCVIR), in their Quality Improvement Guidelines for Percutaneous Management of the Thrombosed or Dysfunctional Dialysis Access, recommends a threshold rate of 0.5% for *major* complications associated with vascular rupture or perforation (10). A major complication was defined in these guidelines as a perforation or rupture requiring blood transfusion or emergent surgery or one leading to limb-threatening ischemia.

When venous rupture occurs during PTA intervention, it does not necessarily result in a poor outcome. Treatment can result in a resolution of the adverse event and restoration of graft function. The classic response in the acute management of angioplasty-induced venous ruptures is an immediate manual compression of the injured site. Alternatively, repositioning of the angioplasty balloon across the injured segment and reinflation of balloon to tamponade the bleeding may be effective in "tacking up" the vascular wall. In the past, an unsuccessful outcome with these two maneuvers led to an abandonment of the procedure or to an immediate occlusion of the rupture to stop uncontrollable bleeding. In recent years, however, reports indicate that deployment of metallic endovascular stents across the area of extravasation may be useful in such cases to treat the vascular rupture and provide patency for the access graft (11,12). Indeed, the rupture of outflow vein or venous anastomotic stricture from balloon angioplasty is typically treated by tacking up the vein with repeat angioplasty or stent placement. When all such management options fail, an alternative is to occlude the affected graft, reconstruct a new AVG, and insert a new hemodialysis catheter for interim hemodialysis.

The treatment of arterial lesions is no different from standard arterial balloon angioplasty. Rupture of artery from a balloon angioplasty is likewise treated by tacking up the artery with repeat balloon angioplasty or surgery. A patient with an arterial rupture that remains uncontrolled following manual maneuvers, for example, can be controlled with surgical ligation of graft and placement of an arterial bypass graft (13).

D. Endovascular Stents

The role of endovascular stent placement in the management of AVG stenosis is not completely clear. The unassisted patency of stents in hemodialysis access is not different from that following PTA except in elastic stenoses (3,14). Thus, stents may be used to salvage additional AVGs but may not provide any additional advantage in terms of prolonging patency duration. They should be reserved for surgically inaccessible stenoses that fail PTA or used in patients who have limited remaining access sites. When deployed, they must never overlap major side veins and obviate the potential for the creation of future access sites (Fig. 1A and B).

Stent deployment appears to be safe, with procedural success rates of 96–100% reported with both Brescia-Cimino and polytetrafluoroethylene (PTFE) grafts (15,16).

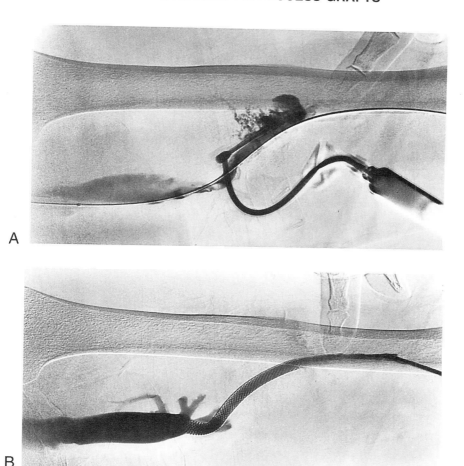

Figure 1   Case study of an immediate venous anastomotic recoil refractory to PTA and with an expanding hematoma at the sheath entry site due to outflow obstruction; it was treated with stent placement over the vein/graft anastomosis. The patient was a 40-year-old, HIV-positive male who had undergone nephrectomy for renal cell carcinoma. He had a history of a failed left radiocephalic AVF and a left forearm loop AVG that had been declotted several times and surgically revised. The patient presented with a left-upper-arm AVG that was placed 3 months earlier and had thrombosed. The AVG was declotted using 1.2 U of reteplase and 3000 U of heparin (22). A 7-mm high-pressure angioplasty balloon was used to treat the venous anastomotic stricture. However, immediate recoil was noted. An 8-mm high-pressure angioplasty balloon was then used to treat the venous anastomotic stricture. Immediate recoil was also noted with the larger balloon. This case was complicated by an expanding hematoma at sheath entry site (Fig. 1A). Finally, immediate patency of the graft/venous junction was established by placement of an 8 mm Wallstent. No further extravasation was seen after antegrade flow was reestablished (Fig. 1B). Return of 'thrill' to the AVG was noted and the patient underwent successful hemodialysis following the procedure.

Both Wallstent and intragraft metallic stents have been used safely in hemodialysis grafts. No consistent complications have been associated with their use although there is a potential for stent migration. Stent-related pseudoaneurysm has also been described in the literature (15). Stent migration can be treated with either retrieval (if possible) and repositioning or placement of an additional stent to treat the underlying lesion. As with PTA, restenosis may occur and necessitate repeat procedures. Causes of recurrence include intimal hyperplasia in or near the stent, stent slippage, and remote stenoses (15).

Several authors have documented that restenosis remains a significant problem when initial balloon angioplasty is employed to treat venous stenotic disease caused by neo-intimal hyperplasia (6,17,18). In such patients, insertion of a stent may be indicated when stenoses of graft venous anastomoses have recurred twice in less than 6 months and has been shown to increase mean restenosis interval (17). A variety of stents have been used for this purpose, including Wallstent, Craggstent, and Passager stent. More recently, flexible self-expanding stents have been used in clinical trials. However, neointimal hyperplasia can still recur through the stent interstices and at the ends of such stents (19). Preliminary results from a multicenter phase 1 trial of a PTFE stent for hemodialysis graft venous anastomotic stenoses show that the PTFE encapsulated stent graft is safe and provides promising patency results for treatment of venous anastomotic stenoses (20). Indicated for the treatment of tracheobronchial strictures, the Viabahn endoprosthesis is constructed from an expandable PTFE tubular lining with a helical nitinol (a flexible alloy) reinforcement exoskeleton. Although not currently indicated for vascular applications, the flexibility and radial strength of this device are being exploited for salvaging stenotic AVGs (21) (Fig. 2A to D). Further studies are needed to determine whether their use can replace traditional surgical patch angioplasty and help combat the long-term complication of balloon angioplasty-namely, restenosis.

E. Thrombus Removal

Removal of any occlusive thrombus is an integral part of the management of AVG-related complications. This can be achieved by thrombolysis (pharmacological or pharmacomechanical) or thrombectomy. There are a variety of percutaneous thrombectomy techniques, including suction thrombectomy, balloon thrombectomy, clot maceration, and mechanical thrombectomy. Thrombolysis, likewise, can be achieved via a percutaneous thrombolytic device, pulse-spray pharmacomechanical thrombolysis, or lyse-and-wait techniques.

1. Complications

Complications reported in various series of patients undergoing hemodialysis graft thrombectomy include major and minor bleeding, venous rupture, arterial embolism, acute respiratory arrest, contrast reaction, sepsis or infection, and death (Table 1). In a recent retrospective analysis of 935 thrombectomy procedures (74% mechanical device–mediated) that compared different thrombectomy techniques and devices, an overall complication rate of 3.3% was found, with the most commonly used interventions of thrombectomy—percutaneous thrombolytic device, Amplatz thrombectomy device, AngioJet, Oasis—having comparable rates of complications (9). The complications were similar to those reported in earlier series. The SCVIR Quality Improvement guidelines suggest threshold rates of 0.5% for major bleeding, venous rupture, acute respiratory arrest, and death and a threshold of 2% for arterial emboli (Fig. 3A to D) (10). Note that the most common complication in these studies was venous rupture, induced by PTA-related

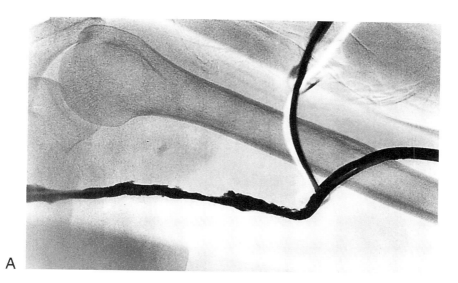

A

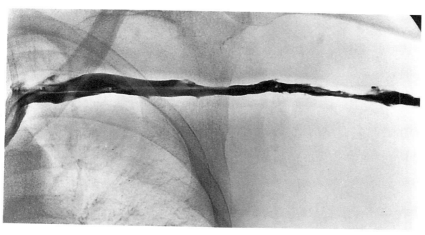

B

Figure 2 Case study of restenoses at the venous anastomosis and within several sites in the outflow vein (to the level of the axillary vein) in an AVG that was treated three times previously with balloon angioplasty; the poor angioplasty result was subsequently treated with a PTFE stent-graft using endovascular techniques. The patient was a 52-year-old HIV-positive male with a 6-month-old left upper arm AVG. At 3.5 months, the patient presented with high venous pressures and was referred for intervention. At that time, three sites of focal stenoses—one at the venous anastomosis, one in the high brachial vein, and one in the axillary vein—were identified and treated with a 9-mm angioplasty balloon. The patient presented again at 6 months with a thrombosed AVG. Following declotting, balloon angioplasty was performed once again using a 9-mm angioplasty balloon. The same three sites of stenosis were identified and the AVG rethrombosed in 2 days. After discussion with the vascular surgeon and nephrologist, it was decided to place a PTFE stent-graft (VIABAHN Endoprosthesis, W.L. Gore and Associates, Flagstaff, AZ). The AVG was declotted again and the outflow vein was found to be irregular and sclerotic from the level of the graft/vein anastomosis through the axillary vein following balloon angioplasty with a 9-mm balloon (Figs. 2A and B). A 7-mm by 15-cm Viabahn stent-graft extension was placed and dilated to 7 mm, reestablishing excellent flow across the diseased venous segment (Fig. 2C). A magnified view of the stent-graft is shown in Figure 2D.

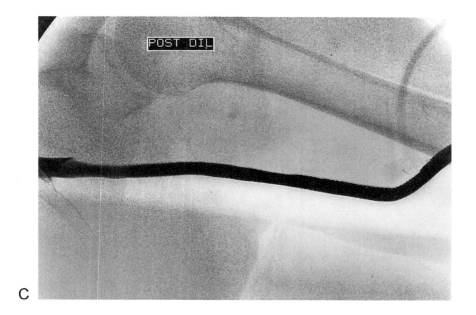

C

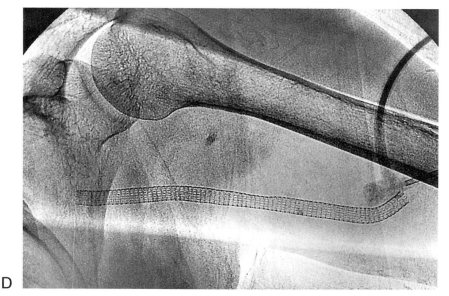

D

Figure 2 Continued.

procedures that were performed in conjunction with thrombectomy or thrombolysis and not directly related to the latter. The cardiopulmonary complications is likely related to dislodgement of arterial plugs and subsequent embolization of thrombotic material to pulmonary arteries, a risk that would be greater if the volume of the thrombosed plug exceeded the diameter of the pulmonary vasculature. Although, in most cases, the size of the thrombosed plugs are reported to be small and safe during pulmonary circulation,

Table 1 Comparison of the Complications Rates Reported in Published Series Versus Threshold Levels Recommended by the SCVIR Quality Improvement Guidelines (10)

Complication	Published series	SCVIR guidelines
Major bleeding	0.7–1.7 %	0.5%
Minor bleeding	2.8–11.1 %	
Venous rupture/dissection	1.2–7.0 %	0.5%
Arterial emboli	1.2–9.3 %	2.%
Acute respiratory arrest	1.6–2.3 %	0.5%
Contrast reaction	0.7–1.4 %	
Sepsis, infection	1.2–2.0 %	
Death	0–1.5%	0.5%

Source: Ref. 9.

the long-term consequences of such silent emboli remain uncertain and care should be taken to minimize embolization. Patients with severe cardiopulmonary disease may be at high risk for complications during thrombectomy, and this should be a contraindication for that procedure. Finally, residual stenosis may be expected in >85% of cases of thrombosis. In all cases, the access should be evaluated with a fistulogram at the end of the procedure and any residual stenosis corrected by angioplasty or surgery.

Thrombolysis can be complicated by pulmonary embolism, cerebral embolism (in the presence of a patent foramen ovale), septic emboli, or local bleeding. The last commonly

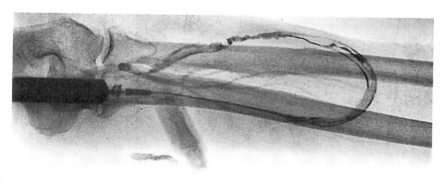

A

Figure 3 Embolization of thrombus into distal brachial artery, treated with Fogarty balloon catheter thrombectomy. The patient was an 87-year-old hypertensive male with a 7-month-old left forearm loop AVG. This was the patient's first access site. The AVG was previously declotted at 4 months after placement, with no complications. At 7 months, the patient presented with a rethrombosed AVG. A standard declotting procedure was performed using 1.2 U reteplase and 3000 U heparin. Initially, the distal brachial, ulnar, and radial arteries were noted to be patent (Fig. 3A). The procedure was complicated by embolization of thrombus into the distal brachial artery, obstructing flow to the radial and ulnar arteries (Fig. 3B). The thrombus was retrieved with a 3F over-the-wire Fogarty balloon catheter (Baxter Healthcare Corporation, Deerfield, IL) (Fig. 3C). As seen here, patency of distal brachial, radial, and ulnar arteries was reestablished (Fig. 3D).

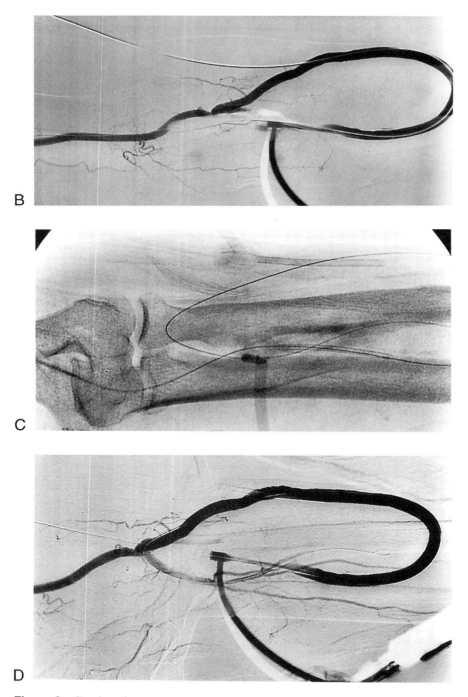

Figure 3 Continued.

occurs from old puncture sites and can be conservatively treated with manual compression. Because the lytic agent is administered into a closed space and not into the patient's circulation, there is minimal risk of systemic bleeding complications. Embolization to radial and ulnar arteries may be treated with a Fogarty balloon and heparinization (21). Anticoagulation may be discontinued following confirmation of normal pulses.

IV. SUMMARY

Complications associated with interventions that salvage dysfunctioning or stenotic hemodialysis grafts are typically related to the type of intervention used and the presence or absence of thrombus within the affected region of the graft. Overall, nonthrombosed grafts have better outcomes than thrombosed grafts. Balloon angioplasty or PTA is a well-accepted intervention for the correction of stenosis. The most common complication associated with PTA intervention of stenotic AVGs is venous rupture, caused largely by the high pressures needed to dilate vessels against the strong intimal hyperplastic walls. Fortunately, the incidence of such complications is low and most complications can be managed with manual compression, repositioning of the balloon and prolonged inflation, stent deployment, or possibly surgical revision. In patients in whom lesions have progressed to thrombosis, additional intervention must resolve the clot. In general, complication rates associated with pharmacomechanical thrombolysis are slightly higher than those with mechanical thrombectomy. Complications associated with various thrombectomy procedures and devices include major and minor bleeding, venous rupture, arterial embolism, acute respiratory arrest, contrast reaction, sepsis or infection, and death. Caution should be exercised in using thrombolytic agents, and thrombectomies should not be performed in patients with severe cardiopulmonary disease. In patients who receive stents as endovascular interventions, complication rates are low. Restenosis appears to be the major problem, necessitating repeat procedures. In summary, endovascular interventions can be safe provided that there is appropriate patient selection and proper technique. Such interventions contribute to prolongation of the long-term patency of vascular access grafts.

REFERENCES

1. Sidawy AN, Gray R, Besarab A, Henry M, Ascher E, Silva M Jr, Miller A, Scher L, Trerotola S, Gregory RT, Rutherford RB, Kent KC. Recommended standards for reports dealing with arteriovenous hemodialysis accesses. J Vasc Surg 2002; 35(3):603–610.
2. Roy-Chaudhry P. Hemodialysis access dysfunction from bedside to bench to bedside. Vascular Access for Hemodialysis VIII. The Eighth Biannual Symposium, Rancho Mirage, CA, May 9–10, 2002.
3. NKF-K/DOQI Clinical Practice Guidelines for Vascular Access: update 2000. Am J Kidney Dis 2001; 37(1 suppl 1):S137–S181.
4. Beathard GA. Percutaneous angioplasty for the treatment of venous stenosis: A nephrologists view. Semin Dial 1995; 8:166–170.
5. Morcos SK, Thomsen HS, Webb JA. Contrast Media Safety Committee of the European Society of Urogenital Radiology. Prevention of generalized reactions to contrast media: A consensus report and guidelines. Eur Radiol 2001; 11(9):1720–1728.
6. Kanterman RY, Vesely TM, Pilgram TK, Guy BW, Wndus DW, Picus D. Dialysis access grafts: anatomic location of venous stenosis and results of angioplasty. Radiology 1995; 195(1):135–139.

7. Katz SG, Kohl RD. The percutaneous treatment of angioaccess graft complications. Am J Surg 1995; 170(3):238–242.

8. Gray RJ, Sacks D, Martin LG. Trerotola SO and the members of the Technology Assessment Committee. Reporting standards for percutaneous interventions in dialysis access. J Vasc Intervent Radiol 1999; 10:1405–1415.

9. Vesely TM. Complications related to percutaneous thrombectomy of hemodialysis grafts. Manuscript submitted to AJKD.

10. Aruny JE, Lewis CA, Cardella JF, Cole PE, Davis A, Drooz AT, Grassi CJ, Gray RJ, Husted JW, Jones MT, McCowan TC, Meranze SG, Van Moore A, Neithamer CD, Oglevie SB, Omary RA, Patel NH, Rholl KS, Roberts AC, Sacks D, Sanchez O, Silverstein MI, Singh H, Swan TW, Towbin RB, Trerotola SO, Bakal CW, for the Standards of Practice Committee of the Society of Cardiovascular & Interventional Radiology. Quality improvement guidelines for percutaneous management of the thrombosed or dysfunctional dialysis access. J Vasc Intervent Radiol 1999; 10:491–498.

11. Rundback JH, Leonardo RF, Poplausky MR, Rozenblit G. Venous rupture complicating hemodialysis access angioplasty: Percutaneous treatment and outcomes in seven patients. Am J Roentgenol 1998; 171(4):1081–1084.

12. Welber A, Schur I, Sofocleous CT, Cooper SG, Patel RI, Peck SH. Endovascular stent placement for angioplasty-induced venous rupture related to the treatment of hemodialysis grafts. J Vasc Intervent Radiol 1999; 10(5):547–551 (Comment in: J Vasc Intervent Radiol 1999; 10(8):1135–1136.

13. Falk A, Mitty H, Guller J, Teoderescu V, Uribarri J, Vassalotti J. Thrombolysis of clotted hemodialysis grafts with tissue-type plasminogen activator. J Vasc Intervent Radiol 2001; 12:305–311.

14. Patel RI, Peck SH, Cooper SG, Epstein DM, Sofocleous CT, Schur I, Falk A. Patency of Wallstents placed across the venous anastomosis of hemodialysis grafts after percutaneous recanalization. Radiology 1998; 209:365–370.

15. Gray RJ, Horton KM, Dolmatch BL, Rundback JH, Anaise D, Aquino AO, Currier CB, Light JA, Sasaki TM. Use of Wallstents for hemodialysis access-related venous stenoses and occlusions untreatable with balloon angioplasty. Radiology 1995; 195(2):479–484.

16. Zaleski GX, Funaki B, Rosenblum J, Theoharis J, Leef J. Metallic stents deployed in synthetic arteriovenous hemodialysis grafts. Am J Roentgenol 2001; 176(6):1515–1519.

17. Turmel-Rodrigues L, Pengloan J, Blanchier D, Abaza M, Birmele B, Haillot O, Blanchard D. Insufficient dialysis shunt: Improved long-term patency rates with close hemodynamic monitoring, repeated percutaneous balloon angioplasty, and stent placement. Radiology 1993; 187:273–278.

18. Beathard GA. Percutaneous transvenous angioplasty in the treatment of vascular access stenosis. Kidney Int 1992; 42:1390–1397.

19. Schurmann K, Vorwerk D, Kulisch A, Rosenbaum C, Biesterfeld S, Gunther RW. Puncture of stents implanted into veins and arateriovenous fistulas: an experimental study. Cardiovasc Intervent Radiol 1995; 18(6):383–390.

20. Vesely T, Dammers R, Planken R, Pouls K, van Det R, Burger H, van de Sande F, Tordoir J. Multicenter phase I results of a PTFE stent graft for hemodialysis graft venous anastomotic stenoses. Vascular Access for Hemodialysis VIII. The Eighth Biannual Symposium, Rancho Mirage, CA, May 9–10 2002.

21. Belville J, Borzatta M. Covered stents for treatment of AV graft stenosis. Vascular Access for Hemodialysis VIII. The Eighth Biannual Symposium, Rancho Mirage, CA, May 9–10, 2002.

22. Falk A, Guller J, Nowakowski FS, Mitty H, Teoderscu V, Uribarri J, Vassalotti J. Reteplase in the treatment of thrombosed hemodialysis grafts. J Vasc Interv Radiol 2001; 12:1257–1262.

35

Complications of Vena Cava Filters

Enrico Ascher, Anil Hingorani, and William R. Yorkovich

Maimonides Medical Center, Brooklyn, New York, U.S.A.

I. INTRODUCTION

The impact of pulmonary embolism (PE) on patient morbidity is significant. A study of 5000 autopsies reported that 55% had evidence of gross PE and that 18% of all deaths were directly attributable to PE (1). It has been estimated that PE occurs in as many as 630,000 patients annually in the United States, and the diagnosis of pulmonary embolism will have been missed in 71% (450,000) of these patients (2,3). Those fortunate enough to survive an 11% (69,300 deaths) first-hour mortality rate are then subjected to a 23.8% first-year mortality (150,000 deaths) (4). With an increasing population (general and aged), these numbers can only be expected to increase.

Lower extremity deep venous thromboses (LEDVT) accounts for 88–92% of pulmonary emboli, and upper extremity deep venous thromboses (UEDVT) account for the remaining 8–12% (5,6). It has also been shown that PE occurs in up to 30–50% of patients with LEDVT of iliac origin who are not anticoagulated. Additionally, when compared to LEDVT, UEDVT is associated with higher morbidity and mortality rates (7), and there is evidence that the incidence of PE of UEDVT origin is rising due to the increased use of central venous catheters (8).

II. INDICATIONS

Anticoagulation has been long proven and continues to be the most effective way of preventing of pulmonary embolism (9,10). However, many occasions arise where this protocol is not appropriate; an alternative treatment must therefore be made available to those patients at risk for developing PE. In the presence of deep venous thrombosis (DVT) in patients for whom anticoagulation has either failed or is contraindicated or who have sustained or are at risk for a complication of anticoagulation (i.e., hemorrhage, thrombocytopenia), the implantation of one or more filtration devices in either or both the inferior and/or superior vena cava to prevent pulmonary embolism is indicated. Filtration is also indicated in the presence of large free-floating vein thrombi in the inferior vena cava or iliac arteries. In those patients in whom there exists either a history or a high risk for the development of DVT, prophylactic implantation of one or more filtration devices may be indicated (11,12). This includes high-risk patients who will be undergoing hip or knee replacement surgery, or gastric bypass for morbid obesity as well as those who are pregnant, in whom anticoagulation is contraindicated.

Prophylactic placement of one or more vena cava filters is also indicated in situations of high-risk trauma, such as a spinal cord injury with an associated severe head injury and complex pelvic fractures or multiple long bone fractures. In patients with DVT, expanded indications for the placement of caval filters may include the presence of cor pulmonale, or metastatic disease, syncope in elderly persons, and or the risk of sustaining falls.

As the use and indications of vena cava filters increases, so does the frequency of associated complications. It is imperative that physicians performing filter placement be familiar with the myriad of potential complications related to the use of these filters. This chapter provides an overview of those complications.

III. DEVICES IN USE TODAY

The most widely placed vena cava filters are the Greenfield (titanium and "over-the-wire" stainless steel), the Bird's Nest, the Vena Tech–LGM, and the Simon-Nitinol (Table 1). Significant data are available in the literature for indications and techniques of placing these devices. Three more recent devices are the Gunther-Tulip, Cordis TrapEase, and Vena Tech LP; for all of which limited experience has been published.

While all of these transvenous filters are effective in preventing pulmonary embolism in the majority of patients, each device has its own characteristics, advantages, disadvantages, and complication rate. Considerations for selection of the appropriate filtration device will include patency, luminal diameter of the vena cava, introducer sheath size, selection of the venous access site, anatomical variations affecting ease of placement, filter stability and migration tendencies, efficacy in clot trapping, rate of vena cava and access vein thromboses, PE recurrence rate, and artifact producing ferromagnetic properties that may affect future magnetic resonance imaging (MRI) examinations. The techniques necessary to deploy these devices into optimal position successfully has been previously described in detail elsewhere (13–15). It can also be noted that there is increasing experience with the successful placement of superior vena cava filters (16–18).

Table 1 Comparison of Key Vena Cava Filter Attributes

Filter	Titanium Greenfield	OTW SS Greenfield	Bird's Nest	Simon Nitinol	Vena Tech LGM	Vena Tech LP	Gunther Tulip	Trap Ease
Introducer size OD diameter (F)	15	15	14	9	13.6	9F	8.5	8
Insertion site thrombosis (%)	13.1–28	9.6–23	7.4–23	11.5–31	16.7–36	–	–	0
Filter migration (%)	–	11.0	12.0	1.7	18.4	–	–	0
DVT (%)	22.7	5.9	36	8–9	–	3	–	–
Maximum caval diameter (mm)	28	28	40	28	28	30	30	30
IVC thrombosis (%)	1–9	4	3–8	4–25	4.5–30	–	–	4.5
PE recurrence (%)	3–5	3–5	2.7–4.1	< 1–4.8	2–3.8	–	–	0
MRI	Safe	Safe	Not recommended	Safe	Safe	Safe	Safe	Safe

IV. COMPLICATIONS

A. Filter Misplacements and Migration

Correct placement of the filter requires careful preoperative planning and meticulous technique. The use of contrast venography to identify the optimal discharge site is essential and will reduce the possibility of misplacing a filter. Intraoperative venography may reveal errant catheter placement, as into the mesenteric vein through the portal system (Fig. 1A). Identification of the malposition and redirection of the catheter for ideal filter deployment from its delivery system may then result in proper placement of the filter into the vena cava (Fig. 1B). Failure to correctly identify and verify catheter positioning prior to filter discharge has resulted in discharge of the filter into the aorta and necessitated use of a second, correctly placed filter (Fig. 2).

Rapid yet precise extrusion of the filter reduces the incidence of leg asymmetry, incomplete opening, and filter tilting and lessens the chance of "caudal drop." Even so, misplacement of the filter at operation may occur, either through inadequate identification of the discharge site, suboptimal technique, or inappropriate device selection. A filter that is tilted or incompletely expanded is at increased risk for migration (Fig. 3). Accidental guideline manipulations or central line placement have also contributed to the dislodgement of previously successfully placed filters (19,20). Migrations are most frequently observed in the immediate postoperative period but may also occur many years later. Either fractured components or the entire device may migrate (21).

Filters may be inadvertently ejected into the right atrium at the time of the procedure, and subsequent proximal migrations have been reported to the right ventricle and the pulmonary artery in addition to the right atrium. Intracardiac migration of a Greenfield filter, with stenting open of the tricuspid valve and wide-open regurgitation has also been reported (22).

B. Perforation of the Vena Cava Wall

The incidence of erosion or perforation of the inferior vena cava (IVC) wall by vena cava filters, injuring adjacent retroperitoneal and abdominal structures, is rare, and symptoms are reported infrequently by patients with these complications (23). Perforations with or without filter migration are often a result of filter angulation or tilting, and filter struts may put adjacent structures in danger of penetration. Perforations of the vena cava by a filter may extend into the abdominal aorta (24–27). Temporary vena cava filters may also be culpable, and incorporation into the caval wall has been reported (28).

C. Gastrointestinal Complications

Besides bleeding, other serious complications of vena cava filter migration and perforation are possible, some extremely urgent. Gastrointestinal complications include small bowel volvulus (29) and duodenal perforation. Duodenal-caval fistulas may be caused by migrating filters and early abdominal surgery after filter placement and may present as upper gastrointestinal bleeding when bleeding ulcers are induced by local strut trauma (30,31).

D. Guidewire Mishaps

Guidewire-related mishaps are potential complications of inferior vena cava filters, and it has been postulated that they may be underreported (32–34). An entrapped guidewire may be impossible to remove following placement of the filter, and endoscopic or operative

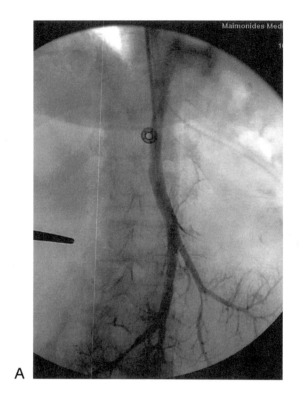

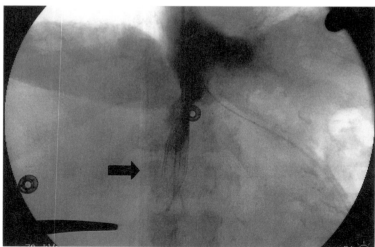

Figure 1   A. Intraoperative venography reveals catheter placement into the mesenteric vein through the portal system. Misplacement was identified and the catheter was repositioned. B. Correctly placed TrapEase filter in the inferior vena cava.

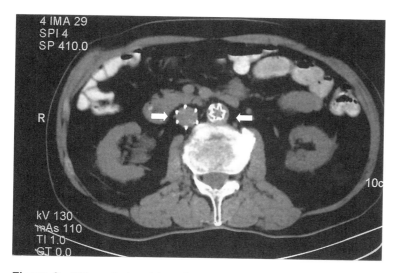

Figure 2 Filter misplaced into the aorta. Also shown is the second filter, placed correctly into the vena cava.

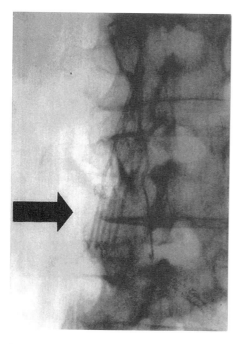

Figure 3 Incomplete expansion of a Greenfield filter.

intervention may be warranted. The guidewire may become entangled and fluoroscopic examination will reveal entanglement of the J-tip guidewire in the IVC filter (Fig. 4).

E. Recurrent Embolism

Pulmonary embolism, despite the presence of a filter and adequate anticoagulation, may recur (35,36). In patients with existing thromboembolic disease, recurrent DVT is not an unexpected event. When possible, anticoagulation is used in conjunction with the filter to treat existing DVT, reduce the progression of thrombus, and potentially reduce subsequent complications. However, anticoagulation does not seem to reduce the rate of recurrent DVT (37). Paradoxical cerebral embolism must be considered in patients with DVT who have new-onset neurological deficits even in the presence of a caval filter (38–40).

F. Renal Complications

Due to the risk of renal vein thrombosis, IVC filter placement above the renal veins may not be appropriate in advanced-stage cancer patients who have a single functional kidney, renal insufficiency, or prior renal vein thrombosis. Suprarenal filter placement should be performed only after analysis of predicted survival, after detailed discussions with the patient, and—most importantly—after renal function evaluation (41). Obstructive uropathy due to a pelviureteric obstruction resulting from vena cava wall perforation may occur (42), and penetration by an IVC filter may also cause ureteral injury (43) or symptomatic hydronephrosis (44).

G. Other Miscellaneous Complications

Less frequently reported complications of vena cava filter mishaps have included penetration of a vertebral body by a filter strut (45) and phlegmasia cerulea dolens (46).

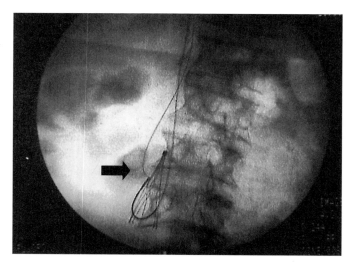

Figure 4   Guidewire entrapped in filter.

V. PREVENTING AND CORRECTING VENA CAVA FILTER COMPLICATIONS

Imaging before, during, and after a procedure can help to reduce or prevent some potential problems. A preprocedural venacavogram is required for measuring the vein's diameter, which is necessary for proper device selection. Pertinent anatomical variations, such as a megacava or dual inferior vena cavas, can be also be identified, as can the presence of IVC thrombosis. In the case of a superior vena cava (SVC) procedure, a venogram is performed to assess the innominate vein, in which placement of the filter is critical because of the vein's short length. Postprocedural venacavograms will assist in the assessment of filter placement and degree of tilting or asymmetry. Continuous fluoroscopy whenever a filter is being placed from the right internal jugular to the IVC to prevent puncture of the right atrium should be used.

Techniques for minimizing the effects of misplaced or migrated vena cava filters are varied and unique for each situation. Successful operative extractions utilizing cardiopulmonary bypass and incision for intracardiac misplaced filters or for those that have migrated to the heart have been reported (47). A vena cava wrapping technique for bleeding from a vena cava perforation, rather than surgical removal of the filter, has been performed because of the still present risk for recurrent PE (48).

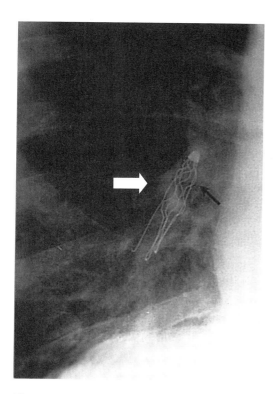

Figure 5 Migrated Greenfield filter into the right inferior pulmonary artery.

Emergent laparotomy may be required to retrieve a broken filter wire projecting into the duodenum. The offending wire/strut/hook may be transected and the vessel wall closed, leaving remaining filter in place if not otherwise contraindicated.

Several techniques have been successfully applied to correct guidewire mishaps, which may often be corrected by the introduction of a snare-tip catheter alone or in conjunction with myocardial biopsy forceps (49). Successful filter retrieval has also been achieved by using a combination of a guidewire and a snare (50). Several techniques of percutaneous retrievals of vena cava filters have also been described with minimal risk, including a "rail and reins" technique (51) and a transfemoral retrieval (52).

Because of the risk for arrhythmias and valvular insufficiency, intracardiac filter retrievals need not be attempted if no other indications are present. Not all retrieval attempts are successful. In one series, attempts at removal with a wire loop and sheath in two cases failed and resulted in the migration of one filter to the right inferior pulmonary artery (53) (Fig. 5).

The balloon of a 6F Fogarty catheter was successfully used to dilate the distal legs in an incomplete filter expansion, adequately expanding the filter base to inhibit the clots and prevent possible migration (54). An additional filter, either above or below a partially expanded filter as appropriate, may also be considered to complete the objective of clot entrapment. Such placement could also conceivably reduce the severity of a migration of an incompletely expanded filter.

VI. CONCLUSION

With careful preoperative planning, proper patient and device selection, and meticulous operative technique, the placement of vena cava filters by a properly trained surgeon is most often a straightforward procedure with minimal adverse consequences. However, the procedure is not without risk of complications and the observations presented here underscore that fact.

In the presence of a suspected complication, computed tomography, aortography, and ascending cavography may be used to demonstrate inferior vena cava penetration by filter struts into the infrarenal aorta. Scanning electron microscopy can reveal structural defects or corrosion in retrieved filters. Energy-dispersive radiographic analysis may demonstrate impurities in the metal composition.

Recent studies have found that duplex ultrasound–directed IVC filter placement is safe, cost-effective, and convenient and that intravascular ultrasound is a more accurate method, than contrast venography for localizing renal veins and measuring vena cava diameter (55,56). Use of this technology can help to limit the incidence of misplaced filters and reduce the chance of subsequent migrations due to suboptimal operative technique.

The need to monitor patients with IVC filters over the long term, preferably using computed tomography, should be considered in those patients in whom misplacement, migration, or other filter abnormalities have either occurred or are at risk for occurring. Complications are rare, but the physician must remain aware of their potential appearance in order to minimize their incidence.

REFERENCES

1. Havig O. Deep vein thrombosis and pulmonary embolism. An autopsy study with multiple regression analysis of possible risk factors. Acta Chir Scand Suppl 1977; 478:1–120.

2. Braverman SJ, Battey PM, Smith RB III. Vena caval interruption. Am Surg 1992; 58(3):188–192.

3. Alpert JS, Dalen JE. Epidemiology and natural history of venous thromboembolism. Prog Cardiovasc Dis 1994; 36:417–422.

4. Juni JE, Abass A. Lung scanning in the diagnosis of pulmonary embolism: The emperor re-dressed. Semin Nucl Med 1991; 21:282–296.

5. Horattas MC, Wright DJ, Fenton AH, Evans DM, Oddi MA, Kamienski RW, Shields EF. Changing concepts of deep venous thrombosis of the upper extremity—Report of a series and review of the literature. Surgery 1988; 104(3):561–567.

6. Gloviczki P, Kazmier FJ, Hollier LH. Axillary-subclavian venous occlusion: The morbidity of a nonlethal disease. J Vasc Surg 1986; 4(4):333–337.

7. Hingorani A, Ascher E, Hanson J, Scheinman M, Yorkovich W, Lorenson E, DePippo P, Salles-Cunha S. Upper extremity versus lower extremity deep venous thrombosis. Am J Surg 1997; 174(2):214–217.

8. Monreal M, Lafoz E, Ruiz J, Valls R, Alastrue A. Upper-extremity deep venous thrombosis and pulmonary embolism. A prospective study. Chest 1991; 99(2):280–283.

9. Alexander P, Giangola G. Deep venous thrombosis and pulmonary embolism: Diagnosis, prophylaxis, and treatment. Ann Vasc Surg 1999; 13(3):318–327.

10. Arcasoy SM, Kreit JW. Thrombolytic therapy of pulmonary embolism: A comprehensive review of current evidence. Chest 1999; 115(6):1695–1707.

11. Langan EM III, Miller RS, Casey WJ III, Carsten CG, Graham RM, Taylor SM. Prophylactic inferior vena cava filters in trauma patients at high risk: Follow-up examination and risk/benefit assessement. J Vasc Surg 1999; 30(3):484–490.

12. Hingorani A, Ascher E, Ward M, Mazzariol F, Gunduz Y, Ramsey PJ, Yorkovich W. Combined upper and lower extremity deep venous thrombosis. Cardiovasc Surg 2001; 9(5):472–477.

13. Ascher E, Hingorani AP, Yorkovich WR. Vena cava filter placement. In: Cameron J, ed. Current Surgical Therapy. 7th ed. St Louis: Mosby, 2001.

14. Ascher E, Hingorani AP, Yorkovich WR. Inferior vena cava filter placement. In: Ahn S, Moore WS, eds. Endovascular Surgery. 3rd ed. Philadelphia: Saunders, 2000.

15. Yorkovich WR, Ascher E. Vena cava filter placement. In: Ahn S, Moore WS, eds. Endovascular Surgery For Venous Disease: Handbook of Endovascular Surgery. 3rd ed. Sec XI. Philadelphia: Karger-Landes, 1999.

16. Ascher E, Hingorani AP, Tsemekhin B, Yorkovich WR, Gunduz Y. Lessons learned from a 6-year clinical experience with superior vena cava Greenfield filters. J Vasc Surg 2000; 32(5):881–887.

17. Ascher E, Hingorani A, Mazzariol F, Jacob T, Yorkovich WR, Gade P. Clinical experience with superior vena cava Greenfield filters. J Endovasc Surg 1999; 6(4):365–369.

18. Ascer E, Yorkovich WR. Superior vena cava Greenfield filters: Indications, techniques and results. Eur Phlebol Digest, 1996.

19. Granke K, Abraham FM, McDowell DE. Vena cava filter disruption and central migration due to accidental guidewire manipulation: A case report. Ann Vasc Surg 1996; 10(1):49–53.

20. Rogers F, Lawler C. Dislodgement of an inferior vena cava filter during central line placement in an ICU patient: A case report. Injury 2001; 32(10):787–788.

21. Ferreiro C, Abad-Cervero JF, Lopez-Pino MA. Fracture and migration of an Antheor vena cava filter. J Vasc Intervent Radiol 1996; 7(1):149–150.

22. James KV, Sobolewski AP, Lohr JM, Welling RE. Tricuspid insufficiency after intracardiac migration of a Greenfield filter: Case report and review of the literature. J Vasc Surg 1996; 24(3):494–498.

23. Feezor RJ, Huber TS, Welborn MB III, Schell SR. Duodenal perforation with an inferior vena cava filter: An unusual cause of abdominal pain. J Vasc Surg 2002; 35(5):1–3.

24. Dabbagh A, Chakfe N, Kretz JG, Demri B, Nicolini P, Fuentes C, Mettauer B, Epailly E, Muster D, Eisenmann B. Late complication of a Greenfield filter associating caudal migration and perforation of the abdominal aorta by a ruptured strut. J Vasc Surg 1995; 22(2):182–187.

25. Seita J, Sakakibara Y, Jikuya T, Shigeta O, Nakata H, Tsunoda H, Mitsui T. Surgical management of a penetrated Greenfield inferior vena cava filter. Thorac Cardiovasc Surg 2001; 49(4): 243–244.

26. Bochicchio GV, Scalea TM. Acute caval perforation by an inferior vena cava filter in a multitrauma patient: Hemostatic control with a new surgical hemostat. J Trauma 2001; 51(5): 991–992; discussion, 993.

27. Bochicchio GV, Scalea TM, Adams R. Acute caval perforation by an inferior vena cava filter in a multitrauma patient: Hemostatic control with a new surgical hemostat. J Trauma 2001; 51(5): 991–992; discussion 993.

28. Burbridge BE, Walker DR, Millward SF. Incorporation of the Gunther temporary inferior vena cava filter into the caval wall. J Vasc Interv Radiol 1996; 7(2):289–290.

29. Lok SY, Adkins J, Asch M. Caval perforation by a Greenfield filter resulting in small-bowel volvulus. J Vasc Interv Radiol 1996; 7(1):95–97.

30. al Zahrani HA. Bird's nest inferior vena caval filter migration into the duodenum: A rare cause of upper gastrointestinal bleeding. J Endovasc Surg 1995; 2(4):372–375.

31. Guillem PG, Binot D, Dupuy-Cuny J, Laberenne JE, Lesage J, Triboulet JP, Chambon JP. Duodenocaval fistula: A life-threatening condition of various origins. J Vasc Surg 2001; 33(3): 643–645.

32. Loehr SP, Hamilton C, Dyer R. Retrieval of entrapped guide wire in an IVC filter facilitated with use of a myocardial biopsy forceps and snare device. J Vasc Intervent Radiol 2001; 12(9):1116–1119.

33. Sing RF, Adrales G, Baek S, Kelley MJ. Guidewire incidents with inferior vena cava filters. J Am Osteopath Assoc 2001; 101(4):231–233.

34. Duong MH, Jensen WA, Kirsch CM, Wehner JH, Kagawa FT. An unusual complication during central venous catheter placement. J Clin Anesth 2001; 13(2):131–132.

35. Vandemergel X. Extensive vena cava thrombosis and massive pulmonary embolism despite the presence of a vena cava filter and an optimal anticoagulant. Rev Med Liege 2001; 56(12):807–808.

36. Barreras JR, Agarwal DM, Maximin ST, Friedman A. Recurrent pulmonary embolism despite the use of a Greenfield filter. Clin Nucl Med 2001; 26(12):1040–1041.

37. Greenfield LJ, Proctor MC. Recurrent thromboembolism in patients with vena cava filters. J Vasc Surg 2001; 33(3):510–514.

38. Kinney TB, Rose SC, Lim GW, Auger WR. Fatal paradoxic embolism occurring during IVC filter insertion in a patient with chronic pulmonary thromboembolic disease. J Vasc Intervent Radiol 2001; 12(6):770–772.

39. Ionita C, Giglio P, Isayev E, Alberico R, Pullicino P. Paradoxical brain embolism from thrombus associated with vena caval filter in a patient with cancer. J Neuroimaging 2002; 12(1):69–71.

40. Georgopoulos SE, Chronopoulos A, Dervisis KI, Arvanitis DP. Paradoxical embolism. An old but, paradoxically, under-estimated problem. J Cardiovasc Surg (Torino) 2001; 42(5):675–677.

41. Marcy PY, Magne N, Frenay M, Bruneton JN. Renal failure secondary to thrombotic complications of suprarenal inferior vena cava filter in cancer patients. Cardiovasc Intervent Radiol 2001; 24(4):257–259.

42. Flanagan D, Creasy T, Chataway F, Kerr D. Caval umbrella causing obstructive uropathy. Postgrad Med J 1996; 72(846):235–237.

43. Goldman HB, Hanna K, Dmochowski RR. Ureteral injury secondary to an inferior vena caval filter. J Urol 1996; 156(5):1763.

44. Berger BD, Jafri SZ, Konczalski M. Symptomatic hydronephrosis caused by inferior vena cava penetration by a Greenfield filter. J Vasc Intervent Radiol 1996; 7(1):99–101.

45. Wambeek ND, Frazer CK, Kumar A. Penetration of a vertebral body by a limb of the Greenfield filter. Australas Radiol 1996; 40(3):364–366.

46. Phlegmasia cerulea dolens: A complication of use of the filter in the vena cava. J Bone Joint Surg Am 1995; 77(11):1783; Comment, J Bone Joint Surg Am 1995;77(3):452–454.

47. Defraigne JO, Vahdat O, Lacroix H, Limet R. Proximal migration of vena caval filters: Report of

two cases with operative retrieval. Ann Vasc Surg 1995; 9(6):571–575; Comment, Ann Vasc Surg 1997;11(1):106.

48. Seita J, Sakakibara Y, Jikuya T, Shigeta O, Nakata H, Tsunoda H, Mitsui T. Surgical management of a penetrated Greenfield inferior vena cava filter. Thorac Cardiovasc Surg 2001; 49(4): 243–244.

49. Loehr SP, Hamilton C, Dyer R. Retrieval of entrapped guide wire in an IVC filter facilitated with use of a myocardial biopsy forceps and snare device. J Vasc Intervent Radiol 2001; 12(9):1116–1119.

50. Lin M, Soo TB, Horn LC. Successful retrieval of infected Gunther Tulip IVC filter. J Vasc Intervent Radiol 2000; 11(10):1341–1343.

51. Liddell RP, Spinosa DJ, Matsumoto AH, Angle JF, Hagspiel KD. Guidewire entrapment in a Greenfield IVC Filter: "Rail and reins technique." Clin Radiol 2000; 55(11):878–881.

52. Salamipour H, Rivitz SM, Kaufman JA. Percutaneous transfemoral retrieval of a partially deployed Simon-Nitinol filter misplaced into the ascending lumbar vein. J Vasc Intervent Radiol 1996; 7(6):917–919.

53. Gelbfish GA, Ascer E. Intracardiac and intrapulmonary Greenfield filters: A long-term follow-up. J Vasc Surg 1991; 14(5):614–617.

54. Danikas D, Constantinopoulous GS, Stratoulias C, Ginalis EM. Use of a Fogarty catheter to open an incompletely expanded Vena Tech-LGM vena cava filter—A case report. Angiology 2001; 52(4):283–286.

55. Conners MS III, Becker S, Guzman RJ, Passman MA, Pierce R, Kelly T, Naslund TC. Duplex scan-directed placement of inferior vena cava filters: A five-year institutional experience. J Vasc Surg 2002; 35(2):286–291.

56. Ashley DW, Gamblin TC, Burch ST, Solis MM. Accurate deployment of vena cava filters: Comparison of intravascular ultrasound and contrast venography. J Trauma 2001; 50(6):975–981.

36

Complications of Percutaneous Treatment of Arteriovenous Malformations

Robert J. Rosen and Thomas Maldonado

New York University Medical Center, New York, New York, U.S.A.

Congenital vascular malformations are among the most difficult lesions to treat in all of vascular surgery. Even in the most experienced hands, the results of treatment are often more palliative than curative, and the risk of significant complication is always present. The risks cannot be eliminated but can be minimized by carefully defining the nature of the lesion, educating the patient and family as to the natural history, and determining the type of treatment indicated, if any. Many of the complications of treatment in these cases are due to initial misdiagnosis—a common problem in this confusing group of disorders. Some of these lesions follow a benign clinical course, while others can produce life-threatening complications and still others involute spontaneously and completely in childhood. It behooves the clinician caring for these patients to correctly identify the problem; only then can an appropriate risk-benefit decision be made regarding therapy.

This chapter deals primarily with complications of percutaneous treatment of vascular malformations. These can be divided into complications related to technique, those related to specific anatomic regions, and complications related to specific embolic agents or devices. Prior to discussing these issues, it is necessary to briefly review the basic types of vascular anomalies in order to avoid the most fundamental mistake of misdiagnosis.

I. TYPES OF VASCULAR ANOMALIES

There are many systems of classification of vascular anomlies, most unnecessarily complex and exhaustive for the purpose of this chapter. We have found that a simple division of these lesions into four major types is sufficient to make clinical decisions regarding the natural history of the condition and the type of treatment required. This classification is derived from the work of Mulliken, Folkman, and Glowacki (1–3) and includes:

1. Hemangioma
2. Arteriovenous fistula

3. Arteriovenous malformation
4. Venous and lymphatic malformation

Hemangiomas are not malformations but benign vascular tumors encountered at birth or in early infancy. They may occur on the skin, where they present as the classic "strawberry birthmark," or elsewhere in the body, including the viscera (Fig. 1A and B). They may be single or multiple and are much more common in females than males. From a clinical point of view, the most important aspect of these lesions is their natural tendency to involute spontaneously during childhood, so that only a minority of these patients will require specific treatment. Often, education and reassurance of the parents are the only interventions required. There are unusual cases where treatment is required during the proliferative phase, particularly where the lesion involves respiratory or digestive structures or interferes with visual development. Rarely, extensive hepatic hemangiomas may cause high-output congestive heart failure and require urgent intervention (4,5).

The vast majority of arteriovenous fistulas (AVF) are acquired, although congenital types do exist, primarily in the central nervous system. An AVF, by definition, consists of a direct communication between artery and vein, generally resulting in high flow with secondary findings of arterial and venous dilation, venous hypertension, and often distal ischemia due to the proximal steal phenomenon. It has long been known that these lesions are curable, but only by directly interrupting or isolating the fistula itself. This principle is still violated on a regular basis by both vascular surgeons and interventional radiologists who occlude proximal feeding vessels using either ligation or embolic devices. Both will invariably result in persistence of the fistula with almost instantaneous recruitment of collateral feeding vessels, producing a lesion that is much more difficult to treat (Fig. 2). Some of these initially simple fistulas recruit so many new collaterals that they are indistinguish-

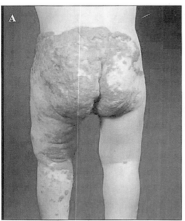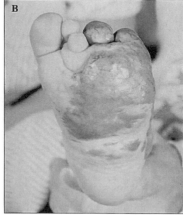

Figure 1 Misdiagnosis of vascular lesions can lead to serious errors in treatment. On a single physical examination, many biologically distinct lesions can have a superficially similar appearance. A. This 10-month-old child has an extensive hemangioma over the buttock and leg, which is starting to show early signs of spontaneous involution. No specific treatment is required. B. Another child with a similar appearing lesion on the foot. This is a venous malformation, which will grow with the child and will never show spontaneous involution.

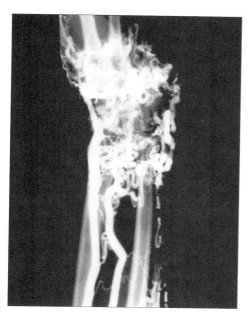

Figure 2 This 48-year-old carpenter sustained a penetrating injury to the palm 4 years previously, resulting in an arteriovenous fistula. Rather than occluding the fistula itself, the radial artery was ligated, leading to recruitment of numerous collaterals and a series of secondary procedures, eventually resulting in amputation of a significant portion of the hand. This angiogram demonstrates profuse collateral development resulting in a lesion as difficult to treat as a complex congenital malformation. This fundamental error in treatment can result from proximal embolization as well as ligation.

able from complex congenital malformations. As in most surgical scenarios, the best chance of cure comes with the initial procedure, which must be directed at obliteration of the fistula itself.

True arteriovenous malformations (AVM) are functionally similar to fistulas, in the effect of a shunt between artery and vein, although the communication is more complex and represents a continuum from microfistulous connections just above capillary level to macrofistolous types. These are congenital lesions that are present at birth by definition and generally grow at the same rate as the individual. They may or may not cause symptoms or even be detected, but they never involute spontaneously. As some of these lesions in children can resemble hemangiomas, the potential for confusion in terms of prognosis and treatment planning is evident. Experienced observers can usually distinguish between the two, but some children must be followed over time before a correct diagnosis can be made confidently. AVMs are notoriously difficult to treat due to their complex blood supply and tendency to recur; since these are slow-growing lesions, there should be no rush to treat, and a careful risk-benefit analysis should be made in conjunction with the patient and family. Lesions may require intervention due to mass effect, distal ischemia, venous hypertension, growth disturbance, or, more rarely, hemorrhage or high-output states. The latter two situations, while often the major concern of parents and referring physicians, are actually quite uncommon, and prophylactic treatment is not warranted.

Treatment failures and complications in patients with AVMs are similar to those outlined above for AVFs. That is, treatment must be directed at eradicating the actual arteriovenous communication, rather than occluding or ligating feeding vessels, which will only result in rapid collateral recruitment. It is obviously much more difficult to interrupt a complex network of feeding vessels than a simple fistula, particularly when there may be no clear delineation between those vessels feeding the AVM and those required for nutritive blood flow to a region. It is this complexity that makes many interventions palliative rather than curative. Only the most localized and accessible AVMs are amenable to complete surgical resection. Partial resections are often complicated by hemorrhage and rapid recurrence, often with exacerbation of the patient's clinical symptoms. Similarly, surgical "skeletonization," meticulous ligation of all feeding vessels in the region, is rarely effective in the long term and often sacrifices transvascular access, making subsequent treatment more difficult (6–8) (Fig. 3A and B).

Venous and lymphatic malformations present clinically in a variety of ways, depending on the anatomical location and depth of the lesion. Superficial venous malformations have a typical bluish discoloration, are soft and compressible, and demonstrate no pulsation or bruits on physical examination. If in an extremity, they may show dramatic enlargement when placed in a dependent position. While these lesions are usually painless, patients may complain of periodic pain and tenderness due to spontaneous thrombosis, or they may experience discomfort due to distension of the lesion after activity or in certain positions. Klippel-Trenaunay syndrome is one of the most common venous anomalies encountered clinically, generally presenting as venous varicosities involving a single extremity, usually the leg (Fig. 4A and B). A significant number of patients with this syndrome have aplasia or hypoplasia of the deep venous system, such that essentially all of the venous drainage from the extremity is via the superficial veins. Venous stripping in these patients can cause a dramatic worsening of symptoms. Any patient with purely unilateral varicosities should

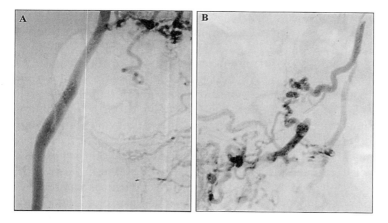

Figure 3 Surgical "skeletonization" is another form of proximal vessel occlusion that is generally ineffective in treating vascular malformations. This 22-year-old patient with a high-flow AVM of the left pelvis and thigh underwent an extensive skeletonization procedure 4 months previously. After studies for recurrent symptoms, the angiogram shows successful ligation of all right iliac and femoral branches (*A*) but resupply of the lesion via multiple enlarged middle sacral and lumbar collaterals (*B*).

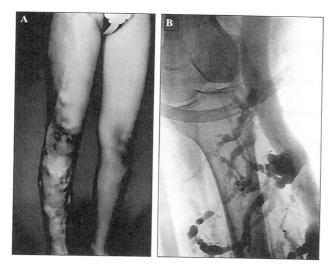

Figure 4 Klippel-Trenaunay syndrome (*A*) is one of the most commonly encountered venous malformations. The distinctive triad includes unilateral varicose veins, hypertrophy of the involved extremity, and cutaneous pigmented lesions in the same area. A serious potential error is to strip or sclerose the varicose veins without initially performing a venogram, as a significant percentage of these patients will have aplasia or hypoplasia of the deep venous system (*B*). Occlusion or removal of the superficial veins may result in acute venous insufficiency.

therefore be investigated with detailed contrast venography prior to any treatment. In extreme cases, the malformation may extend to the pelvis or retroperitoneum. Lymphatic malformations are less common and range from cutaneous lesions with vesicle formation to large soft tissue masses like the cystic hygroma. One of the distinctive features of lymphatic malformations is their tendency to recurrent infection (9,10).

II. EMBOLIZATION TECHNIQUES

Many techniques have been described for the percutaneous treatment of vascular malformations. The two major approaches are transcatheter embolization, used in lesions with a significant arterial component, and direct puncture techniques, mainly used in low-flow venous or lymphatic malformations. Transcatheter treatment involves percutaneous access to the arterial system, selective catheterization of arterial branches feeding the malformation, and the injection of occluding devices or agents. Complications may occur related to the catheterization procedure itself, the anatomical region involved, or the specific embolic device or agent used.

Complications related to arterial access and selective catheterization should be unusual in experienced hands but can occur, particularly in pediatric patients. Problems can include vasospasm, dissection of an artery, and arterial thrombosis, either at the entry site or in arterial branches being selectively catheterized during the procedure. Entry site problems can be minimized by routinely using vascular sheaths, which protect the vessel during catheter manipulation, especially when multiple catheter exchanges may be required. The pulse should always be checked after gaining vascular access; if it is no longer palpable, antispasm agents should be administered (e.g., intra-arterial nitroglycerine) and the patient should be heparinized. This is a problem encountered most often in pediatric patients and young females. The pulse will generally return following sheath removal but may be delayed for several hours, during which time the extremity must be observed closely. Management of the patient whose pulse does not return is controversial—a problem, again, seen mostly in infants and children. While these patients will rarely show signs of ischemia, there is literature documenting the possibility of future growth disturbance and leg-length discrepancy (11). The increased risk of arterial injury in very young patients should be taken into consideration in making the decision on the timing of intervention.

The actual embolization procedure may be complicated by occluding a feeding vessel too proximally or too distally or occluding the wrong vessel altogether. Proximal occlusion of arterial feeders to an AVM, while simple to perform, virtually always results in long-term failure. This is entirely analogous to the proximal ligation of an artery supplying an AVF; collateral vessels will be recruited almost immediately, leading to a recurrence with a much more complex blood supply which is much more refractory to subsequent treatment (12). Just as the goal in surgically treating an AVF is closure of the fistula itself, the goal of embolization in an AVM must be penetration and eradication of the nidus. This goal often cannot be completely achieved in practice, but at the very least, proximal occlusions are to be avoided. Thus, embolic devices such as coils, detachable balloons, or large pledgets of Gelfoam have no role in the treatment of complex lesions other than as protective devices for normal branches in the region.

Conversely, embolic materials that are too small or fine can cause other problems. If the material is smaller than the arteriovenous connections, it will shunt through to the venous circulation and ultimately to the lungs (13–15). The otherwise healthy lung actually has a remarkably high tolerance for this type of embolization, and the patient will rarely demonstrate any signs, symptoms, or changes in pulmonary function studies. Nevertheless, this should be avoided by choosing the appropriate embolic agent. Materials that are extremely penetrating, such as Gelfoam powder, may cause damage to normal tissues if they enter normal parts of the arterial circulation. Nontarget embolization may occur through a variety of mechanisms, including reflux of the embolic material, catheter recoil, device migration, insecure catheter position, and failure of the agent to be completely extruded from the catheter tip. Experience, the use of coaxial microcatheter systems, and scrupulous technique can reduce but not eliminate this type of complication. Depending on the location of the nontarget embolization, the clinical result may range from completely unapparent to an ischemic digit and even to stroke (16). Large embolic devices such as coils can often be retrieved from a nontarget vessel using either interventional or surgical techniques, but most of the agents used in AVM treatment are not retrievable.

Following aggressive embolization of especially large arteriovenous malformations, blood flow may be redistributed toward other circulation beds. The sudden increased pressure in these previously less perfused vessels may result in rupture and significant hemorrhage. This relatively unusual but potentially devastating complication is common to all embolic agents in treating large AVMs.

III. SPECIFIC EMBOLIC AGENTS AND PROBLEMS RELATED TO THEIR USE

A variety of embolic agents have been employed in the treatment of vascular malformations over the past 30 years. Some of these agents remain in common use, others have been abandoned, and still others remain investigational. Some of the features and problems of these agents are considered below.

A. Autologous Tissue or Clot

Among the earliest agents described for the intentional occlusion of blood vessels, these materials are no longer in clinical use due to the unpredictable location and duration of vascular occlusion (17).

B. Gelfoam

Gelfoam is available in a variety of preparations, from sponges to powder. While these are still used as embolic agents in some institutions for the control of gastrointestinal bleeding and traumatic hemorrhage, the have little use in treating AVMs due to their variable duration of occlusion. Gelfoam powder can be extremely dangerous when injected intra-arterially, as the small particle size often leads to tissue necrosis (18).

C. Particles and Microspheres

Two of the most common embolic agents in use are polyvinyl alcohol (PVA) particles and microspheres. These agents are available in graded sized from 50–1000 μm and are injected as a suspension, generally in radiographic contrast. They are thus quite simple to use and can be injected through almost any catheter or microcatheter. The major difference between these two agents is that standard PVA particles are irregularly shaped, being ground mechanically from a sponge material, while the microspheres are smoothly spherical. Both of these agents are non-resorbable, but PVA particles are often associated with early recanalization and AVM recurrence, as the irregular particles are incorporated into vessel walls and new channels are formed (19,20). The experience with microspheres is too limited at this point in determining whether the long-term results will be superior, although this should theoretically be true. In addition, new preparations of spherical PVA have recently been introduced.

Depending on the vascular bed being treated, the risks of particulate embolization primarily relate to improper sizing of the particles or spheres. Particles that are smaller than the AV communication will obviously be shunted through the lesion and lodge in the pulmonary circulation. Since the particles and spheres are themselves radiolucent, this complication may not be immediately apparent. Although experience has shown that inadvertent pulmonary embolization is remarkably well tolerated in the normal lung, large amounts of embolic material or smaller amounts in patients with previously compromised pulmonary function may have significant consequences (21). Extremely small particles (less than 50 μm) that reach normal nontarget vessels may also cause significant ischemic complications, particularly in the gastrointestinal tract (22). Particles that are too large to enter the nidus of the malformation will act as proximal occlusions, resulting in early recurrence of the lesion.

D. Detachable Balloons

These devices consist of latex or silicone balloons with a self-sealing valve that are mounted on a microcatheter and are available (in certain countries) in a variety of shapes and sizes. They offer both distinct advantages and disadvantages. They can be flow-guided fluoroscopically to a high-flow lesion and then inflated and deflated until optimal positioning is attained, at which point they are detached by applying traction to the microcatheter. They are used primarily to treat high-flow fistula-type lesions such as pulmonary AVMs and carotid-cavernous fistulas. The major disadvantages of this device are its complexity, cost, and the occasional premature deflation of the balloon, which can result in reopening of the fistula and possible paradoxical embolization (23). At the present time they are available only on an investigational basis in the United States.

E. Embolization Coils

Coils have been used for transcatheter embolization for over 20 years. They consist of stainless steel or platinum and are supplied in straightened form inside a cartridge; they are pushed through the catheter with a wire or injected with a push of saline, and reassume their coiled shape as they exit the catheter tip. Most coils have fibers attached to increase their occlusive properties. They are available in a wide range of sizes and shapes, including microcoils, which can be passed through microcatheters. More sophisticated coils have recently been introduced that have specialized properties, including extreme flexibility, allowing the coil to behave almost like a liquid (useful in aneurysms), and complex detachment systems that allow for precise positioning prior to releasing the device. Standard coils are relatively inexpensive and easy to use but are not suitable for AVM embolization, as they are equivalent to a vessel ligation and recurrence is virtually guaranteed while access has been sacrificed. In certain anatomical situations, proximal coil occlusion may actually be performed to protect normal branches from distal liquid or particulate embolization. Probably the commonest complication associated with coil embolization is misplacement or migration of the device; this can be minimized by ensuring a stable catheter position prior to extruding the coil as well as using coaxial catheter systems. When the catheter tip is near the ostium of a vessel, the extruding coil may push the catheter tip backward and allow the coil to embolize distally into the normal circulation. Miniature snares are now widely available that usually but not always allow a misplaced coil to be retrieved transluminally.

F. Absolute Ethanol

Ethanol has been used in both arterial and venous malformations, both via transcatheter injection and direct puncture techniques (21,24,25). Essentially a sclerosing agent, ethanol causes intravascular thrombosis and endothelial damage, leading to occlusion, inflammation, and fibrosis. When ethanol is used in venous lesions by direct injection, these properties are desirable, but when it is injected intra-arterially, the risk of complications is considerable. Its direct tissue toxicity can result in sloughing, nerve damage, and mucosal ulceration or perforation (26,27) (Fig. 5A and B). Acute systemic reactions to ethanol may also occur (see Sec. IV.E, below). Since ethanol is nonviscous and radiolucent, extreme care must be exercised to control its distribution and avoid normal structures.

G. Liquid Adhesives

Acrylic adhesives were first introduced 30 years ago for the surgical management of solid-organ trauma, particularly the liver. They were subsequently used to occlude blood vessels supplying vascular malformations, although these agents have been available only intermittently in the United States. The only agent of this type currently available is N-butyl cyanoacrylate (NBCA), which received approval from the U.S. Food and Drug Administration in 2000 for use in central nervous system lesions. The agent is supplied in liquid form and is generally mixed with an oily radiographic contrast agent (ethiodol) that provides radiopacity and slows the polymerization time, which would otherwise be virtually

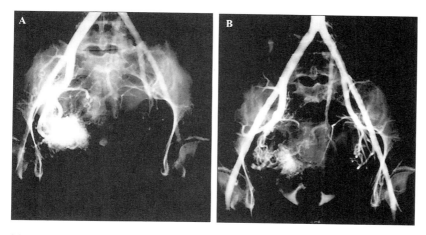

Figure 5 Pelvic angiogram of 32-year-old woman with right pelvic discomfort, which was found to be caused by a high-flow AVM supplied by the right hypogastric artery (*A*). Repeat angiography following intra-arterial absolute ethanol embolization (*B*) shows marked reduction in flow to the lesion. The patient developed colon and bladder perforations requiring colostomy and partial bladder resection as well as permanent nerve injury with foot drop and chronic leg pain. Ethanol is extremely tissue-toxic and may be associated with severe complications when injected intra-arterially.

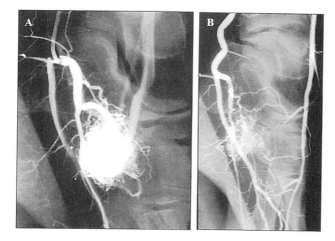

Figure 6 A 35-year-old male with a high-flow arteriovenous malformation in the plantar aspect of the foot, causing steal, with resultant pain and chronic ulceration of the toes (*A*). Repeat study (*B*) following superselective embolization with *N*-butyl cyanoacrylate (NBCA) tissue adhesive shows marked reduction in flow to the nidus with improved distal flow. The patient's pain and ulceration resolved within 3 weeks. Although there is a residual nidus, the clinical problem was successfully resolved. NBCA adhesive has little or no tissue toxicity and can be used safely in almost any part of the circulation.

instantaneous. NBCA polymerizes on contact with any ionic media, including blood, tissue, saline, and contrast agents. Its use therefore requires considerable training and experience as well as scrupulous attention to technique. The theoretical advantage of this type of agent is its ability to penetrate the nidus of an AVM and form a cast, preventing ingrowth of new collaterals. Complete obliteration of the nidus is, in fact, rarely achieved, but a significant reduction in flow can generally be accomplished (Fig. 6A and B). We have used this agent as our primary embolic material for high-flow AVMs for over 20 years and have been impressed with the clinical results and relative freedom from adverse effects (28,29).

There has been ongoing concern regarding possible long-term toxicity or even carcinogenicity with this agent, but there has never been any report of such an effect in humans despite many years of use. Problems and complications with these adhesives have been primarily mechanical and technical in nature, including nontarget embolization and gluing a catheter to the vessel wall. This latter event, while frequently mentioned, rarely occurs in clinical use and is nearly always associated with intracranial lesions where extremely small, fragile microcatheters are used; these have less tensile strength than the glue cast (30). A potential limitation of these cyanoacrylates is the possibility for dissolution and subsequent recanalization of the AVM on long-term follow-up. Resorption and recanalization appears to be more likely if the AVM nidus is incompletely casted with adhesive (31,32).

IV. COMPLICATIONS ASSOCIATED WITH SPECIFIC ANATOMIC REGIONS

Certain anatomic regions are associated with potential complications from percutaneous treatment of vascular malformations due to the nature of the vascular bed or the end organ involved. Neuroembolization procedures obviously carry significant risk, but these are beyond the scope of this chapter and are not discussed here.

A. Pulmonary AVM

Most pulmonary AVMs are asymptomatic and constitute one of the few lesions that are treated prophylactically to eliminate the risk of paradoxical embolization, which may result in stroke or brain abscess (33,34). Complications related to embolization of pulmonary AVMs consist of those involving the lung and those related to paradoxical embolization during the procedure itself. Pulmonary complications related to embolization are unusual due to the dual blood supply of the lung, so that pulmonary infarction is uncommon. When this does occur, it is manifest as pleuritic pain, infiltrate, atelectasis, and pleural effusion. These problems are nearly always self-limited, resolving in days. Passage of the embolic material or device through the malformation is a much more serious risk, presenting the possibility of stroke—the very problem the procedure was intended to protect against. This event is fortunately rare and usually associated with improper sizing of the coil or balloon, premature balloon detachment, or premature balloon deflation. Interestingly, the only patient in whom we encountered this complication had none of the above problems during the procedure but awoke the morning following the procedure with a stroke (unpublished data). The hypothesis was that, after balloon occlusion, thrombus accumulating in the pulmonary artery branch proximal to the occluded AVM was swept through another smaller, angiographically undetected AVM.

B. Gastrointestinal Tract

Other than in patients with Rendu-Osler-Weber syndrome, most vascular malformations in the gastrointestinal (GI) tract are angiodysplasias found in the colon, generally in older patients with intermittent bleeding. While most of the GI tract is so well collateralized that the risk of ischemia is slight, the colon is sparsely vascularized and presents a significant risk of mucosal ischemia with subsequent stricture or even infarction following embolization (22,35,36). The appropriate level of occlusion is controversial, as the occlusion must be distal enough to stop the bleeding but not so distal that there is insufficient collateral flow to maintain viability. NBCA and PVA particles may be used safely, and this is one of the few locations where microcoils may be an acceptable alternative. Ethanol should never be used intra-arterially in the GI tract.

An unusual complication that we have encountered twice is portal vein thombosis following embolization of a high-flow AVM in the small intestine with shunting into the portal system. Both of these patients presented with symptoms of severe portal hypertension (variceal bleeding, intractable ascites) necessitating treatment. Both were treated with superselective NBCA adhesive with an excellent angiographic result and no loss of the agent into the portal system. Both did well initially, but within a week they thrombosed their entire portal system and subsequently expired (unpublished data).

C. Liver, Spleen, and Kidney

As in the lung, the dual blood supply of the liver generally permits safe embolization of vascular malformations. The risk of ischemia is increased in the presence of severe portal hypertension as well as portal vein and biliary obstruction (37).

The spleen is a rare location for vascular malformations but presents a risk that is unusual elsewhere in the body following embolization—the complication of infarction followed by infection with abscess formation (38). For this reason, any patient undergoing splenic embolization should be placed on prophylactic intravenous antibiotics, which should be continued for at least a week following the procedure. Another potential complication is pancreatitis or pancreatic infarction due to embolic material that has entered the small pancreatic branches originating from the splenic artery (39). This complication has occurred primarily when liquid agents have been used. Renal vascular malformations tend to be of two main types. The first is the small angiomatous lesion associated with intermittent gross hematuria; it is usually found in the right kidney of adult females. These lesions are supplied by small intrarenal end vessels; therefore they can be completely cured by embolization. However, a small renal infarction will generally occur, with the patient experiencing flank pain and fever (40,41) (Fig. 7A). This "postembolization syndrome" is virtually always self-limited and resolves in a matter of days. The second type is the large congenital intrarenal fistula, which may present with flank pain, hematuria, a bruit, and occasionally a high-output state. Interestingly, this lesion also appears to favor the right kidney and is often misdiagnosed on imaging studies, because of the massive dilation of the draining veins, as a giant intrarenal aneurysm. This lesion is also curable with embolization, but the patient may experience considerable postoperative discomfort due to the thrombosis of the draining veins.

D. Extremities

Extremity lesions can be among the most difficult malformations to treat, with a significant risk of complications (27,42,43). This is due to the difficulty in separating the

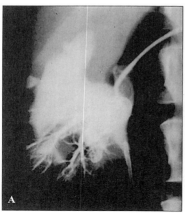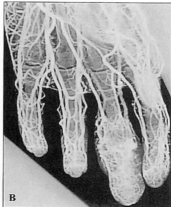

Figure 7 Vascular malformations involving "end vessels" such as the kidney (*A*) or digits (*B*) are extremely difficult to treat without causing ischemia of normal tissues. In the kidney, the segmental infarction that would follow embolization of this small AVM, causing hematuria, would be well tolerated, while in the finger (*B*), embolization carries a real risk of tissue loss.

vessels supplying the malformation from those necessary for maintaining distal viability. This is particularly true in patients who have undergone previous surgical ligations (as many have) or embolizations (Fig. 7A and B). The more distal the lesion, the higher the difficulty in terms of both the catherization technique and preserving distal flow (Fig. 7B). Thus hand and foot lesions are particularly refractory to achieving a satisfactory result (28). The end-vessel digital circulation is also unforgiving of any nontarget embolization, presenting the real risk of loss of the digit. Infants and young children appear to have a better chance of reperfusion than adult patients in this situation.

Ulceration is not uncommon in high-flow extremity malformations; it is related to both tissue ischemia from a steal phenomenon as well as venous hypertension. Particularly in previously treated patients, it can sometimes be diffcult to determine which mechanism is predominantly responsible for the ulceration. If ischemia is the primary mechanism, further embolization may actually worsen the clinical problem, while venous hypertension will be improved by embolization, which reduces the shunt.

E.   Venous Malformations

Venous malformations range from focal cavernous lesions to diffuse intramuscular lesions to anomalous venous channels such, as those seen in Klippel-Trénaunay syndrome. By definition, they show little or no arteriovenous shunting on angiography. Embolization of the arterial branches supplying the area of these venous lesions has been tried in the past, and—not surprisingly—has had no beneficial effect. As with any vascular malformation, treatment is indicated only for significant symptoms or complications; the mere presence of a venous lesion, once its nature has been determined, is not an indication for treatment. Symptoms may include the presence of a soft tissue mass, pain—particularly after activity or when the lesion is in a dependent position, ulceration, secondary signs of venous hypertension, and, rarely, bleeding.

Treatment options (aside from the usual conservative measures) include surgical resection and direct embolization. Surgical resection is often more difficult than anticipated, as the visible or palpable component of the lesion may only be the "tip of the iceberg," with extension into deep tissues and surrounding structures. Detailed imaging studies are mandatory prior to attempted resection, with magnetic resonance imaging (MRI) studies providing the most accurate depiction of the extent of the lesion. Only the most localized of these malformations are suitable for surgical resection, and recurrence after surgery is common (44).

Direct embolization of venous malformations is a form of sclerotherapy. Using radiological guidance [ultrasound, fluoroscopy, computed tomography, or MRI], the lesion is entered directly with a sheathed needle. Contrast material is then injected to outline the lesion and determine the approximate volume, with specific attention to the route of venous drainage. Some cavernous lesions are almost completely isolated from the normal deep veins in the region, while others show large, relatively rapid communication with the systemic venous circulation. Particularly when there is significant communication with normal veins, the lesion must be isolated, using either tourniquet or cuff compression or direct compression of the draining vein. When a lesion is in an extremity, the deep venous system is generally flushed continuously with a heparinized saline solution to reduce the risk of deep venous thrombosis from the sclerosing agent. The commonest sclerosing agents are absolute ethanol and sotradecol solution, both of which are quite tissue-toxic. Leakage of the agent from the lesion out to a skin or mucosal surface may result in ulceration; the entry tract is generally injected with a collagen suspension as the catheter is withdrawn to reduce this risk. Venous malformations in the calf or forearm may be associated with compartment syndromes following embolization. Inflammation and resulting edema can be reduced by administering steroids before and after treatment. Furthermore, in the case of extensive lesions, embolizations should be staged and performed slowly.

Major complications have been reported during ethanol embolization when a significant amount of the agent escapes into the venous circulation (25). The most severe is cardiovascular collapse, which may occur with little warning and is thought to be related to an acute direct vasospastic response of the central pulmonary vasculature to the ethanol. In some cases, a large bolus of ethanol soaked thrombus may also embolize centrally and cause a similar clinical picture. While in our institution virtually all of these procedures are performed under general anesthesia with close physiological monitoring, some authors have advocated routine placement of Swan-Ganz catheters to monitor pressures throughout the procedure (25). We have found that using radiographic contrast, fluoroscopic monitoring, and limiting the total volume of ethanol used in a single procedure (generally 0.5 mL/kg maximum) makes this type of complication exceedingly rare.

V. PEDIATRIC ISSUES

A significant number of patients being diagnosed and treated for vascular malformations will be in the pediatric age range. In this group of patients, a team approach to the problem is particularly important. The need for intervention and its timing is often an issue. The first critical step is making an accurate diagnosis, which may sometimes be quite difficult in infants and children; in them, some hemangiomas and vascular malformations have a similar appearance. Many of these situations can be clarified on imaging studies, while others may need to be followed over a period of time. Hemangiomas will typically show the classic pattern of proliferation followed by involution, while vascular malformations tend to grow at the same rate as the child. Unless there are severe functional disturbances related to the lesion (impaired feeding, breathing, or vision), a rush to treatment is rarely necessary. While the vast majority of hemangiomas will resolve without specific treatment, some authorities now advocate more aggressive early intervention for lesions that are cosmetically disfiguring in order to avoid adverse effects on psychosocial development (45). Timing may also be critical in some extremity vascular malformations that affect limb length, either accelerating or retarding normal bone growth. This problem can be encountered both in venous lesions (Klippel-Trénaunay type) and arterial lesions, specifically high-flow lesions involving the epiphyseal plate. The limb-length discrepancy is usually treated by epiphyseodesis in the venous type, and superselective embolization in the arterial type. Obviously, a careful orthopedic assessment of expected bone growth is critical in the timing of intervention to minimize the ultimate limb-length discrepancy.

VI. SUMMARY

Congenital vascular anomalies constitute a complex and disparate group of conditions. Some of these are benign incidental findings that require no treatment, some will resolve spontaneously, and some are life-threatening conditions requiring urgent intervention. Caring for these patients requires familiarity with this range of conditions and the ability to make an accurate diagnosis. Probably the most common complications are related to initial misdiagnosis followed by misguided attempts at therapy. A multidisciplinary approach is strongly recommended to achieve optimum clinical results. Percutaneous management of these lesions has assumed a primary role in the care of these patients, either as stand-alone therapy or in conjunction with surgery. The two primary approaches are transcatheter embolization, generally employed in the treatment of high flow arteriovenous malformations, and direct embolization, where a sclerosing agent is directly injected into the lesion. Complications of percutaneous procedures are uncommon but include those related to faulty technique, inherent problems with many of the embolic devices and agents, and the complex physiology of vascular malformations.

REFERENCES

1. Mulliken JB, Zetter BR, Folkman J. In vitro characteristics of endothelium from hemangiomas and vascular malformations. Surgery 1982; 92(2):348–353.
2. Mulliken JB, Glowacki J. Hemangiomas and vascular malformations in infants and children: A classification based on endothelial characteristics. Plast Reconstr Surg 1982; 69(3):412–422.
3. Mulliken JB, Glowacki J. Classification of pediatric vascular lesions. Plast Reconstr Surg 1982; 70(1):120–121.
4. Linderkamp O, Hopner F, Klose H, et al. Solitary hepatic hemangioma in a newborn infant complicated by cardiac failure, consumption coagulopathy, microangiopathic hemolytic anemia, and obstructive jaundice. Case report and review of the literature. Eur J Pediatr 1976; 124(1):23–29.
5. Berdon WE, Baker DH. Giant hepatic hemangioma with cardiac failure in the newborn infant. Value of high-dosage intravenous urography and umbilical angiography. Radiology 1969; 92(7):1523–1528.
6. Griffin JM, Vasconez LO, Schatten WE. Congenital arteriovenous malformations of the upper extremity. Plast Reconstr Surg 1978; 62(1):49–58.
7. Olcott Ct, Newton TH, Stoney RJ, Ehrenfeld WK. Intra-arterial embolization in the management of arteriovenous malformations. Surgery 1976; 79(1):3–12.

8. Trout HH, III. Management of patients with hemangiomas and arteriovenous malformations. Surg Clin North Am 1986; 66(2):333–338.

9. Padwa BL, Hayward PG, Ferraro NF, Mulliken JB. Cervicofacial lymphatic malformation: Clinical course, surgical intervention, and pathogenesis of skeletal hypertrophy. Plast Reconstr Surg 1995; 95(6):951–960.

10. Raveh E, de Jong AL, Taylor GP, Forte V. Prognostic factors in the treatment of lymphatic malformations. Arch Otolaryngol Head Neck Surg 1997; 123(10):1061–1065.

11. Perry MO. Iatrogenic injuries of arteries in infants. Surg Gynecol Obstet 1983; 157(5):415–418.

12. Szilagyi DE, Smith RF, Elliott JP, Hageman JH. Congenital arteriovenous anomalies of the limbs. Arch Surg 1976; 111(4):423–429.

13. Carapiet DA, Stevens JE. Pulmonary embolism following embolization of an arteriovenous malformation. Paediatr Anaesth 1996; 6(6):491–494.

14. Coard K, Silver MD, Perkins G, et al. Isobutyl-2-cyanoacrylate pulmonary emboli associated with occlusive embolotherapy of cerebral arteriovenous malformations. Histopathology 1984; 8(6):917–926.

15. Kjellin IB, Boechat MI, Vinuela F, et al. Pulmonary emboli following therapeutic embolization of cerebral arteriovenous malformations in children. Pediatr Radiol 2000; 30(4):279–283.

16. Purdy PD, Batjer HH, Risser RC, Samson D. Arteriovenous malformations of the brain: choosing embolic materials to enhance safety and ease of excision. J Neurosurg 1992; 77(2): 212–217.

17. Barth KH, Strandberg JD, White RI Jr. Long term follow-up of transcatheter embolization with autologous clot, oxycel and gelfoam in domestic swine. Invest Radiol 1977; 12(3):273–280.

18. Nakano H, Igawa M. Complication after embolization of internal iliac artery by gelatin sponge powder. Hiroshima J Med Sci 1986; 35(1):21–25.

19. Standard SC, Guterman LR, Chavis TD, Hopkins LN. Delayed recanalization of a cerebral arteriovenous malformation following angiographic obliteration with polyvinyl alcohol embolization. Surg Neurol 1995; 44(2):109–112; discussion 112–113.

20. Sorimachi T, Koike T, Takeuchi S, et al. Embolization of cerebral arteriovenous malformations achieved with polyvinyl alcohol particles: Angiographic reappearance and complications. AJNR 1999; 20(7):1323–1328.

21. Yakes WF, Haas DK, Parker SH, et al. Symptomatic vascular malformations: Ethanol embolotherapy. Radiology 1989; 170(3 Pt 2):1059–1066.

22. Rosenkrantz H, Bookstein JJ, Rosen RJ, et al. Postembolic colonic infarction. Radiology 1982; 142(1):47–51.

23. DeSouza NM, Reidy JF. Embolization with detachable balloons—Applications outside the head. Clin Radiol 1992; 46(3):170–175.

24. Yakes WF, Luethke JM, Parker SH, et al. Ethanol embolization of vascular malformations. Radiographics 1990; 10(5):787–796.

25. Yakes WF, Rossi P, Odink H. How I do it. Arteriovenous malformation management. Cardiovasc Intervent Radiol 1996; 19(2):65–71.

26. Yakes WF, Luethke JM, Merland JJ, et al. Ethanol embolization of arteriovenous fistulas: A primary mode of therapy. J Vasc Intervent Radiol 1990; 1(1):89–96.

27. Dickey KW, Pollak JS, Meier GH III, et al. Management of large high-flow arteriovenous malformations of the shoulder and upper extremity with transcatheter embolotherapy. J Vasc Intervent Radiol 1995; 6(5):765–773.

28. Sofocleous CT, Rosen RJ, Raskin K, et al. Congenital vascular malformations in the hand and forearm. J Endovasc Ther 2001; 8(5):484–494.

29. Jacobowitz GR, Rosen RJ, Rockman CB, et al. Transcatheter embolization of complex pelvic vascular malformations: Results and long-term follow-up. J Vasc Surg 2001; 33(1):51–55.

30. Pollak J, White RI. The use of cyanoacrylate adhesives in peripheral embolization. J Vasc Intervent Radiol 2001; 12:907–913.

31. Vinters HV, Lundie MJ, Kaufmann JC. Long-term pathological follow-up of cerebral arterio-

venous malformations treated by embolization with bucrylate. N Engl J Med 1986; 314(8): 477–483.

32. Rao VR, Mandalam KR, Gupta AK, et al. Dissolution of isobutyl 2-cyanoacrylate on long-term follow-up. AJNR 1989; 10(1):135–141.

33. Faughnan ME, Lui YW, Wirth JA, et al. Diffuse pulmonary arteriovenous malformations: Characteristics and prognosis. Chest 2000; 117(1):31–38.

34. Brydon HL, Akinwunmi J, Selway R, Ul-Haq I. Brain abscesses associated with pulmonary arteriovenous malformations. Br J Neurosurg 1999; 13(3):265–269.

35. Mitty HA, Efremidis S, Keller RJ. Colonic stricture after transcatheter embolization for diverticular bleeding. AJR 1979; 133(3):519–521.

36. Hemingway AP, Allison DJ. Colonic embolisation: Useful but caution required. Gut 1998; 43(1): 4–5.

37. Schwartz RA, Teitelbaum GP, Katz MD, Pentecost MJ. Effectiveness of transcatheter embolization in the control of hepatic vascular injuries. J Vasc Intervent Radiol 1993; 4(3):359–365.

38. Trojanowski JQ, Harrist TJ, Athanasoulis CA, Greenfield AJ. Hepatic and splenic infarctions: Complications of therapeutic transcatheter embolization. Am J Surg 1980; 139(2):272–277.

39. Raat H, Stockx L, De Meester X, et al. Percutaneous embolization of a splenic arteriovenous fistula related to acute necrotizing pancreatitis. Eur Radiol 1999; 9(4):753.

40. Clouse ME, Levin DC, Desautels RE. Transcatheter embolotherapy for congenital renal arteriovenous malformations. Long-term follow-up. Urology 1983; 22(4):360–365.

41. Nakamura H, Uchida H, Kuroda C, et al. Renal arteriovenous malformations: Transcatheter embolization and follow-up. AJR 1981; 137(1):113–116.

42. Gomes AS, Busuttil RW, Baker JD, et al. Congenital arteriovenous malformations. The role of transcatheter arterial embolization. Arch Surg 1983; 118(7):817–825.

43. White RI Jr, Pollak J, Persing J, et al. Long-term outcome of embolotherapy and surgery for high-flow extremity arteriovenous malformations. J Vasc Intervent Radiol 2000; 11(10):1285–1295.

44. Noel AA, Gloviczki P, Cherry KJ Jr, et al. Surgical treatment of venous malformations in Klippel-Trenaunay syndrome. J Vasc Surg 2000; 32(5):840–847.

45. Demiri EC, Pelissier P, Genin-Etcheberry T, et al. Treatment of facial haemangiomas: The present status of surgery. Br J Plast Surg 2001; 54(8):665–674.

37

Endovascular Complications of Angioplasty and Stenting

Gary M. Ansel

Riverside Methodist Hospital, Columbus, Ohio, U.S.A.

As in every therapeutic procedure, endovascular procedures such as angioplasty and stenting carry an inherent risk of complication to the patient. Though with the proper training these complications can usually be successfully managed endovascularly, improper management may lead to emergency surgery, limb loss, functional disability, and death. It is paramount that physician operators have the proper training and ability to anticipate, recognize, and treat complications as they arise during endovascular procedures.

In a recent review (1), the occurrence of a major morbidity such as myocardial infarction, renal failure, and stroke from elective endovascular procedures has been reported in up to 2.3% of patients. An amputation rate of 0.6% was also seen, though only in patients with preexisting critical limb ischemia.

The incidence of major complications at the site of intervention during balloon angioplasty procedures varies widely depending on the type of procedure and patient population. Prior to the widespread utilization of stents, a large review by Gardiner et al. (2) reported major complications at the angioplasty site in approximately 3% of procedures. Though the addition of stent placement has historically shown an increased complication rate, this most likely represented a learning curve phenomenon combined with the large French size of the early stent equipment (3,4). More recent randomized data comparing balloon angioplasty to stenting in the femoral artery appears to show decreased complications with stent utilization (5). Complex lesions such as occlusions, associated with longer procedure times and frequent equipment manipulations, may predispose to higher rates of complication than those seen in the treatment of simple stenotic lesions (6–9). Limb-salvage patients have also shown a higher procedural complication rate than have claudicants (10). When endovascular complications do occur, over 86% are usually evident in the angiographic suite and almost all are evident within 5 h postprocedure (11,12). As in all procedures, it is proper training and anticipation of the potential for a complication that will be most likely to prevent it.

I. PROCEDURE SITE COMPLICATIONS

Acute vascular complications at the endovascular procedure site include arterial perforation, dissection, thrombosis, spasm, side branch occlusion, and equipment failure. Subacute complications include aneurysm formation, infection, and arteriovenous fistula formation (13–16).

II. ARTERIAL PERFORATION

Arterial perforation can occur both at the site of balloon angioplasty and distally from the guidewire. Perforation has been reported in 0–2.3% of patients (10,17,18). Guidewire perforations are usually related to the use of hydrophilic wires and failure to visualize the distal wire during equipment manipulation. Perforations at the angioplasty site appear to be related to the presence of significant vessel calcification, tortuosity of the vessel, high balloon inflation pressures, and utilization of a balloon that is larger than the native arterial vessel. Lowering the risk of arterial perforation at the angioplasty site can be accomplished by undersizing the angioplasty balloon for the first arterial dilation or utilizing intravascular ultrasound for assessment of arterial size and extent of calcification. Evaluating the patient's symptoms of discomfort during balloon inflation, which is related to stretching of the vessel's adventitie, may also also decrease the risk of perforation during balloon angioplasty and stenting. Discomfort should signal to the operator that they have reached the maximum safe dilation size has been reached and should not be exceeded, as otherwise arterial rupture may occur.

The treatment of distal guidewire perforations is usually conservative. However, in a few vascular beds—such as the deep pelvic and renal areas—small vessel perforations may lead to life-threatening hemorrhage. In these cases transcatheter coil embolization will usually control the hemorrhage (Fig. 1) (19). Vascular perforations at the site of balloon angioplasty may be controlled with prolonged balloon inflation while anticoagulation is reversed. However, more significant perforations may require the placement of covered vascular stents (Fig. 2) or surgical repair (16,20). The choice of treatment is often influenced by the vessel size and location, extent of perforation, and patient's comorbidities. Regardless of the perforation size, the initial treatment is to reinflate the angioplasty balloon to control the hemorrhage. The operator should then evaluate the angiogram to assess the extent of perforation, presence of complicating arterial side branches, and procedural options. Small perforations are often successfully treated simply by inflating the angioplasty balloon to the lowest pressure that will allow for sealing of the perforation. Systemic anticoagulation should be reversed. After a balloon inflation time of approximately 15 min, repeat angiography is completed. Once the perforation is sealed, the patient can usually be safely observed until discharge. Large perforations or vascular ruptures appear to be extremely rare. However, when a rupture occurs in a large vessel, life-threatening hemorrhage can occur. For example, if a rupture should occur during angioplasty of an iliac artery, successful treatment requires control of the hemorrhage by balloon reinflation. Placement of a second balloon into the aorta or proximal iliac artery from another vascular access site is often required. This second balloon is placed proximal to the rupture site to control the hemorrhage that may occur during definitive repair at the original site of intervention. After control of the hemorrhage is obtained, the use of a covered stent is often successful in sealing the perforation. The covered stent should be long enough to fully cover the arterial perforation. Sealing of the perforation with a stent-

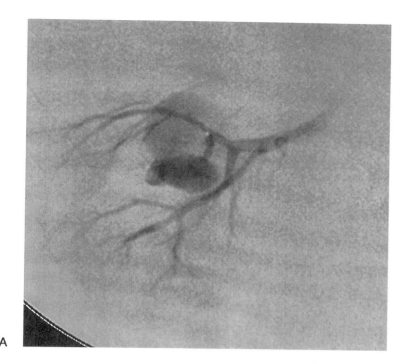

A

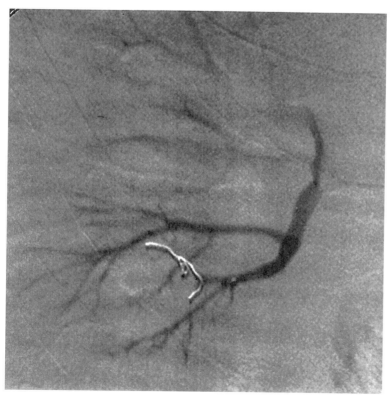

B

Figure 1 A. Angiogram demonstrating contrast extravasation from a guidewire perforation of a renal artery branch vessel. B. Repeat angiogram after thrombotic coil placement.

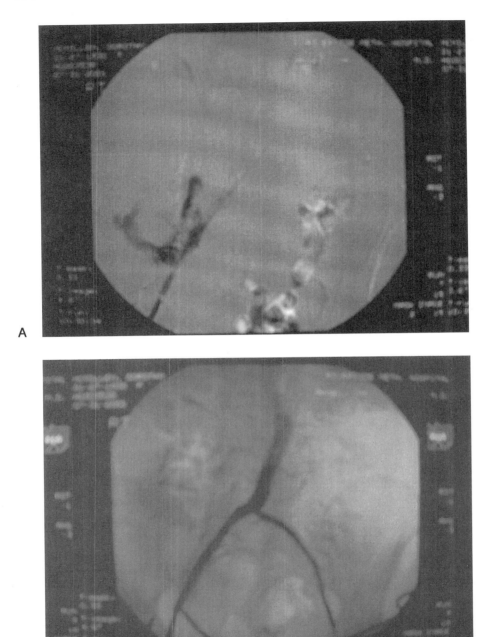

Figure 2   A. Right iliac artery perforation with contrast extravasation. B. Repeat angiogram after placement of two covered stents.

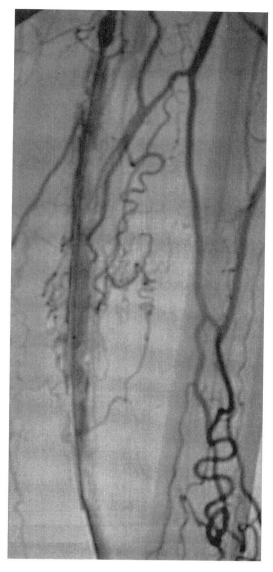

A

Figure 3   A. Extensive femoral artery guidewire perforation. B. Selective femoral artery angiogram after placement of a Nitinol stent.

graft may not occur if severe eccentric calcification is present or if a significant branch vessel such as the hypogastric artery arises from within the area of perforation. Large side branch vessels located at the site of perforation may lead to delayed bleeding as collaterals dilate. After stent-graft placement, delayed thrombosis of the stent-graft is a concern if it is placed in smaller vessels, as in the femoropopliteal regions (21,22). Very large perforations or those that cannot be successfully treated by either prolonged balloon inflation or a

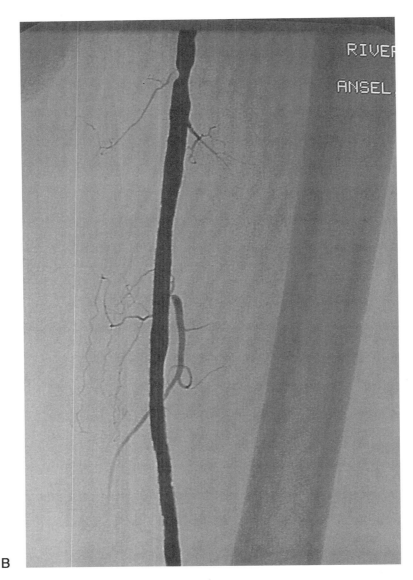

B

Figure 3 Continued.

covered stent will require surgical repair. Continued control of the hemorrhage should be maintained by ongoing balloon inflation. The balloon is deflated only after the affected artery has been surgically exposed in the operating suite. Various balloon expandable and self-expanding covered stents may be utilized. Currently however, a covered stent approved for arterial perforation by the U.S. Food and Drug Administration (FDA) is available only for the coronary vasculature Covered stents used in the peripheral vasculature are utilized "off label."

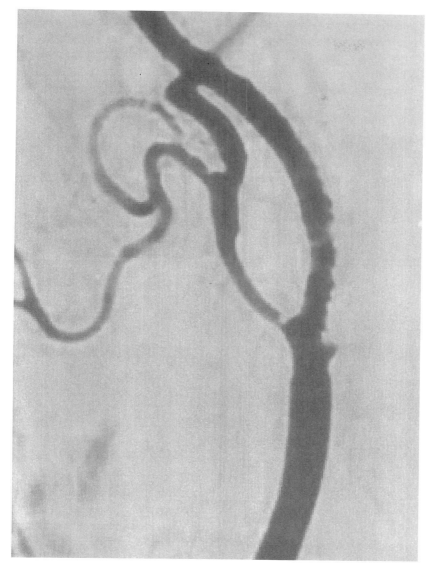

A

Figure 4 A. Carotid stent with intraprocedural thrombus formation. B. Repeat angiogram after treatment with an intravenous IIb/IIIa antiplatelet agent.

III. ARTERIAL DISSECTION

Endovascular stents have diminished the clinical impact of even large intimal dissections (Fig. 3). Since stents can effectively treat a dissection, most clinically relevant dissections occur either during guide wire placement, or from unrecognized and untreated dissection after wire removal. Wire dissections that cannot be crossed from the original acess site can often be crossed and treated from the opposite end of the dissection. Unrecognized

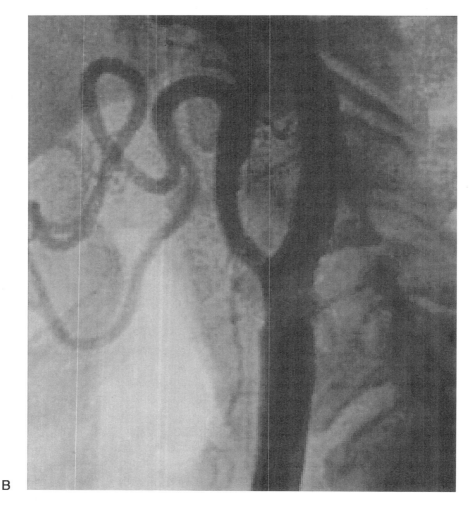

B

Figure 4 Continued.

wire dissections that go from true lumen into false lumen and back into true lumen after an important branch vessel are also important causes of complication from dissection. This true-false-true phenomenon most frequently occurs during the treatment of total occlusions.

IV. ARTERIAL THROMBOSIS

Arterial thrombosis during angioplasty or stenting is usually due to inadequate anti-coagulation or antiplatelet therapy, inadequate balloon angioplasty result, dissection, or unrecognized hypercoagulable condition. Thrombosis may also occur due to blood stasis if the endovascular device is large and obstructs arterial flow in the setting of inadequate anticoagulation. An activated clotting time (ACT) should be obtained after heparin administration and during long cases every 60 min. The size of the endovascular equipment relevant to the arterial vessel and the restriction of arterial flow as well as the length of the procedure determine what constitutes an adequate ACT.

The prevention of subacute thrombosis has been studied best in the coronary intervention literature. Previous aggressive anticoagulation regimens utilized in early coronary artery stenting usually consisted of aspirin, dypyridamole, dextran, heparin, and warfarin. These regimens were associated with considerable bleeding complications, especially at the sheath insertion sites, at rates of 3–6% (23). However, subacute thrombosis rates of over 7% were still seen (24). In the largest study to date, 1652 cardiac patients were randomized to aspirin plus warfarin, aspirin plus ticlopidine, or asprin alone after coronary stenting. The aspirin-plus-ticlopidine group had a significantly lower subacute thrombosis rate (0.6%) than either of the other groups (both 2.4%) (25). It would appear prudent to recommend the use of aspirin plus ticlopidine or clopidogrel for peripheral angioplasty/stenting procedures to decrease the risk of subacute thrombosis. The formation of visible thrombus (Fig. 4), usually platelet-mediated, during an endovascular procedure should prompt the consideration of an intravenous IIb/IIIa antiplatelet agent such abciximab (26).

V. ARTERIAL SPASM

Arterial spasm rarely leads to a serious complication during angioplasty. However, severe symptoms of pain may occur. The occurrence of arterial vessel spasm appears to be more common in younger patients (18). It has also been our experience that small vessels or vessels supplying an organ are more prone to spasm than the large vessels supplying the limbs. Though prolonged spasm could lead to thrombosis, the major risk of spasm is often the difficulty with differentiating it from dissection (Fig. 5). Spasm should be prevented by routinely administering a vasodilator agent (nitroglycerine, papaverine, verapamil) prior

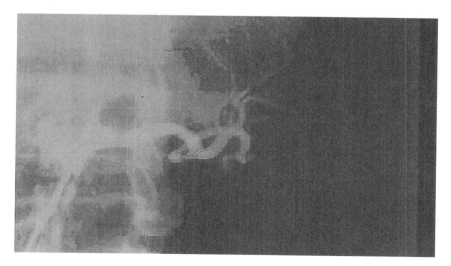

A

Figure 5 A. Left renal artery angiogram. B. Severe arterial spasm after balloon angioplasty. C. Final angiogram after stent placement and intra-arterial nitroglycerin.

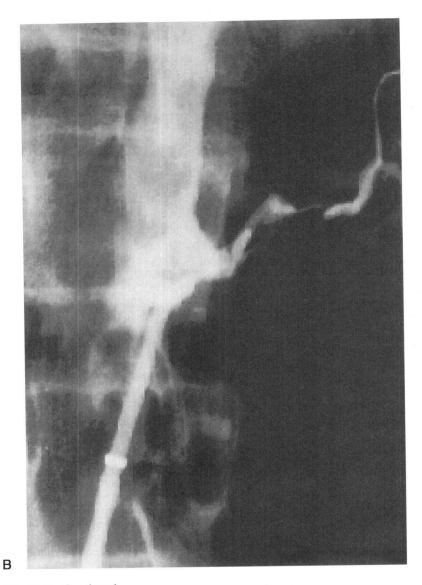

B

Figure 5 Continued.

to vessel manipulation. Occasionally, a guidewire may have to be removed to distinguish refractory spasm from dissection.

VI. EQUIPMENT FAILURE

Another source of procedural complication is related to device failure. This includes angioplasty balloon rupture prior to stent expansion, stent embolization, guidewire fracture, and catheter fracture.

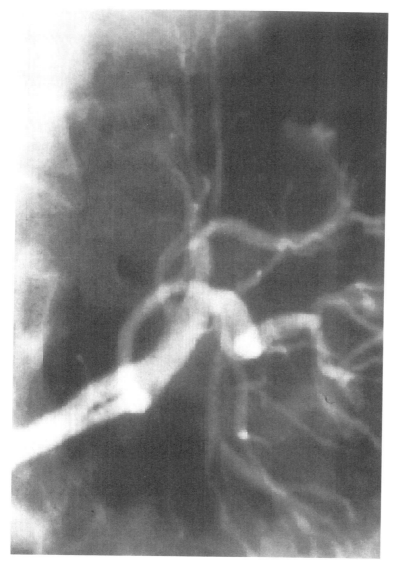

C

Figure 5 Continued.

Angioplasty balloon rupture prior to stent expansion has decreased as technology has improved. Most balloon rupture currently seen is due to the utilization of a balloon that is longer than the stent (Fig. 6). During early balloon inflation on the ends, the stent edges may lead to balloon puncture. Another source of balloon rupture is arterial calcification. A small number of balloons are defective from the time of manufacturing; these should be noted when negative pressure is applied during balloon preparation. Negative pressure should always be repeated after hand-mounting stents on to a previously inflated balloon.

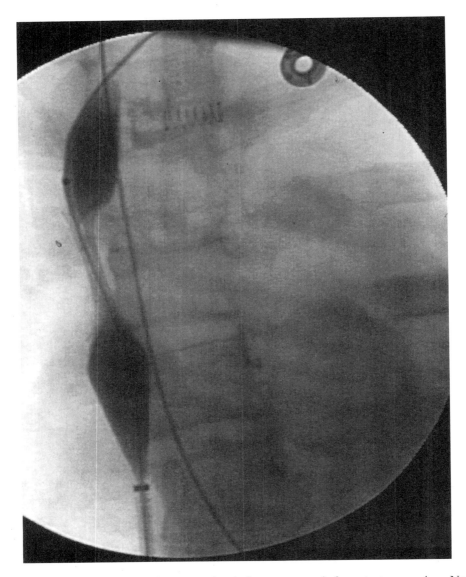

Figure 6 Fluoroscopy demonstrating balloon rupture before stent expansion. Note the excess balloon material beyond the ends of the stent.

When a balloon rupture occurs prior to stent expansion, several strategies may allow for successful completion of stent deployment. Rapid inflation of the balloon with hand pressure will often expand the stent enough to allow for balloon removal and replacement with a new balloon. However, occasionally hand inflation is not adequate and another method of balloon inflation, by connecting the balloon port to the contrast power injector filled with saline, will be necessary for adequate stent expansion. An injection larger than the balloon capacity at a flow rate of approximately 5 mL/s is usually successful. Other strategies include the following: if a 0.035 wire based system has been used, replacing the 0.035 wire with a 0.014/0.018 wire to utilized a coronary balloon for initial stent expansion, bringing the sheath or guide catheter to the end of the stent for support while te balloon is removed, or advancing the balloon out of the stent and advancing a coronary wire and balloon beside the original balloon shaft and enlarging the stent to allow for balloon removal.

VII. DEVICE EMBOLIZATION

There are multiple ways for whole devices such as stents or parts of devices such as wires and catheters, to embolize and complicate an angioplasty or stent procedure. Balloon material, wires, or ends of catheters can become embedded on the ends of the stent and be torn free (Fig. 7). Rarely is surgical exploration and removal the proper method of dealing

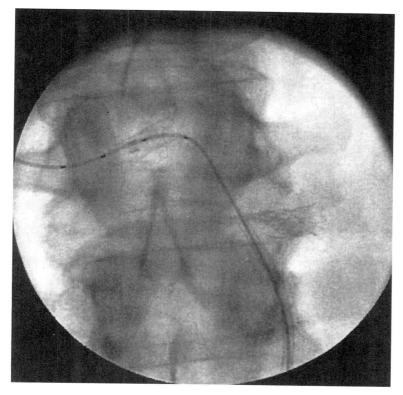

A

Figure 7 A. Fluoroscopy demonstrating the tip of an angiographic catheter that has been sheared off at the end of a renal artery stent. B. Fluoroscopy after placement of a 0.014 guidewire and coronary balloon to allow for removal of the catheter tip to the abdominal aorta. C. Fluoroscopy showing the catheter tip secured against the wall of the iliac artery by a balloon expandable stent.

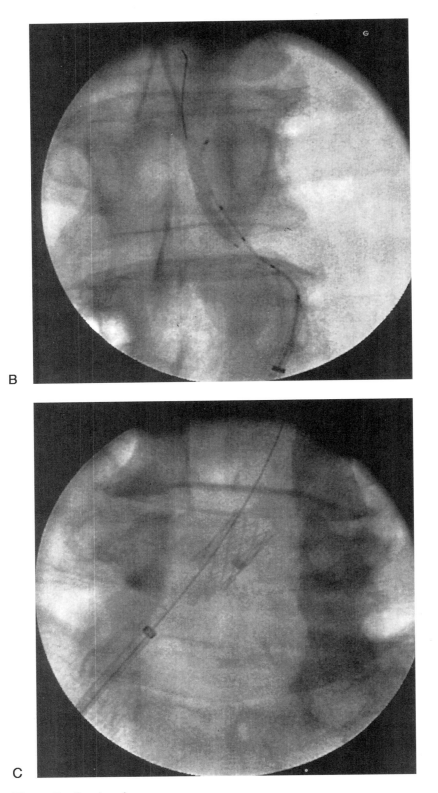

B

C

Figure 7 Continued.

with these events. The basis of treatment is controlling the embolized material for removal or trapping the material within another stent to allow for endothelialization. There are a number of devices and maneuvers for capturing loose stents or fractured catheters or wires (27). Vascular snare (Fig. 8) and grasping forceps are the most commonly used tools for capturing debris. The decision must then be made as to whether the debris can be removed without snagging on the arterial wall or the extravascular tissue. If the embolized material is flexible and smooth, such as a wire or catheter, it can usually be removed. However, stents that have become embolized should first be captured and then expanded in a more proximal vessel such as the iliac artery or trapped against the side of the aorta with a large self-expanding stent (Fig. 9).

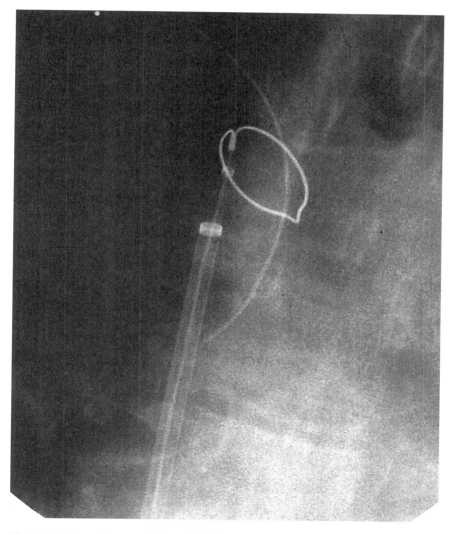

Figure 8 Vascular snare being utilized to secure a guidewire.

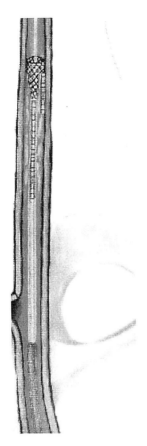

Figure 9 Schematic of a self-expanding stent being utilized to secure a embolized, nonexpanded stent against the arterial wall.

VIII. CONCLUSION

Though uncommon, complications of endovascular angioplasty and stenting may have devastating outcomes that can threaten limb and life. Adequate awareness of the complications inherent to specific vascular beds, as well as the ability and training to promptly recognize and treat complications as they arise, will allow the endovascular specialist to achieve excellent clinical outcomes.

ACKNOWLEDGMENT

I would like to thank Dr. Mark H. Wholey, UPMC Shadyside, Pittsburgh, PA, and Dr. Mark Burket, Medical College of Toledo, Toledo, OH, for graciously allowing the use of case examples.

REFERENCES

1. Axisa B, Fishwick G, Bolia A, et al. Complications following peripheral angioplasty. Ann R Coll Surg Engl 2002; 84:39–42.
2. Gardiner GA Jr, Meyerovitz MF, Stokes KR, et al. Complications of transluminal angioplasty. Radiology 1986; 159:201–208.
3. Henry M, Amor M, Ethevenor G, Henry I, Amicabile C, Beron R, et al. Palmaz stent placement in iliac and femoropopliteal arteries: Primary and secondary patency in 310 patients with 2–4 year follow-up. Radiology 1995; 197:167–174.
4. Gray BH, Olin JW. Limitations of percutaneous transluminal angioplasty with stenting for femoropopliteal arterial occlusive disease. Semin Vasc Surg 1997; 10:8–16.
5. Food and Drug Administration IntraCoil data: Cardiovascular and Radiological Health Advisory Board.
6. Tegtmeyer CJ, Hartwell GD, Selby JB, et al. Results and complications of angioplasty in aortoiliac disease. Circulation 1991; 83(suppl I):I-53–I-56.
7. Jorgensen B, Skovgaard N, Norgard J, et al. Percutaneous transluminal angioplasty in 226 iliac artery stenoses: Role of the superficial femoral artery for clinical success. Vasa 1992; 21:382–386.
8. Blum U, Gabelmann A, Redecker M, et al. Percutaneous recanalization of iliac artery occlusions: results of a prospective study. Radiology 1993; 189:536–540.
9. Gupta AK, Ravimandalam K, Rao VR, et al. Percutaneous balloon angioplasty for arteriosclerosis obliterans: Long term results. In: Yao JST, Perarce WH, eds. Techniques in Vascular Surgery. Philadelphia: Saunders, 1992:329–345.
10. Matsi PJ, Manninen HI. Complications of lower-limb percutaneous transluminal angioplasty: A prospective analysis of 410 procedures on 295 consecutive patients. Cardiovasc Intervent Radiol 1998; 21:361–366.
11. Burns BJ, Phillips AJ, Gox A, et al. The timing and frequency of complications after peripheral percutaneous transluminal angioplasty and iliac stenting: Is a change from inpatient to outpatient therapy feasible? Cardiovasc Intervent Radiol 2000; 23:452–456.
12. Kruse JR, Cragg AH. Safety of short stay observation after peripheral vascular intervention. J Vasc Intervent Radiol 2000; 11:45–49.
13. Bortslap A, Lampmann L. Balloon rupture and arteriovenous communication: A rare complication of transluminal angioplasty. Vasa 1993; 22:352–354.
14. Hunter D, Simmons R, Hulbert J. Antibiotics for radiology interventional procedures. Radiology 1988; 166:572–573.
15. Paddon AJ, Nicholson AA, Eltles DF, et al. Long-term follow-up of percutaneous balloon angioplasty in adult aortic coarctation. Cardiovasc Intervent Radiol 2000; 23:364–367.
16. Scheinert D, Ludwig J, Steinkamp HJ, et al. Treatment of cath induced iliac artery injuries with self-expanding endografts. J Endovasc Ther 2000; 7:213–220.
17. Lederman RJ, Mendelsohn FO, Santos R, et al. Primary renal artery stenting: Characteristics and outcomes after 363 procedures. Am Heart J 2001; 142:314–323.
18. Morris CS, Bonnevie GJ, Najarian KE. Nonsurgical treatment of acute iatrogenic renal artery injuries occurring after renal artery angioplasty and stenting. Am J Roentgenol 2001; 177:1353–1357.
19. Oltaenu B, Oltaenu C, Borelli C. Embolization of a perforation of a cortical renal artery occurring during percutatneous renal angioplasty. Eur Radiol 2000; 10:1357.
20. Ragg JL, Biamino G. Perforations in recanalization of arterial occlusions of the femoropopliteal area. Zentralbl Chir 2000; 125:34–41.
21. Beregi JP, Prat A, Willoteaux S, et al. Covered stents in the treatment of peripheral arterial aneurysms: Procedural results and mid term follow-up. Cardiovasc Intervent Radiol 1999; 22:13–19.

22. Bauermeisto G. Endovascular stent-grafting in the treatment of superficial femoral artery occlusive disease. J Endovasc Ther 2001; 8:315–320.

23. Schatz RA, Baim DS, Leon M, et al. Clinical experience with the Palmaz-Schatz coronary stent: Initial results of a multicenter study. Circulation 1991; 83:148–161.

24. Karrillon GJ, Morice MC, Benveniste E, et al. Intracoronary stent implantation without ultrasound guidance and with replacement of conventional anticoagulation by antiplatelet therapy: 30-day clinical outcome of the French Multicenter Registry. Circulation 1996; 94:1519–1527.

25. Zidar JP. Rationale for low-molecular weight heparin in coronary stenting. Am Heart J 1997; 134(suppl):S81–S87.

26. Tong FC, Cloft HJ, Joseph GS, et al. Abciximab rescue in acute carotid stent thrombosis. Am J of Neuroradiol 2000; 21:1750–1752.

27. Bartorelli AL, Fobbiocchif, Montarsi F, et al. Successful transcatheter management of Palmaz stent embolization after superior vena cava stenting. Cathet Cardiovasc Diagn 1995; 34:162–166.

38

Complications of Carotid Stenting

Ramtin Agah

University of Utah, Salt Lake City, Utah, U.S.A.

Patricia Gum and Jay S. Yadav

The Cleveland Clinic Foundation, Cleveland, Ohio, U.S.A.

I. INTRODUCTION

Stenting of the carotid artery is rapidly making the transition from an investigational tool to the primary treatment modality for symptomatic and asymptomatic carotid lesions. A key impetus behind this drive has been the significant reduction in the periprocedural complication rate associated with this technique. The most significant sequela of carotid stenting is the development of neurological deficit, described as small reversible deficits to frank large strokes. With more experience, the development of dedicated angioplasty equipment for the carotid bed and technological advances—including the development and utilization of embolic protection devices—the periprocedural complication rate (death, major and minor stroke) of 5–9% reported in the early series has been reduced to 2–3% currently (1–15). This significant reduction of neurological events associated with carotid artery stenting (CAS) is best understood by an in-depth review of the nature and causes of these complications.

II. PROCEDURAL COMPLICATIONS

A. Access-Related

1. Access

Early in the carotid stenting experience, the direct antegrade carotid approach was used in some patients to establish access (4,16). Even though this approach simplified the ability to access and intervene in the lesion, it had significant limitations, most significantly compression hematoma and a nidus for thrombus formation close to the stent. With the evolution of guide catheter technology specifically for percutaneous carotid intervention, the direct carotid access site has by and large been abandoned for the retrograde femoral approach.

Furthermore, the refinement in equipment has caused the access-size requirement to decrease over the past decade, with standard 9F sheath giving way to a 6F sheath or 8F guides for carotid stenting using the femoral approach. The initial experience with these larger sheaths was tainted with more frequent vascular complications, including arteriovenous fistulas, large hematomas, and retroperitoneal bleeding; but these have decreased in frequency and severity with the adoption of the smaller sheaths (4,5).

2. Guide Catheters

One of the major influences in the technical success of carotid stenting has been the evolution of the guide catheter. Indeed, the most common reason for "technical failure" early on was the inability to deliver a guide across a tortuous aortic arch. These technical limitations resulted in both lower success rates (5–15% failure rate) and also more complications due to plaque embolization and or dissection in the common carotid in the process of delivering the guide (1,4,15,17). The development of new guide catheters has minimized these issues, with recent series reporting a 98–100% technical success rate with minimal to no procedural complications related to guide delivery by the experienced operator (3,8,9,18) (Figs. 1 and 2).

B.   Lesion-Related Complications

1.   Cerebral Ischemia

Most patients tolerate transient occlusion of the blood flow to the respective hemisphere very well. This is especially true with present protocols of short balloon inflation during percutaneous transluminal angioplasty (PTA) and stenting. However, reports of episodes of loss of consciousness, seizure, and or transient ischemic attack (TIA) during balloon inflation still range from 1.5 to 6.2% (1,5,6). These events appear to be more common in patients with an incomplete circle of Willis and/or multiple stenotic and/or occlusive lesions in the contralateral supra-aortic territory (2) (Fig. 3). No long-term sequelae from these transient episodes of ischemia have been reported.

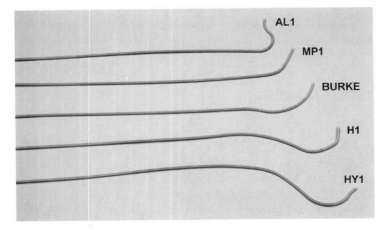

Figure 1   Guide catheters for carotid intervention.

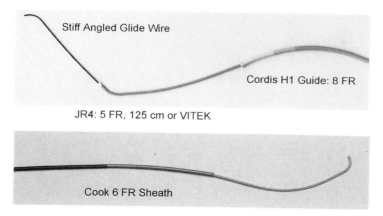

Figure 2 Telescoping diagnostic catheters through guide catheters.

2. Bradycardia and Hypotension

This is a relatively common phenomenon, reported in as many as half of all the patients undergoing CAS (5,19,20). The mechanism of this phenomenon is stimulation of the vagal nerve via the glossopharyngeal afferent fibers emanating from the carotid baroreceptors. Patients with previous carotid endarterectomy (CEA), who have commonly lost these neuroreceptors, are less susceptible to this reflex during carotid stenting for restenotic lesions. Furthermore, it has been suggested that this reflex is more common with inflation

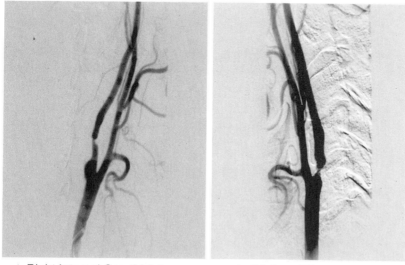

Right Internal Carotid Artery   Left Internal Carotid Artery

Figure 3 Severe bilateral carotid stenosis. Treatment of right internal carotid artery resulted in transient seizure and neurological deficit in patient.

of the balloon at the carotid bifurcation or the ostium of the internal carotid and utilization of larger balloons (20,21) (Fig. 4).

Early on in the CAS experience, transvenous pacemakers were routinely used to obviate these episodes of bradycardia (1). In the more recent series, atropine has been used primarily to treat these patients. Most of these episodes are self-limited and as such require no further treatment beyond atropine. However, in 10–19% of the patients, there can episodes of prolonged hypotension requiring pressor therapy beyond the initial 12 h (19, 20). In only one reported case has there been a need for placement of a permanent pacemaker after CAS in a patient with preexisting sick sinus syndrome (5). Again, even though most of these episodes are self-limited and relatively transient, the operator must be vigilant for such episodes and ready to treat them in patients with multiple supra-aortic lesions, who may be more susceptible to the consequences of cerebral ischemia with transient hypotension.

3. Acute Vessel Closure

These episodes, not unlike interventions in the coronary bed, are secondary to spasms, thrombosis, and dissections. Even though infrequent, the consequence of acute vessel closure in the carotid vascular bed can be catastrophic due to the relatively short period of ischemia that brain parenchyma can tolerate prior to irreversible injury. With routine stenting of the carotid lesion, better conformity of stent design to carotid architecture, and more optimal antiplatelet and antithrombotic regimen, the frequency of acute vessel closure has been significantly reduced, from 5 to 7% in the initial experience to below 1% in the current series (2,4,5,18).

4. Embolization

With the development of self-expanding stent technology for carotid applications, guide catheters, and optimization of the antiplatelet regimen, the number of neurological com-

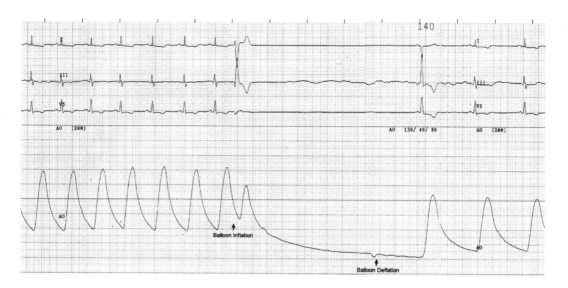

Figure 4 Rhythm and pressure recordings during postdilatation of a carotid artery stent.

plications due to carotid artery dissection, vasospasm, and stent thrombosis has declined; in the current era, distal embolization remains the major cause of neurological sequelae with CAS (Fig. 5).

It is estimated that routine PTA and stenting is associated with a 5% rate of embolization in most vascular beds. However, even though this rate of embolization may be acceptable in other vascular beds, the clinical sequelae of these events in the carotid vasculature is much more troublesome due to the nature of the target organ. Vascular surgeons have long recognized that patients with atherosclerosis often harbor a friable and unstable plaque at the carotid bifurcation, poised to shower the brain distally with microemboli (22,23). Several studies using transcranial Doppler have reported episodes of embolization during revascularization (22–26). In a study of 301 patients undergoing CEA, Ackerstaff et al. demonstrated that although microembolization is noticed in the majority (69%) of the patients, the overall rate of clinical sequelae in this cohort was only 5.7% (23). A smaller study of 39 patients undergoing CAS has also revealed a similar incidence of embolization to be operative with CAS, especially during balloon inflation and stent deployment (25).

At best, these noninvasive measures for microembolization appear sensitive but not specific for predicting clinical neurological events; as in all these studies, the incidence of clinical neurological sequelae is much lower than the rate of embolization (23,25). As such, the suggestion has been made that microembolization may have a threshold effect. Hence, even though the majority of patients may have embolization with a routine carotid procedure, it is only when these events reach a certain threshold that they may cause clinical sequelae. In favor of this hypothesis are data showing that there is a direct correlation between the frequency of embolization and the size of emboli and the rate of clinical neurological events (27).

Regardless of its exact pathophysiological mechanism, there has been a concerted effort to prevent and reduce the risk of embolization with carotid stenting. Initial pharmacological attempts included use of glycoprotein IIB-IIIa (GPIIB-IIIa) antagonist. However, this approach has had mixed results (28,29). In cases where intraprocedural embolization is associated with signs of a neurological event, the efficacy of intra-arterial

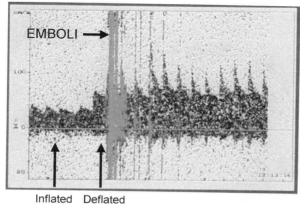

Figure 5 Transcranial Doppler recording of the middle cerebral artery during carotid angioplasty.

Table 1 The Results of Series Before and After Utilization of Emboli Protection Devices in CAS

| Study | Without protection | | With protection | |
	Stroke	Stroke/Death	Stroke	Stroke/Death
Al-Mubarak (18)			1% ($n = 162$)	2%
Reimers (8)			1.2% ($n = 84$)	1.2%
Tybler (27)			2.0% ($n = 54$)	2%
Henry (7)			2.2% ($n = 184$)	2.7%
Vitek (10)	6.0% ($n = 350$)	7.0% +		
Wholey (6)	4.2% ($n = 4757$)	5.1%		
Diethrich (4)	6.4% ($n = 110$)	7.4%		

fibrinolytic agents has not been demonstrated. In small case series there is no evidence of clinical benefit with such an approach, likely due to the plaque-like rather thrombotic nature of the emboli (30). In turn, mechanical means to prevent and "capture" these embolic particles have come of age. The number of these prevention devices is rapidly expanding; some that are currently in clinical use include the PercuSurge balloon wire, filter wire EX, the Angiogaurd basket device, and Neuro shield filters (7,8,18).

The results of the few published series using a variety of these distal protection devices have consistently reported a stroke rate (minor and major) of 1.2–2.0%, which is less than half the event rates commonly reported prior to the utilization of these devices (4.2–60%), as shown in Table 1 (7,8,18). However, the ability of these devices to reduce neurological sequelae of carotid stenting can only be conclusively determined when the results of current trials become available. Furthermore, the superiority of one device over another is hard to assess at the present time, but devices that do not totally occlude cerebral blood flow during deployment seem to be associated with higher procedural success rate, as patients with bilateral disease and an incomplete circle of Willis do not tolerate transient occlusion of the carotid artery (Fig. 6).

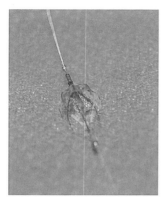 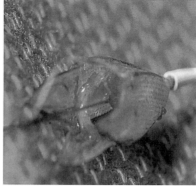

Figure 6 Two examples of an Angioguard filter with a large amount of embolic debris that resulted in slow flow through the filter during a carotid artery stenting procedure.

In addition, these prevention devices may not completely eliminate embolic events, since the embolization via external carotid to internal carotids and collaterals is possible in patients with severe stenosis, as suggested in at least one case report (31).

III. POSTPROCEDURAL

A. Stent Thrombosis

The incidence of stent thrombosis with carotid stenting has been declining since the early published series (5,15,26,32). The technical changes leading to this improvement can be summarized as follows.

1. Stent Apposition and Type

Early in the experience, most stents used in the carotid setting were hand-mounted balloon-expandable Palmaz stents. Although these stents offered radial strength, they were more susceptible to incomplete deployment and malposition, especially in the presence of calcification, tissue rigidity, and significant variations in diameter between the internal and common carotid arteries. These mechanical issues produced a substrate with higher subacute stent thrombosis rates (33). With the introduction of self-expanding nitinol stent technology, the ability to adequately appose stents in most if not all cases has significantly improved.

2. Anticoagulation Regimen

Early experience with carotid stenting preceded the current regimen of clopidogrel or ticlodopine to prevent subacute stent thrombosis. As such, the early experience with carotid intervention, like that with coronary intervention, suffered from episodes of subacute stent thrombosis due to lack of an optimized anticoagulation regimen. The present regimen of clopidogrel or ticlodopine dosing followed by a maintenance dose for a minimum of 1 month has significantly reduced such events.

B. Stent Deformation or Collapse

The Palmaz balloon-expandable stent had an incidence of stent deformation or collapse ranging from 8 to 16% (5,33–35). Equally alarming was the fact that most patients were asymptomatic and that these findings could not be discerned by noninvasive means such as ultrasound (33). This mechanical failure of the stent was attributed to external compression and plastic deformation of the stainless steel structure. The transition to self-expanding stents has overcome this problem, and balloon-expandable stents are no longer used in the carotid bifurcation (Fig. 7).

C. Neck Pain

Up to 4% of patients have developed neck pain postprocedure due to stretching of the carotid adventitia; furthermore there have also been reports of pain in the posterior aspect of the scalp, likely secondary to irritation of the greater auricular nerve (1). Most these episodes are self-limited and require only oral analgesics until the symptom subsides.

D. Hyperperfusion Cerebral Hemorrhage

Cerebral hyperperfusion syndrome is a recognized complication of CEA (36,37). There have been several case and small series reports of this complication also occurring with

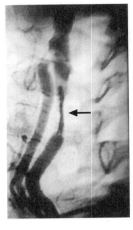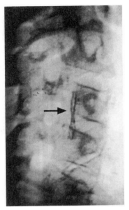

Figure 7 A crushed balloon-expandable Palmaz stent in the internal carotid artery and evidence of luminal compromise secondary to the stent deformity.

carotid stenting (38–40). By alleviating a high-grade symptomatic stenotic lesion, hyper-perfusion may occur as a result of a sudden, rapid increase in cerebral blood flow. This transient cerebral hyperemia can lead to headache, vomiting, arterial hypertension, confusion, seizures, focal neurological deficits, and subarachnoid hemorrhage. The exact predisposition is not known, but some have suggested risk factors including lesions with a significant pressure gradient across the stenosis with poor distal flow to the ipsilateral hemisphere, poor collateral blood flow, contralateral carotid occlusion, perioperative hypertension, and the use of anticoagulant and antiplatelet agents. The worst complica-tion associated with this syndrome is cerebral hemorrhage, occurring in less than 0.5% of the cases, based on a small series (40).

IV. LATE EVENTS

Remarkably there has been a minimal incidence of late events associated with carotid stenting. Early on with the predominant use of Palmaz stents, late events (TIA, death, stroke) beyond the initial 30 days were reported in 2.5% of the patients, possibly as a direct consequence of the frequent crush injuries with this stent (4,32). In more recent series with self-expanding stents, this complication has been reduced to 1.0% (6).

The rate of restenosis ranges from 2 to 5%. This rate is significantly lower than that in other vascular beds, likely due to the more focal nature of the lesion (bifurcation) and the large size of the arterial lumen (3–6). Most cases of restenosis are amenable to repeat angioplasty with good results, and there have even been case reports of gamma radiation therapy for refractory in-stent restenosis in this setting (41).

V. CONCLUSIONS

The dramatic rapid progress in CAS in the last decade has transformed this investigational tool into a viable treatment strategy. This transformation has been driven by technical and technological improvements in CAS, which, in turn, have resulted in the reduction of complications associated with this procedure. Ultimately results of ongoing trials will allow objective assessment of the safety and efficacy of this technique in everyday practice.

REFERENCES

1. Wholey MH, et al. Endovascular stents for carotid artery occlusive disease. J Endovasc Surg 1997; 4(4):326–338.
2. Theron JG, et al. Carotid artery stenosis: Treatment with protected balloon angioplasty and stent placement. Radiology 1996; 201(3):627–636.
3. Bonaldi G. Angioplasty and stenting of the cervical carotid bifurcation: Report of a 4-year series. Neuroradiology 2002; 44(2):164–174.
4. Diethrich EB, Ndiaye M, Reid DB. Stenting in the carotid artery: Initial experience in 110 patients. J Endovasc Surg 1996; 3(1):42–62.
5. Yadav JS, et al. Elective stenting of the extracranial carotid arteries. Circulation 1997; 95(2):376–381.
6. Wholey MH, et al. Global experience in cervical carotid artery stent placement. Catheter Cardiovasc Intervent 2000; 50(2):160–167.
7. Henry M, et al. Benefits of cerebral protection during carotid stenting with the PercuSurge GuardWire system: Midterm results. J Endovasc Ther 2002; 9(1):1–13.
8. Reimers B, et al. Cerebral protection with filter devices during carotid artery stenting. Circulation 2001; 104(1):12–15.
9. Cremonesi A, Castriota F. Efficacy of a nitinol filter device in the prevention of embolic events during carotid interventions. J Endovasc Ther 2002; 9(2):155–159.
10. Vitek J, Iyer S, Roubin G. Carotid stenting in 350 vessels: Problems faced and solved. J Invas Cardiol 1998; 10(5):311–314.
11. Laird JS, Pompa J. Procedural results and early clinical outcomes after carotid stent-supported angioplasty in high-risk patients. J Am Coll Cardiol 1997; 29(suppl):362A.
12. Iyer SR, Dorros G. Clinical significance of neurological events associated with carotid stenting. J Am Col Cardiol 1997; 29(suppl):362A.
13. Henry MA, Henry I. Endovascular treatment of atherosclerotic stenosis of the internal carotid. J Vasc Intervent Radiol 1998; 9(suppl):162.
14. Henry M, Amor M, Henry I. Endovascular treatment of atherosclerotic stenosis of the internal carotid. J Am Coll Cardiol 1997; 29(suppl):221a.
15. Iyer SSR, Yadav GS, Diethrisch EB. Angioplasty and stenting for extracranial carotid stenosis: Multicenter experience. Circulation 1996; 94(8):I-58.
16. Bergeron P, et al. Percutaneous stenting of the internal carotid artery: The European CAST I Study. Carotid Artery Stent Trial. J Endovasc Surg 1999; 6(2):155–159.
17. Dietz A, et al. Endovascular treatment of symptomatic carotid stenosis using stent placement: Long-term follow-up of patients with a balanced surgical risk/benefit ratio. Stroke 2001; 32(8): 1855–1859.
18. Al-Mubarak N, et al. Multicenter evaluation of carotid artery stenting with a filter protection system. J Am Coll Cardiol 2002; 39(5):841–846.
19. Gray WWH, Barret D. Hemodynamic consequences of carotid stenting. Circulation 1997; 96 (suppl):I-284.
20. Mendelsohn F, Weissman N, Crowley J. Hypotension associated with carotid stenting (HAWCS). Circulation 1997; 96(suppl):I-307.
21. Sivaguru ASG, Venables J. Blood pressure changes after carotid endarterectomy and angioplasty. Br J Surg 1997; 84:562–578.
22. Gaunt ME, et al. Clinical relevance of intraoperative embolization detected by transcranial Doppler ultrasonography during carotid endarterectomy: A prospective study of 100 patients. Br J Surg 1994; 81(10):1435–1439.

23. Ackerstaff RG, et al. The significance of microemboli detection by means of transcranial Doppler ultrasonography monitoring in carotid endarterectomy. J Vasc Surg 1995; 21(6):963–969.

24. Markus HS, et al. Carotid angioplasty. Detection of embolic signals during and after the procedure. Stroke 1994; 25(12):2403–2406.

25. Al-Mubarak N, et al. Effect of the distal-balloon protection system on microembolization during carotid stenting. Circulation 2001; 104(17):1999–2002.

26. McCleary AJ, et al. Cerebral haemodynamics and embolization during carotid angioplasty in high-risk patients. Br J Surg 1998; 85(6):771–774.

27. Tubler T, et al. Balloon-protected carotid artery stenting: relationship of periprocedural neurological complications with the size of particulate debris. Circulation 2001; 104(23):2791–2796.

28. Kapadia SR, et al. Initial experience of platelet glycoprotein IIb/IIIa inhibition with abciximab during carotid stenting: a safe and effective adjunctive therapy. Stroke 2001; 32(10):2328–2332.

29. Hofmann R, et al. Abciximab bolus injection does not reduce cerebral ischemic complications of elective carotid artery stenting: a randomized study. Stroke 2002; 33(3):725–727.

30. Wholey MH, et al. Management of neurological complications of carotid artery stenting. J Endovasc Ther 2001; 8(4):341–353.

31. Al-Mubarak N, et al. Embolization via collateral circulation during carotid stenting with the distal balloon protection system. J Endovasc Ther 2001; 8(4):354–357.

32. Roubin GS, et al. Carotid stent-supported angioplasty: a neurovascular intervention to prevent stroke. Am J Cardiol 1996; 78(3A):8–12.

33. Mathur A, et al. Palmaz stent compression in patients following carotid artery stenting. Cathet Cardiovasc Diagn 1997; 41(2):137–140.

34. Mathur AR, Dorros G, Iyer SJ. Palmaz stent collapse in patinets following carotid artery stenting. J Am Coll Cardiol 1997; 29(suppl):363a.

35. Johnson SP, et al. Stent deformation and intimal hyperplasia complicating treatment of a post-carotid endarterectomy intimal flap with a Palmaz stent. J Vasc Surg 1997; 25(4):764–768.

36. Jorgensen LG, Schroeder TV. Transcranial Doppler for detection of cerebral ischaemia during carotid endarterectomy. Eur J Vasc Surg 1992; 6(2):142–147.

37. Magee TR, Davies AH, Horrocks M. Transcranial Doppler evaluation of cerebral hyperperfusion syndrome after carotid endarterectomy. Eur J Vasc Surg 1994; 8(1):104–106.

38. McCabe DJ, Brown MM, Clifton A. Fatal cerebral reperfusion hemorrhage after carotid stenting. Stroke 1999; 30(11):2483–2486.

39. Chamorro A, et al. A case of cerebral hemorrhage early after carotid stenting. Stroke 2000; 31(3):792–793.

40. Meyers PM, et al. Cerebral hyperperfusion syndrome after percutaneous transluminal stenting of the craniocervical arteries. Neurosurgery 2000; 47(2):335–343; discussion 343–345.

41. Chan AW, et al. Carotid brachytherapy for in-stent restenosis. Catheter Cardiovasc Intervent 2003; 58(1):86–92.

39

Endovascular Access Complications

Mark A. Farber and Robert Mendes

University of North Carolina, Chapel Hill, North Carolina, U.S.A.

Since receiving approval by the U.S. Food and Drug Administration in 1999, endovascular treatment of abdominal aortic aneurysms has been increasingly performed, especially in high-risk patients. Despite this new approach, a significant number of patients are excluded for various reasons, including unacceptable anatomy and challenging access issues (1–4). Current delivery systems are designed with outer diameters in excess of 18 F (Table 1) for introduction of the primary device, and despite the recognized need for smaller, more flexible delivery catheters (5), they remain unavailable except in clinical trials and design stages. Therefore the current stiff introducer systems may result in access complications that need to be addressed during or after endovascular device implantation. Many times these complications are directly related to the extent of atherosclerotic occlusive disease within the iliac system. These complications fall into three categories: access failure, vessel compromise, and hemodynamic compromise; they result in conversion to open repair in 1–4% of procedures (6–8).

I. ACCESS FAILURE

Access complications may occur in as many as 20–30% of all implantations (9–11). Many of these events can be avoided by careful preoperative planning and patient selection. Iliac arteries less than 7.5 mm in diameter, which may be more difficult to traverse (12), are more common in women (13,14). Fairman (10) has reported that the incidence of these complications increases as the case difficulty and anatomic complexity increases. However, adjuvant maneuvers and procedures can, in many instances, result in endovascular salvage (10,15). Three characteristics that should be identified during planning to help minimize complications include (a) the caliber of access vessels (common iliac, external iliac, and common femoral); (b) the degree, location, extent and circumferential nature of calcium present; and (c) vessel tortuosity. Critical assessment of the iliac vessels should be undertaken with noncontrasted and contrast-enhanced computed tomography (CT) scans. By comparing these images, the degree of calcification can best be appreciated. Three-dimen-

Table 1 Catheter Sizes for Endovascular Device Delivery

Device	Outer diameter (F)[a]
Vanguard	20.5
Ancure	23.5
AneuRx	21
Talent	24–27
Excluder	18
Zenith	21
MEGS[b]	18

[a] 3F = 1 mm.
[b] Montefiore Endovascular Graft System.

sional reconstructions of CT scans or angiography can also be extremely useful in further evaluating the extent of aortoiliac occlusive disease and tortuosity of the vessels. Vessel tortuosity often compounds access issues even when stiffer wires—such as an Amplatz Super Stiff (Boston Scientific) or Lunderquist (Cook)—are employed.

Access issues may also be device-specific. Knowledge of device-specific characteristics such as flexibility, tip shape, hydrophilic nature, and delivery system profile is an integral part of becoming proficient at device insertion without complications. It is rare, however, that a single iliac vessel or device characteristic leads to an access failure. More commonly, the cause is a combination of factors acting synergistically to prevent device insertion—factors that were not appreciated at the time of initial evaluation.

When access failure occurs, there are several options to facilitate device insertion. These include dilatation, angioplasty, wire manipulation, conduits, and extra-anatomic bypass. One must keep in mind, however, that the goal is to completely exclude the aneurysm while providing adequate inflow for the extremity. In an attempt to limit the need for unnecessary associated procedures, the larger, straighter iliac vessel should be used as the primary site for deployment.

A. Stenosis Management

Access vessel stenosis is best addressed during endovascular prosthesis implantation. If angioplasty is attempted prior to stent-graft insertion, it may be difficult to obtain access across the lesion. In addition, dissections or complications may arise from the angioplasty itself, preventing future access and deployment of an endoprosthesis. This philosophy also applies to the use of stents, which may decrease the functional luminal diameter of the vessel or become dislodged during deployment of the device. Our approach is to treat iliac artery lesions with sequential dilatation with Coons (Cook) hydrophilic dilators at the beginning of the procedure to facilitate passage of the endoprosthesis and/or introducer sheaths. This is typically performed by gently advancing a 16F dilator through the lesion and then sequentially inserting larger dilators until the desired size is reached (usually 22–24F). Renal fascial dilators have been used in some cases; however, they are stiffer and constructed with a more abrupt tapered profile, rendering them less effective. Once the vessel has been successfully dilated, the device is inserted. After device deployment, angioplasty, if necessary, can be undertaken in a more protected environment with the stent-graft in place.

When recoil of the stenotic lesion exists, angioplasty may be necessary. When this is performed, vessel integrity and strength are compromised and can lead to vessel avulsion with removal of the sheath or delivery catheter. This occurs more frequently with iliac bifurcation lesions resulting in external iliac avulsion. Vessel disruption can occur in performing these dilatations or after device insertion, even though extreme care is taken. For this reason, detailed completion angiograms of the entire iliac system should be performed with small ($\leq$8F) sheaths in place to evaluate for residual hemodynamic lesions, dissection, or vessel rupture. Larger sheaths may occlude ruptures or mask a dissection that could be present. In addition, access wires should be the last intravascular component removed from the patient prior to closure of the femoral vessels. It is customary to leave the wire in place for several minutes after sheath removal and to monitor the patient for signs of bleeding from an undiagnosed access vessel complication.

When residual problems of dissection or stenosis exist, placement of a stent may be necessary to ensure stent-graft patency and viability of the extremity. If extravasation of contrast exists, then a covered stent or modular stent-graft extension should be deployed to prevent ongoing hemorrhage (see Sec. III, below).

B. Tortuosity

Vessel tortuosity is best negotiated by employing stiffer wires, as mentioned above. It is helpful to provide slow countertension on the wire while inserting the stent-graft. This reduces the potential for wire kinking, typically encountered with tortuous vessels. However, it should be noted that even though the vessel straightens with the use of stiff wires, the vessel will return to its original conformation after the wire is removed. This may influence exact endoprosthesis deployment and positioning. When tortuosity is felt to be the primary cause of access failure, several options exist to circumvent it. Many times insertion of an introducer sheath will alter the anatomy of the vessel and allow for passage of the device. If this is unsuccessful, Yano (16) has reported that digital dissection and straightening of the iliac artery has been successful in device insertion and reduces the risk of vessel rupture. Closed iliac endarterectomy with or without endoluminal bypass, brachofemoral access ("body-flossing"), or an iliac conduit can also be utilized to facilitate device insertion (16–18). Each of these options carries its own risks.

C. Iliac Conduits

The use of iliac conduits has been previously described (16,19) and is typically reserved to facilitate device insertion in patients who have both severe occlusive disease and tortuosity. Retroperitoneal exposure of the iliac vessel can be accomplished under regional anesthesia if necessary. After exposure of the common and external iliac vessels an 8- or 10-mm prosthetic graft is sewn onto the iliac artery above the level of the critical stenosis or tortuosity. Generally Dacron is preferred for the prosthetic material, since it can more easily be secured around the device or introducer sheath. Because of pelvic anatomy, insertion of the device directly through the retroperitoneal incision is difficult and involves maneuvering at awkward angles. To overcome this problem, the conduit is typically routed to the groin and brought out under the inguinal ligament. In this way it can also be used as an iliofemoral bypass if desired. Care must be taken in traversing the anastomosis to avoid disruption, and it is generally preferred to place a large introducer sheath at the onset of device deployment to prevent excess manipulation of the anastomosis.

D. Brachial Artery Catheterization

The brachial approach is an alternative option. When vessels cannot be traversed in a retrograde fashion, a wire and protection catheter can be placed from the left brachial approach (17). The wire is typically snared and brought out of the ipsilateral common femoral artery. By placing the wire under tension at both ends, the endoprosthesis is inserted more easily through tortuous vessels. While the brachial approach allows insertion of devices that may otherwise never have been placed, it is not without risks. Left brachial artery trauma and avulsion have been reported, and it also subjects the patient to a higher risk of stroke, although there is no report of this in the literature associated with endovascular aneurysm repair (20).

II. VESSEL COMPROMISE

Vessel rupture can occur after attempted angioplasty or subsequent to device insertion. Avulsion of an iliac vessel is associated with larger introducers and introducer withdrawal. In inserting these large devices, it is important to use fluoroscopic guidance of the iliac vessels to avoid inadvertent perforation. When resistance is encountered, forcing the device should be avoided. If avulsion or rupture occurs, it is important to maintain wire access across the region of concern. Immediate availability of aortic and large iliac balloons is a necessary part of safe endovascular abdominal aortic aneurysm (AAA) procedures. Over-the-wire balloon insertion is used to convert an emergent situation into a controlled one. The balloon should be centered across the injury and dilute contrast should be used for balloon inflation. This allows for visualization of the balloon placement while still allowing for a rapid deflation of the balloon. Hypogastric artery avulsion is rare but typically requires exposure and either ligation or reimplantation.

Once control of the situation has been obtained, management can proceed with careful consideration to the sizes and types of devices needed. For vessel disruption, either modular stent-graft components or covered stents (Wallgrafts, Boston Scientific; or ViaBahn, W. L. Gore & Associates) can be used. Wallgrafts seem better suited for more tortuous vessels and external iliac lesions. When an avulsion occurs, the status of the hypogastric artery and potential for common iliac seal must be evaluated. Of note, hypogastric artery avulsion may be difficult to control with simple balloon tamponade. Often, placement of the primary stent-graft may exclude the injured vessel segment. If an adequate seal has occurred above the perforation, the stent-graft can be extended down to the common femoral vessels and an endoluminal anastomosis performed. If this is not feasible, the vessels can be exposed with a retroperitoneal incision and bypass grafting performed as needed. When a bypass graft cannot be performed due to a severely damaged or aneurysmal vessel, then ligation with a femorofemoral bypass can be employed to reestablish limb blood flow.

Advanced techniques for endovascular placement of a common iliac occlusion device and crossover femorofemoral bypass exist; however this option should be reserved for the more experience user until commercially available occlusion device are available.

III. HEMODYNAMIC COMPROMISE

Although hemodynamic compromise can occur anywhere within the limbs of an endovascular endoprosthesis, it arises most commonly within the native iliac vessels. Unsupported devices may kink within tortuous vessels and require placement of intragraft stents. The reported use intragraft stents for unsupported devices approaches 30% (21,22). For supported devices, molding and angioplasty should be performed when necessary. If needed, bilateral pull-through or groin pressures can be measured to help determine whether a hemodynamic lesion exists. In addition, multiple views of the iliac vein can help to localize residual stenosis. Sometimes limitation of flow is caused by dissections distal to the endograft. It is important to evaluate the iliac vessels without large sheaths in place to avoid obscuring an iliac vessel complication. Dissections and vessel stenosis that are resistant to angioplasty are typically best treated with stent placement. Choice of stent type is determined by the length of the lesion, vessel tortuosity, and vessel size.

A. Common Femoral Artery Disease

Most patients with aortic aneurysms have associated atherosclerotic disease of the common femoral vessels, which predisposes them to injury during endovascular aneurysm repair (23). Injury to the femoral artery can occur in many of patients from repeated insertion, withdrawal, and deployment of devices and sheaths. Disease is often worse at the femoral bifurcation than at the level of the inguinal ligament. For this reason a high exposure of the common femoral artery as it emerges from underneath the inguinal ligament is preferred. As a result, femoral artery reconstructions may be necessary, requiring standard vascular techniques. For device insertion, the choice of a longitudinal versus transverse arteriotomy is dictated by the extent of atherosclerotic disease present. For vessels in this region that are heavily diseased, a longitudinal arteriotomy is preferred, so that patch closure with or without endarterectomy can be performed more easily. Focal dissections of the common femoral vessel occur occasionally, and careful inspection of the posterior wall of the vessel should be performed prior to closure. If necessary, tacking stitches should be placed or endarterectomy performed to ensure adequate lower extremity blood flow. In rare cases of severe disease or concomitant femoral aneurysmal disease, interpostion grafting can be used for reconstruction. This approach, instead of routine or patch closure, may also be necessary when large or multiple components are inserted through the femoral vessels. Prosthetic material is often used for these conditions; however, autologous vein is also an option.

When inflow or common femoral repairs are performed, it is advisable to follow patients closely for vessel occlusion or stenosis during the postoperative period. May has reported a 9% incidence of acute lower extremity ischemia associated with endovascular aneurysm repair (24). Acceleration times (25) and duplex inspection are an invaluable tool in this region and can help detect problems before a clinical emergency develops.

Percutaneous approaches for contralateral limb management have been described (26) with complications. Complications include vessel occlusion or disruption, embolic complications, and pseudoaneurysm formation. These may occur at the completion of the procedure or during follow-up. In light of the minimal complication rate from common femoral artery exposure, we prefer to perform bilateral femoral artery exposures to avoid these complications. As newer smaller devices are introduced, this philosophy may need to be reevaluated.

Embolic complication can occur from the access vessels; however, this is rare. Decreased distal perfusion is more often the result of a dissection or common femoral artery complication. If embolic complications do occur, lower extremity angiography and thrombectomy can be performed at the completion of the procedure. Adequate heparinization should be maintained to avoid thrombotic complications during the procedure.

IV. CONCLUSION

Access complications usually involve a combination of iliac calcification, tortuosity, and stenosis, which can be identified with preoperative imaging. While the presence of any one of these aspects can easily be overcome, their combination can lead to technical failure and misadventures during the procedure. Carefully planned endovascular techniques should be employed to allow for safe device insertion. High-quality angiography and analysis of the iliac vessels allows for early recognition of these complications. Safe repair can often be achieved using endovascular techniques; however, conversion to open surgical intervention may occasionally be required.

REFERENCES

1. Blum U, Voshage G, Lammer J, Beyersdorf F, Tollner D, Kretschmer G, Spillner G, Polterauer P, Nagel G, Holzenbein T. Endoluminal stent-grafts for infrarenal abdominal aortic aneurysms. N Engl J Med 1997; 336:13–20.
2. Collin J. Transluminal aortic aneurysm replacement. Lancet 1995; 346:457–458.
3. Moore WS. The role of endovascular grafting technique in the treatment of infrarenal abdominal aortic aneurysm. Cardiovasc Surg 1995; 3:109–114.
4. Armon MP, Yusuf SW, Latief K, Whitaker SC, Gregson RH, Wenham PW, Hopkinson BR. Anatomical suitability of abdominal aortic aneurysms for endovascular repair. Br J Surg 1997; 84:178–180.
5. Carpenter JP, Baum RA, Barker CF, Golden MA, Mitchell ME, Velazquez OC, Fairman RM. Impact of exclusion criteria on patient selection for endovascular abdominal aortic aneurysm repair. J Vasc Surg 2001; 34:1050–1054.
6. Buth J, Laheij RJ. Early complications and endoleaks after endovascular abdominal aortic aneurysm repair: Report of a multicenter study. J Vasc Surg 2000; 31:134–146.
7. Stelter W, Umscheid T, Ziegler P. Three-year experience with modular stent-graft devices for endovascular AAA treatment. J Endovasc Surg 1997; 4:362–369.
8. Jacobowitz GR, Lee AM, Riles TS. Immediate and late explantation of endovascular aortic grafts: The endovascular technologies experience. J Vasc Surg 1999; 29:309–316.
9. Zarins CK, White RA, Schwarten D, Kinney E, Diethrich EB, Hodgson KJ, Fogarty TJ. AneuRx stent graft versus open surgical repair of abdominal aortic aneurysms: Multicenter prospective clinical trial. J Vasc Surg 1999; 29:292–305; discussion, 306–308.
10. Fairman RM, Velazquez O, Baum R, Carpenter J, Golden MA, Pyeron A, Criado F, Barker C. Endovascular repair of aortic aneurysms: Critical events and adjunctive procedures. J Vasc Surg 2001; 33:1226–1232.
11. Wolf YG, Fogarty TJ, Olcott CI, Hill BB, Harris EJ, Mitchell RS, Miller DC, Dalman RL, Zarins CK. Endovascular repair of abdominal aortic aneurysms: Eligibility rate and impact on the rate of open repair. J Vasc Surg 2000; 32:519–523.
12. Naslund TC, Edwards WH Jr, Neuzil DF, Martin RS III, Snyder SO Jr, Mulherin JL Jr, Failor M, McPherson K. Technical complications of endovascular abdominal aortic aneurysm repair. J Vasc Surg 1997; 26:502–509; discussion 509–510.
13. Fleischmann D, Hastie TJ, Dannegger FC, Paik DS, Tillich M, Zarins CK, Rubin GD. Quantitative determination of age-related geometric changes in the normal abdominal aorta. J Vasc Surg 2001; 33:97–105.
14. Velazquez OC, Larson RA, Baum RA, Carpenter JP, Golden MA, Mitchell ME, Pyeron A, Barker CF, Fairman RM. Gender-related differences in infrarenal aortic aneurysm morphologic features: Issues relevant to Ancure and Talent endografts. J Vasc Surg 2001; 33:S77–S84.
15. Chuter TA, Reilly LM, Kerlan RK, Sawhney R, Canto CJ, Ring EJ, Messina LM. Endovascular repair of abdominal aortic aneurysm: Getting out of trouble. Cardiovasc Surg 1998; 6:232–239.
16. Yano OJ, Faries PL, Morrissey N, Teodorescu V, Hollier LH, Marin ML. Ancillary techniques to facilitate endovascular repair of aortic aneurysms. J Vasc Surg 2001; 34:69–75.
17. Criado FJ, Wilson EP, Abul-Khoudoud O, Barker C, Carpenter J, Fairman R. Brachial artery

catheterization to facilitate endovascular grafting of abdominal aortic aneurysm: Safety and rationale. J Vasc Surg 2000; 32:1137–1141.

18. Wain RA, Lyon RT, Veith FJ, Marin ML, Ohki T, Suggs WA, Lipsitz E. Alternative techniques for management of distal anastomoses of aortofemoral and iliofemoral endovascular grafts. J Vasc Surg 2000; 32:307–314.

19. White GH, May J, McGahan T, Yu W, Waugh RC, Stephen MS, Harris JP. Historic control comparison of outcome for matched groups of patients undergoing endoluminal versus open repair of abdominal aortic aneurysms. J Vasc Surg 1996; 23:201–211; discussion 211–212.

20. Lin PH, Bush RL, Weiss VJ, Dodson TF, Chaikof EL, Lumsden AB. Subclavian artery disruption resulting from endovascular intervention: Treatment options. J Vasc Surg 2000; 32:607–611.

21. Amesur NB, Zajko AB, Orons PD, Makaroun MS. Endovascular treatment of iliac limb stenoses or occlusions in 31 patients treated with the ancure endograft. J Vasc Intervent Radiol 2000; 11:421–428.

22. Parent FN GV III, Meier GH III, et al. Endograft limb occlusion and stenosis after Ancure endovascular abdominal aneurysm repair. J Vasc Surg 2002; 35:686–690.

23. Henretta JP, Karch LA, Hodgson KJ, Mattos MA, Ramsey DE, McLafferty R, Sumner DS. Special iliac artery considerations during aneurysm endografting. Am J Surg 1999; 178:212–218.

24. May J, White GH, Waugh R, Stephen MS, Chaufour X, Yu W, Harris JP. Adverse events after endoluminal repair of abdominal aortic aneurysms: A comparison during two successive periods of time. J Vasc Surg 1999; 29:32–37; discussion 38–39.

25. Burnham SJ, Jaques P, Burnham CB. Noninvasive detection of iliac artery stenosis in the presence of superficial femoral artery obstruction. J Vasc Surg 1992; 16:445–451; discussion 452.

26. Traul DK, Clair DG, Gray B, O'Hara PJ, Ouriel K. Percutaneous endovascular repair of infrarenal abdominal aortic aneurysms: A feasibility study. J Vasc Surg 2000; 32:770–776.

40

Device Failure

Tikva S. Jacobs and Michael L. Marin

Mount Sinai School of Medicine, New York, New York, U.S.A.

Larry H. Hollier

Louisiana State University Health Sciences Center School of Medicine, New Orleans, Louisiana, U.S.A.

I. INTRODUCTION

Parodi performed the first endovascular repair of an abdominal aortic aneurysm over a decade ago (1). More than 25,000 aortic stent grafts have since been deployed worldwide, and preliminary results have been promising. However further follow-up and close monitoring to determine the long-term safety and efficacy of these devices has been recommended (2–6). Problems with deployment, stent-graft migration, endoleak, material failure, and aneurysm rupture have all been reported (7–11). Many of these problems were seen with first-generation stent grafts, suggesting parallel learning curves between the surgeons, device engineers, and manufacturers. Technical and mechanical device problems have been addressed and individual implants improved. However, new problems continue to be discovered as patients with second-generation stent grafts approach midterm follow-up. As an increasing number of explanted grafts become available for analysis, new and device-specific material failure is being identified.

Device fatigue remains one of the most concerning modes for potential procedure failure, encompassing the breakdown of the intrinsic mechanical parts of the stent graft. It is often difficult to identify device fatigue, as patients are typically asymptomatic at the time of presentation. Many of the first identified stent fractures were initially recognized within explanted stent-graft devices that had been removed for evidence of aneurysm expansion or recovered at autopsy. The challenges of identifying material failure have made a true understanding of the magnitude of the problem difficult. Moreover the clinical significance of many identified failures is unknown.

The purpose of this chapter is to familiarize the reader with the more common modes of material failure associated with individual devices and to dicuss the frequency, cause, and significance of such material failures, as we have learned about these through our institution's own experience.

Multiple devices have been implanted in patients worldwide; even though some are no longer available for clinical use, it is important to educate oneself about them so that their failure can be recognized early and monitored closely. Prior to discussing endovascular stent-graft failure, this chapter first offers a short review of the techniques used for endovascular repair and a description of the actual devices used, so as to help the reader understand where and why these devices fail.

II. BACKGROUND

A. Techniques for Endovascular AAA and TAA Repair

The four techniques used to deploy endovascular stent grafts in the repair of abdominal aortic aneurysms (AAAs) are described in detail elsewhere (12–17). In brief, they are aortoaortic, aorto-uni-iliac, bifurcated-modular, and bifurcated-unibody (Fig. 1A to E). Although the aortoaortic tube graft is seldom used for primary AAA repair today, it is used to repair thoracic aortic aneurysms (TAAs). The technique chosen for such repairs is dependent on the anatomy of the aorta and the iliac arteries as well as the patient's clinical presentation and its relevance to specific protocols. A variety of devices are deployed using these four techniques. Some of these devices are no longer available for clinical use, while others are currently under investigation by the U.S. Food and Drug Administration (FDA) and still others are being developed. What these devices have in common is the combination of a metallic stent and a material graft. However, how they differ helps to explain not only why some become subject to fatigue but also where and how.

B. Devices for AAA and TAA Repair

1. Individually Fabricated Endovascular Graft

The first endovascular stent grafts were "homemade" devices, fabricated by individual vascular surgeons. The first abdominal aortic aneurysm treated with an endovascular stent-graft repair was constructed by Parodi using a custom-made device comprising a Palmaz stent attached to a polyester tubular graft (Barone Industries, Buenos Aires, Argentina) (18). Similar endovascular stent-graft devices were individually constructed throughout the world using components designed for other purposes, including the Chuter device, Sydney endovascular graft and the Volodos/Kharkov Institute Device (19,20). At our institution, a modified Parodi endovascular AAA device was fabricated. It was constructed from a thin-walled, funnel-shaped polytetrafluoroethylene (PTFE) graft sutured to a stainless steel Palmaz stent (Cordis Endovascular, a Johnson & Johnson Company) (Fig. 2). The Palmaz stents used for device anchoring are balloon-expandable and made of 316L stainless steel (20).

2. Commercially Fabricated Endovascular Devices

As endovascular repair of aortic aneurysms began to gain acceptance in the vascular community, commercially fabricated stent-graft devices were developed and FDA trials began. Discussing the components needed for the "ideal" endovascular stent graft seems relatively straightforward; however, turning those ideas into reality is more challenging (21,22). Through the years, multiple devices were introduced for experimental use and individual devices underwent numerous revisions. The first stent graft to undergo clinical trials in the United States was the EVT/Guidant Endovascular stent graft.

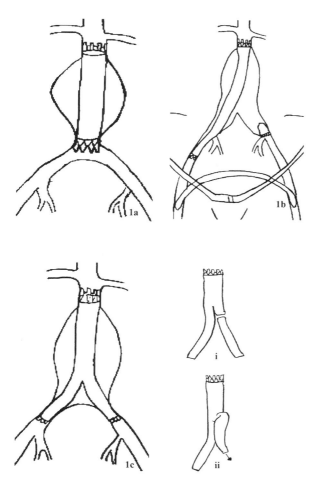

Figure 1 Artist illustration of techniques for endovascular repair of abdominal aortic aneurysms. a. Aorto-aortic tube graft. b. Aortouni-iliac reconstruction. An aortouni-common or external iliac graft is inserted. A femorofemoral bypass combined with a contralateral common iliac artery occluder is used to complete the reconstruction. c. Endovascular bifurcated aortic graft reconstruction. Two techniques are suggested. i. Modular bifurcated reconstruction employing an aortic body and contralateral limb inserted separately; ii. Unibody bifurcated reconstruction employing a single endograft and a cross femoral wire to bring one limb to the contralateral extremity.

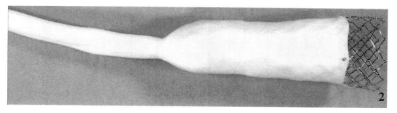

Figure 2 A Parodi-type handmade balloon expandable stent grafting system. This graft is composed of a Palmaz balloon expandable stent sutured to a tapered polytetrafluoroethylene graft.

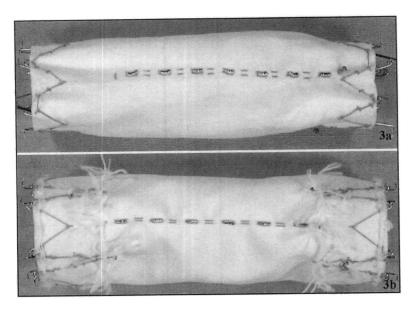

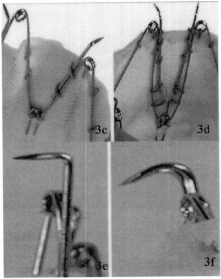

Figure 3 The Guidant Ancure endovascular grafting system. a. The first generation device produced by the Endovascular Technologies Corporation was composed of a polyester woven graft with an attachment apparatus at either end. The attachment devices are constructed, of elgiloy metal bent to form Z configured hooks. b. The device was later modified into its current form employing a varied attachment system with the same principle of Z configured metal coupled with penetrating hooks for aortic fixation. Loose polyester fibers were left on the outside of the revised graft to stimulate endoluminal sealing. c. The initial EVT graft permitted the fixation hooks to be laser welded onto the Z-configured stent spring. d. Separation of the hooks from the Z stent resulted in a design modification where by each hook was sutured onto the surface of the graft directly (see also Fig. 10). e. The original EVT hook had an acute angle at its junction point with the main hook shaft. f. Fractures occurred at this angle necessitating a more gradual curve in the hook structure.

EVT (Endovascular Technologies)/Guidant-Ancure Device.   The EVT stent graft comprises a polyester fabric vascular graft hand-sewn to self-expanding Z-configured elgiloy (cobalt-chromium and nickel) metal stents at the proximal and distal attachment sites (Fig. 3). The aortic attachment portion of this device has eight angled hooks to aid in the fixation of the graft to the aortic wall. In the initial model, eight individual shanks with hooks at the distal end were laser-welded to the zigzag stent rings (Fig. 3C). Hook fractures were encountered during the phase 2 trial, prompting modification of this design. Presently there are four V-shaped shanks containing two hooks each, which are sewn to the polyester graft (Fig. 3D). The shape of the hook has been modified as well to incorporate a gradual angle rather than a sharp right angle, which is prone to fracture (15,23, 24) (Fig. 3E and F). This device is available in bifurcated, aorto-uni-iliac, and tubular configurations.

Vanguard Device.   The Vanguard (Boston Scientific Inc., Nadile, MA) endovascular stent graft is a modification of the Stentor stent-graft system (25). It is modular graft available for tube or bifurcated repairs. It comprises a flexible, self-expanding prosthesis constructed of a nitinol wire frame coverd by a thin-walled woven polyester fabric. The Vanguard stent is composed of independent rows of zigzag nitinol wires that are held together by polypropylene suture ties. These ties are located at the apex of the metal bends, allowing movement of the individual nitinol stent rows to accommodate for arterial angulation. The graft is a seamless low-porosity polyester fabric attached at the proximal and distal ends of the device by polyester sutures (Fig. 4). There are small barbs on the proximal end of the graft to assist in anchoring the device to the aortic wall (2,6,26).

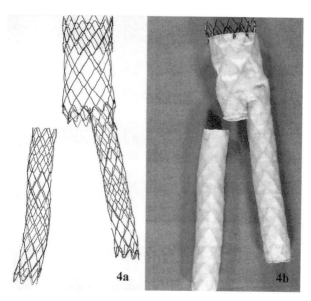

Figure 4   The Boston Scientific Vanguard endovascular grafting system. a. The endoskeleton of the Vanguard system is composed of Z configured nitinol wire fixed at the apices by polypropylene sutures. An aortic body and ipsilateral limb are displayed with a contralateral iliac stent limb. b. The nitinol skeleton is covered with a thin walled polyester graft in the complete prosthesis for clinical use.

Talent Device. The Talent (Medtronic AVE/World Medical Manufacturing, Minn., MN) device is composed of a series of self-expanding serpentine nitinol stents, several of which are connected to a longitudinal nitinol bar. Each stent is sutured over its entire length to a polyester graft. The fabric material is fixed to the outside of the nitinol stents in the aortic body, while the stents are on the outside of the graft, on the limbs. The proximal aortic fixation device can be an uncovered nitinol stent, allowing for transrenal fixation (Fig. 5). The Talent endovascular stent-graft system has a configuration designed for tube, aorto-uni-iliac, or bifurcated graft use and can be manufactured in custom-made sizes designed on the basis of computed tomographic (CT) or angiographic measurements (26,27).

The AneuRx Device. The AneuRx (Medtronics) endovascular device is a self-expanding modular bifurcated stent-graft system (Fig. 6). The modular component consists of a thin-walled noncrimped woven polyester graft supported by suture-fixed individual 1-cm nitinol rings, forming an exoskeleton. The nitinol stents are laser-cut out of nitinol hypotubing and sewn to the graft with polyester sutures (4,20).

Gore Device. The Gore Excluder (W.L. Gore Associated, Inc.) is a modular system with a self-expanding Nitinol exoskeleton attached to an ePTFE graft internally (Fig. 7). Angled wired barbs are attached to the proximal end of the main device to assist in anchoring the device to the aortic wall. Polyethelene tape attaches the ePTFE graft to the nitinol exoskeleton to avoid sutures or suture holes in the graft material (5,20).

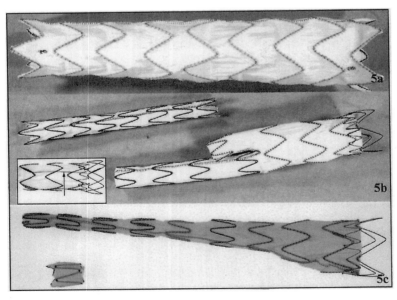

Figure 5 The Talent endovascular grafting system. a. The Talent endovascular tube graft is composed of Z configured nitinol stents covered on the external surface with a polyester graft. Each Z shaped stent is sutured completely to the surface of the fabric material with suture material. b. The Talent modular bifurcated stent graft system. A main aortic body containing an ipsilateral limb is joined with a contralateral limb to reconstruct the aortic bifurcation. Note in the inset the longitudinal bar present in the aortic body seen with trans-illuminated imaging. c. Aortouni-iliac stent graft system. A tapered Talent endograft is displayed along with a single complete polyester encapsulated Z stent, which is used for the contralateral common iliac occlusion.

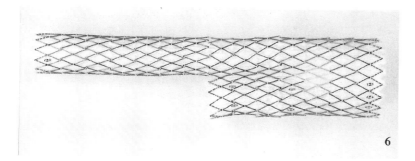

Figure 6 The AneuRx endovascular graft. The AneuRx graft is composed of individual rings of nitinol laser cut into nitinol hypotubing. Each of the Z rings is sutured to the fabric graft by a blanket stitch. A modular bifurcated device is demonstrated.

The Cordis LP Device. The modular Cordis LP bifurcated endvascular stent graft consists of a nitinol stent sutured within a seamless woven polyester bifurcated graft (Fig. 8A). The senitinol stents are laser-cut from seamless nitinol hypotubing and heat-treated to achieve proper thermal properties. The nitinol is attached to the fabric using multiple polyester point and blanket sutures. The transrenal attachment device has broad open spaces that permit stent-graft fixation across the renal arteries, and six to eight fixation barbs angled caudad at its base at the proximal end of the graft fabric to penetrate the aortic wall

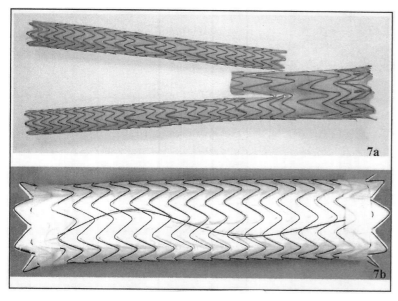

Figure 7 The W.L. Gore TAG™ endovascular graft for thoracic aortic aneurysms. This endovascular graft is constructed of expanded polytetrafluoroethylene fabric with external Z configured nitinol wire support. The nitinol wire frame is fixed to the outer surface of the polytetrafluoroethylene graft by means of ePTFE membrane.

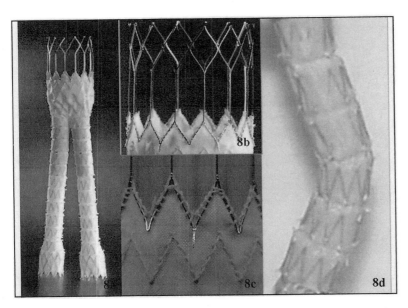

Figure 8 The Cordis Quantum LP™ bifurcated endvascular stentgraft system. a. The Quantum LPTM is comprised of nitinol stents sutured within a seamless woven polyester bifurcated graft. The nitinol stents are laser cut from seamless nitinol hypotubing and heat-treated to achieve proper thermal material properties. The nitinol is attached to the fabric using multiple polyester point and blanket sutures. b. The transrenal attachment device has broad open spaces that permit stentgraft fixation across the renal arteries. c. Six to eight fixation barbs angled caudad at its base at the proximal end of the graft fabric to assist in aortic fixation. d. Along the length of the stump the graft has circumferential crimps or fabric hinges that form five discrete pockets for fixation of the sinusoidal nitinol Z-stents. This configuration allows flexibility without kinking and allows the legs to absorb cyclic motion in the unstented areas.

below the renal arteries and firmly anchor the stent graft in position (Fig. 8B,C). There are two 5-cm equal-length stumps at the end of the aortic body stent into which the iliac leg prostheses are inserted and permanently fixed. Along the length of the stump, the graft has circumferential crimps or fabric hinges that form five discrete pockets for fixation of the short sinusoidal nitinol Z stents. This configuration allows flexibility without kinking and allows the legs to absorb cyclic motion in the unstented areas (Fig. 8D). The iliac limbs are designed to overlap with in the stump legs of the aortic prosthesis a minimum of 2 cm and a maximum of 5 cm (28).

Thoracic Aortic Stentgrafts. Two thoracic stent grafts are commonly used, the Talent device (Medtronic AVE/World Medical Manufacturing, Minn., MN) and the TAG (W.L. Gore Associates, Inc.). The Talent stentgraft is a tubular device that is identical in design to the one previously described (see above). The TAG consists of self-expanding Z-shaped nitinol stents covered internally by ePTFE material. The stent members are fixed to the graft without sutures by means of a continuous ePTFE membrane. Both designs have a longitudinal bar running the length of the stent graft. Multiple overlapping stent grafts may be used with either device to achieve adequate length to exclude an aneurysm (29–31).

C. Evaluation of Material Failure

Material failure has been a problem since early first-generation stent-graft trial. In 1996, Moore reported metal fractures in the EVT device. The patient had a persistent endoleak 12 months postimplantation and underwent open repair. At exploration, proximal and distal hook fractures were found. Review of this patient's follow-up plain films revealed evidence of hook fracture at the 6-month follow-up. This fracture led to a retrospective review of all plain films at that institution. Nine patients were found to have fractures in one or more of the metal components of the attachment system. Of these, only one patient went on to require open conversion 18 months after initial implantation (24).

In 1997, Blum et al. and Mialhe et al. reported early results of the Stentor endovascular stent graft. During this time, "leaks" caused by tears in the polyester graft along its suture line were found at angiography. While some of these leaks sealed spontaneously, others required secondary procedures and were corrected with a second stent graft (25,32). Both of these first-generation stent-graft devices underwent redesign. EVT was acquired by Guidant, who redesigned the metal fixation device as described earlier. Boston Scientific took over Stentor and introduced a low-water-permeability polyester fabric that did not require suturing. Ancure and Vanguard were, respectively the new models introduced, in hopes that they would succeed where their predecessors failed. Although material failure was discovered by persistent endoleaks, these findings prompted a closer surveillance of stent-graft devices and closer attention to design, since material failure was now a known entity that could be identified on plain film x-rays.

III. MODES OF FAILURE

Over the last 10 years, reports of device failure have been scattered throughout the literature in the form of case reports or follow-up results of FDA trials (6,9,33–35). These isolated reports prompted our institution to review its own experience with endovascular stent grafts and device fatigue.

686 patients underwent endovascular aortic aneurysm repair (over a ten-year period) and were followed prospectively in a database. Of these, 404 had a full complement of follow-up analyses for review and formed the study set for our investigation. A total of 60 patients (15%) of this subset demonstrated stentgraft fatigue as identified by x-ray studies or the analysis of an explanted stentgraft device. Forty-nine (81%) of those patients had been treated for an AAA, while 11(19%) had a TAA repair. Patients were variably followed at 1, 3, 6, and 12 months and annually thereafter with physical exam, plain film abdominal or chest x-rays, duplex ultrasonography, and spiral CT scans. Of the 60 patients with stentgraft failure, 55 were identified with x-ray analysis and 5 were found on inspection of explanted stent grafts (36).

The 60 fatigued stent grafts in this study were distributed among seven different graft types (Table 1). The average time to fatigue for all devices combined was 19 months (range 1–48 months), the average follow-up since fatigue identification being 8 months. A marked variation in the time to failure was seen depending upon the type of fatigue, — i.e., suture fracture, graft holes, or stent fractures (Table 2). Of the 60 patients followed with graft fatigue, 11 expired during follow-up and 1 was lost to folow-up 2 years after his fatigue was identified. Of the 11 deaths, 3 were device-related and 1 patient died on post-op day 15 secondary to complications suffered after an open surgical conversion. A second patient's death was device-related, caused by an aneurysmal rupture in the presence of a type I

Table 1 Distribution of Stent-Graft Fatigue by Device

Device for aortic aneurysm repair	Total implanted	X-rays reviewed	Total fatigue/ fracture (%)	Average time to fracture/fatigue (range)	Average follow-up since fracture/fatigue (range)[b]
Abdominal					
Vanguard	26	22 (85%)	16 (72%)	26 months[b] (3–48)	13 months (1–39) out of 13 pts
Talent	337	232 (69%)	24 (10%)	13 months (1–31)	5 months (1–12) out of 22 pts
MEG	164	24 (21%)	5 (15%)	38 months (33–48)	6 months (1–8)
EVT/Ancure	9/20	7/6	1/0 (14%)	12 months	24 mo and then lost to follow-up
AneuRx	39	33 (85%)	3 (10%)	10 months (1–24)	3 months (1–6)
Gore	18	18 (100%)	0		
Teramed	10	10 (100%)	0		
Thoracic					
Gore-TAG	22	19 (86%)	7 (37%)	24 months (3–38)	12 months (1–42 out of 6 pts)
Talent	41[c]	33 (80%)	4 (12%)	9.5 months (1–24)	4 months (2–7)
Total	686	404	60	19 months	8 months

[a] Excluding those patients that underwent open conversion and endograft explantation.
[b] Excluding the patient with an acute conversion.
[c] Including emergent use not part of a clinical study.
Source: Ref. 36. Copyright© 2003 Elsevier Inc. Reprinted with permission.

Table 2 Time to Diagnosis of Device Fatigue Based on Failure Type

Device	Type of fracture	Number of failures	Average time to fatigue (range)
AAA			
Vanguard	Suture disruption	14	25 months (3–48)
	Graft hole	2	Intraoperative and 36 months
Talent	Metal fracture	23	13 months (1–31)
	Graft hole	1	16 months
AneuRx	Metal fracture	3	10 months (1–24)
MEGs	Metal fracture	5	38 months (33–48)
EVT	Metal fracture	1	8 months
TAA			
Gore	Metal fracture	7	24 months (3–38)
Talent	Metal fracture	4	9.5 months (1–24)

endoleak. The stent fracture was in the proximal region of the graft, while the endoleak occurred at the distal attachment site. The endoleak was not amenable to endovascular exclusion and the patient was not a candidate for open repair. The third patient died 31 months after stent-graft implantation from a ruptured aneurysm. The patient had been noncompliant after his 12-month follow-up and, in the interim, developed a type I endoleak that became symptomatic at the time of rupture. The remaining 8 patients died of causes unrelated to their aortic aneurysms (Table 3). Excluding the one early postoperative death, the average time to expiration was 29 months (range of 17–52 months) postimplantation and

Table 3 Mortality of Patients with Stent-Graft Device Fatigue

Patient	Cause	Time from operating room device implantation	Time from fracture	Device[a]	Device-related
1	Congestive heart failure	27 months	4 months	Vanguard	No
2	Emphysema	34 months	26 months	Vanguard	No
3	Colon cancer	24 months	9 months	Vanguard	No
4	Lung cancer	30 months	26 months	Vanguard	No
5	Post-op from open surgical conversion	POD #5	NA	Vanguard	Yes
6	Myocardial infarction	17 months	12 months	Vanguard	No
7	Cardiac arrest	23 months	20 months	Vanguard	No
8	Cardiac arrythmia	52 months	4 months	MEG's	No
9	Prostate cancer/MI	26 months	2 months	Talent	No
10	Ruptured AAA	31 months	NA	Talent	Yes
11	Rupture of type I Endoleak[b]	23 months	NA	Talent-TAA	Yes

Abbreviations: OR, POD, post-operative day.
[a] Vanguard devices were implanted 2 years prior to the Talent device and therefore have had longer follow-up.
[b] Leak diagnosed prior to rupture; however, patient was not a candidate for open surgery.

13 months (2–26 months) after fatigue was first identified. The remaining patients continue to be followed for clinical sequelae of their stent-graft fatigue (36).

A. Stentgraft Failure Analyzed by Device

Of the 60 patients with device fatigue, 16 had Vanguard AAA stent grafts inserted (Table 4); 9 failures occurred in bifurcated grafts and 7 in aortic tube grafts. There were 14 suture disruptions, 5 proximal row separations, and 9 body separations. Two explanted devices were found to have multiple wear holes through the graft fabric (Fig. 9) (36).

Twenty-four material failures occurred in Talent stentgrafts. Sixteen Talent patients had bifurcated grafts while 6 fatigues occurred in aorto-uni grafts and two in a tube graft. Fatigue was recognized within several different regions of the endovascular graft devices. Twenty-three patients had fractured stents. Fourteen occurred along the longitudinal bar of the graft (7 in the aortic body proximal bar, 1 in the aortic body distal bar, and 6 in an iliac limb) (Fig. 10A to C). Nine fractures were detected in the serpentine nitinol wire of the Talent device (4 in the body and 5 within the proximal transrenal stent) (Fig. 10D and E). One patient had a wear hole detected in an explanted prosthesis at the site of graft-to-stent fixation (Fig. 10F) (36).

The nine remaining fatigued stent grafts occurred in three different device designs, the MEGS, the EVT, and the AneuRx. Metallic fractures occurred in 5 patients with MEGS stent grafts, all after at least 33 months of follow-up. Four occurred within the proximal diamond row portion of the Palmaz stainless steel stent in the setting of maximal stent dilatation (Fig. 11) and one in the second row. The EVT device was noted to have distal hooks and proximal shank fractures approximately 6 months after insertion (Fig. 12). Three patients had fractures of their AneuRx device (Fig. 13). Metal fatigue within

Table 4 Failure Mode Analysis by Device

Device	Number failed	Location	Number
AAA	**49**		
Talent	24	Graft hole	1
		Longitudinal bar	14
		Aortic body, proximal	7
		Aortic body, distal	1
		Iliac	6
		Proximal transrenal stent	5
		Z-shaped body stent	4
Vanguard	16	Row separation	5
		Body separation	9
		Graft hole	2
EVT	1	Hooks and shanks	1
MEGS	5	Top row of stent	4
		Second row	1
AneuRx	3	Stent fracture	3
TAA	**11**		
Gore	7	Isolated longitudinal bar	3
		Longitudinal bar and Z stent	2
		Z stent	2
Talent	4	Longitudinal bar	1
		Z stent	3

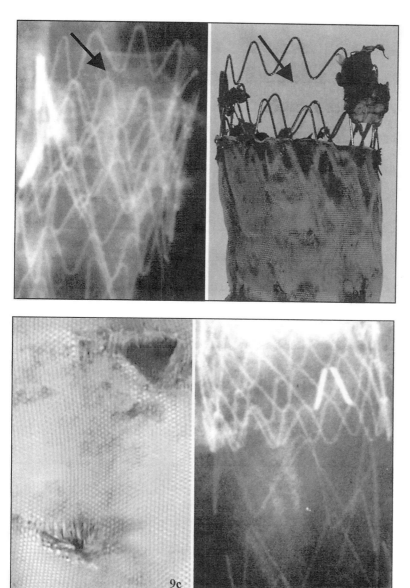

Figure 9 Clinical examples of fatigue in the Boston Scientific Vanguard endovascular graft. A 69 year old man had a tube graft inserted for the repair of an abdominal aortic aneurysm. a. Proximal row separation was defined on this graft along with a distal endoleak secondary to retraction of the prosthesis. b. The graft was explanted and a conventional repair was done at 36 months. Arrow points to the site of the proximal row separation. c. High-powered magnification of the graft depicted in 9b demonstrates fabric fatigue and wear holes on the prosthesis surface. d. A 79-year-old man had an endovascular tube graft placed for the repair of an AAA. On surveillance abdominal x-rays suture fractures in the body of the graft are detected (arrow). This patient remains in a surveillance program (From Ref. 36. Reprinted with permission.).

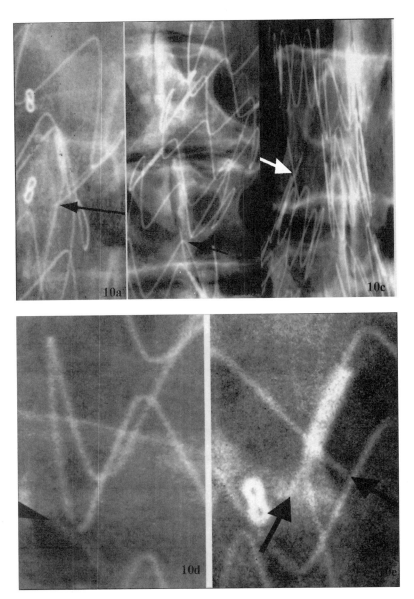

Figure 10 Clinical examples of fatigue in the Talent endovascular system. a. A proximal longitudinal bar fracture in a Talent endovascular graft (arrow). b. A distal aortic longitudinal bar fracture (arrow). c. An ipsilateral limb longitudinal bar fracture in a Talent endovascular graft. d. A midbody Z-stent fracture (arrow). e. A proximal transrenal stent fracture in a Talent endovascular graft. Note the fracture has occurred adjacent to the site of the nitinol wire crimp, which contains the two ends of the Z-configured stent. f. Following a persistent Type I endoleak a 70 year old man had his endovascular graft explanted and a conventional repair completed. The explanted graft demonstrated signs of graft wear with frayed fabric yarns and the creation of a defined hole (arrow). (From Ref. 36. Reprinted with permission.).

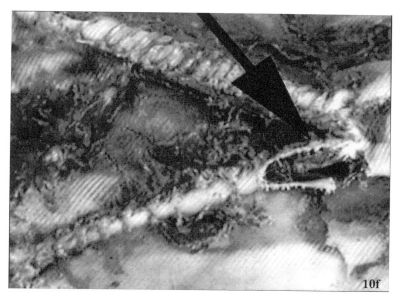

Figure 10 Continued.

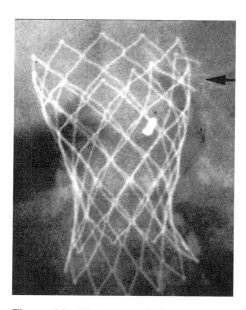

Figure 11 The Palmaz balloon expandable proximal stent attachment device of the handmade Parodi-Palmaz system. Note a fracture of the proximal diamond row (arrow) (From Ref. 36. Reprinted with permission.).

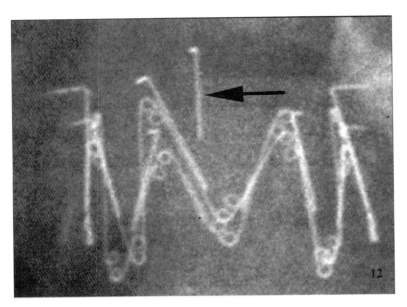

Figure 12 Attachment system of the EVT endovascular grafting system. Note fracture of the hook shank at the site of its laser weld on the Z-configured attachment system (arrow) (From Ref. 36. Reprinted with permission.).

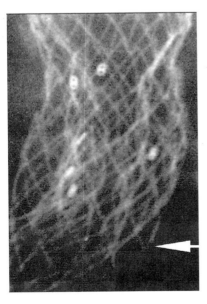

Figure 13 An abdominal X-ray of a patient who underwent AneuRx stentgrafting of an abdominal aortic aneurysm. Arrow denotes site of a fracture in one of the nitinol rings on the stent strut (From Ref. 36. Reprinted with permission.).

AneuRx grafts was extremely difficult to identify conclusively on plain film examination secondary to overlapping metal densities of the stent and the relatively close diamond pattern (36).

Eleven patients with thoracic aortic stent-graft devices were identified that had device material failure. Seven Gore TAG prostheses were found to have stent fractures and four Talent thoracic grafts demonstrated evidence of metal fatigue. One TAG graft had a strut fracture seen on chest x-ray films 3 months postimplantation and subsequently developed a second fracture of a longitudinal nitinol bar detected at 32 months. Two patients (one Talent and one TAG) presented with a sudden onset of pain and were diagnosed with enlarging aneurysms and new type I endoleaks on CT scan. The patient who had the TAG prosthesis underwent open conversion and device explantation (Fig. 14). The patient with the Talent graft was not a candidate for open surgery and ultimately died of aneurysmal rupture. The remaining 8 patients had stent fractures detected in the longitudinal bar (3) and z stents (5) of the stent graft (36).

B. Metallic Fracture

The 42 metallic stent fractures analyzed at our institution occurred in devices fabricated by six different manufacturers. Thirty-six fractures were documented in superelastic Nitinol stents, 5 fractures in stainless steel, devices and 1 in an elgiloy stent. Of the 686 devices implanted in this investigation, 493 (72%) were fabricated from nitinol, 24% were stainless steel, and 4% were elgiloy.

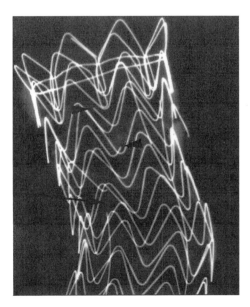

Figure 14   A high resolution explant radiograph of a W.L. Gore TAG stentgraft that was used to repair a thoracic aortic aneurysm. This patient presented 32 months after endovascular repair of a thoracic aneurysm with a new endoleak. The endoprosthesis was explanted and a conventional reconstruction was successfully accomplished. Explanted examination of the endograft using a plain film x-ray demonstrates Z-configured wire fractures (arrow-heads) and a longitudinal bar fracture (full arrow) (From Ref. 36. Reprinted with permission.).

As mentioned previously, elgiloy metal fractures were first reported in the early EVT devices. Eight of the 39 patients enrolled in that trial were found to have hook fractures (24). This device was withdrawn from clinical use and has since been redesigned to the improved Ancure/Guidant device. Even though the hooks were remodeled to decrease the stress on the metal, Najibi et al. recently reported two cases of delayed isolated hook fractures that occurred at 36 months postimplantation in the proximal attachment system of the Ancure device (34). Both patients were asymptomatic and the clinical relevance of their fracture for the device as a whole has yet to be determined. Although the EVT device at our institution had similar fractures to those reported in the literature, there was no evidence of metallic fracture in those devices implanted using the remodeled Ancure system. However, the mean follow-up for Ancure patients at our institution was only 13 months.

Although stress fatigue has been suggested as the likely cause of metallic fracture in the EVT and later Ancure devices, other forms of failure including metal corrosion have been postulated as the cause for the nitinol fractures in early explanted Stentor grafts (35,37). Heintz et al. found evidence of corrosion on scanning electron microscope (SEM) studies of Stentor explants, with more severe irregularities detected in those stents implanted for longer time periods. The explanted stents reviewed in our study failed to show significant signs of corrosion, even in high-risk regions of the metal, and did reveal a relatively uniform surface oxide layer, which may provide resistance to corrosion (Fig. 15A to D). The lack of

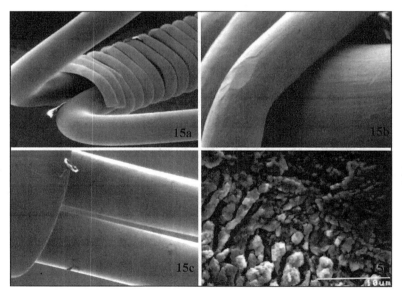

Figure 15 Scanning electron microscopy (SEM) of explanted endovascular grafts for AAA. a. The Vanguard endovascular graft has platinum wire wound around the proximal and distal portions of the attachment system to improve x-ray visualization (×40). b. Despite the suspected increased potential for metal fatigue and corrosion at the interface of these two metals no such fatigue was found in the nitinol in this 36 month old implant (200×) c. A SEM of a Talent stent explanted 15 months after insertion. The site depicts the crimped region of the two ends of the metal bar. No significant wear or pitting was detected on the surface of the nitinol stent at this presumably high risk area for fatigue (×40). d. High powered (4K) magnification of the surface of a Talent nitinol spring after explantation. A rough appearing, uniform oxide layer is discerned (From Ref. 36. Reprinted with permission.).

corrosion on the explanted devices in this study compared to the results of the earlier Stentor models may reflect an improved understanding of nitinol processing. Surface treatments such as electropolishing (38), TiN annealing (39), heat treatments, and nitric acid passivation (40) have all been shown to improve the corrosion resistance of nitinol by enhancing the formation of a thin, uniform oxide layer on the surface of the metal (41).

With improvements in corrosion resistance and the absence of significant evidence of corrosion identified on the newer stent grafts explanted at our institution, other causes of metallic fracture should be considered. Studies have shown that structural changes in the morphology of the stent graft, such as foreshortening of the aneurysm after exclusion (42), or the impact of aortic pulsations and the associated cyclic loading during systole and diastole (43), may result in accelerated endovascular stent graft fatigue. Harris et al. found kinking responsible for complications such as limb occlusion and migration or separation of the modular components in the Stentor/Vanguard device (42). Although the investigation by Harris and associates did not show evidence of metallic fracture, one can postulate that those structural changes that occur secondary to tortuosity of the aorta and cyclic loading could ultimately result in fracture. Umschied et al. reported kinking in stentgrafts resulting in similar complications with the Stentor/Vanguard devices. That study also reported metallic fracture in the longitudinal bar of Talent stentgraft devices (43). At our institution, 18 fractures occurred in the longitudinal nitinol bars of Talent or Gore stentgrafts. These events were associated with tortuosity of the implant vessels with presumed increased stress across the nitinol wire.

Microcracks, which are material irregularities produced commonly during metal laser cutting, together with the pulsatile aorta, may ultimately result in surface disruption and crack propagation. At the present time limited in vivo information exists on fatigue crack propagation for endovascular stents. The majority of studies have been done on larger implants for orthopedic applications or heart valve replacements (44). These applications experience very different loads, and endovascular stents are manufactured with much thinner metal strut widths, approximating 250 µm. At these tolerances, even if the material used has a high threshold for crack propagation, there is a very small distance in the stent structure for the crack to propagate prior to fracture (45). In our review the metallic fractures in the diamond row portion of the Palmaz stainless steel stents, or in the zizzag portion of the nitinol ring stents, could have been due to a combination of the causes mentioned above, which emphasizes the importance of further studies in vivo of fatigue crack propagation for endovascular stent grafts.

C. Fabric Fatigue

The polyester material used in stent grafts today is similar to the material used in conventional AAA repairs. Degradation of the polyester fabric is known to take place after 10–20 years following conventional surgical implantation (46). However, the fabric wear seen in implanted endovascular stents is reported much earlier. Fabric fatigue can be accelerated when mechanical stresses combine with the extrinsic forces and electrochemical properties of the intravascular environment. Fabric fatigue was one of the first reported causes of aneurysmal rupture and stent-graft failure in the earlier Stentor graft (6). External abrasions of the fabric on the metal stent as well as frank graft holes have been described in the literature (37,47). Both can be related to a combination of pulsatile flow of the aorta and the geometric characteristics of the stent itself. Movement between the stent graft and the arterial wall can cause fabric wear and surface breakdown, resulting in external abrasions (47). The graft holes are probably caused by micromotion of the individual stents against the polyester fabric, causing abrasion of the material and a likely type III endoleak (6). At our institution, 5 explanted stent grafts had evidence of fabric fatigue: 2 in Vanguard grafts, 2 in a Talent AAA stent graft, and the last in a Gore TAG.

In the Stentor and Vanguard devices, polypropylene ties fasten the individual stent rows to each other. The stent itself is attached to the graft only at the proximal and distal ends, allowing for continuous motion between the stent and the graft. Fewer examples of graft fenestrations have been reported with the Talent design, which could be secondary to complete fixation of the graft by sutures to the stent, thereby decreasing the amount of movement between the graft and the metallic nitinol stents. Material fatigue can also occur during manufacturing and packaging. In our study, one patient was found to have a type III endoleak immediately after deployment; on explantation fabric fatigue was seen. This can occur when the stent graft is drawn into the catheter from the opposite direction from which it will be deployed. Then the angled points of the stents can press firmly against the graft fabric, potentially causing a small tear or hole (36).

D. Suture Breakage

The polypropylene sutures used to assemble the Stentor/Vanguard device may also be subject to fatigue and contribute to device failure. Micromotion of the nitinol endoskeleton secondary to the pulsatile flow of the aorta causes friction and wear of the sutures, with ultimate suture fracture and stent row separation. As of January 2001, there has been a 21% prevalence of row separation reported in the Vanguard model (48). Riepe et al. found that the most movement took place in the large frames of the body middle ring in the Stentor model (7). The twisting motion often caused by micromovements and circulation can lead to wear and finally rupture of the sutures of the body of the frame. Of the 14 suture disruptions that were identified at our institution, 5 were row separations and 9 occurred in the body, corroborating Riepe's hypothesis of increased motion in the body of the stent.

Fracture of sutures linking individual stents may also play a role in secondary graft failure. As more sutures break along the length of a graft, the longitudinal strength of the graft is decreased, causing instability of the stent graft as a whole. This results in kinking and morphological changes in the stent graft that can ultimately lead to separation from the aorta and device migration (7).

IV. ETIOLOGY OF FAILURE

Device fatigue is not the result of one single event. Most likely a combination of causes results in ultimate device fatigue. Besides intrinsic properties of the materials used for stent-graft fabrication—i.e., strength of a metal, corrosion resistance, or flexibility of a fabric—and the extrinsic hostile environment of the native aorta, other factors can play a role in the ultimate fatigue/failure of a device.

A. Endoleaks

Endoleaks and their clinical application have been discussed at length in the literature (49–54). In brief, there are four types of endoleaks that have been described. A type I endoleak involves leakage at the stentgraft attachment sites, either the distal or proximal end. A type II endoleak results from retrograde filling of the sac from arteries arising from the aneurysm. A type III endoleak is a disruption of the stent-graft device either from graft tears or modular separation, and a type IV endoleak refers to leakage from a porous stent graft. It seems obvious that increased pressure of the aneurysmal sac by lack of complete exclusion could potentially be a cause of rupture; however, the interaction of endoleaks and device failure is less clear.

In the literature, endoleaks are reported to occur in 10–44% of endovascular repairs (50). At our institution, the overall endoleak rate is approximately 35%. In our study population, 24 (40%) of the 60 patients with stent-graft device fatigue were diagnosed with an endoleak at some point after graft implantation (Table 5) Device fatigue was identified prior to endoleak in 5 patients (21%). One patient had proximal and distal metallic fractures in a first generation EVT stent graft and the second had a row separation secondary to suture fracture of a Vanguard device, which later developed a type I endoleak from dislodgment of the distal left limb. The third patient was noted to have a body separation of a Vanguard device at his 17 month x-ray, and 7 months later was noted to have a small endoleak. One year later, at his 36-month follow-up, an angiogram was done, which noted distal and proximal dislodgement as well as an increase in aneurysmal size, and the patient was treated with a Talent stentgraft. The fourth patient was noted to have a body separation at his 3-month follow-up. Nine months later, a CT scan revealed a type I distal endoleak and enlargement of the aneurysmal sac. The patient was treated with an endovascular limb with resolution of the endoleak. The last patient was noted at 6-month follow-up to have a stent fracture of the third row of metallic stents in the AneuRx stent graft and 18 months later developed a type II endoleak. In 4 of the 5 cases where an endoleak developed after identification of device fatigue the 2 events were unrelated (36).

Table 5 Incidence of Endoleaks in Grafts with Device Fatigue

Device	Number of endoleaks	Time of diagnosis in relation to fatigue			Management
		Before	After	Same time	
AAA					
Vanguard	9	2	3	4	Endovascular repair (5) Open repair (2) Observation (2)
Talent	7	5		2	Embolization of type II endoleak (2) Open repair (3) Resolved spontaneously (2) Observation (1)
EVT	1		1		MEGS A-I-F (1)
MEGS	1	1			Endovascular repair (1)
AneuRx	2		1	1	Endovascular repair (1) Observation (1)
TAA					
Gore	2			2	Open repair (1) Observation (1)
Talent	2			2	Refused surgery, died from rupture (1) Observation (1)

However; the contrary may not be true. Eight patients (33%) developed stent-graft fatigue after the endoleak was diagnosed, and 11 fatigued grafts (46%) were identified at the same time as the endoleak (36). Endoleaks have been shown to maintain pressure and turbulent flow in the aneurysmal sac, leading to eventual enlargement of the aneurysm and risk of rupture (3,49). Residual aneurysmal sac pressure may be communicated to the stent graft itself in the form of increased device pulsatility, which can lead to metal fracture, suture disruption, and fabric wear, resulting in material failure. Although type I and III endoleaks are usually treated immediately to prevent aneurysmal expansion and rupture, type II endoleaks are more common and are usually followed (55,56). In our study, six of the endoleaks that were diagnosed prior to device fatigue were type II endoleaks. All six were observed on average 20 months (range 6–32) prior to diagnosis of the stent-graft fracture. One can hypothesize that although a type II endoleak may not generate enough pressure to cause aneurysmal dilatation and eventual rupture, there is enough pulsatile flow to expose the stent graft to excess micromotion, which, in turn, could lead to device failure in metal fracture, suture disruption, or fabric wear.

Several authors have shown that even aneurysms that do not show evidence of endoleak still have pressure transmitted through the mural thrombus or the aortic wall, which may contribute to aneurysmal rupture—a concept known as endotension (57,58). This transmitted pressure can also be responsible for micromotion between the stentgraft components, thus increasing the likelihood of abrasion, corrosion, or fabric wear.

V. CLINICAL SIGNIFICANCE

Although fractures were found in 60 patients with endovascular stent grafts, the majority have been asymptomatic and have not required secondary intervention. It appears that endoleaks and aneurysm size are more important than material failure in determining the risk of rupture. While three patients developed symptomatic aneurysms in the setting of stent fractures, these events did not appear to be related to the fatigued stents. The one device related death was in a patient who had an immediate type III leak (graft hole) after implantation and died after open conversion as a consequence of that leak. Since concern regarding stent erosion through the fabric of stent grafts remains, we recommend that if a patient is asymptomatic and there is no evidence of aneurysm enlargement, rupture, or a type I or III endoleak, observation of the device for fatigue is acceptable in the setting of increased graft surveillance.

VI. CONCLUSION

Endovascular grafts have been used clinically to treat aortic aneurysms for over 10 years. A significant growth in our understanding of the failure modes of the materials used to fabricate these devices as well as respect for the relatively harsh environment into which they must function has led to the development of improved stent-graft designs. However, these devices may still experience metal fatigue, fabric fatigue, and ultimately device fatigue. Improved manufacturing practices can decrease the frequency of these events; however, the clinical implications of many forms of device fatigue remains to be defined.

REFERENCES

1. Parodi JC, Palmaz JC, Barone HD. Transfemoral intraluminal graft implantation for abdominal aortic aneurysms. Ann Vasc Surg 1991; 5:491–499.

2. Becquemin JP, Lapie V, Favre JP, Rousseau H. Mid-term results of a second generation bifurcated endovascular graft for abdominal aneurysm repair: The French Vanguard trial. J Vasc Surg 1999; 30:209–218.
3. Zarins CK, White RA, Hodgson KJ, Schwarten D, Fogarty TJ. Endoleak as a predictor of outcome after endovascular aneurysm repair: AneurRx multicenter clinical trial. J Vasc Surg 2000; 32:90–107.
4. Zarins CK, White RA, Moll FL, Crabtree T, Bloch DA, Hodgdon KJ, et al. The AneuRx stent graft: Four-year results and worldwide experience 2000. J Vasc Surg 2001; 33:S135–S145.
5. Bush RL, Lumsden AB, Dodson TF, Salam AA, Weiss VJ, Smith RB, et al. Mid-term results after endovascular repair of the abdominal aortic aneurysm. J Vasc Surg 2001; 33:S70–S76.
6. Beebe HG, Cronenwett JL, Katzen BT, Brewster DC, Green RM. Results of an aortic endograft trial: Impact of device failure beyond 12 months. J Vasc Surg 2001; 33:S55–S63.
7. Riepe G, Heilberger P, Umschield T, Chakfe N, Raithel D, Stelter W, Morlock M, Kretz JG, Schroder A, Imig H. Frame dislocation of body middle rigs in endovascular stent tube grafts. Eur J Vasc Endovasc Surg 1999; 17:28–34.
8. Bohm T, Soldner J, Rott A, Kaiser WA. Perigraft leak of an aortic stent graft due to material fatigue. AJR 1999; 172:1355–1357.
9. Norgren L, Jernby B, Engellau L. Aortoenteric fistula caused by a ruptured stent-graft: A case report. J Endovasc Surg 1998; 5:269–272.
10. Maleux G, Rousseau H, Otal P, Colombier D, Glock Y, Joffre F. Modular component separation and reperfusion of abdominal aortic aneurysm sac after endovascular repair of the abdominal aortic aneurysm: A case report. J Vasc Surg 1998; 28:349–352.
11. Holzenbein TJ, Kretschmer G, Thrunher S, Schoder M, Aslim E, Lammer J, Polterauer P. Midterm durability of abdominal aortic aneurysm endograft repair: A word of caution. J Vasc Surg 2001; 33:S46–S54.
12. Parodi JC, Marin ML, Veith FJ. Transfemoral, endovascular stented graft repair of an abdominal aortic aneurysm. Arch Surg 1995; 130:549–552.
13. Marin ML, Hollier LH, Avrahami R, Parsons R. Varying strategies for endovascular repair of abdominal and iliac artery aneurysms. Surg Clin North Am 1998; 78(4):631–645.
14. Ohki T, Veith FJ, Sanchez LA, Marin ML, Cynamon J, Parodi JC. Varying strategies and devices for endovascular repair of abdominal aortic aneurysms. Semin Vasc Surg 1997; 10(4): 242–256.
15. Moore WS. The EVT tube and bifurcated endograft systems: Technical considerations and clinical summary. J Endovasc Surg 1997; 4:182–194.
16. Dake MD, Miller C, Semba CP, Mitchell S, Walker PJ, Liddell RP. Transluminal placement of endovascular stent-grafts for the treatment of descending thoracic aortic aneurysm. N Engl J Med 1994; 331:1729–1734.
17. Temudom T, D'Ayala M, Marin ML, Hollier LH, Parsons R, Teodorescu V, Mitty H, Ahn J, Falk A, Kahn R, Griepp R. Endovascular grafts in the treatment of thoracic aortic aneurysms and pseudoaneurysms. Ann Vasc Surg 2000; 14:230–238.
18. Parodi JC, Barone A, Piraino R, Schonholz C. Endovascular treatment of abdominal aortic aneurysms: Lessons learned. J Endovasc Surg 1997; 4:102–110.
19. Chuter TA, Green RM, Ouriel K, Fiore WM, Deweese JA. Transfemoral aortic graft placement. J Vasc Surg 1993; 18:185–197.
20. Faries PL. Endovascular grafts for the treatment of abdominal aortic aneurysm. In: Marin ML, Hollier LH, eds. Endovascular Grafting: Advanced Treatment for Vascular Disease. Armonk, NY: Futura, 2000.
21. Allen RC, White RA, Zarins CK, Fogarty TJ. What are the characteristics of the ideal endovascular graft for abdominal aortic aneurysm exclusion? J Endovasc Surg 1997; 4:195–202.
22. Chuter TAM. Stent-graft design: The good, bad and the ugly. Cardiovasc Surg 2002; 10:7–13.
23. Broeders IAMJ, Blankensteijn JD, Wever JJ, Eikelboom BC. Mid-term fixation stability of the endovascular technologies endograft. Eur J Vasc Endovasc Surg 1999; 18:300–307.

24. Moore WS, Rutherford RB. Transfemoral endovascular repair of abdominal aortic aneurysm: Results of the North American EVT phase 1 trial. J Vasc Surg 1996; 23:543–553.

25. Mialhe C, Amicabile C, Becquemin JP. Endovascular treatment of infrarenal abdominal aneurysms by the Stentor system: Preliminary results of 79 cases. J Vasc Surg 1997; 26:199–209.

26. May J, White GH, Harris JP. Devices for aortic aneurysm repair. Surg Clin North Am 1999; 79(3):507–527.

27. Criado FJ, Wilson EP, Fairman RM, Abdul-Khoudoud O, Wellons E. Update on the Talent aortic stent-graft: A preliminary report from United States phase I and II trials. J Vasc Surg 2001; 33:S146–S149.

28. Brener BJ, Faries P, Connelly T, Sefranek V, Hertz S, Kirksey L, Hollier L, Marin M. An in situ adjustable endovascular graft for the treatment of abdominal aortic aneurysms. J Vasc Surg 2002; 35:114–119.

29. Mitchell RS, Miller DC, Dake MD. Stent graft repair of thoracic aortic aneurysms. Semin Vasc Surg 1997; 10:257–271.

30. Mitchell RS, Dake MD, Semba CP, Fogarty TJ, Zarins CK, Liddell RP, et al. Endovascular stent graft repair of thoracic aortic aneurysms. J Thorac Cardiovasc Surg 1996; 11:1054–1062.

31. D'Ayala M. Endovascular grafting for thoracic aortic aneurysms. In: Marin ML, Hollier LH, eds. Endovascular Grafting: Advance Treatment for Vascular Disease. Armonk, NY: Futura, 2000.

32. Blum U, Voshage G, Lammer J, Beyersdorf F, Tollner D, Kretschmer G, Spillner G, Polterauer P, Nagel G, Holzenbein T, Thurnher S, Langer M. Endoluminal stent-grafts for infrarenal aortic aneurysms. N Engl J Med 1997; 336:13–20.

33. Breek JC, Hamming JF, Lohle PNM, Lampmann LEH, Van Berge Henegouwen DP. Spontaneous perforation of an aortic endoprosthesis. Eur J Vasc Endovasc Surg 1999; 18:174–175.

34. Najibi S, Steinberg J, Katzen BT, Zemel G, Lin PH, Weiss VJ, Lumsden AB, Chaikof EL. Detection of isolated hook fractures 36 months after implantation of the Ancure endograft: A cautionary note. J Vasc Surg 2001; 34:353–356.

35. Heintz C, Riepe G, Birken L, Kaiser E, Chakfe N, Morlock M, Delling G, Imig H. Corroded nitinol wires in explanted aortic endografts: An important mechanism of failure? J Endovasc Ther 2001; 8:248–253.

36. Jacobs TS, Won J, Gravereaux EC, Faries PL, Morrissey N, Teodorescu VJ, Hollier LH, Marin ML. Mechanical failure of prosthetic human implants: A ten-year experience with aortic stent graft devices. J Vasc Surg 2003; 37:16–26.

37. Guidoin R, Marios Y, Douville Y, King MW, Castonguay M, Traore A, Formichi M, Staxrud LE, Norgen L, Bergeron P, Becquemin JP, Egana JM, Harris PL. First generation aortic endografts: Analysis of explanted Stentor devices from the EUROSTAR registry. J Endovasc Ther 2000; 7:105–122.

38. Trepanier C, Leung TK, Tabrizian M, Yahia L, Bienvenu JG, Tanguay JF, Piron DL, Bilodeau L. Preliminary investigations of the effects of surface treatments biological response to shape memory NiTi stents. J Biomed Mater Res (Appl Biomater) 1999; 48:165–171.

39. Starosvetsky E, Gotman I. Corrosion behavior of titanium nitride coated Ni-Ti shape memory surgical alloy. Biomaterials 2001; 22:1853–1859.

40. Trepanier C, Tabrizian M, Yahia L, Bilodeau L, Piron DL. Effect of modification of oxide layer on NiTi stent corrosion resistance. J Biomed Mater Res (Appl Biomater) 1998; 43:433–440.

41. Duerig TW, Pelton AR, Stockel D. An overview of nitinol medical applications. Mater Sci Eng A273–A275 1999; 5:149–160.

42. Harris P, Brennan J, Martin J, Gould D, Bakaran A, Gilling-Smith G, Buth J, Gevers E, White D. Longitudinal aneurysm shrinkage following endovascular aortic: A source of intermediate and late complications. J Endovasc Surg 1999; 6:11–16.

43. Umschied T, Stelter WJ. Time-related alterations in shape, position, and structure of self-expanding modular aortic stent-grafts: A 4 year single center follow-up. J Endovasc Surg 1999; 6:17–32.

44. Teoh SH. Fatigue of biomaterials: A review. Int J Fatigue 2000; 22:825–837.
45. McKelvey AL, Ritchie RO. Fatigue-crack propagation in nitinol, a shape-memory and superelastic endovascular stent material. J Biomed Mater Res 1999; 47:301–308.
46. Riepe G, Loos J, Imig H, Schroder A, Schneider E, Peterman J, et al. Long-term in vivo alterations of polyester vascular grafts in humans. Eur J Vasc Endovasc Surg 1997; 13(6):540–548.
47. Alimi YS, Chakfe N, Rivoal E, Slimane KK, Valerio N, Riepe G, Kretz JG, Juhan C. Rupture of an abdominal aortic aneurysm after endovascular graft placement and aneurysm size reduction. J Vasc Surg 1998; 28:178–183.
48. Device Alert. Vanguard endoprosthesis. Upper stent row separation with or without nitinol wire fracture 2001. Available from: http://www.medical-devices.gov.uk/da2001(01).htm.
49. Wain RA, Marin ML, Ohki T, Sanchez LA, Lyon RT, Rozenblit A, Suggs WD, Yuan JG, Veith FJ. Endoleaks after endovascular graft treatment of aortic aneurysms: Classification, risk factors, and outcome. J Vasc Surg 1998; 27:69–80.
50. White GH, Yu W, May J, Chaufour X, Stephens MS. Endoleak as a complication of endoluminal grafting of abdominal aortic aneurysms: Classification, incidence, diagnosis and management. J Endovasc Surg 1997; 4:152–168.
51. Schurink GWH, Aarts NJM, van Baalen JM, Shultze Kool LJ, van Bockel JH. Experimental study of the influence of endoleak size on pressure in the aneurysm sac and the consequences of thrombosis. Br J Surg 2000; 87:71–78.
52. White GH, May J, Petrasek P, Waugh R, Stephen M, Harris J. Endotension: An explanation for continued AAA growth after successful endoluminal repair. J Endovasc Surg 1999; 6:308–315.
53. Schurink GWH, Aarts NJM, Wilde J, van Baalen JM, Chuter TAM, Schultze Kool LJ, van Bockel JH. Endoleakage after stent-graft treatment of abdominal aneurysm: Implications on pressure and imaging—An in vitro study. J Vasc Surg 1998; 28:234–241.
54. Parodi JC, Berguer R, Ferreira LM, La Mura R, Schermerhorn ML. Intra-aneurysmal pressure after incomplete endovascular exclusion. J Vasc Surg 2001; 33:909–914.
55. Deaton DH, Makaroun MS, Fairman RM. Endoleak: Predictive value for anueryms growth at 3 years. Ann Vasc Surg 2002; 16:37–42.
56. Resch T, Ivancev K, Lindh M, Nyman U, Brunkwall J, Malina M, Lindblad B. Persistant collateral perfusion of abdominal aortic aneurysm after endovascular repair does not lead to progressive change in aneurysm diameter. J Vasc Surg 1998; 28:242–249.
57. Gilling-Smith G, Brennan J, Harris P, Bakaran A, Gould D, McWilliams R. Endotension after edovascular aneurysm repair: Definition, classification, and strategies for surveillance and intervention. J Endovasc Surg 1999; 6:305–307.
58. Kato N, Shimono T, Hirano T, Mizumoto T, Suzuki T, Ishida M, Fujii H, Yada I, Takeda K. Aneurysm expansion after stent-graft placement in the absence of endoleak. J Vasc Intervent Radiol 2002; 13:321–326.

41

Endoleak

Hugh G. Beebe

Jobst Vascular Center, Toledo, Ohio, and Dartmouth–Hitchcock Medical Center, Hanover, New Hampshire, U.S.A.

I. INTRODUCTION

The understanding of endoleaks and their management is critically important in the endovascular repair of abdominal aortic aneurysm (AAA). The goal of all elective AAA treatments is to protect the patient from the life-threatening potential of aneurysm rupture and resultant hemorrhage. Thus an endovascular prosthesis can eliminate the potential for such hemorrhage if it succeeds in achieving total exclusion of circulation within the aneurysm. This dichotomous view of success, either the AAA has no circulation within the sac or it has circulation, was held to be the primary criterion of treatment success in the early days of endografts.

However, another way of thinking about endograft success derives from the accumulating experience of the past decade. Restated, it can be said that the goal of all elective AAA treatments is to provide the best prevention of aneurysm-related death. This is a more sophisticated concept that involves including risk of the treatment itself and inclusion of a range of late problems that may occur with either conventional open surgery or endografts. Viewing the goal of endovascular AAA treatment in this way diminishes the impact of endoleak per se on evaluating results. This view seems appropriate now because of the still emerging understanding of different types of endoleaks with unequal potential effects, differences among device types in relation to endoleak and the complex influence of imaging methods used to identify them.

Some experts have the opinion that endoleak is a poor predictor of aneurysm growth even though it is statistically associated with AAA enlargement. Absence of endoleak is not a reliable predictor of aneurysm shrinkage since many apparently excluded AAA remain unchanged in size after stent grafting. It has recently been stated that while endoleak is a risk factor for aneurysm enlargement, it cannot be used as an endpoint for effective endovascular aneurysm treatment (1).

659

This chapter summarizes what is presently understood about endoleaks, emphasizes prevention or avoidance, and discusses endoleak management. It also indicates where incomplete understanding and controversial issues remain. Endovascular aneurysm treatment is still a young endeavor having come into general use less than a decade ago, and it is expected that added experience will produce changes that clarify and improve endoleak prevention and management.

II. ENDOLEAK TYPES

The term *endoleak* was only first introduced in 1996, when the leadership group in Sidney, Australia, at the Royal Prince Alfred Hospital, wrote a letter to the editor suggesting its use to differentiate this type of AAA exclusion failure from hemorrhage due to AAA rupture (2). At that time, endoleaks were still being lumped together regardless of cause, but not long thereafter, the same group suggested differentiating endoleaks in two publications that formed the basis for our current classification scheme (3,4). At the same time, opinion articles appeared that opened the discussion about the clinical implication of the various types of endoleak (5). The following classification combines a description of endoleak types and summarizes their significance or potential significance in clinical terms.

A. Type I

This endoleak is defined simply as flow into the aneurysm sac around either the proximal attachment zone or distal attachment, whether a straight graft in the aorta or either of two limb attachments within the iliac arteries. Proximal type I endoleak is a clear failure of endografting with implications for ongoing AAA rupture risk. The systolic blood pressure in the sac from this type of endoleak is always assumed to be equal to systemic levels. Distal type I endoleak is perhaps less threatening to the success of endograft treatment in some special cases, but not clearly so. Recognition of type I endoleak during the operative procedure requires immediate additional steps to eliminate it. Endoleak detection and management are taken up below (Fig. 1).

B. Type II

This is the most complex and controversial endoleak type. The definition of type II is circulation within the sac from aortoiliac anatomical branches. These most commonly are lumbar and inferior mesenteric arteries, but type II endoleaks can also arise from accessory renal arteries, horseshoe kidney arteries, internal iliac arteries, and occasional aberrant pelvic branches of the iliolumbar, uterine, or middle sacral vessels.

It is probably going to be necessary in the future to subclassify type II endoleaks, because including them all together in a single category has resulted in conflicting reports about their behavior and significance. The ideal classification would be to stratify them according to their physiology, but data on flow and pressure, presently requiring direct measurement, are not often available. At present it seems useful to attempt to classify type II endoleaks according to whether they appear to have separate anatomical inflow and outflow tracts. It is probably true that lumbar branch endoleaks not associated with another vessel will usually occlude spontaneously (Fig. 2).

C. Type III

This is also a very serious, life-threatening type of endoleak that should prompt immediate treatment. It is defined as a direct endoleak arising from loss of physical integrity of the

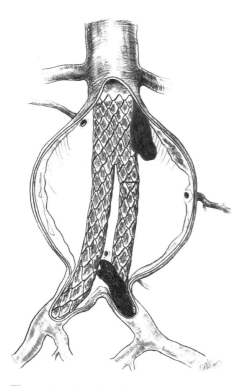

Figure 1 Type I endoleak, shown both proximally and distally, occurs when there is inadequate sealing at the stent-graft attachment zones.

endograft prosthesis. There are several ways in which this can arise. One way is through perforation of the prosthesis fabric by an adjacent metallic stent. This is caused by relative motion between these two parts of the endograft caused by a variety of influences that include inherent looseness of the fabric, lack of fabric strength, and odd angulation of the endograft usually associated with AAA sac shrinkage that presents an apex of stent metal in direct contact with fabric. Another is through loss of attachment between modular components such that they separate where an iliac limb contralateral to the main endograft trunk has been inserted. This type of endoleak typically occurs late in follow-up after endografting. It is for this reason that it appears to represent such a special danger to the patient, as discussed below (Fig. 3).

D. Type IV

This is a somewhat vague type of endoleak that is device-specific in its occurrence and unclear in its several implications. It is defined as a direct endoleak occurring through porous fabric of the intact endoprosthesis. This kind of bleeding is commonly seen in conventional open surgery, especially where knitted fabric grafts are used. The practice of preclotting is a common remedy and various types of coated grafts that address this type of problem are commercially available.

In endovascular therapy there is uniquely a requirement to use arteriography right after endograft deployment to determine the procedure's success. Thus one significance of

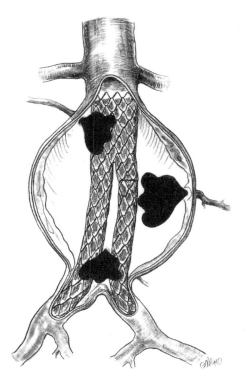

Figure 2 Type II endoleak can arise from various branches of the aortoiliac segment, most commonly from lumbar arteries and the inferior mesenteric artery.

type IV endoleak is that it may make detection of a more serious endoleak unclear or lead to wrong assumptions in interpreting completion arteriography during the endograft procedure. Some investigators have questioned whether such porous fabric might be capable of transmitting pressure within the sac even after flow has ceased from thrombus forming in the fabric interstices (Fig. 4).

E. Type V

This type of endoleak is not really an endoleak at all in the strict sense because it is not associated with blood flow. Type V is defined as "endotension," a name proposed by Gilling-Smith and his colleagues (6) to express the important concept that even though blood flow might not exist, a thrombus is fully capable of transmitting pressure into the AAA sac. There are both clinical and experimental data to support this concept, and the topic serves to stimulate fundamental and skeptical reflection on how much we actually know about the behavior of excluded AAA. The great variable in the literature addressing endotension is the quality of images used to rule out endoleak in AAA that enlarge after stent grafting. Meier et al. (7) found only 2 of 17 cases with AAA expansion among 658 receiving Ancure stent grafts that did not show endoleak in a clinical trial setting with core lab review. They marshaled an argument that the concept is flawed and only represents missed endoleak. Several authors have reported AAA sac expansion following endografting with repeated lack of apparent flow on follow-up contrast imaging (8–10). Zarins et al. (11) even reported post–stent-graft

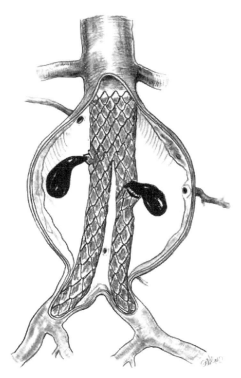

Figure 3 Type III endoleak, dangerously associated with rapid aneurysm expansion and rupture, is shown here caused by fabric erosion from physical contact with a metal stent (right) and by disconnection of the left iliac limb of a modular bifurcation endograft.

rupture in five patients who did not show evidence of endoleak, as have others (12). Experimentally, the Montefiore group demonstrated conclusively that endoleaks, produced in a prosthetic in vivo model and subsequently excluded by coil embolization proven to stop flow, still result in a pressurized sac at almost systemic levels (13).

III. DIAGNOSIS OF ENDOLEAK

A. Intraprocedural

Assessment of endoleak at the completion of an aortic stent graft procedure is almost exclusively done by arteriography unless there is a strong contraindication to contrast use. Completion arteriography should always involve use of a power injector of contrast, concurrent use of cine loop and frame-by-frame review, and—as some have recommended—multiple arteriograms taken at several intervals along the endograft length (14). The use of steep oblique views will sometimes add important information about endoleak source. A slightly prolonged imaging run will allow the late filling of a type II endoleak by iliolumbar branches that may occur several seconds after contrast has left the endograft (Fig. 5A and B).

Unfortunately, in many institutions, the practice of completion arteriography is limited to a single anteroposterior (AP) injection. The result of this may be the discovery on the first

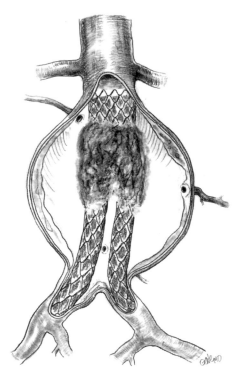

Figure 4 Type IV endoleak, illustrated schematically here, through interstices of the graft fabric in certain specific endograft types may make assignment of endoleak source difficult on completion arteriography.

postoperative computed tomography (CT) images of a posterior midline type I endoleak, which was probably present from the beginning and might have been resolved by adjunctive measures at the time if more careful completion arteriography had identified it. If an endograft procedure has been long and difficult, the combination of a tired team feeling the lead apron's weight and a higher than usual cumulative fluoroscopy time may limit interest in detailed imaging. But it is often the difficult case that is more liable to have the important type I endoleak. A disciplined approach to completion arteriography will yield benefits. As mentioned above, the presence of a type IV endoleak from porous fabric or other construction details of certain stent graft types may produce confusing findings on completion arteriography. Reversing heparin and waiting for an interval to repeat the arteriogram may be helpful.

Some centers have investigated the use of intraoperative pressure monitoring by placing small catheters into the AAA sac alongside the stent graft so as to be able to mea-

Figure 5 A. This arteriogram was obtained at the end of a short run time upon completion of an aortic endograft. The full length of the endograft and renal and mesenteric branches can be seen. No endoleak is apparent. B. This arteriogram was obtained in the same patient shown in Figure 5A using the same position and power injection of contrast but with a longer run time. The iliolumbar artery (ILA) filling a type II endoleak is now apparent (arrows).

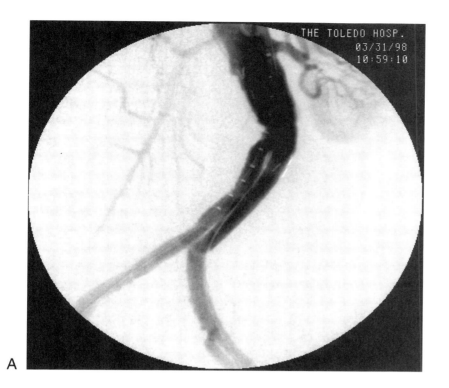

A

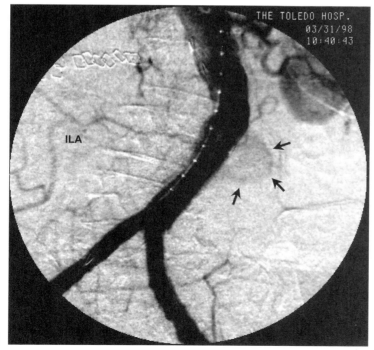

B

sure pressure changes upon completion of the procedure and, in some cases for a short interval postoperatively, before withdrawing the catheter. Stelter and Umscheid (15) were pioneers in this physiological approach to assessing whether a satisfactory endpoint of the endograft procedure had been achieved and reported summary information on 201 patients. But they concluded that correlation between pressure changes observed during stent-graft deployment and the "fate of the aneurysm over time" was not known. Thus the use of pressure monitoring was considered to be an adjunct to endoleak detection by arteriography. This type of monitoring was studied by Bell and colleagues (16), who found that AAA sac pressure monitoring operatively and for 24 h postoperatively showed evidence of higher pressures and pulsatility in 5 of 15 patients with endoleaks. However, these endoleaks were also seen on arteriography. Given the uncertain meaning of the pressure data, the likelihood that significant endoleak can be found with careful arteriography and the theoretical added risk of complications such as infection, it would seem that pressure monitoring, at least by this method, would not be advisable outside of a clinical trial.

B. Postoperative Follow-Up

The diagnosis of endoleak during follow-up is presently made exclusively through various types of imaging, CT scanning most commonly, duplex ultrasound, arteriography when the source is unclear or when a therapeutic attempt by endovascular occlusion is made, and, far less commonly, by magnetic resonance arteriography.

C. CT Scan

The quality of imaging is a large variable in determining the presence of endoleak and the incidence of its occurrence. CT scanning done with thick acquisition protocols that allow collimation greater than 5 mm or with poor timing of contrast can fail to show evidence of an endoleak that is found to be present on closely timed arteriography. The ideal CT scan for endograft follow-up is done with 1:1.5 pitch, 3–5 mm collimation, and timing to ensure that the 150 mL of intravenously injected contrast arrives in the aortoiliac segment at the right time. This matter of the right time for detecting endoleak is not quite the same as for preoperative evaluation of morphology. It has been observed that delayed CT will show some endoleaks that are missed without an interval of time, allowing low-flow volumes to be seen. Usually these are type II endoleaks, as types I and III come directly from the aortic flow lumen. When the aorta is heavily calcified or contains unusual calcified projections into the lumen, it may be important to obtain a CT image acquisition before and after contrast injection, allowing one to distinguish between calcified vascular tissue and endoleak. It may also be difficult on occasion to decide about a small or subtle endoleak in the presence of prominent metallic flare artifact on the CT image. The quality of CT scans for endograft follow-up requires high standards of excellence in technique and interpretation, as with any diagnostic test being used to rule out a potentially serious finding.

Three-dimensional (3D) postprocessing of CT scans for follow-up assessment of aortic stent grafts is a large subject beyond the scope of this chapter. However, in discussing endoleak, one aspect ought to be mentioned—the use of volume measurement of the infrarenal aorta. This procedure, from the lowermost renal artery to the aortic bifurcation, can be readily done using postprocessing of CT scan data, enabling serial comparison of an indicator of aneurysm size change that is more sensitive than diameter (B Kritpracha and H Beebe, unpublished data) (17).

White and colleagues (18) demonstrated that significant variation in measuring AAA size occurs with variation in CT scan technique and concluded that volumetric analysis is very useful in the follow-up of patients whose AAA do not shrink. When the CT images fail to show contrast within the sac but AAA volume is increasing, an undetected endoleak should be suspected. This may present an indication for further diagnostic imaging by arteriography. Another use of volume measurement from 3D postprocessing that may be useful in following type II endoleaks is to measure the volume of the endoleak separately from that of the AAA. Anecdotal evidence from our imaging laboratory suggests that declining endoleak volume predicts eventual spontaneous closure (Fig. 6).

The assignment of endoleak type by CT scan is probably inaccurate in as many as 20% of cases, although well-controlled data on this matter are limited. In one report specifically related to endoleak type, Parent et al. (19) detected the source artery in all of 36 patients with type II endoleak using color duplex ultrasound but in only 7 of the same patient cohort using CT scan. There is a tendency for observers to make a value judgment about endoleaks from CT scan appearance, but there are no physiological data to be found on these images. Thus comments sometimes seen in published reports about "major" or "minor" endoleaks based on the size of the contrast-filled space in the aorta and its contrast density are wholly theoretical.

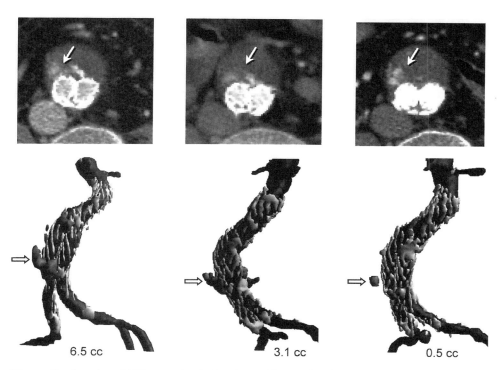

6.5 cc   3.1 cc   0.5 cc

Figure 6 A series of CT scans (top) showing evidence of endoleak (arrows) obtained over a total span of 12 months. Below the CT scan are views of a 3D model made from the CT scan showing the endoleak (open arrow). Serial calculations of the type II endoleak volume (numbers below model) showed progressive decrease and the endoleak closed spontaneously. (Medical Media Systems, West Lebanon, NH.)

D. Duplex Ultrasound Scanning

The appeal of color-flow duplex scanning for follow-up evaluation of stent grafts comes from its low cost, patient acceptance, and risk-free repeatability. The drawbacks, however, are significant. As with all ultrasound examinations, there is an influence of operator variability, and this is heightened in abdominal studies. Additionally, body habitus, intestinal gas, and the lower resolution of the required low-frequency transducers may all adversely affect quality. There is also the need for patient preparation for the examination, which constitutes a nuisance factor (Fig. 7).

McLafferty et al. (20) reported correlation between duplex and CT scans in 79 patients after stent graft, including 7 with endoleak, and concluded that it was an accurate test. They also summarized a complex literature from other centers evaluating the role of duplex scanning. One of those reports from highly experienced French authors emphasized the accuracy of ultrasound in detecting endoleak in a study of 54 patients without and 35 with endoleak by CT (21). There was poor correlation between ultrasound and CT determination of AAA diameter. Wolf et al. (22) found discordant results in 8% of 100 endograft patients with 11 endoleaks seen on CT but not on duplex. They concluded that duplex scanning, if of assured high quality, was comparable to CT scanning in practical clinical value since those not seen by duplex scan were not associated with AAA expansion. The general value of such a conclusion will need to be validated by additional larger studies. The use of ultrasound contrast agents has been shown to enhance the value of ultrasound in stent graft follow-up (23,24) (Fig. 8).

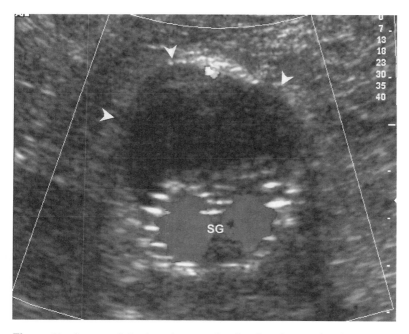

Figure 7 A normal duplex ultrasound color-flow image showing the aneurysm sac (arrowheads) and the stent graft (SG) within it. There was no color-flow evidence of endoleak throughout the entire aortoiliac segment.

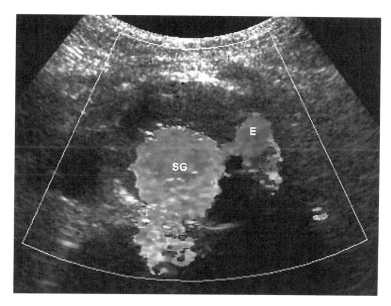

Figure 8 A color-flow ultrasound image, printed in gray scale, showing flow within stent graft (SG) and a type II endoleak (E) elsewhere within the AAA sac.

E. Arteriography

Standard contrast arteriography is used for endoleak evaluation when the source is unclear and a therapeutic maneuver is undertaken to stop the endoleak. Examples include expanding AAA without demonstrated endoleak or after determining that an endoleak is present but its type is not clear. The clinical setting is an important part of judging the need for arteriography. If an AAA is stable in size and the endoleak is highly likely to be a type II or an apparently small endoleak from a distal type I, observation without being entirely certain of the source may be appropriate for an interval of time. However, when an AAA is enlarging after stent-grafting and the endoleak source is presumed to be a type II, an arteriogram to establish this conclusively is indicated and may provide an opportunity for concurrent treatment as discussed below (Fig. 9A and B).

Technical details are of value in getting the most information from this type of examination and most often involve thoughtful projection angles to reveal endoleak origins and use of balloon occlusion to isolate or augment small sites of endoleak blood flow. For example, Matsumura et al. (25) were able to demonstrate microleaks arising from an endograft, that were not clearly shown on routine CT views by using balloon occlusion arteriography.

F. Magnetic Resonance Arteriography (MRA)

This imaging method (MRA) varies quite widely in quality from one center to the next largely because of variation in equipment, especially the software used to process magnetic resonance images and local expertise in its use. However, gadolinium-enhanced MRA has been shown to be of value in endoleak detection, and it does not confuse calcium with contrast in the AAA sac, as occasionally happens in CT scans (26). MRA also offers

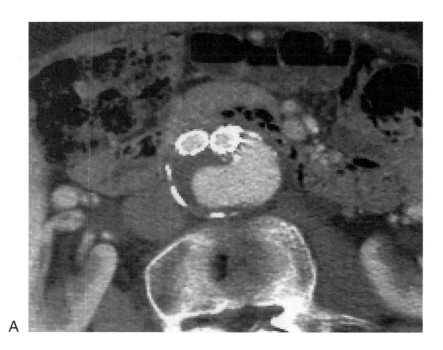

A

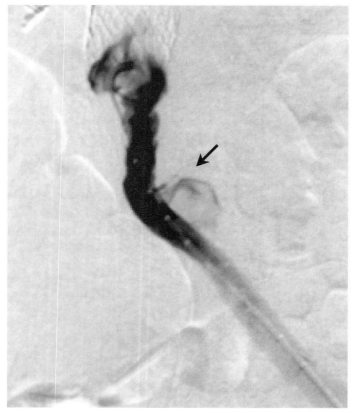

B

benefit in patients with mild chronic renal insufficiency who should not receive large volumes of contrast for CT scanning.

G. Adjuncts to Imaging Methods

The usefulness of physical findings in endograft follow-up has seldom been emphasized. In patients whose AAA can be palpated, detection of pulsatility by simple but skilled examination should not be dismissed in this era of highly technical imaging. The finding of a quiet AAA after stent-grafting is reassuring, and a change in later follow-up to an AAA that has a definite pulsatile quality is a valid index of concern. Some very experienced clinicians have emphasized the importance of physical findings in deciding which patients with endoleaks may require treatment (27).

An interesting and creative approach to endoleak detection was suggested by the work of Serino and colleagues (28), who explored changes in D-dimer levels, a fibrin degradation product, after endografting in a well-controlled study of 74 patients. They found highly significantly increased D-dimer levels in those with type I endoleak and concluded that this may prove to be a useful marker for fixation problems after endovascular AAA repair.

H. Pseudoendoleak

Endoleak evidence is mostly derived from imaging data. The appearance of an area of radiodensity within the treated AAA sac that is outside the endoprostheses and of increased density compared to the rest of the sac is a fair description of the criteria for diagnosis of endoleak. However, there are at least three ways in which CT scans can meet these criteria and yet not be associated with endoleak. One is specific to endografts constructed with the fabric on the outside of the stent. If the fabric bulges out or away from the underlying stent during contrast CT, it can have the false appearance of endoleak. This misleading finding is most often seen in follow-up images of the Vanguard stent graft (Boston Scientific Corp., Natick MA), which is no longer used. However, many patients with this endograft remain in follow-up. Another source of confusion may result from odd calcifications in the AAA sac, sometimes quite far into the lumen and perhaps from old areas of dissection. If the available images are not duplicated before and after contrast injection, that additional step may be needed to resolve the question on subsequent exams. Last, the persistence of contrast trapped in the AAA during the insertion of the endograft has been reported as a source of pseudoendoleak (29).

IV. TIME OF ENDOLEAK OCCURENCE

If one considers all endoleaks regardless of type, they are most common in the immediate postoperative period, as might be imagined. But if one considers *persistent* endoleak, a more significant endpoint descriptor, then endoleaks continue to accumulate during follow-up. The reasons for this are many and include the timing and quality of imaging, characteristics of specific endograft types, morphology changes in excluded AAA, and device structural failures.

Figure 9 A. This CT scan image clearly shows an endoleak, but does not identify the source which remained unclear after reviewing the entire scan. B. The patient whose CT image was seen in Figure 9A had an arteriogram with selective injections done to localize the endoleak source. As seen here, a type II endoleak is proven to be arising from a focal structural defect in the endograft (arrow).

An example is the increasing endoleak problem during an endograft trial reported by the Vanguard IDE investigators (30). These results were presented as presence of persistent endoleak by follow-up interval. In that way, inspection of a life table provides the trend of endoleak development or resolution and patterns that may be revealed by the shape of the curve. It is also simplifies results reporting because of the problem of individual patients whose endoleaks seal and recur.

The Eurostar registry, which collates data from 87 European centers, showed increasing endoleaks over length of follow-up in data on 2463 patients who received stent grafts of eight types with 171 (6.9%) endoleaks detected at 1 month and 317 occurring later as new-onset endoleaks (31). The Eurostar analysis was primarily in the form of clinical effects that could reasonably be associated with endoleak, such as increase in AAA size, late rupture, and, less clearly, secondary intervention. These clinical endpoints were correlated with endoleak status and defined by three groups: (a) type II endoleak, (b) type I or type III endoleak, and (c) no direct imaging evidence of endoleak. Analysis of effect on AAA growth showed surprising enlargement of AAA in group A, which caught up with group B by 36 months. Unfortunately, the Eurostar analysis did not separate early and late new-onset endoleaks.

Reports on type II endoleaks both early and late are conflicting in many respects. Resch and colleagues (32) observed a decrease in AAA size in endoleak-free patients, but those with type II endoleak showed no statistically significant change in aortic diameter on follow-up, and this has been found repeatedly in other studies (33,34). Also, AAA with type II endoleaks have been observed to shrink (35) and, on occasion, to expand and rupture (36,37). Some authors have concluded that this variable behavior may be explained by time of occurrence in addition to the probable differences in blood pressure between sources of type II endoleaks.

It has long been noted anecdotally that late-onset type III endoleaks usually cause dramatically rapid AAA expansion, leading to speculation that this reflects atrophy of the aortic wall during the interval of sac depressurization between stent-graft exclusion and endoleak development. Wolf et al. (38,39) reported interesting observations on AAA diameter in four patients with late-onset endoleak, some increasing by 16 mm over 20 days and 10 mm over 10 days. Ohki and associates (40) reported the seriousness of eight type I and III endoleaks occurring 10–55 months after stent-grafting that required prompt open conversion or secondary stent graft. Carpenter et al. (41) found endoleak treatment to be significantly the most common indication for readmission after endografting in a population of 337 patients, with only a 71% readmission-free survival at one year.

In summary, review of diverse and often conflicting literature on the subject of endoleak occurrence time suggests that type I endoleak is a serious threat and especially dangerous if it is proximal or occurs late. Type II is not predictable in behavior and must be observed for its effect on AAA size. Type III usually occurs late and suddenly, though not always. Its presence requires immediate intervention. Type IV should be restricted to periprocedural time interval by definition. Type V or endotension is discussed separately below but is best thought of in the same way as type II because it is a diagnosis of exclusion.

V. AVOIDING ENDOLEAK

Even though endoleak is of limited value as a criterion for judging endograft success, absolute exclusion of blood flow within an AAA is a desirable outcome and thus makes endoleak prevention a goal (42). The main focus of prevention has been case selection based on anatomical factors. It should be realized that case selection is driven by consideration of device limitations and therefore will evolve and change in response to the characteristics of new stent-graft devices. Perhaps the influence of difference among various stent-graft devices is the main reason for the lack of agreement in analyses of risk factors for endoleak and a wide range of early postoperative occurrences.

Proximal type I endoleak, generally considered a clear failure of stent-grafting, has usually been thought to be associated with adverse case selection involving anatomical features of the proximal infrarenal attachment zone, such as severe angulation, short length, conical shape, luminal thrombus, or dense calcification. Conflicting reports disclose lack of agreement on all of these factors. Neck angulation was associated with proximal type I endoleak in a report of results in 184 patients from Albertini et al. (43). However, the Eurostar data from 2146 endografts showed no correlation with aortic neck angulation (44). That same report did show that neck length was a highly significant ($p = 0.0001$) risk factor for proximal type I endoleak. But another report from four endograft centers showed no effect on endoleak of neck length less than 10 mm in 55 patients who received suprarenal stent grafts, thus suggesting the possible influence of device characteristics (45). Petrik and Moore (46) studied 100 endograft patients with a surprisingly high 44% incidence of endoleak and concluded that they were unable to demonstrate endoleak predictive value to anatomical factors that included neck angulation, neck thrombus or calcification, and number of patent lumbar arteries or the inferior mesenteric artery. They did not examine neck length, however.

Type II endoleaks have generally been thought to be predicted by a larger number of patent lumbar arteries, particularly when associated with a patent inferior mesenteric artery, but not all reports have found that correlation (47,48). This led to investigation of preventive branch embolization prior to endografting, which proved unsuccessful in a study involving 25 of 72 patients but illustrated the difficulties of this technically involved method (49). Another approach has been to prevent type II endoleak using insertion of thrombogenic material into the sac. Walker and colleagues (50) injected an absorbable gelatin sponge material into AAA sacs during stent-graft procedures when aortic side branches were seen on arteriography. Forty-eight of 93 (52%) patients had the test treatment. Excluding 15 patients with type I endoleaks, no patient treated with the sponges or those who did not show patent branch vessels and did not receive sponge injection had evidence of endoleak on median follow-up of 4 months. This "broad brushstrokes" approach to eliminating type II endoleaks has much theoretical appeal because it could form the basis for a selective approach to follow-up that might simplify the process, make duplex scan more useful, and reduce the overall cost of surveillance. Type III and IV endoleaks are fundamentally a design or device characteristics problem that presents management challenges for clinicians. These complications may be preventable by better device selection when problems become evident in retrospective analyses.

VI. MANAGEMENT OF ENDOLEAKS

The complexity of endoleaks is increased by including type II endoleaks together with all other types in some reports of endograft outcomes. In the analysis of endoleak significance provided by Zarins et al. (34), the conclusion was reached that "The presence or absence of endoleak on CT scan before hospital discharge does not appear to predict patient survival or aneurysm rupture rate after endovascular aneurysm repair." Many theoretical reasons could be advanced to account for this surprising result: a relatively small study cohort, a short follow-up interval (only 61% had CT images available for analysis at 1 year), differences in follow-up imaging protocols among institutions, and the definition of primary success endpoints that also had an aggregating effect. The understanding of whether different types of endoleak are also different in their implications for the patient is unlikely to be improved by treating them equally.

Among experienced clinicians, consensus was recently expressed that "type I and type III endoleaks will have serious consequences, even if sealing appears to have occurred" (51). They also believed that based on current data, most but certainly not all type II endoleaks appear to have a benign course; they frequently seal but probably should be separated into different types. It would be of obvious value to identify type II endoleaks destined to produce continued AAA enlargement. But current methods depend on anatomical differences as a surrogate for direct information about physiological parameters such as peak pressure, pulse pressure, and mean pressure.

The proposed anatomical basis for classifying type II endoleaks is to separate those with only a single vessel source (no outflow and somewhat similar conceptually to pseudoaneurysm) from those with inflow and outflow. The implications of this for the importance of pressure levels and flow volumes is unclear, but many believe that type II endoleaks with named vessel inflow and outflow are more likely to result in sac enlargement than the common "lumbar only" endoleak that often disappears. This does not align well with the observations made by several investigators that small endoleaks with only an inflow source may produce high pressures within the AAA sac. Schurink et al. (52) found that even a small endoleak causes considerable pressure in the aneurysm sac, and this was independent of endoleak size. In their in vitro experiment, systolic pressure was considerably reduced, but diastolic pressure was similar to that in the sac or even higher than in the systemic circulation because thrombus could cause a valve phenomenon. Parodi and colleagues (53) used an in vitro model to provide data of compelling interest by showing that small endoleaks could produce sac pressures higher than systemic levels but also went on to show the effect of providing an outflow vessel. When both inflow and outflow were simulated, there was a flow volume-related fall in pressure, and mean sac pressure became systemically lower than systemic.

It would be desirable to base the management of endoleak on observed physiological data, and perhaps that goal can be achieved when implantable pressure-sensing devices are available for guidance. But presently the exercise of clinical judgment about whether to intervene and what to do is based on anatomical and device imaging.

A. Type I

Most practitioners of experience act to remedy a proximal type I endoleak as soon as it is observed, and its presence is a clear indication for intervention. When the endoleak is recognized during the primary procedure, a variety of methods from forceful balloon dilation to insertion of additional stents or stent-graft extensions have been successfully employed (54,55). The use of large-diameter balloon-expanded stents, such as the Palmaz (Cordis Endovascular, Warren, NJ), has proven to be a successful adjunct to close a type I endoleak and is probably used more often than the few reports in the literature suggest (56). Short-length large-diameter stent grafts, so-called extender cuffs, have been provided by device manufacturers and are frequently used to resolve proximal type I endoleaks. It has been observed, however, that short-term success does not always yield long-term success. A well-documented example of proximal stent extension failure serves to heighten awareness that no controlled observations on late results of proximal cuff extensions have yet appeared (39). Disturbing observational evidence of proximal extender cuff use to manage primary endograft migration with failure in three of six cases has been reported (57).

The primary onset of a late proximal type I endoleak almost always is associated with stent-graft migration. The cause of the migration should be sought, since this will be the primary determinant of appropriate treatment. Three general causes for late migration are (a) enlargement of the aortic attachment zone; (b) traction on the upper endograft by a change in AAA morphology, causing severe angulation; and (c) loss of frictional attachment from changes in the device such as stent fracture.

Distal type I endoleak—nowadays virtually limited to iliac limbs, since straight aortic endograft use is rare—is approached in a similar way with use of increasingly involved measures from simple balloon angioplasty to stents and stent-graft extensions. The blood pressure implications of any endoleak communicating directly with the aortic lumen are important, but the decision to manage a small distal type I endoleak that persists after various measures, initially by observation, may sometimes be appropriate depending on the procedural circumstances.

B. Type II

Assigning an endoleak observed by CT the classification of type II is sometimes found to be wrong on subsequent arteriography. Type II endoleak that appears to be limited to lumbar artery branches does not represent a proven threat to endograft treatment success unless later follow-up shows further AAA enlargement. Therefore, most experienced clinicians who elect to observe an endoleak thought to be type II at the completion of the endograft procedure use routine follow-up imaging, anticipating occlusion without further intervention. However, an exception to this may exist in the growing use of endografts for emergency treatment of ruptured AAA. The presence of hemorrhage presents a blood loss problem that is separate from the small potential for late AAA expansion related to type II endoleak.

When the source includes inflow and outflow vessels, a direct approach by endovascular catheterization with insertion of coils to induce thrombosis is often used and has been well described by Baum and colleagues (58) at the University of Pennsylvania who later changed their approach. After observing late endoleak recurrence, they adopted a direct translumbar approach, which has been more successful. Improved late results of endoleak occlusion in 33 cases of proven type II endoleak but without data on AAA sac size change allowed them to conclude that transarterial (in contrast to direct translumbar) coil embolization was "ineffective and should not be performed" (59). This approach must be confirmed and accompanied by data on late AAA size effects. Also, it has not been compared with laparoscopic clipping of endoleak source vessels, a technique described only in anecdotal reports. This report of late failure of transarterial coil insertion correlates with the observations made experimentally by Marty and colleagues (60) at Montefiore Medical Center, who showed that proven coil occlusion of experimental endoleaks in a canine model failed to reduce sac pressure. They concluded that coil embolization failed to interrupt pressure transmission to the aneurysmal wall and therefore may be not a reliable management option for endoleaks. It may also be true that the material used for branch vessel occlusion is an important variable and that coils are not the best for this purpose. Martin et al. (61) used a liquid embolic agent known as Onyx in six patents with documented occlusion and early modest AAA sac shrinkage in five. The injection of thrombin into lumbar branches has been discouraged because of neurological complication risk when this compound extends into remote blood vessels (59). The need for chronic anticoagulation with warfarin has been shown not to influence the occurrence of type II endoleak but to

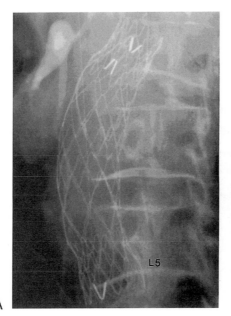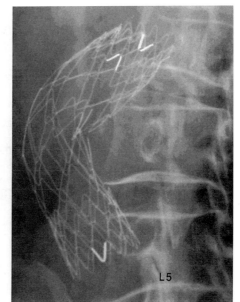

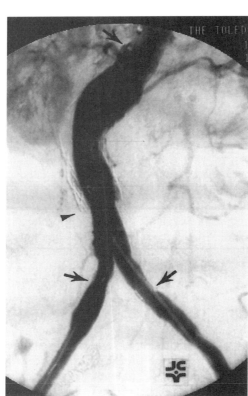

interfere with endoleak resolution and AAA shrinkage (62). Thus, if stopping antico-agulation is an option, at least for an interval of time, it should be considered.

C. Type III

The loss of endograft integrity usually occurs late and is a serious matter. The disconnection of modular components of a bifurcation endograft is usually due to either operator error in placing the limb into the aortic trunk for too short a distance or when morphology change puts physical stress on the junction of the two parts of the endograft. Often this can be remedied by getting a guidewire across the space and into both distracted components and using this as a basis for insertion of an additional stent graft (63). But angulation and thrombosis may make this impossible. Alternatives to consider include maneuvers to achieve an aorto-uni-iliac configuration together with femorofemoral bypass and contralateral occlusion of the disconnected limb or direct open repair using the proximal portion of the endograft as inflow to the disconnected side. Employment of a preplaced balloon through the patent intact limb facilitates this procedure. Other type III endoleaks arising from a stent graft in good position but with loss of fabric integrity due to stent perforation have been treated successfully by insertion of an entirely new endograft within the failed one (Fig. 10A and B).

Although endovascular repair of late endoleaks is usually possible, one should review whether the original decision to attempt endograft repair of an aneurysm was appropriate in the first place. If the patient's anatomical features are very adverse it may be that the endograft failure cannot be treated by further endografting and is best managed by conversion to conventional open surgery (64,65).

VII. A VIEW TOWARD THE FUTURE OF ENDOLEAK

Despite opinions to the contrary, most clinicians remain vigilant and concerned about endoleak. Yet the practical difficulty and cost of endlessly pursuing a series of contrast CT scans is recognized by all as undesirable. It seems easy to predict that alternative imaging methods such as duplex ultrasound, perhaps together with plain abdominal x-rays, and criteria for selecting which patients need more intensive imaging follow-up protocols will be an active subject of clinical investigation in the near term.

It may be that use of computerized postprocessing yielding sophisticated 3D images and sensitive measurements of volume, angulation, and diameter change that are automatically processed and made available by Internet access with graphic plots of change that are now becoming available (Medical Media Systems, West Lebanon, NH) will make follow-up easier. A broad database resulting from that approach could be used to identify categories that benefit from specific types of follow-up or early intervention to prevent clinical events from endoleaks rather than waiting to react to them after the fact.

Investigation of various pressure-sensing devices to be inserted into the AAA sac at the time of stent-grafting or as a part of the endograft is being pursued. If these come into

---

Figure 10   A. These two plain abdominal x-rays of an aortic straight endograft taken 12 months apart demonstrate upward migration of the distal end of the endograft after expansion of the distal aortic attachment zone. The border of the L5 vertebral body is marked for reference (L5). A late occuring distal type I endoleak resulted. B. The patient was treated by a secondary endograft in a bifurcated configuration (arrows) inserted through the original straight endograft (arrowhead), which resulted in sealing.

clinical application, validation work to understand the effects, if any, of variable thrombus patterns within the sac over time will be important. Possibly a semiautomatic method of evaluating endoleak status will result. However, in this regard, it would seem that such a pressure-measuring device would be analogous to the smoke detector fire alarm that tells you when a problem has arisen but does not anticipate its occurrence.

Adjunctive means of attaching an endoluminal prosthesis to the vascular wall have been described, suggesting the possibility that methods such as endovascular stapling or other physical attachments could be used in the future management of endoleak (66).

In an effort to simplify the concern over endoleaks of all types, it has been proposed that a preemptive approach by injecting an agent that will solidify the AAA sac as an adjunct to endografting would beg the question of endoleak significance (67). This intriguing idea should provide a stimulus to creative thinking but will require extensive work to define materials and indications. Still, given the complex and unsettled nature of endoleak management today, there is great appeal to an approach that prevents them or prevents their adverse effect.

ACKNOWLEDGMENT

The author gratefully acknowledges the medical illustrations contributed by Steven S. Gale, M.D.

REFERENCES

1. Deaton DH, Makaroun MS, Fairman RM. Endoleak: Predictive value for aneurysm growth at 3 years. Ann Vasc Surg 2002; 16:37–42.
2. White GH, Yu W, May J. Endoleak—A proposed new terminology to describe incomplete aneurysm exclusion by an endoluminal graft. J Endovasc Surg 1996; 3:124–125.
3. White GH, May J, Waugh RC, Yu W. Type I and type II endoleaks: A more useful classification for reporting results of endoluminal AAA repair. J Endovasc Surg 1998; 5:189–191.
4. White GH, May J, Waugh RC, Chaufour X, Yu W. Type III and type IV endoleak: Toward a complete definition of blood flow in the sac after endoluminal AAA repair. J Endovasc Surg 1998; 5:305–309.
5. Beebe HG, Bernhard VM, Parodi JC, White GH. Leaks after endovascular therapy for aneurysm: Detection and classification. J Endovasc Surg 1996; 3:445–448.
6. Gilling-Smith G, Brennan J, Harris P, Bakran A, Gould D, McWilliams R. Endotension after endovascular aneurysm repair: Definition, classification, and strategies for surveillance and intervention. J Endovasc Surg 1999; 6:305–307.
7. Meier GH, Parker FM, Godziachvili V, Demasi RJ, Parent FN, Gayle RG. Endotension after endovascular aneurysm repair: The Ancure experience. J Vasc Surg 2001; 34:421–426.
8. White GH, May J, Petrasek P, Waugh R, Stephen M, Harris J. Endotension: An explanation for continued AAA growth after successful endoluminal repair. J Endovasc Surg 1999; 6:308–315.
9. Baum RA, Carpenter JP, Cope C, Golden MA, Velazquez OC, Neschis DG, Mitchell ME, Barker CF, Fairman RM. Aneurysm sac pressure measurements after endovascular repair of abdominal aortic aneurysms. J Vasc Surg 2001; 33:32–41.
10. Gilling-Smith GL, Martin J, Sudhindran S, Gould DA, McWilliams RG, Bakran A, Brennan JA, Harris PL. Freedom from endoleak after endovascular aneurysm repair does not equal treatment success. Eur J Vasc Endovasc Surg 2000; 19:421–425.
11. Zarins CK, White RA, Fogarty TJ. Aneurysm rupture after endovascular repair using the AneuRx stent graft. J Vasc Surg 2000; 31:960–970.

12. Bade MA, Ohki T, Cynamon J, Veith FJ. Hypogastric artery aneurysm rupture after endovascular graft exclusion with shrinkage of the aneurysm: Significance of endotension from a "virtual," or thrombosed type II endoleak. J Vasc Surg 2001; 33:1271–1274.

13. Mehta M, Ohki T, Veith FJ, Lipsitz EC. All sealed endoleaks are not the same: A treatment strategy based on an ex-vivo analysis. Eur J Vasc Endovasc Surg 2001; 21:541–544.

14. White GH, Yu W, May J, Chaufour X, Stephen MS. Endoleak as a complication of endoluminal grafting of abdominal aortic aneurysms: Classification, incidence, diagnosis, and management. J Endovasc Surg 1997; 4:152–168.

15. Stelter W, Umscheid T, Ziegler P. Three-year experience with modular stent-graft devices for endovascular AAA treatment. J Endovasc Surg 1997; 4:362–369.

16. Treharne GD, Loftus IM, Thompson MM, Lennard N, Smith J, Fishwick G, Bell PR. Quality control during endovascular aneurysm repair: Monitoring aneurysmal sac pressure and superficial femoral artery flow velocity. J Endovasc Surg 1999; 6:239–245.

17. Wever JJ, Blankensteijn JD, Th M Mali WP, Eikelboom BC. Maximal aneurysm diameter follow-up is inadequate after endovascular abdominal aortic aneurysm repair. Eur J Vasc Endovasc Surg 2000; 20:177–182.

18. White RA, Donayre CE, Walot I, Woody J, Kim N, Kopchok GE. Computed tomography assessment of abdominal aortic aneurysm morphology after endograft exclusion. J Vasc Surg 2001; 33(2 suppl):S1–S10.

19. Parent FN, Meier GH, Godziachvili V, LeSar CJ, Parker FM, Carter KA, Gayle RG, DeMasi RJ, Marcinczyk MJ, Gregory RT. The incidence and natural history of type I and II endoleak: A 5-year follow-up assessment with color duplex ultrasound scan. J Vasc Surg 2002; 35:474–481.

20. McLafferty RB, McCrary BS, Mattos MA, Karch LA, Ramsey DE, Solis MM, Hodgson KJ. The use of color-flow duplex scan for the detection of endoleaks. J Vasc Surg 2002; 36:100–104.

21. d'Audiffret A, Desgranges P, Kobeiter DH, Becquemin JP. Follow-up evaluation of endoluminally treated abdominal aortic aneurysms with duplex ultrasonography: Validation with computed tomography. J Vasc Surg 2001; 33:42–50.

22. Wolf YG, Johnson BL, Hill BB, Rubin GD, Fogarty TJ, Zarins CK. Duplex ultrasound scanning versus computed tomographic angiography for postoperative evaluation of endovascular abdominal aortic aneurysm repair. J Vasc Surg 2000; 32:1142–1148.

23. McWilliams RG, Martin J, White D, Gould DA, Harris PL, Fear SC, Brennan J, Gilling-Smith GL, Bakran A, Rowlands PC. Use of contrast-enhanced ultrasound in follow-up after endovascular aortic aneurysm repair. J Vasc Intervent Radiol 1999; 10:1107–1114.

24. Heilberger P, Schunn C, Ritter W, Weber S, Raithel D. Postoperative color flow duplex scanning in aortic endografting. J Endovasc Surg 1997; 4:262–271.

25. Matsumura JS, Ryu RK, Ouriel K. Identification and implications of transgraft microleaks after endovascular repair of aortic aneurysms. J Vasc Surg 2001; 34:190–197.

26. Haulon S, Lions C, McFadden EP, Koussa M, Gaxotte V, Halna P, Beregi JP. Prospective evaluation of magnetic resonance imaging after endovascular treatment of infrarenal aortic aneurysms. Eur J Vasc Endovasc Surg 2001; 22:62–69.

27. Greenberg R, Green R. A clinical perspective on the management of endoleaks after abdominal aortic endovascular aneurysm repair. J Vasc Surg 2000; 31:836–837.

28. Serino F, Abeni D, Galvagni E, Sardella SG, Scuro A, Ferrari M, Ciarafoni I, Silvestri L, Fusco A. Noninvasive diagnosis of incomplete endovascular aneurysm repair: D-dimer assay to detect type I endoleaks and nonshrinking aneurysms. J Endovasc Ther 2002; 9:90–97.

29. Lee WA, Rubin GD, Johnson BL, Arko F, Fogarty TJ, Zarins CK. "Pseudoendoleak"—Residual intrasaccular contrast after endovascular stent-graft repair. J Endovasc Ther 2002; 9:119–123.

30. Beebe HG, Cronenwett JL, Katzen BT, Brewster DC, Green RM. Results of an aortic endograft trial: Impact of device failure beyond 12 months. J Vasc Surg 2001 Feb; 33(2 suppl):S55–S63.

31. van Marrewijk C, Buth J, Harris PL, Norgren L, Nevelsteen A, Wyatt MG. Significance of

endoleaks after endovascular repair of abdominal aortic aneurysms: The EUROSTAR experience. J Vasc Surg 2002; 35:461–473.

32. Resch T, Ivancev K, Lindh M, Nyman U, Brunkwall J, Malina M, Lindblad B. Persistent collateral perfusion of abdominal aortic aneurysm after endovascular repair does not lead to progressive change in aneurysm diameter. J Vasc Surg 1998; 28:242–249.

33. Tuerff SN, Rockman CB, Lamparello PJ, Adelman MA, Jacobowitz GR, Gagne PJ, Nalbandian MM, Weiswasser J, Landis R, Rosen RJ, Riles TS. Are type II (branch vessel) endoleaks really benign? Ann Vasc Surg 2002; 16:50–54.

34. Zarins CK, White RA, Hodgson KJ, Schwarten D, Fogarty TJ. Endoleak as a predictor of outcome after endovascular aneurysm repair: AneuRx multicenter clinical trial. J Vasc Surg 2000; 32:90–107.

35. Schunn CD, Krauss M, Heilberger P, Ritter W, Raithel D. Aortic aneurysm size and graft behavior after endovascular stent-grafting: Clinical experiences and observations over 3 years. J Endovasc Ther 2000; 7:167–176.

36. Hinchliffe RJ, Singh-Ranger R, Davidson IR, Hopkinson BR. Rupture of an abdominal aortic aneurysm secondary to type II endoleak. Eur J Vasc Endovasc Surg 2001; 22:563–565.

37. White RA, Walot I, Donayre CE, Woody J, Kopchok GE. Failed AAA endograft exclusion due to type II endoleak: Explant analysis. J Endovasc Ther 2001; 8:254–261.

38. Wolf YG, Hill BB, Rubin GD, Fogarty TJ, Zarins CK. Rate of change in abdominal aortic aneurysm diameter after endovascular repair. J Vasc Surg 2000; 32:108–115.

39. Wolf YG, Hill BB, Fogarty TJ, Cipriano PR, Zarins CK. Late endoleak after endovascular repair of an abdominal aortic aneurysm with multiple proximal extender cuffs. J Vasc Surg 2002; 35:580–583.

40. Ohki T, Veith FJ, Shaw P, Lipsitz E, Suggs WD, Wain RA, Bade M, Mehta M, Cayne N, Cynamon J, Valldares J, McKay J. Increasing incidence of midterm and long-term complications after endovascular graft repair of abdominal aortic aneurysms: A note of caution based on a 9-year experience. Ann Surg 2001; 234:323–334.

41. Carpenter JP, Baum RA, Barker CF, Golden MA, Velazquez OC, Mitchell ME, Fairman RM. Durability of benefits of endovascular versus conventional abdominal aortic aneurysm repair. J Vasc Surg 2002; 35:222–228.

42. Lee WA, Wolf YG, Fogarty TJ, Zarins CK. Does complete aneurysm exclusion ensure long-term success after endovascular repair? J Endovasc Ther 2000; 7:494–500.

43. Albertini J, Kalliafas S, Travis S, Yusuf SW, Macierewicz JA, Whitaker SC, Elmarasy NM, Hopkinson BR. Anatomical risk factors for proximal perigraft endoleak and graft migration following endovascular repair of abdominal aortic aneurysms. Eur J Vasc Endovasc Surg 2000; 19:308–312.

44. Mohan IV, Laheij RJ, Harris PL. Risk factors for endoleak and the evidence for stent-graft oversizing in patients undergoing endovascular aneurysm repair. Eur J Vasc Endovasc Surg 2001; 21:344–349.

45. Greenberg R, Fairman R, Srivastava S, Criado F, Green R. Endovascular grafting in patients with short proximal necks: An analysis of short-term results. Cardiovasc Surg 2000; 8:350–354.

46. Petrik PV, Moore WS. Endoleaks following endovascular repair of abdominal aortic aneurysm: The predictive value of preoperative anatomic factors—A review of 100 cases. J Vasc Surg 2001; 33:739–744.

47. Arko FR, Rubin GD, Johnson BL, Hill BB, Fogarty TJ, Zarins CK. Type-II endoleaks following endovascular AAA repair: Preoperative predictors and long-term effects. J Endovasc Ther 2001; 8:503–510.

48. Gorich J, Rilinger N, Sokiranski R, Soldner J, Kaiser W, Kramer S, Ermis C, Schutz A, Sunder-Plassmann L, Pamler R. Endoleaks after endovascular repair of aortic aneurysm: Are they predictable?—Initial results. Radiology 2001; 218:477–480.

49. Gould DA, McWilliams R, Edwards RD, Martin J, White D, Joekes E, Rowlands PC, Brennan J, Gilling-Smith G, Harris PL. Aortic side branch embolization before endovascular aneurysm repair: Incidence of type II endoleak. J Vasc Intervent Radiol 2001; 12:337–341.

50. Walker SR, Macierewicz J, Hopkinson BR. Endovascular AAA repair: Prevention of side branch endoleaks with thrombogenic sponge. J Endovasc Surg 1999; 6:350–353.

51. Veith FJ, Baum RA, Ohki T, Amor M, Adiseshiah M, Blankensteijn JD, Buth J, Chuter TA, Fairman RM, Gilling-Smith G, Harris PL, Hodgson KJ, Hopkinson BR, Ivancev K, Katzen BT, Lawrence-Brown M, Meier GH, Malina M, Makaroun MS, Parodi JC, Richter GM, Rubin GD, Stelter WJ, White GH, White RA, Wisselink W, Zarins CK. Nature and significance of endoleaks and endotension: Summary of opinions expressed at an international conference. J Vasc Surg 2002; 35:1029–1035.

52. Schurink GW, Aarts NJ, Wilde J, van Baalen JM, Chuter TA, Schultze Kool LJ, van Bockel JH. Endoleakage after stent-graft treatment of abdominal aneurysm: Implications on pressure and imaging—an in vitro study. J Vasc Surg 1998; 28:234–241.

53. Parodi JC, Berguer R, Ferreira LM, La Mura R, Schermerhorn ML. Intra-aneurysmal pressure after incomplete endovascular exclusion. J Vasc Surg 2001; 34:909–914.

54. Fairman RM, Velazquez O, Baum R, Carpenter J, Golden MA, Pyeron A, Criado F, Barker C. Endovascular repair of aortic aneurysms: Critical events and adjunctive procedures. J Vasc Surg 2001; 33:1226–1232.

55. Chuter TA, Reilly LM, Kerlan RK, Sawhney R, Canto CJ, Ring EJ, Messina LM. Endovascular repair of abdominal aortic aneurysm: Getting out of trouble. Cardiovasc Surg 1998; 6:232–239.

56. Dias NV, Resch T, Malina M, Lindblad B, Ivancev K. Intraoperative proximal endoleaks during AAA stent-graft repair: Evaluation of risk factors and treatment with Palmaz stents. J Endovasc Ther 2001; 8:268–273.

57. Cao P, Verzini F, Zannetti S, De Rango P, Parlani G, Lupattelli L, Maselli A. Device migration after endoluminal abdominal aortic aneurysm repair: Analysis of 113 cases with a minimum follow-up period of 2 years. J Vasc Surg 2002; 35:229–235.

58. Baum RA, Carpenter JP, Tuite CM, Velazquez OC, Soulen MC, Barker CF, Golden MA, Pyeron AM, Fairman RM. Diagnosis and treatment of inferior mesenteric arterial endoleaks after endovascular repair of abdominal aortic aneurysms. Radiology 2000; 215:409–413.

59. Baum RA, Carpenter JP, Golden MA, Velazquez OC, Clark TW, Stavropoulos SW, Cope C, Fairman RM, Stavropoulous SW. Treatment of type 2 endoleaks after endovascular repair of abdominal aortic aneurysms: Comparison of transarterial and translumbar techniques. J Vasc Surg 2002; 35:23–29.

60. Marty B, Sanchez LA, Ohki T, Wain RA, Faries PL, Cynamon J, Marin ML, Veith FJ. Endoleak after endovascular graft repair of experimental aortic aneurysms: Does coil embolization with angiographic "seal" lower intraaneurysmal pressure? J Vasc Surg 1998; 27:454–461.

61. Martin ML, Dolmatch BL, Fry PD, Machan LS. Treatment of type II endoleaks with Onyx. J Vasc Intervent Radiol 2001; 12:629–632.

62. Fairman RM, Carpenter JP, Baum RA, Larson RA, Golden MA, Barker CF, Mitchell ME, Velazquez OC. Potential impact of therapeutic warfarin treatment on type II endoleaks and sac shrinkage rates on midterm follow-up examination. J Vasc Surg 2002; 35:679–685.

63. Holzenbein TJ, Kretschmer G, Thurnher S, Schoder M, Aslim E, Lammer J, Polterauer P. Midterm durability of abdominal aortic aneurysm endograft repair: A word of caution. J Vasc Surg 2001; 33(2 suppl):S46–S54.

64. May J, White GH, Waugh R, Petrasek P, Chaufour X, Arulchelvam M, Stephen MS, Harris JP. Life-table analysis of primary and assisted success following endoluminal repair of abdominal aortic aneurysms: The role of supplementary endovascular intervention in improving outcome. Eur J Vasc Endovasc Surg 2000; 19:648–655.

65. May J, White GH, Harris JP. Early and late conversion from endoluminal to open repair. Semin Vasc Surg 1999; 12(3):207–214.

66. Trout HH III, Tanner HM. A new vascular Endostaple: A technical description. J Vasc Surg 2001; 34:565–568.

67. Fry PD, Martin M, Machan L. Endoleaks and the need for a paradigm shift. J Endovasc Ther 2000; 7:521.

42

Complications Following Endovascular Thoracic Aortic Aneurysm Repair

Alfio Carroccio and Sharif H. Ellozy

Mount Sinai School of Medicine, New York, New York, U.S.A.

Larry H. Hollier

Louisiana State University Health Sciences Center School of Medicine, New Orleans, Louisiana, U.S.A.

Complications associated with endovascular stent-graft repair of thoracic aneurysms include anatomical as well as device-related problems. The consequences related to anatomy include issues with access during and following endograft insertion, endoleaks resulting from poor stent-graft fixation or persistent collateral flow within the excluded segment, ischemia following interruption of excluded aortic branch vessels, and the host inflammatory response to the endograft (1–10). Device-related complications include stent fractures as well fabric breakdown, which may ultimately result in device-related endoleak (11). These endovascular-related complications are the focus of this chapter.

I. ANATOMICALLY RELATED COMPLICATIONS

A. Access Vessels

Successful endovascular repair of aortic aneurysms requires access arteries, that will allow safe passage of the endograft device. The iliac arteries, which are the more commonly used access vessels, are often plagued by vessel tortuosity and calcified obstructive occlusive disease. A combination of these variables may, in their worst form, result in vessel disruption, thrombosis, or procedure termination due to failed access. Despite successful deployment, arterial repair may be necessary in nearly a third of such cases (10). This problem becomes even more pronounced with thoracic aortic aneurysms due to the larger-diameter devices required for thoracic aneurysms as compared to abdominal aneurysms. Endograft delivery systems used in thoracic aneurysm repair can range in diameter from 22 to 27F; therefore the avoidance of vessel injury calls for thorough preoperative evaluation.

With preoperative knowledge of the underlying access vessel anatomy (Fig. 1), cases with prohibitive anatomy can be approached by adjunctive measures to enhance success, such as balloon angioplasty, as well as the utilization of accessory conduits (12). Balloon angioplasty can dilate a restrictive arterial lesion to a diameter that can allow passage of the endograft delivery system. Similarly, with multiple occlusive lesions and/or tortuosity, a more prudent approach may be to place an accessory conduit of either polytetrafluoro-ethylene (PTFE) or Dacron to the common iliac artery or distal aorta through which the device can be inserted, thus bypassing the complex diseased area. Following the procedure, the conduit can be removed.

B. Endoleaks

Endoleaks, a complication specific to endovascular therapy, is the persistent blood flow within the aneurysmal sac following endograft placement. Endoleaks can be due to poor exclusion of blood flow at the proximal and distal fixation sites (type I), collateral flow between arterial branches within the excluded aneurysmal sac (type II), leaks at junction sites between sequential grafts, or device failure (type III) (Fig. 2).

Risk for type I endoleak is increased with severe angulation at aortic neck fixation sites, where the currently available, relatively stiff devices may not adequately exclude blood flow on placement as well as risk subsequent migration with delayed endoleak (13). The transition from the aortic arch to the descending thoracic aorta results in angulation, which—when combined with a short segment of normal aorta in which fixation is attempted—may prove problematic. These situations may be approached by increasing the area of fixation by laying

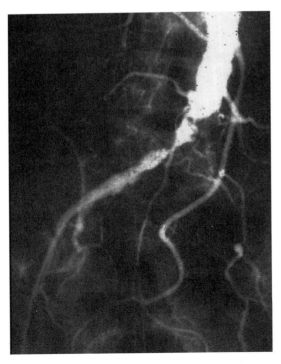

Figure 1   Angiogram in a patient with an aortic aneurysm demonstrating the presence of severe occlusive disease within the iliac arteries.

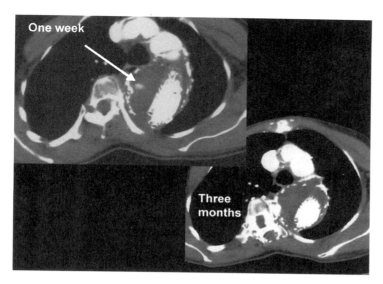

Figure 2 Chest CT scan following endovascular repair of thoracic aneurysm. (upper left) Type II endoleak evident in the early postoperative period (arrow). (lower right) CT scan repeated with no endoleak identified.

the device across the origin of the left subclavian. Ischemic consequences following intentional sacrifice of left subclavian blood flow by endograft deployment across its origin do exist. Alternatively, to avoid the ischemic consequences of subclavian interruption, a transposition of the left subclavian to the common carotid artery or using a conduit for carotid-subclavian bypass may provide a means of ensuring successful exclusion of the aneurysm from luminal blood flow and avoiding a type I endoleak (14,15).

Type II endoleaks resulting from the development of collateral channels devoloping between excluded intercostal or bronchial arteries are likely to thrombose (1,2). Management of type II endoleaks that fail to thrombose on delayed follow-up is considered in the context of aneurysmal size changes. Although there is no general consensus in this regard we feel that aneurysm growth does necessitate intervention to thrombose these collateral channels, while aneurysms that remain stable are observed. Data to support intervention despite the lack of growth remains to be determined.

C. Ischemia

Following endograft exclusion of thoracic aneurysms, intercostal arteries within the excluded segment are likely to thrombose. The clinical consequences following loss of flow within these arteries may range from a benign and clinically silent event to spinal cord ischemia with clinically evident paralysis/paresis.

Paraplegia following endovascular treatment of thoracic aortic aneurysms has been reported in the literature to occur at a rate of 0%–12% (2–4,10,16,17). When it is combined with concomitant or previous open abdominal aneurysm repair, there appears to be an increased risk of paraplegia. In our experience, patients undergoing a repair limited to endovascular means with no previous or concurrent aortic surgery had no paraplegia (16). It seems important, therefore, to discuss the possible mechanisms that may lead to spinal cord ischemia in endovascular repair.

We feel that four mechanisms may explain spinal cord ischemia during or following endovascular repair of thoracic aortic aneurysm:

1. Paraplegia that is immediately evident following occlusion of critical intercostal arteries.
2. Despite sacrifice of intercostal vessels, collateral arterial blood supply maintains spinal cord perfusion in the resting state. Spinal cord ischemia, however, may develop with episodes of hypotension or subsequent loss of collaterals.
3. Coverage of critical intercostal arteries does not result in their occlusion; instead, they are evident as endoleaks. Subsequently intercostal arteries can thrombose with resolution of endoleak, presenting with spinal cord compromise.
4. Visceral ischemia from abdominal repair or visceral embolization results in cytokine release, inducing secondary cord ischemia from a "no reflow" phenomenon.

The lower incidence of spinal cord ischemia during endovascular repair of thoracic aortic aneurysms places emphasis on the role of intercostal arteries and other collateral blood supplies. In a report from Griepp et al., routine intraoperative somatosensory evoked potentials were utilized during thoracoabdominal aortic aneurysm repair (18). They observed no acute changes after serial temporary occlusion of segmental vessels. In their study, with no reattached intercostal or lumbar arteries in any patients, an overall paraplegia rate of 2% was achieved. The absence of evidence of spinal cord ischemia following occlusion of intersegmental arteries during aneurysm resection questions the essential integrity of the "artery of Adamkiewicz" in spinal cord function.

They support there is a functionally continuous anterior spinal artery stretching from the foramen magnum to the cauda equina, with multiple inputs throughout its length, and that no single segmental input is absolutely required for maintenance of spinal cord integrity. Instead, with multiple contributions into the anterior spinal artery, serial sacrifice of segmental vessels can occur without spinal cord ischemia. They identified a risk of paraplegia when the number of sacrificed intercostals was greater than 10 — a scenario more likely with the more extensive type II aneurysms.

The severity of the spinal cord ischemia following endograft deployment can be dependent upon the extent of existing collateral circulation. Where there is adequate collateral preservation after endografting, we do not expect to see clinical evidence of ischemia. If collaterals are absent and critical intercostal arteries are covered, an ischemic event occurs (Fig. 3). If the existing intercostal or lumbar artery collateral supply is marginal, a tenuous cord perfusion more vulnerable to any postoperative hemodynamic insult results. There may exist an incomplete or intermediate cord ischemia in the regional distribution of the excluded intercostal arteries secondary to marginal collateralization. This may present as a delayed-onset neurological deficit in the endograft patients, as the vulnerable cord is more sensitive to decreases in spinal artery perfusion pressure caused by postoperative hemodynamic compromise or delayed thrombosis of previously patent yet covered intercostal arteries.

While intercostal thrombosis can, in its more deleterious form, result in paraplegia, we have noticed a syndrome of back pain following endovascular thoracic aneurysm repair that we propose is also a consequence of intercostal artery thrombosis. We identified a proportion of our patients complaining of paraspinal back pain 24–72 h following endovascular repair of their thoracic aneurysms. This pain persists for 2–14 days without any other clinically evident events. In these instances, we identified occlusion of previously

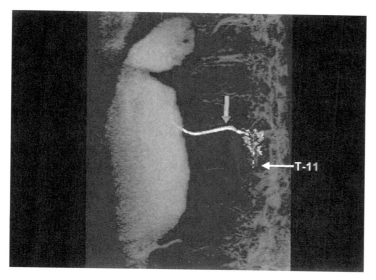

Figure 3 MRA of the thoracic aorta (sagittal view) illustrating a single dominant spinal artery originating from the aneurysmal segment.

patent intercostal arteries when these patients were evaluated with computed tomography (CT) or magnetic resonance angiography (MRA). Paraspinus muscle ischemia from intercostal thrombosis is our proposed etiology of this ischemia. To more accurately quantify these findings, we have instituted a protocol utilizing preoperative MRA to identify the intercostal and spinal artery blood supply in patients undergoing thoracic and thoracoabdominal aneurysm repair. Following their aneurysm repairs, reevaluation of

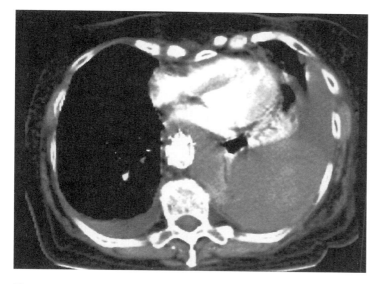

Figure 4 CT scan of the chest following thoracic aneurysm stent-grafting demonstrating the presense of a reactive effusion.

their intercostal and spinal artery blood supply will be evaluated for association with clinical sequelae ranging from paraspinous pain to paraplegia.

D. Inflammatory Response

Reports of a host response to the presence of the endografts as a postimplanatation syndrome has been reported to occur in 43–78% of patients (8,9). The clinical consequences of this phenomenon include pain, fever, leukocytosis, elevated sedimentation rates, and elevated c-reactive protein.

An inflammatory response specific to thoracic aneurysm repairs has been the development of a pleural effusion not present prior to endograft insertion (Fig. 4). We have witnessed this in 10% of our patient population. In its more severe form, it can result in respiratory compromise requiring repeated thoracentesis. Interestingly, despite the lack of evidence of aneurysmal leak or rupture in any of these patients, thoracentesis yields a serosanguinous effusion.

II. DEVICE-RELATED COMPLICATIONS

As with any device, trials and follow-up investigations provide evidence of durability. Stent grafts are no exception to this rule. They are composed of both a metallic frame and a synthetic graft, and repeated stress on these elements can ultimately result in metal fracture and fabric erosion. Concerns in this regard, of course, depend on whether these forces will result in a type III endoleak and thus treatment failure and risk of rupture (Fig. 5).

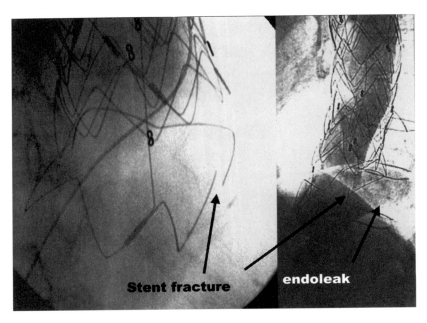

Figure 5   Fluoroscopic image demonstrating stent fracture (arrow).

A. Stent Fracture

In a review by Jacobs et al. reporting device failure rates in endovascular aortic aneurysm repair, a 15% device failure rate as determined by radiographic imaging and or pathologic specimens was identified (11). Of these failures, 23% were suture disruption, 5% were fabric failure, and 72% were metal stent fractures. Approximately 20% of thoracic aneurysms resulted in device failures, all due to metallic stent fractures. This is concerning, as any device failure can potentially result in treatment failure, with patients requiring repeated intervention to exclude the aneurysm sac.

III. SUMMARY

Complications following endovascular repair of thoracic aortic aneurysms are both anatomical and device-related. This suggests a more crucial role for adequate preoperative anatomical assessment as well as modification of devices. Restrictive access vessels, complex aneurysmal disease, and critical collateral blood supply to the spinal cord are areas that need further characterization. Similarly, the creation of devices with increased durability, lower profiles, and increased flexibility may prove successful in overcoming some of the limitations we currently face.

REFERENCES

1. Thompson CS, Gaxotte VD, Rodriguez JA, et al. Endoluminal stent grafting of the thoracic aorta: initial experience with the Gore Excluder. J Vasc Surg 2002; 35(6):1163–1170.
2. Heijman RH, Deblier IG, Moll FL, et al. Endovascular stent-grafting for descending thoracic aortic aneurysms. Eur J of Cardiothorac Surg 2002; 21:5–9.
3. Taylor PR, Gaines PA, McGuinness CL, Cleveland TJ, Beard JD, Cooper G, Reidy JF. Thoracic aortic stent grafts—Early experience from two centers using commercially available devices. Eur J Vasc Endovasc Surg 2001; 22(1):70–76.
4. Dake MD, Miller DC, Mitchell RS, et al. The "first generation" of endovascular stent-grafts for patients with aneurysms of the descending thoracic aorta. J Thorac Cardiovasc Surg 1998; 116:689–704.
5. Dake MD, Kato N, Mitchell RS, et al. Endovascular stent-graft placement for the treatment of acute aortic dissection. N Engl J Med 1999; 340:1546–1552.
6. Mitchell RS, Miller DC, Dake MD. Endovascular stent graft repair of thoracic aortic aneurysms. Semin Vasc Surg 1997; 10:257–271.
7. Mitchell RS. Endovascular stent-graft repair of thoracic aortic aneurysms. Semin Thorac Cardiovasc Surg 1997; 9:257–268.
8. Won JY, Lee DY, Shim WH, et al. Elective endovascular treatment of descending thoracic aortic aneurysms and chronic dissections with stent-grafts. J Vasc Intervent Radiol 2001; 12(5):575–582.
9. Nienaber CA, Fattori R, Lund G, et al. Non surgical reconstruction of thoracic aortic dissection by stent-graft placement. N Engl J Med 1999; 340:1539–1545.
10. White RA, Donayre CE, Walot I, et al. Endovascular exclusion of descending thoracic aortic aneurysms and chronic dissections: initial clinical results with the AneurRx device. J Vasc Surg 2001; 33:927–934.
11. Jacobs T, Won J, Faries P, et al. Device failure following aortic stent grafting. 56th Annual Meeting for the Society of Vascular Surgery, Boston, MA, June 9–12, 2002.
12. Yano OJ, Faries PL, Morrissey N, Teodorescu V, Hollier LH, Marin ML. Ancillary techniques to facilitate endovascular repair of aortic aneurysms. J Vasc Surg 2001; 34(1):69–75.
13. Resch T, Koul B, Dias NV, et al. Changes in aneurysm morphology and stent-graft con-

figuration after endovascular repair of aneurysms of the descending thoracic aorta. J Thorac Cardiovasc Surg 2001; 22(1):47–52.

14. Shigemura N, Kato M, Kuratani T, et al. New operative method for acute type B dissection: Left carotid artery-left subclavian artery bypass combined with endovascular stent-graft implantation. J Thorac Cardiovasc Surg 2000; 120(2):406–408.

15. Moore RD, Brandschwei F. Subclavian-to-carotid transposition and supracarotid endovascular stent graft placement for traumatic aortic disruption. Ann Vasc Surg 2001; 15(5):563–566.

16. Gravereaux EC, Faries PL, Burks JA, Latessa V, Spielvogel D, Hollier LH, Marin ML. Risk of spinal cord ischemia after endograft repair of thoracic aortic aneurysms. J Vasc Surg 2001; 34(6):997–1003.

17. Greenberg R, Resch T, Nyman U. Endovascular repair of descending thoracic aortic aneurysms: An early experience with intermediate-term follow up. J Vasc Surg 2000; 31:147–156.

18. Griepp RB, Ergin MA, Galla JD, Lansman S, Khan N, Quintana C. Looking for the artery of Adamkiewicz: A quest to minimize paraplegia after operations for aneurysms of the descending thoracic and thoracoabdominal aorta. J Thorac Cardiovasc Surg 1996; 112:1202–1215.

43

Complications of Angiogenesis Therapy

Joshua Bernheim, Sashi Kilaru, and K. Craig Kent

New York Presbyterian Hospital–The University Hospitals of Columbia and Cornell, New York, New York, U.S.A.

Cardiovascular disease is the major cause of death in adults in most developed and many developing countries. The mainstay of therapy for coronary and lower extremity ischemia is revascularization, either by catheter-based or surgical techniques. Both approaches have been effective in reducing the morbidity associated with these disease processes. Unfortunately, not all patients with coronary or peripheral ischemia are candidates for intervention. Often, multiple comorbidities associated with diffuse atherosclerosis preclude the use of invasive treatments. Consequently, a less invasive strategy would be a welcome adjunct to current therapeutic alternatives.

Therapeutic angiogenesis—the promotion of new vessel growth using vascular growth factors—is currently one of the more dynamic areas in biomedical research. Reestablishing blood flow to an ischemic region through angiogenesis has the potential to provide a "biological bypass" for patients with atherosclerotic occlusive disease. Studies in animals have suggested that the exogenous administration of angiogenic factors, particularly fibroblast growth factor (FGF) or vascular endothelial growth factor (VEGF), may augment blood flow in regions of arterial ischemia, thereby improving distal tissue perfusion. The successful development of therapeutic angiogenesis as a minimally invasive approach to vascular insufficiency could tremendously expand our ability to treat patients with coronary and limb-threatening ischemia.

Numerous reports have documented, in animals, the potential for a variety of cytokines and growth factors to induce neovascularization and enhance perfusion of ischemic tissues. These investigations have led to a number of pilot clinical trials designed to test the safety and efficacy of therapeutic angiogenesis. In an early study, Isner at al. in 1997 reported the results of a phase 1 clinical trial of VEGF in nine patients with critical limb ischemia (1). The majority of these patients had either rest pain or nonhealing ulcers, and none were considered to be candidates for surgical or percutaneous revascularization. Gene transfer was performed on two occasions separated by 4-week intervals with intramuscular injection into ischemic limbs of naked plasmid DNA encoding $VEGF_{165}$. Successful gene expression in patients was documented by an increase in serum VEGF levels. The investigators noted an improvement in the average ankle-brachial index (ABI) at 12 weeks from 0.33 to 0.48. New collaterals were demonstrated by both MRA and contrast radiography. Limb salvage was achieved in 6 of 9 patients.

Isner's initial report produced a wave of enthusiasm that led to the organization of several prospective clinical trials where VEGF and other growth factors were further tested. In a recently completed phase II randomized, placebo-controlled trial (TRAFFIC, Chiron Corporation), patients with intermittent claudication were randomized to placebo versus one or two doses of intra-arterial recombinant FGF (2). A total of 192 patients were enrolled. A positive effect on peak walking time was observed at 90 days in one treatment arm. At 180 days, however, treatment with FGF did not alter claudication severity, stair climbing, walking speed, or walking distance. The findings of this study were generally discouraging.

In a recently completed phase I multicenter trial, Comerota et al. tested the safety and tolerability of an increasing single dose of plasmid DNA encoding FGF (NV1FGF) in patients with limb-threatening peripheral occlusive disease (3). Fifty-one patients were enrolled, and doses ranging from 500 to 4000 g of NV1FGF were injected intramuscularly into the thighs and calves of ischemic extremities. No serious adverse events were noted during the course of this study. Clinical outcomes for the first 15 patients with 6-month follow-up were reported. A significant decrease in rest pain was noted and the ABI increased in all patients. Moreover, healing was observed in all 9 patients who presented with ulcers. These encouraging results have led to the initiation of a phase II placebo-controlled trial that is currently under way.

Multiple other trials of angiogenesis have either been completed or are currently under way. The results of these trials have in general been mixed, and it is clear at this point that therapeutic angiogenesis is still investigational. However, scientific investigation in this field is advancing at a rapid pace. New growth factors, combinations of growth factors, or new approaches including stem cell therapy are all being evaluated. Over the next few years, advances in these areas may bring this technology to fruition.

The ability to "turn on" growth of new blood vessels can be advantageous. However, angiogenesis can potentially produce complications, such as diabetic retinopathy and the spread of tumors. In recent years, gene therapy—one method of applying angiogenic proteins—has been plagued by a number of untoward events that have dampened enthusiasm for its use. There is clearly a need to fully understand both the benefits of these new techniques and their potential complications. In the remainder of this chapter, we discuss the various potential complications and concerns that have been raised regarding the use of therapeutic angiogenesis.

I. INCREASED VASCULAR PERMEABILITY

Although VEGF is most widely known for its properties as a stimulant of angiogenesis, it was originally described as a vascular permeability factor (4). In fact, VEGF is one of the most effective permeability-enhancing agents yet discovered, with a rapid onset of action and a potency up to 50,000 times greater than that of histamine (5,6). Increased permeability stimulated by VEGF can result in extravasation of plasma proteins into the extravascular space, leading to fibrin deposition and edema. This phenomenon has been well documented in clinical trials. Baumgartner found—in a study where naked plasmid DNA encoding VEGF was used to treat peripheral ischemia—that 24% of patients with rest pain and 60%

of those with gangrene developed significant peripheral edema (7). There were no untoward events in these patients, and in most cases the edema promptly responded to diuretic therapy.

Capillary leakage from increased vascular permeability has the potential to be a life-threatening side effect of angiogenesis when the treatment is systemically applied. In a murine model, Thurston et al. observed lethal consequences related to vascular permeability—including diffuse tissue edema and brain swelling—with systemic adenoviral gene transfer of VEGF (8). In human subjects, however, there have been no reports of life-threatening edema attributable to VEGF therapy. This is likely due to the fact that, in trials thus far, patients have been treated with localized therapy, resulting in low doses of VEGF of short duration. In Thurston's model, the gene transfer regimen was designed to produce circulating levels of VEGF 3–5 logs greater than those seen in any human clinical application (1,8,9). It appears that local delivery results in systemic levels of VEGF that are in the range of picograms per milliliter. This is due to the high affinity of VEGF for matrix proteins. The effect on vascular permeability appears to be specific to VEGF and its homologues. In a Miles assay, an established test to demonstrate the permeability-enhancing effects of substances on the vascular system, other angiogenic factors, such as granulocyte-macrophage colony-stimulating factor, transforming growth factor beta, PDGF, and FGF were not associated with significant vascular permeability (10).

II. HYPOTENSION

Vasodilatation does occur in response to multiple growth factors, including VEGF and FGF. This effect results in part from upregulation of nitric oxide (NO) synthase (11–13); NO is an important mediator of angiogenesis as well as a vasodilator (14–16).

In an early study of angiogenesis in pigs, 4 of 8 animals undergoing intracoronary VEGF administration died of refractory hypotension (17). Hypotension has also been observed in human subjects receiving intra-arterial FGF protein. Lazarous et al. reported a case of hypotension in a study of claudicants receiving recombinant FGF, after which the study was modified to reduce the rate of administration of the drug (18). Unger et al. also reported a patient who developed hypotension after intracoronary administration of 100 µg/kg of FGF (19). Thus far, hypotension has been confined to protocols where the angiogenic protein is administered either intra-arterially or intravenously. Hypotension has not developed following delivery of angiogenic agents via vectors; their gradual expression results in lower circulating levels of growth factors. It is also likely that, even when intravascular proteins are used as the method of delivery, refinements of dosing and rate of administration of growth factors will lessen the potential for this complication.

III. VASCULAR MALFORMATIONS

Growth factors used for therapeutic angiogenesis have the potential to stimulate disorganized proliferation of normal vessels, leading to the formation of hemangiomas or other vascular malformations. Hemangiomas have been observed in animals when there has been prolonged exposure of skeletal muscle or myocardium to high concentrations of VEGF (20–22). To date, no association has been made between VEGF and vascular malformations in human clinical trials with the doses and durations of therapy used. There is only a single case report of telangectasia formation in a leg following VEGF gene transfer (23). Despite detailed examination of autopsy specimens, amputated limbs, and explanted hearts, vascular neoproliferation has not been demonstrated in other studies of clinical angiogenesis (10,24–30).

IV. RETINOPATHY

The high incidence of diabetes mellitus in patients with peripheral vascular disease has raised concern over the possibility that angiogenic growth factors might exacerbate proliferative diabetic retinopathy, which results from the abnormal proliferation of retinal arterioles and is exceedingly common in patients with diabetes. Levels of VEGF and FGF-2 are increased in the neovascular membrane and ocular fluid of patients with diabetic retinopathy (31–33). Moreover, subretinal administration of adenoviral vectors expressing VEGF results in the development of retinopathy (34).

Thus far, in clinical trials of angiogenesis, this complication has not occurred. Close monitoring of patients with careful, routine ophthalmological examinations has been a required part of most angiogenesis protocols. Isner et al. reported their findings in 44 diabetic patients undergoing VEGF gene transfer for a variety of indications. All patients underwent detailed retinal evaluation with fluorescin before the introduction of the vector and at 3, 6, and 12 months after gene transfer. No patient with preexisting retinopathy had progression of his or her proliferative disease, and no patient with a normal examination prior to therapy developed retinopathic changes. Moreover, none of the nondiabetic patients developed retinal pathology in the first year following gene transfer (10). Thus, at this point, the risk of developing retinopathy remains theoretical.

V. NEPHROTOXICITY

Nephrotoxicity is a side effect angiogenic therapy. Rats receiving 4 weeks of high-dose basic FGF developed glomerular pathology that included both vacuolization of the glomerular cells regulating filtration, and hyperplasia of Bowman's capsule epithelium (35). Thus, renal toxicity appears to be related to a direct toxic effect of FGF, resulting in structural changes in the glomerulus, and not as a consequence of the angiogenic properties of FGF. Nephrotoxicity has been observed in clinical trials where FGF is the angiogenic agent. In a recently conducted phase II trail sponsored by Scios Corporation, 5 of the 16 subjects who received FGF intravenously developed significant proteinuria, leading to early termination of the trial. Though a worrisome occurrence, it should be noted that patients in this trial were receiving systemic therapy with recombinant protein. Intramuscular or even intra-arterial administration of FGF, when this growth factor is applied through a genetic vector, can lessen systemic toxicity and result in more focused targeting of ischemic tissues.

VI. NEOPLASIA

In many of the initial studies of angiogenesis, the focus was its important role in tumor progression (36,37). As such, antiangiogenic proteins have been extensively evaluated as tools for treating cancer. It follows that attempts to provoke angiogenesis for therapeutic purposes has the potential to stimulate the growth or spread of preexisting tumors. This is particularly concerning since patients with vascular insufficiency are usually elderly and at high risk for developing cancer. Although solid tumors require angiogenesis to grow, angiogenic proteins do not appear to directly produce neoplastic changes. FGF can stimulate proliferation of multiple cell types. VEGF can also stimulate growth of several non-endothelial tumors (i.e., those that express VEGFR-1 and VEGFR-2 receptors) (38). Neurolipin, a third receptor for VEGF, has also been found in many neoplastic cells.

Despite this theoretical concern, in neither animal nor human studies has there been any definitive evidence that patients developed or had progression of cancer. In the VIVA (Vascular Endothelial Growth Factor in Ischemia for Vascular Angiogenesis) trial (39), where recombinant VEGF protein was used to treat myocardial ischemia, and the TRAFFIC (Therapeutic Angiogenisis with Recombinant Fibroblast Growth Factor-2 for Intermittent Claudication) trial (2), where VEGF was used to treat claudication, the only patients diagnosed with new neoplasms were in the control groups. Given the potential for tumors to remain silent for extended period of time, the verdict is still out. Large, randomized trials of angiogenesis with long-term follow-up will be required before any final determination can be made.

VII. ATHEROSCLEROSIS

Angiogenesis proteins not only promote new vessel formation but their effects on existing vessels may lead to the development or progression of atherosclerotic lesions. Multiple studies have demonstrated that the development of atherosclerotic plaque is associated with proliferation of the vasa vasorum (39–41). Treating hypercholesterolemic mice with endostatin, a potent angiogenesis inhibitor, for 16 weeks reduced plaque development by 85% (42). Moreover, VEGF has been identified as a monocyte chemoattractant (43,44); experiments have also shown that activated macrophages present within atherosclerotic lesions have a profoundly deleterious effect on plaque evolution, stability, and rupture (45).

Inhibition of angiogenesis retards plaque formation. However, it does not necessarily follow that angiogenesis-promoting factors will accelerate atherosclerosis. Human studies to date have not demonstrated progression of atherosclerotic disease as a complication of angiogenisis. Balloon injury of rat and rabbit arteries followed by application of VEGF using a variety of vectors did not result in accelerated restenosis or disease progression. On the contrary, reduced intimal thickening and mural thrombus were observed in these animals, likely as a result of VEGF's ability to stimulate endothelial regeneration (46–49). Vale et al. conducted similar studies in humans. After angioplasty of diseased femoral arteries, balloon catheters impregnated with a hydrogel coating were used to deliver naked DNA encoding VEGF. These patients experienced no significant increase in restenosis up to 48 months after gene transfer and showed no evidence of new lesion formation (50).

VIII. COMPLICATIONS ASSOCIATED WITH VIRAL VECTORS

Adenoviral vectors have been used in over half of the trials of therapeutic angiogenesis. Inflammation and cell toxicity are virus-related side effects that can develop regardless of the gene expressed. First-generation adenoviral vectors can stimulate expression of viral proteins in target cells, resulting in the production of cytotoxic T lymphocytes. This immune response prevents repeated application of the same vector. In addition, high titers of adenoviruses can damage cells and produce an inflammatory response that results in systemic toxicity and damage to tissues. The most widely publicized complication of gene therapy to date was the death of a young man at the University of Pennsylvania who underwent hepatic arterial infusio of large doses of adeno viral vector. The patient's presenting condition was a relatively mild form of ornithine transcarboxylase deficiency, a rare hereditary metabolic disorder in which the liver is unable to process ammonia. The gene replacement protocol was designed to treat this deficiency (51). This event prompted intense scrutiny into the potential complications of gene therapy. The field has since rebounded from this incident, and multiple studies are currently under way. However, issues related to viral vectors remain, and new, less toxic and antigenic vectors are under development.

IX. MORTALITY

Patients with peripheral vascular disease have diminished survival and are prone to developing complications related to their multiple comorbidities. This has led to difficulty in classifying adverse events in angiogenesis trials, since it is not readily possible to determine which events are due to the actual intervention versus the underlying disease process. The 2-year mortality for patients with critical limb ischemia can be as high as 30–35% (52). The small sample size and nonrandomized design of most trials performed to date compounds this problem. Isner reported that among the 100 patients enrolled in gene therapy trials at his institution, 9 deaths occurred over a 7-year period (10). Although none of these deaths were directly attributable to gene therapy, the presence of comorbidities complicates the determination of outcome.

X. CONCLUSIONS

Angiogenic agents that are currently under study have potent biological effects and the potential to produce a wide array of complications. However, analysis of available data in ongoing phase I and II trails is very encouraging. There is little evidence that these proteins produce major morbidity or mortality. Once the size and number of trials increases and more randomized studies are initiated, a better safety profile can be generated for these angiogenic agents. The future of angiogenesis therapy lies in the development of growth factors and methods of their delivery that allow tissues to be specifically targeted with sufficient selectivity that systemic complications do not occur. The outcome will likely be safe and effective new therapies for the treatment of atherosclerosis.

REFERENCES

1. Baumgartner I, Pieczek A, Manor O, Blair R, Kearney M, Walsh K, Isner JM. Constitutive expression of ph VEGF165 after intramuscular gene transfer promotes collateral vessel development in patients with critical limb ischemia. Circulation 1998; 97(12):1114–1123.
2. Lederman RJ, Mendelsohn FO, Anderson RD, Saucedo JF, Tenaglia AN, Hermiller JB, Hillegass WB, Rocha-Singh K, Moon TE, Whitehouse MJ, Annex BH. Therapeutic angiogenesis with recombinant fibroblast growth factor-2 for intermittent claudication (the TRAFFIC study): A randomised trial. Lancet 2002; 359(9323):2053–2058.
3. Comerota AJ, Throm RC, Miller KA, Henry T, Chronos N, Laird J, Sequeira R, Kent KC, Bacchetta M, Goldman C, Salenius JP, Schmieder FA, Pilsudski R. Naked plasmid DNA encoding fibroblast growth factor type 1 for the treatment of end-stage unreconstructible lower extremity ischemia: preliminary results of a phase I trial. J Vasc Surg 2002; 35(5):930–936.
4. Senger DR, Galli SJ, Dvorak AM, Perruzzi CA, Harvey VS, Dvorak HF. Tumor cells secrete a vascular permeability factor that promotes accumulation of ascites fluid. Science 1983; 219:983–985.

5. Dvorak HF, Brown LF, Detmar M, et al. Vascular permeability factor/vascular endothelial growth factor, microvascular hyperpermeability, and angiogenesis. Am J Pathol 1995; 146:1029–1039.

6. Brown LF, Detmar M, Claffey K, et al. Vascular permeability factor/vascular endothelial growth factor: A multifunctional angiogenic cytokine. EXS 1997; 79:233–269.

7. Baumgartner I, Rauh G, Pieczek A, Wuensch D, Magner M, Kearney M, Schainfeld R, Isner JM. Lower-extremity edema associated with gene transfer of naked DNA vascular endothelial growth factor. Ann Intern Med 2000; 132:880–884.

8. Thurston G, Suri C, Smith K, McClain J, Sato TN, Yancopoulos GD, McDonald DM. Leakage-resistant blood vessels in mice transgenically overexpressing angiopoietin-1. Science 1999; 286:2511–2514.

9. Isner JM, Baumgartner I, Rauh G, Schainfeld R, Blair R, Manor O, Razvi S, Symes JF. Treatment of thromboangiitis obliterans (Buerger's disease) by intramuscular gene transfer of vascular endothelial growth factor: preliminary clinical results. J Vasc Surg 1998; 28:964–975.

10. Isner JM, Vale PR, Symes JF, Losordo DW. Assessment of risks associated with cardiovascular gene therapy in human subjects. Circ Res 2001; 89:389–400.

11. van der Zee R, Murohara T, Luo Z, Zollmann F, Passeri J, Lekutat C, Isner JM. Vascular endothelial growth factor (VEGF)/vascular permeability factor (VPF) augments nitric oxide release from quiescent rabbit and human vascular endothelium. Circulation 1997; 95:1030–1037.

12. Cuevas P, Carceller F, Ortega S, Zazo M, Nieto I, Gimenez-Gallego G. Hypotensive activity of fibroblast growth factor. Science 1991; 254:1208–1210.

13. Fulton D, Gratton JP, McCabe TJ, Fontana J, Fujio Y, Walsh K, Franke TF, Papapetropoulos A, Sessa WC. Regulation of endothelium-derived nitric oxide production by the protein kinase akt. Nature 1999; 399:597–601.

14. Murohara T, Asahara T, Silver M, Bauters C, Masuda H, Kalka C, Kearney M, Chen D, Symes JF, Fishman MC, Huang PL, Isner JM. Nitric oxide synthase modulates angiogenesis in response to tissue ischemia. J Clin Invest 1998; 101:2567–2578.

15. Ziche M, Morbidelli L, Choudhuri R, Zhang H-T, Donnini S, Granger HJ, Bicknell R. Nitric oxide synthase lies downstream from vascular endothelial growth factor–induced but not fibroblast growth factor-induced angiogenesis. J Clin Invest 1997; 99:2625–2634.

16. Babaei S, Teichert-Kuliszewska K, Monge J-C, Mohamed F, Bendeck MP, Stewart DJ. Role of nitric oxide in the angiogenic response in vitro to basic fibroblast growth factor. Circ Res 1998; 82:1007–1015.

17. Hariawala M, Horowitz JR, Esakof D, Sheriff DD, Walter DH, Chaudhry GM, Desai V, Keyt B, Isner JM, Symes JF. VEGF improves myocardial blood flow but produces EDRF-mediated hypotension in porcine hearts. J Surg Res 1996; 63:77–82.

18. Lazarous DF, Unger EF, Epstein SE, Stine A, Arevalo JL, Chew EY, Quyyumi AA. Basic fibroblast growth factor in patients with intermittent claudication: results of a phase I trial. J Am Coll Cardiol 2000; 36:1339–1344.

19. Unger EF, Goncalves L, Epstein SE, et al. Effects of a single intracoronary injection of basic fibroblast growth factor in stable angina pectoris. Am J Cardiol 2000; 85:1414–1419.

20. Springer ML, Chen AS, Kraft PE, Bednarski M, Blau HM. VEGF gene delivery to muscle: Potential role of vasculogenesis in adults. Mol Cell 1998; 2:549–558.

21. Lee RJ, Springer ML, Blanco-Bose WE, Shaw R, Ursell PC, Blau HM. VEGF gene delivery to myocardium: Deleterious effects of unregulated expression. Circulation 2000; 102:898–901.

22. Schwarz ER, Speakman MT, Patterson M, Hale SS, Isner JM, Kedes LH, Kloner RA. Evaluation of the effects of intramyocardial injection of DNA expressing vascular endothelial growth factor (VEGF) in a myocardial infarction model in the rat—Angiogenesis and angioma formation. J Am Coll Cardiol 2000; 35:1323–1330.

23. Isner JM, Pieczek A, Schainfeld R, Blair R, Haley L, Asahara T, Rosenfield K, Razvi S, Walsh K, Symes J. Clinical evidence of angiogenesis following arterial gene transfer of ph VEGF165. Lancet 1996; 348:370–374.

24. Symes JF, Losordo DW, Vale PR, Lathi K, Esakof DD, Maysky M, Isner JM. Gene therapy with vascular endothelial growth factor for inoperable coronary artery disease: Preliminary clinical results. Ann Thorac Surg 1999; 68:830–837.

25. Tabata H, Silver M, Isner JM. Arterial gene transfer of acidic fibroblast growth factor for therapeutic angiogenesis in vivo: Critical role of secretion signal in use of naked DNA. Cardiovasc Res 1997; 35:470–479.

26. Tsurumi Y, Takeshita S, Chen D, Kearney M, Rossow ST, Passeri J, Horowitz JR, Symes JF. Direct intramuscular gene transfer of naked DNA encoding vascular endothelial growth factor augments collateral development and tissue perfusion. Circulation 1996; 94:3281–3290.

27. Witzenbichler B, Asahara T, Murohara T, Silver M, Spyridopoulos I, Magner M, Principe N, Kearney M, Hu J-S, Isner JM. Vascular endothelial growth factor-C (VEGF-C/VEGF-2) promotes angiogenesis in the setting of tissue ischemia. Am J Pathol 1998; 153:381–394.

28. Laitinen M, Makinen K, Mannienen H, Matsi P, Kossila M, Agrawal RS, Pakkanen T, Luom-Viita H, Hartikainen J, Alhava E, Laakso M, Yla-Herttuala S. Adenovirus-mediated gene transfer to lower limb artery of patients with chronic critical leg ischaemia. Hum Gene Ther 1998; 9:1481–1486.

29. Mack CA, Patel SR, Schwarz EA, Zanzonico P, Hahn RT, Ilercil A, Devereux RB, Goldsmith SJ, Christian TF, Sanborn TA, Kovesdi I, Itackett N, Isom OW, Crystal RG, Rosengart TK. Biologic bypass with the use of adenovirus-mediated gene transfer of the complementary deoxyribonucleic acid for vascular endothelial growth factor 121 improves myocardial perfusion and function in the ischemic porcine heart. J Thorac Cardiovasc Surg 1998; 115:168–176.

30. Giordano FJ, Ping P, McKirnan D, Nozaki S, DeMaria AN, Dillmann WH, Mathieu-Costello O, Hammond HK. Intracoronary gene transfer of fibroblast growth factor-5 increases blood flow and contractile function in an ischemic region of the heart. Nat Med 1996; 2:534–539.

31. Frank RN, Amin RH, Eliott D, Puklin JE, Abrams GW. Basic fibroblast growth factor and vascular endothelial growth factor are present in epiretinal and choroidal neovascular membranes. Am J Ophthalmol 1996; 122:393–403.

32. Aiello LP, Avery RL, Arrigg PG, Keyt BA, Jampel HD, Shah ST, Pasquale LR, Theme H, Iwamoto MA, Parke JE, Nguyen MD, Aiello LM, Ferrara N, King GL. Vascular endothelial growth factor in ocular fluids of patients with diabetic retinopathy and other retinal disorders. N Engl J Med 1994; 331:1480–1487.

33. Adamis AP, Miller JW, Bernal M-T, D'Amico DJ, Folkman J, Yeo T-K, Yeo K-T. Increased vascular endothelial growth factor levels in the vitreous of eyes with proliferative diabetic retinopathy. Am J Ophthalmol 1994; 118:445–450.

34. Baffi J, Byrnes G, Chan CC, Csaky KG. Choroidal neovascularization in the rat induced by adenovirus mediated expression of vascular endothelial growth factor. Invest Ophthalmol Vis Sci 2000; 41:3582–3589.

35. Mazue G, Bertolero F, Garafano L, Brughere M, Carminati P. Experience with the preclinical assessment of basic fibroblast growth factor. Toxicol Lett 1992; 64/65:329–338.

36. Folkman J. Tumor angiogenesis: Therapeutic implications. N Engl J Med 1971; 285:1182–1186.

37. Hanahan D, Folkman J. Patterns and emerging mechanisms of the angiogenic switch during tumorigenesis. Cell 1996; 86:353–364.

38. Herold-Mende C, Steiner HH, Andl T, et al. Expression and functional significance of vascular endothelial growth factor receptors in human tumor cells. Lab Invest 1999; 79:1573–1582.

39. Kwon HM, Sangiorgi G, Ritman EL, McKenna C, Holmes DR, Schwartz RS, Lerman A. Enhanced coronary vasa vasorum neovascularization in experimental hypercholesterolemia. J Clin Invest 1998; 101:1551–1556.

40. Williams JK, Armstrong ML, Heistad DD. Vasa vasorum in atherosclerotic coronary arteries: Responses to vasoactive stimuli and regression of atherosclerosis. Circ Res 1988; 62:515–523.

41. Barger AC, Beeuwkes R III, Lainey LL, Silverman KJ. Hypothesis: vasa vasorum and neovascularization of human coronary arteries: A possible role in the pathophysiology of atherosclerosis. N Engl J Med 1984; 310:175–177.

42. Moulton KS, Heller E, Konerding MA, Flynn E, Palinski W, Folkman J. Angiogenesis inhibitors endostatin and TNP-470 reduce intimal neovascularization and plaque growth in apolipoprotein E-deficient mice. Circulation 1999; 99:1726–1732.

43. Barleon B, Sozzani S, Zhou D, et al. Migration of human monocytes in response to vascular endothelial growth factor (VEGF) is mediated via the VEGF receptor flt-1. Blood 1996; 87:3336–3343.

44. Clauss M, Gerlach M, Gerlach H, et al. Vascular permeability factor: A tumor-derived polypeptide that induces endothelial cell and monocyte procoagulant activity and promotes monocyte migration. J Exp Med 1990; 172:1535–1545.

45. Libby P, Geng YJ, Aikawa M, et al. Macrophages and atherosclerotic plaque stability. Curr Opin Lipidol 1996; 7:330–335.

46. Van Belle E, Tio FO, Couffinhal T, Maillard L, Passeri J, Isner JM. Stent endothelialization: Time course, impact of local catheter delivery, feasibility of recombinant protein administration, and response to cytokine expedition. Circulation 1997; 95:438–448.

47. Van Belle E, Tio FO, Chen D, Maillard L, Kearney M, Isner JM. Passivation of metallic stents following arterial gene transfer of ph VEGF165 inhibits thrombus formation and intimal thickening. J Am Coll Cardiol 1997; 29:1371–1379.

48. Asahara T, Chen D, Tsurum Y, Kearney M, Rossow S, Passeri J, Symes J, Isner J. Accelerated restitution of endothelial integrity and endothelium-dependent function following phVEGF165 gene transfer. Circulation 1996; 94:3291–3302.

49. Asahara T, Bauters C, Pastore CJ, Kearney M, Rossow S, Bunting S, Ferrara N, Symes JF, Isner JM. Local delivery of vascular endothelial growth factor accelerates reendothelialization and attenuates intimal hyperplasia in balloon-injured rat carotid artery. Circulation 1995; 91:2793–2801.

50. Vale PR, Wuensch DI, Rauh GF, Rosenfield K, Schainfeld RM, Isner JM. Arterial gene therapy for inhibiting restenosis in patients with claudication undergoing superficial femoral artery angioplasty [abstr]. Circulation 1998; 98(suppl I):I-66.

51. Stolberg SG. FDA officials fault Penn team in gene therapy death. New York Times, December 9, 1989.

52. TransAtlantic Inter-Society Consensus (TASC). Management of peripheral arterial disease (PAD). J Vasc Surg 2000; 31:S1–S296.

Index

About the Editors

JONATHAN B. TOWNE is Professor of Surgery and Chief of Vascular Surgery, Medical College of Wisconsin, Milwaukee. He received the M.D. degree (1967) from the University of Rochester School of Medicine and Dentistry, New York. He obtained vascular surgery training under Dr. Jesse Thompson in Dallas, Texas.

LARRY H. HOLLIER is Professor of Surgery and Dean of the Louisiana State University Health Sciences Center School of Medicine, New Orleans, Louisiana. He previously served as President of the Mount Sinai Hospital and Chairman of the Department of Surgery at the Mount Sinai School of Medicine, New York, New York. The author of more than 300 articles in medical literature, he serves on the editorial boards of 14 surgical journals. Dr. Hollier received the M.D. degree (1968) from Louisiana State University School of Medicine, New Orleans. He obtained vascular surgery training under Dr. Jesse Thompson in Dallas, Texas.

ISBN 0-8247-4776-3

9 780824 747763

90000